FUNCTIONAL BRAIN MAPPING AND THE ENDEAVOR TO UNDERSTAND THE WORKING BRAIN

Edited by **Francesco Signorelli**
and **Domenico Chirchiglia**

Functional Brain Mapping and the Endeavor to Understand the Working Brain
http://dx.doi.org/10.5772/50860
Edited by Francesco Signorelli and Domenico Chirchiglia

Contributors

Nobuko Yamada-Goto, Mirko Avesani, Peter Lin, Ou Bai, Bruna Velasques, Pedro Ribeiro, Roberto Piedade, Mauricio Cagy, Michelle Yongmei Wang, Jürgen Dammers, Lukas Breuer, Giuseppe Tabbì, Markus Axer, Mikael Lundqvist, Pawel Herman, Anders Lansner, Jennifer Rodger, Tenelle Wilks, Alan Harvey, Teodora-Adriana Perles-Barbacaru, Hana Lahrech, Braun, Meghan Healey, Andres Antonio Gonzalez-Garrido, Fabiola Gómez-Velázquez, Julieta Ramos-Loyo, Francisco Mercado, Marisa Fernández-Sánchez, Paloma Barjola, Francisco Gómez-Esquer, Virginia Guerra, Mitsuru Kashiwagi, Hiroshi Tamai, Ana Karla Jansen-Amorim, Bruss Lima, Cecilia Ceriatte, Mario Fiorani, Ricardo Gattass, Juliana Soares, Mark Murphy, J. Guiomar Niso Galán, Ricardo Gutiérrez, Ernesto Pereda, Fernando Maestú, Francisco Del Pozo, David Papo, María Gudín, Sira Carrasco, Todd Richards, Virginia Berninger, Kazuo Nishimura, Ren, Francis McGlone, Anna Bartels, Laura Teune, Klaus Leenders, Leah Jappe, Bonnie Klimes-Dougan, Kathryn Cullen, Francesco Signorelli

Published by InTech

Janeza Trdine 9, 51000 Rijeka, Croatia

Publishing Process Manager Oliver Kurelic

Technical Editor InTech DTP team

Cover InTech Design team

First published June, 2013

Printed in Croatia

A free online edition of this book is available at www.intechopen.com

Additional hard copies can be obtained from orders@intechopen.com

Functional Brain Mapping and the Endeavor to Understand the Working Brain, Edited by Francesco Signorelli and Domenico Chirchiglia

p. cm.

ISBN 978-953-51-1160-3

Contents

Preface IX

Section 1 **Functional Neuroimaging of Attention, Sensorimotor Integration and Speech 1**

Chapter 1 **Sensorimotor Integration and Attention: An Electrophysiological Analysis 3**
Bruna Velasques, Mauricio Cagy, Roberto Piedade and Pedro Ribeiro

Chapter 2 **A High Performance MEG Based BCI Using Single Trial Detection of Human Movement Intention 17**
Peter T. Lin, Kartikeya Sharma, Tom Holroyd, Harsha Battapady, Ding-Yu Fei and Ou Bai

Chapter 3 **Brain Mapping of Developmental Coordination Disorder 37**
Mitsuru Kashiwagi and Hiroshi Tamai

Chapter 4 **Shared Neural Correlates for Speech and Gesture 61**
Meghan L. Healey and Allen R. Braun

Chapter 5 **Brain Mapping of Language Processing Using Functional MRI Connectivity and Diffusion Tensor Imaging 77**
Todd L. Richards and Virginia W. Berninger

Chapter 6 **Pre-Attentive Processing of Mandarin Tone and Intonation: Evidence from Event-Related Potentials 95**
Gui-Qin Ren, Yi-Yuan Tang, Xiao-Qing Li and Xue Sui

Chapter 7 **Exploring the Effect of Verbal Emotional Words Through Event-Related Brain Potentials 109**
Andrés Antonio González-Garrido, Fabiola Reveca Gómez-Velázquez and Julieta Ramos-Loyo

Section 2 Functional Neuroimaging in Vision, Mood and Cognition 133

Chapter 8 **Genetic Marker Mice and Their Use in Understanding Learning and Memory 135**
Mark Murphy, Yvette M. Wilson and Christopher Butler

Chapter 9 **Attractor Hypothesis of Associative Cortex: Insights from a Biophysically Detailed Network Model 155**
Mikael Lundqvist, Pawel Herman and Anders Lansner

Chapter 10 **Multi-Scale Information, Network, Causality, and Dynamics: Mathematical Computation and Bayesian Inference to Cognitive Neuroscience and Aging 181**
Michelle Yongmei Wang

Chapter 11 **The Crossmodal Influence of Odor Hedonics on Facial Attractiveness: Behavioural and fMRI Measures 209**
Francis McGlone, Robert A. Österbauer, Luisa M. Demattè and Charles Spence

Chapter 12 **Seeing with Two Eyes: Integration of Binocular Retinal Projections in the Brain 227**
Tenelle A. Wilks, Alan R. Harvey and Jennifer Rodger

Chapter 13 **The Role of Cortical Feedback Circuitry on Functional Maps of V2 in Primates: Effects on Orientation Tuning and Direction Selectivity 251**
Ana Karla Jansen-Amorim, Cecilia Ceriatte, Bruss Lima, Juliana Soares, Mario Fiorani and Ricardo Gattass

Chapter 14 **Ceasing Thoughts and Brain Activity: MEG Data Analysis 267**
Takaaki Aoki, Michiyo Inagawa, Kazuo Nishimura and Y,oshikazu Tobinaga

Chapter 15 **Brain Imaging and the Prediction of Treatment Outcomes in Mood and Anxiety Disorders 279**
Leah M. Jappe, Bonnie Klimes-Dougan and Kathryn R. Cullen

Chapter 16 **Mental Function and Obesity 301**
Nobuko Yamada-Goto, Goro Katsuura and Kazuwa Nakao

Section 3 **Experimental and Clinical Applications of Functional Neuroimaging 343**

Chapter 17 **Surgical Resection of Tumors Infiltrating Left Insula and Perisylvian Opercula — Utility of Anatomic Landmarks Implemented by Intraoperative Functional Brain Mapping 345**
Francesco Signorelli, Domenico Chirchiglia, Rodolfo Maduri, Giuseppe Barbagallo and Jacques Guyotat

Chapter 18 **Optimized Signal Separation for 3D-Polarized Light Imaging 355**
Jürgen Dammers, Lukas Breuer, Giuseppe Tabbì and Markus Axer

Chapter 19 **Causal Relationships and Network Parameters in Effective Brain Connectivity 375**
Guiomar Niso, Ernesto Pereda, Fernando Maestú, María Gudín, Sira Carrasco and Francisco del-Pozo

Chapter 20 **Neuroimaging of Epilepsy: EEG-fMRI in the Presurgical Evaluation of Focal Epilepsy 393**
Mirko Avesani, Silvia Giacopuzzi and Antonio Fiaschi

Chapter 21 **Brain Function in Fibromyalgia: Altered Pain Processing and Cognitive Dysfunction 431**
Francisco Mercado, Paloma Barjola, Marisa Fernández-Sánchez, Virginia Guerra and Francisco Gómez-Esquer

Chapter 22 **FDG- PET Imaging in Neurodegenerative Brain Diseases 463**
L. K. Teune, A. L. Bartels and K. L. Leenders

Chapter 23 **Quantitative Mapping of Angiogenesis by Magnetic Resonance Imaging 477**
Teodora-Adriana Perles-Barbacaru and Hana Lahrech

Preface

Brain mapping is nowadays a well established field of functional neuroscience that has a high clinical impact, sustained by incessant advancements of basic and clinical research.

The world-class group of neuroscientists gathered together to elaborate this book has done a skillful job: apart from delineating their area of expertise they managed to give the reader an accurate hint about what are the current implications of brain mapping both in research and clinic. Ideal for researchers and clinicians involved in functional neurosciences, this book is a valuable reading for anyone, student, resident or seasoned specialist, seeking to keep up to date with the latest developments in functional brain mapping.

By dividing the book in three chapters we intended to give the reader an inkling of the main topics studied, namely sensorimotor integration, speech, vision, mood and cognition, as well as the central research and clinical applications of brain mapping. These are the stepping stones from which further developments will arise and contribute to improve our understanding of brain function and our capacity to enhance, preserve and restore it in case of impairment or loss.

Prof. Francesco Signorelli
Associate Professor of Neurosurgery
University "Magna Græcia", Catanzaro, Italy
Consultant Neurosurgeon
Hospices Civils de Lyon, Hôpital Neurologique et Neurochirurgical,
Department of Neurosurgery, Lyon, France

Prof. Domenico Chirchiglia
Aggregate Professor of Neurosurgery
University "Magna Græcia", Catanzaro, Italy

Section 1

Functional Neuroimaging of Attention, Sensorimotor Integration and Speech

Chapter 1

Sensorimotor Integration and Attention: An Electrophysiological Analysis

Bruna Velasques, Mauricio Cagy,
Roberto Piedade and Pedro Ribeiro

Additional information is available at the end of the chapter

http://dx.doi.org/10.5772/55199

1. Introduction

Selective attention is fundamental for the information processing. The perceptive system receives different external and internal stimuli at all times and our organism needs to be capable to perceive environmental stimuli, in order to discriminate the difference among these stimuli and, thus, archive relevant information in the brain. In such manner, the attention process becomes a determinant mechanism in the sensorimotor integration.

In the last decades, researchers in sensorimotor integration have been concerned in establishing the relevant and fundamental elements that better explain the relation among individual, task and environment in the motor action production. The maintenance of movement stability is the main goal of the central nervous system (CNS) in dealing with visual stimuli. In the CNS, the sensorimotor integration is subdivided into three different levels: the most inferior level, considered the first stage, is the spinal cord; the second level regards several subcortical areas, such as reticular formation, vestibular nuclei, superior colliculus, cerebellum and basal ganglia. These areas receive information from the spinal cord and assist in the postural stability control; the last stage, considered the superior level, is associated with the cerebral cortex and is responsible for movement refinement and gesture diversification. The main objective of the present chapter is to investigate and to present the findings that point to a relation between the attention and sensorimotor integration, highlighting the participating electrophysiology and the cortical areas.

Hence, the present chapter will describe some cortical structures and the electrophysiological processes that occur during the sensorimotor integration, focusing on the role of attention. Moreover, this chapter will analyze the recent findings in sensorimotor integration highlighting how attention participates in this mechanism, it will describe the electrophysiological data around the cortical information processing, explain the main electrophysiological characteristics of attention, and it will illustrate the experiments involving brain mapping, attention and sensorimotor integration.

2. Cortical structures and sensorimotor integration: The role of attention

The sensorimotor integration is the process that organizes all types of sensory information and transforms it into a motor command. Attention is a cognitive function that underlies the sensorimotor integration process with its three stages: stimuli identification and selection; motor command organization; and motor execution. In this sense, it is observed that cortical areas involved in sensorimotor integration and attention overlap. The cortical structures most associated with sensorimotor integration and attention are the parietal, occipital, frontal, motor and somatomotor cortices.

The parietal cortex is widely involved in visuospatial sensorimotor integration. Particularly, the lateral intraparietal area (LIP) is an important region, which is connected with frontal areas that participate in the control and programming of eye movements (frontal eye field) and receive visual inputs from multiple visual areas [1]. The high amount of connections with other cortical and subcortical areas makes this region a relevant zone of association.

Attention is a cognitive process responsible for selecting and focusing on one or more features of the environment, while others are ignored, and for establishing the relationship among these features [2, 3]. It is a multidimensional capacity and it is directly related to memory and learning. Furthermore, attention processes are involved in the different information processing stages [4].

Neural mechanisms involved in attention interact among themselves, and we can highlight two main ones: top-down (i.e., voluntary attention) and bottom-up (i.e., reflexive attention). The top-down mechanism is based on the integration among previous knowledge, expectations and individual goals, in order to make a decision associated with attention shifting [4,5,6]. This mechanism influences the direction of sensorial, perceptual and decision processes. Specifically, the frontal and parietal cortices are involved in the voluntary mechanism [7,8]. The classic paradigm to study voluntary attention consists of the presentation of information as a signal (for example, a visual cue) that enables the subject to predict relevant features of the experimental set, such as the location and direction of the target stimulus [9]. In contrast, the bottom-up mechanism, or reflexive attention, is triggered by the physical features of the stimulus; in other words, the attention orientation is not directly controlled by the voluntary systems [8,9]. For example, a red flower will stand out more in a green field than in a colored flowers field. The ability to identify the flower depends on its difference or similarity in relation to other distractors. In another example, a sudden movement in the peripheral vision is immediately perceived, and this stops the action that was being executed in order to direct the attention to the new stimulus (sudden movement). Likewise, an individual crossing a busy street will be attracted by a sudden braking car, even if the vehicle was not coming his/her way. This effect of interruption and exogenous direction is based on the stimulus features and it is considered integrant part of the defense system [8,10,11]. The top-down and bottom-up mechanisms interact among them and sometimes compete for control of the neural processing and, consequently, execute the movement [3]. Recent investigations demonstrate an overlapping among the cortical areas involved in top-down and bottom-up attention. The task execution requiring both kinds of attention demonstrates activation of the parietal cortex and the premotor areas [5].

However, the voluntary attention condition also presents right prefrontal cortex activity. This area is associated with working memory, which may indicate that it is engaged voluntarily. In addition, the temporal-parietal junction activation is slightly different between the two kinds of attention, with a high involvement of the lateral, anterior and superior portion when reflexive attention is used [12]. Despite these small differences in the activated regions, in general an overlapping occurs among the areas participating in the two kinds of attention. Specifically, both attentions present activation of premotor region, frontal eye field (FEF) and superior parietal cortex, even if this last region exhibits more participation in the reflexive attention [8,12]. Despite these findings, few studies have shown how these areas interact with each other.

Thus, the mechanisms involved in attention process depend on the organization and integration of multiple cerebral centers. In this context, the participation of several structures and neural circuits demonstrates that attention is a process organized in a complex way related to the network integration of these components [8,13]. In particular, an experiment was conducted in which subjects were exposed to two initial conditions: presentation of visual images on a screen and a blank screen presentation. The subjects were instructed to maintain gaze in a central point in both conditions. During the visual presentation, four colored complex images were showed. These images could appear in different ways: in a sequential manner, each image on a different screen, or the four images on the same screen simultaneously. Moreover, two conditions were tested: i) no attention paid to the stimulus condition, where the subjects were instructed to maintain the gaze on a fixed point and to ignore the peripheral visual stimuli; ii) attention paid to the stimulus condition, where the subjects were instructed to direct the attention covertly to the place next to the fixation point and count the occurrence of these images [14]. The task begins with the presentation of a reference point near the fixed point, and the subjects were oriented to direct their attention to the target location immediately after the reference point presentation and to wait for the stimulus appearance (expectation period). Hence, attention effects could be studied in the presence and absence of visual stimuli. The authors verified a cortical activity increase during both conditions; attention directed to a specific location and expectation of visual stimuli occurrence. In particular, they found greater activation in frontal and parietal cortices when compared to the visual areas. This suggests that parietal and frontal cortices influence the early stages of scene scanning and they act as primary sources in the voluntary attention mechanism [13,15].

In this manner, attention can be classified according to its shifting nature: overt or covert attention. The overt attention is defined as an act to direct the sensory organs toward the stimuli and it is associated with both reflexive and voluntary attention [8,16]. On the other hand, covert attention is the act of mentally focus on one of the possible sensorial stimuli (vision, kinesthesia, hearing, etc) and it is associated with voluntary attention. Covert attention is the ability to attend a location or set without executing eye movements [11,17]. Thus, when staring at a fixed point represented by an asterisk (*), you perceive that it is possible to read the words around the point or to detect the objects' colors without moving your eyes. This kind of shifting is voluntary or endogenously controlled, because the attention direction depends only on the observer. Studies suggest that covert visual attention is a mechanism used to explore the visual field of interest [17]. For example, when someone is driving or maintaining their eyes on the road, even if the eyes do not move, the attention could shift from the road to their thoughts. The eyes maintain the focus on the object attended previously – the road, though attention has shifted [18]. In the last 30 years, researches based on a paradigm developed by Posner et al [19] have dominated the studies of oriented attention. This paradigm examines the advantage in indicating, by the use of a visual cue, the location where the target is more likely to appear. The participants are instructed to not perform any kind of overt attention, i.e. eye movement. The subjects are oriented to respond to the target as soon as detected. Two kinds of visual cues are presented: central and peripheral. The central cue is displayed directly on the fovea and indicates if the target will appear on the right or left portion of the screen. This condition is called central because of two reasons: it is centered in the visual field and it requires a central processing to interpret a symbol in a direction towards which the attention could be endogenously guided [20,21]. The peripheral cue is presented in the peripheral visual field on the screen portion where the target will appear, and it is represented by a flash of light. In the control group, none of the cues are presented. The results using this paradigm show that subjects responded faster to the target presented in the same location of the cue than when the target is showed in a different location from the cue. This demonstrates that visual attention is oriented in a covert way, with the absence of overt eye movement [22].

Despite an early distinction between overt and covert attention, recent findings point to an overlapping of cortical areas related to the shifting gaze – overt attention – and of those areas which participate in the covert attention mechanism. In particular, these studies verified an activity of the frontal cortex, especially of the pre-central sulcus, of the intraparietal cortex and of the lateral occipital cortex [23]. Experiments using Functional Magnetic Resonance Imaging (fMRI) investigated shifting attention tasks, both covert and overt, and verified an activation in the same areas – frontal, parietal and temporal cortices. Moreover, they demonstrated a higher activation during covert attention when compared to overt attention [14,24]. However, the right dorsolateral frontal cortex was activated only during covert attention shift, and this region is typically associated with voluntary attention and working memory [24]. Beauchamp et al. [23] reproduced these results through the execution of an experiment using both conditions: covert and overt attention. The results found were in agreement with previous studies, that is, Beauchamp et al. [23] verified that the same neural mechanisms were involved in overt and covert attention shifting.

Several studies involving covert attention orientation task revealed the involvement of cortical and subcortical areas in the control of attention direction toward visual stimuli. In particular, the attention visual model developed by Posner [6] establishes the existence of three distinct systems related to attention that work in directing voluntary attention. The systems are: posterior, anterior and vigilance.

The first one, the posterior system, is responsible for stimulus selection and localization, and for shifting attention between stimuli [22]. Moreover, it is associated with shifting of covert attention and it involves three structures: posterior parietal cortex, superior colliculus and pulvinar thalamic nucleus. The posterior parietal cortex acts in the attention disengagement from a particular stimulus; the superior colliculus is associated with the attention shifting; and the pulvinar thalamic nucleus is responsible for attention engagement with a novel stimulus [20,22].

The anterior system is involved in the detection of relevant stimuli and in the motor response preparation. This system comprises the frontal cortex, the cingulate cortex and the basal ganglia, and it is involved in the attention recruitment for the stimulus detection and in the control of brain areas for the performance of complex cognitive tasks, such as object recognition [25].

The last system proposed by Posner, the vigilance system, is characterized by alertness maintenance, in other words, it keeps the overall responsiveness of the nervous system attentive to external events. This system includes the frontal and parietal cortexes, specifically of the right hemisphere. Furthermore, there is the involvement of the reticular formation and the locus coeruleus, which in general increase the body alertness and attention guidance system modulation.

According to Raz and Buhle [7], the circuits mediating the attention process are associated with three types of networks which modulate attention: alerting, orienting and executive. The alerting network is associated with readiness in preparing the response to an imminent stimulus and can be interpreted as a basic "net" for all other attention functions. Recent data demonstrated that this "net" is represented in cortical and subcortical areas of the right hemisphere, in which the anterior cingulate cortex acts as a central coordinator of alertness structures [14,23]. The orienting network is related to the selection of specific information among multiple sensory stimuli. Finally, the executive network involves planning and decision making, error detection, difficulty or danger judgment, emotion and thought regulation. Despite the description of such model, there is a difficulty in establishing the neural circuits associated with each of these networks.

Knudsen [26] described a general attention model, which could be identified by four fundamental processes: working memory, top-down sensitivity control, competitive selection, and automatic bottom-up filtering for salient stimuli. The working memory acts in the temporary storage of information. The top-down sensitivity control enables higher cognitive information processing in such a way that it controls the intensity of the competing information channels' signals for accessing working memory, and it gives an advantage to the most intense channel in the competitive selection [2,14,27]. This, on the other hand, could be the process determining which information will access the working memory. Finally, the automatic bottom-up filtering for salient stimuli improves the response to rare, or biological relevant - instinctive or learned – information [4,25,28,29]. Thus, we can think in different hierarchical levels in the attention processing. And, according to the nature of the information or the task, the spatial maps may enhance or inhibit the activity in sensory areas, and induce oriented behaviors as well as eye movement.

3. The role of attention on the sensorimotor integration process

During the last decades, researchers that have been investigating sensorimotor integration have been concerned with establishing relevant elements to better explain the relationship among individual, task and environment in the production of the motor action [30]. In this context, theoretical models have been proposed. The models are necessary because they express the main aspects of a phenomenon, and reduce its complexity allowing the understanding of its properties [31,32]. In many sensorimotor integration models the memory system receives special attention, because it composes the comparison system, fundamental for error correction. In particular, the capacity to select, store and recover information is manipulated depending on the type of memory involved, implicit or explicit [33].

The motor control field is divided according to three distinct aspects: postural control, gait and voluntary action [34]. In gait regulation and voluntary action, visual information is essential to guarantee the movement performance [35]. Surely, the ability to walk or take a pen can be performed without light stimuli; for example, the case of an individual with visual deficit or the time when we try to get a glass of water during the night represent our ability to execute tasks without visual information [36]. But, if we consider the system integrity as a whole, vision is important in the motor action production. Specially, the sensorimotor integration models consider that the light stimulus coming from the environment and from the objects is the first stage of a wider process called decision making [37]. Thus, once volition to perform a motor action is removed de from the model,, the visual system is what determines part of this process; or, at least, it is through the vision that the initial stages of information processing are established [38]. The maintenance of the movement stability is the main goal of the central nervous system (CNS) when dealing with visual information [39,40]. Hence, the decision making depends on a repertoire of information that is registered on different cortical and subcortical structures, in order for the gesture stability to be achieved and maintained, especially where the channel input is the visual system [41]. According to Gibson, it is through the visual system that we interpret the relationship among individual, task and environment [42]. The Ecological Theory proposed by Gibson establishes a close relationship between individual and environment [43]. In the years that followed the pioneer ideas of Gibson, the researchers investigated their concepts and hypotheses that explain the functioning between the visual system and its relationship with the environment, in particular, the effect of this relationship on decision making [44].

In 1902, Raymond Dodge found 5 ocular movements responsible for maintaining the fovea in a target: three movements sustain the fovea in the visual target (saccade, smooth pursuit and vergence) and two more stabilize the eye during the head movement (vestibulo-ocular reflex and optokinetic reflex) [3,45]. These five ocular movements are responsible for the coupling relationship integrity among individual, task and environment [46]. As predicted by the sensorimotor integration models, the five ocular movements are not the only elements in the information flow related to information processing [47]; but, they participate in the early stage of information processing.

We know that the early stage of information processing is integrated with all the processing aspects, such as: selection, planning and motor response execution [38]. In this way, when we think about delays and errors in the information flow during the decision making processing, part of it is due to the early stages [48]. As previously mentioned, delays and errors are also related with other stages of processing; in particular, they occur when we compare new, or recent, information with that already stored; when this happens, we can observe indecision in the response selection in a situation that extrapolates normal parameters [33]. Researchers that study sensorimotor integration believe that the extrapolation of these parameters is associated with pathology, specific tasks and with environments which generate difficulty or ambiguity in the repertoire [49]. It is more difficult to control the motor action when tasks are executed in an environment of low stability, or with more unpredictability. Summarizing, the ocular movements are considered to be the gateway to information processing; specifically, these movements play a key role in maintaining the fovea on the target and in the stability of the eye when the head is moving. The combination of eye movements is part of a bigger system that integrates the individual with the environment, considering cognitive and volitional aspects [50].

In this context, the saccade is defined as a very quick movement (± 200 msec) of the eyeball from a fixed point to another, in order to focus the eye on different parts of the visual field in a short time interval [50]. The purpose of the saccade is to move the eyes very rapidly. The saccade occurs in fractions of seconds and at an angular speed of up to 900º/s [3]. This velocity is determined by the distance between the target and the fovea. It is possible to change the amplitude and direction of the saccadic movement, but not its velocity. In general, the saccadic movement is not modified by visual stimuli; this modification only occurs in the posterior saccade. The saccade only slows down under special conditions, such as: fatigue, drug and disease, such as schizophrenia. It is also produced by other stimuli besides the visual ones, such as sounds, information from the somatosensory system, spatial memories and even verbal commands [51,52].

Studies demonstrate that saccade reaction time decreases when other stimuli sources (hearing or touching) are presented in a temporal or spatial proximity to the visual source [53]. These results are found even in conditions where the individuals are instructed to ignore the secondary stimuli in tasks that involve focal attention. Data suggest a spatial-temporal interdependence in the neural structure involved in saccadic eye movement origin, such as the superior coliculus. The coliculus is a fundamental structure in the sensorimotor integration process [54]. Models using neural networks mainly seek to explain multisensorial spatial integration by a convergence process between information coming from vision, hearing and touch, and sensorimotor structures necessary to maintain the coordination between head and eyes. In this context, recent experiments explore stochastic models - time-window-of-integration model – in an attempt to include the temporal aspects of the integration process, since the former models have only approached the spatial issue. Thus, these experiments compare the model prediction with data extracted from visual-tactile tasks involving focused attention [53].

In the Central Nervous System (CNS), the sensorimotor integration process is subdivided into three different levels. In the hierarchical concept, these three levels are integrated. Starting from the bottom, the first stage (inferior level) of sensorimotor integration presents the spinal cord [55]. There we find the final common pathway of the motor neurons which innervate the corresponding muscle fibers. At this stage, there is the first level of integration between the afferents coming from different joints, muscles and skin, and the descendants coming from the cerebral cortex, facilitated by spinal interneurons [56]. At this stage of the sensorimotor integration, standardized events occur, such as: rapid removal (reflex) of one or more members caused by aversive stimuli, or responses that arise while walking [57].

The second stage of the sensorimotor integration takes place in several subcortical structures: reticular formation, vestibular nucleus, superior coliculus, cerebellum and basal ganglia. These structures receive spinal cord information and help in the postural stability control, as well as in the walking process [58]. For example, in the postural control the information from visual and somatosensory stimuli is important to maintain balance.

Finally, the superior stage of movement control is associated with the cerebral cortex [59]. In the cerebral cortex, we found structures that enable movement sophistication, a gesture diversification and a control on the supposed degrees of freedom, a term coined by Nicolai Berstei in 1949. The involvement of different cortical structures contributes to the formation of a sensory frame of reference with the participation of perceptive processes and, consequently, several kinds of memory [60]. As mentioned previously, the beginning of these connection networks and the various stages of sensorimotor integration are activated when the environment is rich in visual stimuli and requests saccadic eye movement.

Sensorimotor integration models, involving vision, are proposed in several situations; for example, Teixeira [61] explores the relationship between the environment information flow and the central nervous system functions. The model describes the sensorial information traffic in the CNS and the stages of information processing [62]. The first stage of this model refers to the stimulus transduction by the sensorial systems; the second one is related to executive function processing; and the third one is associated with substructures coordination in the movement production [40]. In detail, the model divides the information flow into three different stages where the attention affects them directly or indirectly. The first level, also called pre-attentive, refers to the sensorial information reception and to the more elementary perception processes. At this level, the sensorial system as a whole receives information from the internal and external environments [63]. This level is automatic, that is, the sensorial stimuli are not integrated yet to the executive functions, such as memory and attention. On the other hand, at the second level of the model, the attention has a fundamental role, since the internal and external stimuli pass through a conscious process [64]. This level is identified by a pre-thought about small details of the action; in particular, the prefrontal cortex participates in this entire module. A relevant aspect of this level is the comparison between new sensorial stimuli and elements previously stored in the memory [3]. Finally, the third level is called sub-attention and it is the stage where the motor control structures are integrated. This level is characterized by a high degree of sophistication, since the pre-conceived motor pattern becomes real with an originating intention [65].

4. Conclusion

The present chapter described the importance of attention in the sensorimotor integration. Specifically, we addressed the cortical and subcortical structures that are involved in the information processing, and the role of attention in the stages of sensorimotor integration. We emphasized the saccadic eye movement as a behavioral measure used to access the attention and sensorimotor integration. We identified a wide participation of the parietal and frontal cortices in the three mechanisms investigated, i.e., attention, information processing and sensorimotor integration. These cortical structures are considered strategic because of their communication network with other areas. The parietal region is directly associated with sensorial and multisensorial integration and the frontal area coordinates the attention process and the motor planning. The parietal and frontal cortices work together, but their participation is different depending on location or task context; researchers also observed an overlapping between these areas during attention and sensorimotor integration.

These regions influence two main attention mechanisms: top-down (i.e., voluntary attention) and bottom-up (i.e., reflexive attention). They interact between them and sometimes compete for control of the neural processing for the movement execution. Both types of attention also present activation of premotor region, frontal eye field (FEF) and superior parietal cortex. Furthermore, the attention mechanism has different hierarchical levels that depend on the nature of the information or the task. In this sense, the degree of attention in both sensorimotor integration and information processing will also depend on the information nature. In other words, attention is a fundamental element in the sensorimotor integration, and it is a feature that contributes to a better performance of a motor task.

Author details

Bruna Velasques[3,4,5,6*], Mauricio Cagy[1], Roberto Piedade[2] and Pedro Ribeiro[2,4,5]

*Address all correspondence to: bruna_velasques@yahoo.com.br

1 Biomedical Engineering Program, Universidade Federal do Rio de Janeiro, Rio de Janeiro, , Brazil

2 Brain Mapping and Sensory Motor Integration, Institute of Psychiatry of the Federal University of Rio de Janeiro (IPUB/UFRJ), Rio de Janeiro, Brazil

3 Neurophysiology and Neuropsychology of Attention, Institute of Psychiatry of the Federal University of Rio de Janeiro (IPUB/UFRJ), Rio de Janeiro, Brazil

4 Institute of Applied Neuroscience (INA), Rio de Janeiro, Brazil

5 School of Physical Education, Bioscience Department (EEFD/UFRJ), Rio de Janeiro, Brazil

6 Neuromuscular Research Laboratory, National Institute of Traumatology and Orthopedics (NITO), Rio de Janeiro, Brazil

References

[1] Gotlieb, J, & Snyder, L. H. Spatial and non-spatial functions of the parietal cortex. Curr Opin Neurobiol. (2010). , 20(6), 731-40.

[2] Estévez-gonzález, A, García-sánchez, C, & Junqué, C. La attención: una compleja función cerebral. Revista de Neurología.(1997). , 25(148), 1989-97.

[3] Kandel, E, Schwartz, S, & Jessel, T. Principles of Neuroscience. 4. ed. New York: McGraw-Hill; (2000).

[4] Gilbert, C. D, & Sigman, M. Brain states: top-down influences in sensory processing. Neuron. (2007). , 54(5), 677-96.

[5] Esterman, M, Prinzmetal, W, Degutis, J, Landau, A, Hazeltina, E, Verstynen, T, & Robertson, L. Voluntary and involuntary attention affect face discrimination differently. Neuropsychologia. (2008). , 46(4), 1032-40.

[6] Posner, M. I. Orienting of attention. Q J Exp Psychol. (1980). , 1, 3-25.

[7] Raz, A, & Buhle, J. Typologies of attentional networks. Nat Rev Neurosci. (2006). , 7(5), 367-79.

[8] Shipp, S. The brain circuitry of attention. Trends Cogn Sci. (2004). , 8(5), 223-230.

[9] Corbetta, M, & Shulman, G. L. Control of goal-directed and stimulus-driven attention in the brain. Nat Rev Neurosci. (2002). , 3, 201-15.

[10] Kowler, E, Anderson, E, Dosher, B, & Blaser, E. The role of attention in the programming of saccades. Vision Research. (1995). , 35(13), 1897-916.

[11] Sheliga, B. M, Riggio, L, & Rizzolatti, G. Orienting of attention and eye movements. Exp Brain Res. (1994). , 98(3), 507-22.

[12] Mcdowell, J. E, Dyckman, K. A, Austin, B. P, & Clementz, B. A. Neurophysiology and neuroanatomy of reflexive and volitional saccades: evidence from studies of humans. Brain Cogn. (2008). , 68(3), 255-70.

[13] Kastner, S, Pinsk, M. A, De Weerd, P, Desimone, R, & Ungerleider, L. G. Increased activity in human visual cortex during directed attention in the absence of visual stimulation. Neuron. (1999). , 22(4), 751-61.

[14] Corbetta, M, Patel, G, & Shulman, G. L. The reorienting system of the human brain: from environment to theory of mind. Neuron. (2008). , 58(3), 306-24.

[15] Astafiev, S. V, Shulman, G. L, Stanley, C. M, Snyder, A. Z, Van Essen, D. C, & Coerbetta, M. Functional organization of human intraparietal and frontal cortex for attending, looking, and pointing. J Neurosci. (2003). , 23, 4689-4699.

[16] Ignashchenkova, A, Dicke, P. W, Haarmeier, T, & Thier, P. Neuron-specific contribution of the superior colliculus to overt and covert shifts of attention. Nat Neurosci. (2004). , 7(1), 56-64.

[17] Moore, T, Armstrong, K. M, & Fallah, M. Visuomotor origins of covert spatial attention. Neuron.(2003). , 40(4), 671-68.

[18] Hoffman, J. E, & Subramaniam, B. The role of visual attention in saccadic eye movements. Percept Psychophys. (1995). , 57(6), 787-795.

[19] Posner, M. I. Snyder CRR, Davidson BJ. Attention and the detection of signals. J Exp Psychol: General.(1980). , 109, 160-174.

[20] Posner, M. I, & Badgaiyan, R. D. Attention and neural networks. In: RW Parks, DS Levine, DL Long (eds) Fundamentals of Neural Network Modelling. Cambridge, MA: MIT Press; (1998).

[21] Posner, M. I, Walker, J. A, Friedrick, F. J, & Rafal, R. D. Effects of parietal injury on covert orienting of visual attention. J Neurosci. (1984). , 4, 1863-74.

[22] Posner, M. I, & Petersen, S. E. (1990). The attentional system of the human brain. Annu Rev Neurosci. 1990;, 13, 25-42.

[23] Beauchamp, M. S, Petit, L, Ellmore, T. M, Ingeholm, J, & Haxby, J. V. A parametric fMRI study of overt and covert shifts of visuospatial attention. NeuroImage. (2001). , 14(2), 310-21.

[24] Nobre, A. C, Gitelman, D. R, Dias, E. C, & Mesulam, M. M. Covert visual spatial orienting and saccades: overlapping neural systems. NeuroImage. (2000). , 11, 210-6.

[25] Nabas, T. R, & Xavier, G. F. Atenção. In: Andrade, V. M., Santos, F. H. e Bueno, O. F. A. (eds.). Neuropsicologia Hoje. Porto Alegre: Artes Médicas; (2004).

[26] Knudsen, E. I. Fundamental components of attention. Annu Rev Neurosci. (2007). , 30, 57-78.

[27] Allport, A. Attention and control: have we been asking the wrong questions? A critical review of twenty-five years. In: Meyer, D. E. & Kornblum, S. (eds.) Attention and performance. New Jersey: Erlbaum; (1993).

[28] Pierrot-deseilligny, C, Müri, R. M, Nyffeler, T, & Milea, D. The role of the human dorsal lateral prefrontal cortex in ocular motor behavior. Ann N Y Acad Sci.(2005). , 1039, 239-51.

[29] Pierrot-deseilligny, C, Rivaud, S, Gaymard, B, & Agid, Y. Cortical control of reflexive visually-guided saccades. Brain.(1991). , 114, 1473-85.

[30] Bruno, N, & Battaglini, P. P. Integrating perception and action through cognitive neuropsychology (broadly conceived). Cogn Neuropsychol. (2008).

[31] Brozovic, M, Gail, A, & Andersen, R. A. Gain mechanisms for contextually guided visuomotor transformations. J Neurosci. (2007). , 27(39), 10588-96.

[32] Song, D, Lan, N, Loeb, G. E, & Gordon, J. Model-based sensorimotor integration for multi-joint control: development of a virtual arm model. Ann Biomed Eng.(2008). , 36(6), 1033-48.

[33] Krakauer, J. W. Motor learning and consolidation: the case of visuomotor rotation. Adv Exp Med Biol.(2009). , 629, 405-21.

[34] Carver, S, Kiemel, T, & Jeka, J. J. Modeling the dynamics of sensory reweighting. Biol Cyber. (2006). , 95(2), 123-34.

[35] Krieghoff, V, Brass, M, Prinz, W, & Waszak, F. Dissociating what and when of intentional actions. Front Hum Neurosci.(2009).

[36] Magescas, F, Urquizar, C, & Prablanc, C. Two modes of error processing in reaching. Exp Brain Res. (2009). , 193(3), 337-50.

[37] Puga, F, Sampaio, I, Veiga, H, Ferreira, C, Cagy, M, Piedade, R, & Ribeiro, P. The effects of bromazepam on the early stage of visual information processing (Arq de Neuropsiquiatr.(2007). A):955-9., 100.

[38] Proteau, L, Roujoula, A, & Messier, J. Evidence for continuous processing of visual information in a manual video-aiming task. J Motor Behaviour. (2009). , 41(3), 219-31.

[39] Pascolo, P. B, Carniel, R, & Pinese, B. Human stability in the erect stance: alcohol effects and audio-visual perturbations. J Biomech.(2009). , 42(4), 504-509.

[40] Konczak, J. Vander Velden H, Jaeger L. Learning to play the violin: motor control by freezing, not freeing degrees of freedom. J M Behav.(2009). , 41(3), 243-252.

[41] Lu, M. K, Bliem, B, Jung, P, Arai, N, Tsai, C. H, & Ziemann, U. Modulation of preparatory volitional motor cortical activity by paired associative transcranial magnetic stimulation. Hum Brain Mapp. (2009). , 30(11), 3645-56.

[42] Franz, V. H, Hesse, C, & Kollath, S. Visual illusions, delayed grasping, and memory: No shift from dorsal to ventral control. Neuropsychologia. (2009). , 47(6), 1518-31.

[43] Goodale, M. A. Action without perception in human vision. Cogn Neuropsychol. (2008).

[44] Konkle, T, Wang, Q, Hayward, V, & Moore, C. I. Motion aftereffects transfer between touch and vision. Curr Biol. (2009). , 19(9), 745-50.

[45] Tanaka, K, Abe, C, Awazu, C, & Morita, H. Vestibular system plays a significant role in arterial pressure control during head-up tilt in young subjects. Auton Neurosci. (2009).

[46] Fishbach, A, & Mussa-ivaldi, F. A. Seeing versus believing: conflicting immediate and predicted feedback lead to suboptimal motor performance. J Neurosci.(2008). , 28(52), 14140-14146.

[47] Soto, D, Hodsoll, J, Rotshtein, P, & Humphreys, G. W. Automatic guidance of attention from working memory. Trends Cogn Sci.(2008). , 12(9), 342-8.

[48] Kaku, Y, Yoshida, K, & Iwamoto, Y. Learning signals from the superior colliculus for adaptation of saccadic eye movements in the monkey. J Neurosci.(2009). , 29(16), 5266-5275.

[49] Bastian, A. J. Understanding sensorimotor adaptation and learning for rehabilitation. Curr Opin Neurol.(2008). , 21(6), 628-33.

[50] Hutton, S. B. (2008). Cognitive control of saccadic eye movements. Brain Cogn. 2008;, 68(3), 327-340.

[51] Berman, R. A, Joiner, W. M, Cavanaugh, J, & Wurtz, R. H. Modulation of presaccadic activity in the frontal eye field by the superior colliculus. J Neurophysiol.(2009). , 101(6), 2934-42.

[52] Wurtz, R. H. Vision for the control of movement. Invest Ophthalmol Vis Sci.(1996). , 11, 2130-45.

[53] Colonius, H, Diederich, A, & Steenken, R. Time-Window-of-Integration (TWIN) Model for Saccadic Reaction Time: Effect of Auditory Masker Level on Visual-Auditory Spatial Interaction in Elevation. Brain Topogr. (2009).

[54] Stein, B. E, Stanford, T. R, & Rowland, B. A. The neural basis of multisensory integration in the midbrain: Its organization and maturation. Hear Res. (2009).

[55] Hotz-boendermaker, S, Funk, M, Summers, P, Brugger, P, Hepp-reymond, M. C, Curt, A, & Kollias, S. S. Preservation of motor programs in paraplegics as demonstrated by attempted and imagined foot movements. NeuroImage. (2008). , 39(1), 383-94.

[56] Perez, M. A, Lundbye-jensen, J, & Nielsen, J. B. Changes in corticospinal drive to spinal motoneurones following visuo-motor skill learning in humans. J Physiol.(2006). Pt 3):843-55.

[57] Knikou, M. The H-reflex as a probe: pathways and pitfalls. J Neurosci Methods. (2008). , 171(1), 1-12.

[58] Glasauer, S, Amarim, M. A, Viaud-delmon, I, & Berthoz, A. Differential effects of labyrinthine dysfunction on distance and direction during blindfolded walking of a triangular path. Exp Brain Res.(2002). , 145(4), 489-97.

[59] Hattori, N, Shibasaki, H, Wheaton, L, Wu, T, Matsuhashi, M, & Hallet, M. Discrete parieto-frontal functional connectivity related to grasping. J Neurophysiol.(2008).

[60] Chen, T. L, Babiloni, C, Ferretti, A, Perrucci, M. G, Romani, G. L, Rossini, P. M, & Tartaro, A. Del Gratta C. Human secondary somatosensory cortex is involved in the processing of somatosensory rare stimuli: an fMRI study. NeuroImage. (2008). , 40(4), 1765-71.

[61] Teixeira, L. A, & Teixeira, M. C. Shift of manual preference in right-handers following unimanual practice. Brain Cogn.(2007). , 65(3), 238-43.

[62] Schmidt, R. A. Motor schema theory after 27 years: reflections and implications for a new theory. Res Q Exerc Sport.(2003). , 74(4), 366-75.

[63] Salillas, E, El Yagoubi, R, & Semenza, C. Sensory and cognitive processes of shifts of spatial attention induced by numbers: an ERP study. Cortex.(2008). , 44(4), 406-13.

[64] Theeuwes, J, Belopolsky, A, & Olivers, C. N. Interactions between working memory, attention and eye movements. Acta Psychol (Amst). (2009). , 132(2), 106-14.

[65] Royer, A. S, & He, B. Goal selection versus process control in a brain-computer interface based on sensorimotor rhythms. J Neural Eng. (2009). Feb;6(1):016005.

Chapter 2

A High Performance MEG Based BCI Using Single Trial Detection of Human Movement Intention

Peter T. Lin, Kartikeya Sharma, Tom Holroyd,
Harsha Battapady, Ding-Yu Fei and Ou Bai

Additional information is available at the end of the chapter

http://dx.doi.org/10.5772/54550

1. Introduction

Human volitional movement is orchestrated by dynamic changes in brain activity that can be detected by noninvasive electrophysiological recording using electroencephalography (EEG) or magnetoencephalography (MEG). At least two kinds of movement-related brain activity can be observed: movement–related cortical potentials (MRCP) and event-related desynchronization/synchronization (ERD/ERS) in the alpha (8-13Hz) and beta frequency band (16-30Hz) as reviewed in [1-3]. Both have been observed prior to movement onset and represent the activation of widespread sensorimotor networks responsible for the preparation and intention to move. Although it may be more difficult to identify premovement activity from the spatial distribution of MRCP due to the small amplitude of the signal and the need for signal averaging to enhance the signal-to-noise ratio, changes in oscillatory activity may be detectable even on a single trial basis. Functional mapping studies using EEG and MEG have demonstrated that somatotopically restricted motor areas are activated before the actual production of certain limb movements. For example, as assessed by studying movement-related ERD in [4-6], the hand area is activated before the production of hand movements whereas the foot area is activated prior to foot movements. Furthermore, there is a consistent lateralization of activation with right hand movements activated by predominantly left sensorimotor cortex whereas left hand movements are activated by right sensorimotor cortex. If the spatial resolution of the signal is high enough, discrimination of different movement intentions from the spatiotemporal distribution of oscillatory brain activity should be possible on a single trial basis and could be harnessed as a flexible control signal for external devices in the design of brain computer interfaces (BCI).

Brain computer interfaces are neural signal driven systems developed as a means of communication for patients with severe neuromuscular impairment. Although BCI technology can also be used to monitor human attention level or other higher level cognitive tasks such as decision making as detailed in [7,8], the predominant goal of current BCI efforts is the restoration of motor function. Due to neurologic conditions such as spinal cord injury, stroke or Amyotrophic Lateral Sclerosis (ALS), severe motor paralysis may develop and at the extreme, progress to a locked-in state, where there is complete inability to move but retained ability to think. By detecting brain activity associated with specific user intentions and translating thought into action, BCI provides a potential medium for communication and rehabilitation. By providing users with feedback control, BCI systems may be useful in promoting cortical plasticity after conditions including stroke or spinal cord injury.

There are two methodological approaches to BCI: invasive and non-invasive. The invasive approach utilizes intracortical neuronal population activity as detected with microelectrode arrays implanted directly into the brain with the advantage of high signal strength. Several groups in [9-11] have utilized this approach successfully for the prediction of movement trajectory, cursor control or use of a robotic arm. However, due to the inherent technical demands and risks of surgical implantation, non-invasive techniques are generally used. In the non-invasive approach, electroencephalography (EEG) and magnetoencephalography (MEG) have emerged as the most viable options. Any activity in the brain is accompanied by changes in ion concentrations in neurons leading to polarization and depolarization. Such neuronal population activity can be measured by EEG, whereas MEG measures the magnetic field associated with these currents. Both modalities have a time resolution on the order of milliseconds, allowing for the study of the highly dynamic activity of the brain in contrast to slower response time from imaging-based BCI using positron emission topography (PET), optical imaging using near infrared spectroscopy (NIRS) or functional MRI signals as in [12]. EEG is advantageous in that it is portable and cost effective but as magnetic fields suffer far less degradation than electric fields from the spatial blurring effect of the skull, MEG provides a better spatial resolution leading to more accurate decoding, as reviewed in [13]. The advantage of MEG is the more simplified reconstruction of signals into source space leading to reduction of noise and subsequent better feature separation. MEG may have a greater potential to interpret brain activity on a single trial basis instead of utilizing indirect control of brain rhythmic activity or slow cortical potentials as used in current EEG-based BCI and detailed in [14,15]. However, the lack of portability and the costs of MEG instrumentation are impractical for general BCI use.

Optimization of BCI involves the use of technology and design of signal processing algorithms with a fast response time, low error rate, and reduced training time. Due to the need for high temporal precision, electromagnetic signals are the most practical for widespread BCI use. Signal processing algorithms using a combination of spatial and temporal filters or signal averaging extract relevant features, enhance the signal-to-noise ratio and reduce classification error and are an active area of research reviewed in [16,17]. Ideally, BCI operation on a single trial basis is preferred due to the improved response speed and higher information transfer rate, but at the cost of a potentially noisier signal with higher error rate depending on the feature selected. In addition, identifying signal features that represent the activation of biologically realistic sources reduces the likelihood of misclassification from neurophysiologic

http://dx.doi.org/10.5772/54550

artifacts such as eye blinks, scalp muscle activity or cognitive activity unrelated to the task paradigm. Shorter training times reduce the likelihood of mental fatigue and improve the generalizability of use for diverse patient populations. A task paradigm based on movement direction or natural motor behavior may also reduce training time as it may be more intuitive.

In this chapter we present a multi-dimensional prediction based BCI that reliably decodes human movement intention. We previously demonstrated that ERD/ERS changes using a contingent negative variation based four class-paradigm can be reliably discriminated using EEG in [18]. In this study, subjects began to prepare for one of four movements after viewing an initial cue signal. After a period, they performed the movement, but the classification took place during the period of mental preparation. We also demonstrated that spatially distinct movement intentions using the right hand and left hand using an ERD/ERS paradigm can be reliably classified and differentiated with MEG signals in [19]. However, several potential BCI users may have brain injury specifically affecting the structural or functional integrity of the hand area, limiting the ability to generalize from this paradigm. If the prediction/decoding of movement intentions to move the right hand, left hand, leg and tongue before movements occur is robust, the natural behavior of human intentions to move different effectors can be decoded to control a two-dimensional cursor for BCI applications. Our BCI performance critically depends on the reliable decoding of intention from the spatial distribution of brain activity. We adopted synthetic aperture magnetometry (SAM) as a spatial filter for enhancing the spatial resolution of MEG signals. The robustness of the prediction suggests that spatially filtered MEG can be used as a robust BCI method supporting multi-dimensional control.

2. Spatiotemporal filtering in BCI

2.1. Optimizing BCI signals for classification

In order to extract a robust control signal for classification from multichannel EEG or MEG data, various signal processing methods are available. The selection of a simple task paradigm associated with a reliable neurophysiological signal is an important first step prior to data processing and classification. As ERD is a fundamental physiological signal associated with natural movements, it is a logical choice for analysis. Spatial and temporal filters reduce the data load and improve discrimination and classification. As many potential signals including ERD are spatially restricted to the sources of activation from somatotopic representation and lateralization, algorithms that enhance the spatial signal may improve the distinctness of spatial patterns. Restricting the analysis to a subset of electrodes or sensors over areas of interest (i.e., C3 and C4 EEG electrodes over sensorimotor cortical regions) is a simple method of spatial filtering. Computational data-driven spatial filters that have been used in EEG-based BCI include independent component analysis (ICA), common spatial patterns (CSP), surface Laplacian derivation (SLD), and principal component analysis (PCA) in [20-23]. These methods are similar in their ability to enhance the spatial resolution of the feature in order to enhance discrimination. In the temporal domain, frequency filters may be used to reduce dimensionality as different cognitive tasks may be associated with dynamic changes in specific frequency bands. Furthermore, there may be subject-specific dominant frequency band changes associated with the same task, making optimization and selection of temporal filters an adaptive process. Temporal filters that are used include finite impulse response (FIR) filtering, power spectral density (PSD) estimation and discrete wavelet transformation (DWT). Signal averaging is also a commonly used method in the P300 and visual evoked potential (VEP) based BCI systems in [24,25] to enhance signal quality although this may slow down the response time.

The exact choice or combination of signal processing methods may depend on the task paradigm utilized or the subject population studied. Comparison of the combination of various methods including spatial and temporal filtering, feature extraction and pattern classification have been explored by several groups in decoding single trial EEG signals associated with movement in [26,27]. These studies demonstrate the critical point that the selection of computational methods can affect the speed and accuracy of BCI performance.

2.2 Synthetic Aperture Magnetometry (SAM) and Source Space BCI

Synthetic aperture magnetometry (SAM) is a powerful adaptive beamforming approach used in MEG. Beamforming is a technique used in radar or sonar technology that involves estimating the contribution of a single source to a group of sensors by excluding activity from all other sources. SAM is a minimum variance beamformer technique that is designed to pass the signal from a small region of interest with unit gain while blocking signals from outside that area as detailed in [28]. Data from single trials are used to estimate sensor weight matrices which then applied to raw MEG data from sensors yield source images. The number of sources does not need to be specified using this method. SAM takes advantage of the spatial and temporal correlation of MEG sensor arrays and acts as a spatial filter to map three dimensional source power. The spatial distribution of event-related changes in cortical rhythm within a specified frequency range and time window relative to the event can be estimated. Furthermore, using the sensor weight covariance matrices, virtual sensor time series can be generated and used for source based estimates of changes in activation or connectivity. This technique has been demonstrated to be effective in localizing source activation associated with various cognitive tasks including speech, motor and sensory processing in [29-31]. It has been used effectively in various clinical settings including preoperative localization of motor cortex for tumor resection, identification of epileptogenic foci and mapping language areas as demonstrated in [32-35].

Source space analysis methods are a relatively novel avenue in BCI research. Compared with sensor based signals, source based signals should be less noisy and provide better features for classification. High-resolution EEG techniques including source reconstruction have been proposed as a useful method in [36] to improve BCI accuracy. Several EEG studies have used source reconstruction methods in classifying movement related signals in [37-40]. A prior study utilized beamforming techniques as a spatial filter in BCI design using EEG data in [37]. Regions of interest were preselected and beamforming was used to suppress source activity outside of the regions of interest. Results showed better classification accuracy compared to surface Laplacian and comparable to common spatial pattern (CSP) filtering in the setting of large artifacts. Another EEG study used a source reconstruction method with a spherical head model and simple source distribution to demonstrate better classification rate compared to electrodes studying movement related ERD and MRCP in [38]. These studies provide evidence that source localization may help refine accuracy of classification using EEG. However, source localization including beamforming using EEG may be limited by sparse electrode sampling in typical EEG-based BCI compared to the dense whole head sensor coverage with MEG, limiting the ability to estimate sources accurately. Furthermore, the signal-to-noise ratio of EEG signals on a single trial basis is low, making source localization more difficult. The Laplacian spatial filter is commonly used for EEG signals to improve the signal-to-noise ratio. However, due to the more intricate geometry of magnetic fields compared to electric fields, it is not possible to find a general spatial filter that improves the signal-to-noise ratio analogous to Laplacian filtering. For MEG signals, the position and orientation of the sources of interest must be taken into account as well.

Due to the more robust source localization methods with MEG, source space MEG BCI analysis may be a powerful paradigm to enhance signal strength for improving feature classification. Prior MEG based BCI studies have been conducted based on the sensor domain, focusing mainly on the source identification problem [41-43]. In [44], a source based MEG analysis was proposed using a novel blind source separation method called functional source separation (FSS) to identify sources of activation and source time courses for potential BCI use. There are few beamformer based MEG BCI studies despite the robustness of these techniques in mapping movement-related desynchronization as demonstrated in prior studies. As movement-related ERD can be somatotopically restricted as well as lateralized, we hypothesized that using SAM as a spatial filter would give rise to improved separation of spatially distinct patterns for classification.

3. Methods

3.1. Subjects

Eight healthy volunteers, 5 male and 3 female (age: 31±8 years) participated in the experiment. All subjects participating in this study were right-handed according to the Edinburgh inventory in [45]. All subjects had not received prior BCI-related training. The protocol was approved by the Institutional Review Board. All subjects gave written informed consent for the study.

3.2. Experimental paradigm

A visual warning cue randomly selected from a set of four cues: 'right" for right hand extension, 'left' for left hand extension, 'leg' for left foot extension, and 'tongue' for pressing the tongue against the roof of the mouth, was presented on a computer screen placed about 50 cm in front of the subject (see Figure 1). The subjects were instructed to prepare for the movement without physically moving after the initial cue presentation. The duration of the visual cue was 0.5 s. After 2.5sec a 'GO' signal was displayed at which time the subject started physically moving as soon as possible. This continued for another 2.5 sec after which a stop signal was displayed at which time the subject stopped moving and returned to baseline rest. A 4-7 sec rest period was given after which the process was repeated. During the period of visual stimuli the subjects were asked to keep eyes open and reduce blinks as much as possible. The subjects were allowed to become familiar with the paradigm before data recording. The experiment consisted of 6-7 sessions with each session consisting of 30 movement tasks, i.e. about 45 trials for each of four movements. Subjects were asked to keep the head still during recording to reduce head motion. Trials contaminated with EMG activities before the 'GO' cue were excluded both for the classification and analysis.

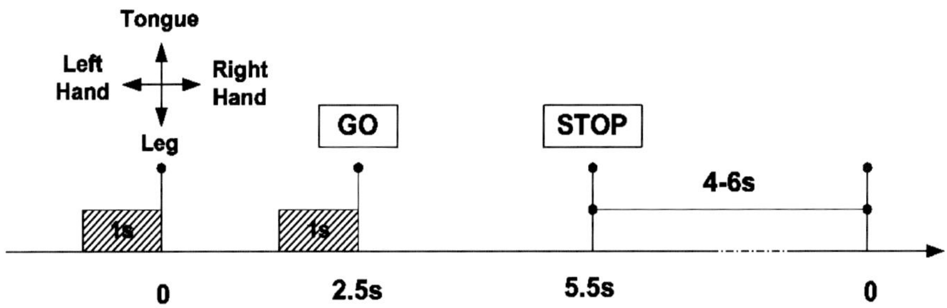

Figure 1. Experimental paradigm. Activation period: -1 second to 0 before 'GO' cue. Control period: -1 second to 0 before warning cue of 'Right Hand', 'Left Hand', 'Foot' and 'Tongue'. At the "GO" cue, subjects began repeated extensions of the right hand, left hand or left foot or tongue movements as per the initial instruction cue. Subjects continued the movements until the "STOP" cue. Data from the activation and control windows were used for SAM analysis, with virtual channels during the activation period used for classification/prediction.

3.3. Data acquisition

MEG data was recorded at 600 Hz using a 275-channel CTF whole head MEG system (VSM MedTech Inc., Coquitlam BC, Canada) in a shielded environment. The CTF MEG system is equipped with synthetic 3rd gradient balancing, an active noise cancellation technique that uses a set of reference channels to subtract background interference.

High-resolution structural MRI images were also acquired for co-registration for each subject using a magnetization-prepared rapid acquisition by gradient echo sequence (MP-RAGE) (TI/TE/TR/FA=725/2.928/7.6/6°, FOV=22 cm, partition thickness=1.2mm, 256 x 256, in-plane voxel size=0.859375).

EMG was recorded using bipolar electrodes over the right and left wrist extensors (extensor digitorum communis), and left ankle dorsiflexors (tibialis anterior). This allowed for the exclusion of any trial with movement prior to the 'GO' cue by monitoring for premature muscular activity. Premature motor execution was monitored by the experimenter by EMG and trials with early activation were excluded from the analysis.

3.4. SAM analysis

Synthetic Aperture Magnetometry (SAM) was used for source localization of MEG signals. "Source localization" implies simplification of the complex activity of a very large numbers of neurons to a few parameters that help describe that activity, as in [46]. During SAM analysis, the SAM images were created for active state vs. control state, i.e. it extracted a dominant modulated source from a background of less pronounced modulation and noise.

MEG analysis software developed at NIMH MEG core facility was used for epoching data, SAM analysis and MRI conversion. For all measurements, fiducial skin markers were placed on subjects' nasion and bilateral preauricular points. The data was epoched according to the marker events for a period of 9 sec starting 1 sec before the instruction cue and continuing 8 sec after. For SAM analysis, all epoched data for each event ('right', 'left', 'leg', or 'tongue') were pooled together to form a grand dataset. Before SAM analysis, a multisphere head model was created for each subject (threshold value about 40% to determine the boundary of shells) based on anatomical images of each subject using MEG analysis software.

For SAM Analysis, single-trial event-related MEG data from the grand datasets were used to compute covariance matrices for each dataset corresponding to each event. The frequency range of interest was the beta band (15-30 Hz). The active state was defined 1 sec before 'GO' cue to 'GO' cue onset (1.5 s – 2.5 s); -1 s to instruction cue onset was set as the control state (-1 s – 0 s) (see Figure 1). These parameters were fed in to compute the covariance between the active and the control state. For ERD analysis a statistical parametric image was computed, on a voxel- by-voxel basis, from the difference in cortical power for the two states, relative to their noise variance. Only voxels displaying statistically significant power changes were displayed in color scale on the individual MRI. Thus an optimal spatial filter was designed which created a 3D source image comparing the source strength for the two states. This image was superposed on the MRI image of the subjects to obtain the source- signal-to-noise ratio image corresponding to each event for all the subjects.

3.5 Virtual channel selection

A *virtual channel* is tuned to a particular source or target. In SAM analysis as described above, a beamformer was calculated for each voxel of the image, and the beamformer was used to calculate a source power estimate. The same beamformer was used to determine coefficients or weights for each channel, and a virtual channel was obtained from a weighted sum of all the MEG channels with those weights. The target location for the present study was the motor cortex area. As previously described, human limb movements are controlled predominantly by the contralateral sensorimotor areas. The source-signal-to-noise ratio image obtained through SAM analysis would have high activity regions in these areas. Consistent with expected somatotopic representations, virtual channels were selected from regions showing strong ERD in the left and right hand, leg and tongue areas respectively. Around 20-30 virtual channels were selected for each subject.

3.6. Time–course analysis of MEG sensor and virtual channel data

The digital MEG signal was sent to a DELL PC workstation and was offline processed using a home-made MATLAB (Math Works, Natick, MA) Toolbox: brain-computer interface to virtual reality or BCI2VR [27,47]. This was used for time-course analysis, feature extraction and classification for MEG-Sensor domain as well as Virtual channel data.

3.6.1. Time–frequency analysis of MEG sensor data

Time-Frequency analysis was performed on the MEG sensor data (See Figure 2) to observe the power (ERD) patterns for each event. The region of interest was selected in the motor cortex areas associated with human movement intention as detailed in [48-50]. The MEG channels constrained to the central MEG sensors associated with the right hand, left hand, leg, or tongue area depending on the event were used for the analysis. It was intended to analyze the power in the beta band, i.e. the ERD patterns with respect to the time-course of the motor tasks. Power in the frequency range 0- 60 Hz, for four movements was calculated using the Welch method described in [51], which was applied with the use of a Hamming window to reduce side-lobe effect and estimation variance. A baseline correction was introduced from -1 s to 0 s. The length of the sliding window was 1 s with a slide increment of 0.1 s. The segment length was 0.25 s with frequency resolution of 4 Hz and there was no overlapping between consecutive segments.

3.6.2. Time–course of event-related power for virtual channel data

An event related power analysis was performed on the virtual channel data obtained through SAM analysis. We intended to observe the ERD patterns over time for each event. The time-course of event-related power was obtained from the variance of virtual channel signal in a sliding window with length of 1s and a slide increment of 0.1 s. These virtual channels were already filtered from the beta band. A baseline correction was introduced from -1 s to 0.5 s. Event related power analysis was performed to verify whether ERD was a dominant pattern for virtual channels selected when subjects were intending to perform the four different movements.

3.7. Feature extraction and classification

The data pool consisted of about 180 trials with 45 samples for each of four classes. The offline performance of multi-class classification was evaluated from 10-fold cross-validation; 90% of data pool was used for training, and the other 10% was used for testing so that the testing dataset was independent from the training dataset. For classification methods using feature evaluation for feature selection, those parameters or features were also determined by training data set only.

3.7.1. Feature extraction for MEG sensors and virtual channels

For MEG -Sensor based classification, the MEG channels were constrained through empirical channel reduction; this covered the entire motor cortex area. Thus the central 52 MEG chan-

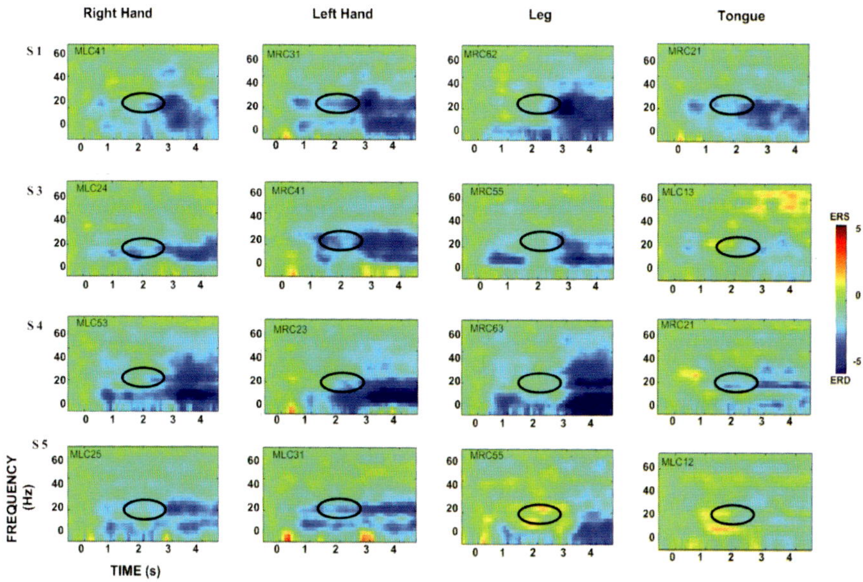

Figure 2. Time-frequency analysis in the sensor domain. Time-frequency map for movements of the right hand, left hand, leg and tongue for subjects S1, S3, S4 and S5 are plotted from the MEG raw sensor domain (left corner of each map, M – MEG, R – right, L – left, and C – central). Power is symbolized by blue for ERD and red for ERS. The region of interest corresponding to the active state period corresponding to movement intention is marked by the black ellipse.

nels were used for sensor based classification (The layout can be found in http:// kurage.nimh.nih.gov/meglab/Meg/Meg). For SAM-filtered virtual channel based classification of movement intensions from MEG data, channel reduction was achieved through the selection of virtual channels. Also, the selection of beta band (15- 30 Hz) to study ERD served as an important parameter for feature reduction. In the MEG-Sensor domain, the power samples were calculated in the beta band (15- 30 Hz) for the active state period when subjects were intending or urging to move (1.5 s – 2.5 s), the segment length was 0.25 s with no overlapping between consecutive segments. For Virtual channels, the beta band power samples were calculated as the variance of the data samples from the active state period before movement occurred.

The SAM-filtered MEG virtual channel signals or MEG sensor domain signals provided high-dimensional features; for example, 25 virtual channels with 16 frequency bins produced 400 features. A subset of features determined by feature selection was determined for classification.

3.7.2. Feature selection and classification

The feature selection was achieved by either Bhattacharyya distance or genetic algorithm.

Bhattacharyya distance: The Bhattacharyya distance is the square of mean difference between two task conditions divided by the averaged variance of the samples in two task conditions so that a larger Bhattacharyya distance will lead to better classification accuracy as described in [52]. The empirically extracted features were ranked by Bhattacharya distance for further classification.

Genetic Algorithm (GA): Genetic algorithms are computational models inspired by evolution as described in [53]. It is a stochastic search in the feature space guided by the concept of inheriting, where at each search step, good properties of the parent subsets found in previous steps are inherited. 10-fold cross-validation was used with a Mahalanobis linear distance (MLD) classifier for feature evaluation as in [54]. The population size used was 20, the number of generations was 100, the crossover probability was 0.8, the mutation probability was 0.01, and the stall generation was 20.

The classification techniques were developed in a home-made MATLAB (Math Works, Natick, MA) Toolbox: brain-computer interface to virtual reality or BCI2VR described in [27,47]. It was intended to use these classification techniques to reliably decode human movement intentions spatially for the four classes. The classifiers selected were based on their performance in previous computational comparison studies in [27,54-56].

GA-based Mahalanobis Linear Distance Classifier (GA-MLD): The Mahalanobis Distance Classifier had proved effective for classification in previous studies [27,57]. It was further optimized using GA-based feature extraction method. The optimal feature subset was selected by GA, and the selected features providing the best cross-validation accuracy were applied to a Mahalanobis Linear Distance Classifier (MLD) as in [52]. The number of features for the subset was 4, which was determined from the 10-fold cross-validation accuracy with feature numbers of 2, 4, 6, and 8.

Direct Decision Tree Classifier (DTC): A Decision tree is a classifier which uses symbolic treelike representations of finite sets of if-then-else questions that are natural, intuitive and interpretable as in [58]. For example, a certain feature subset of channels over the left motor cortex area are associated with right hand movement as shown in [59-61]. Then, these would be the best to discriminate intention to move the right hand, whereas they might operate rather poorly for the discrimination of other movement intentions. We used multistage classification, i.e., decision tree classifier (DTC), to discriminate one intention from others in each successive stage. At each level of DTC, the features for one-to-others classification were ranked by Bhattacharya distance (see detailed method in [27]) and the 4 features with higher rank were used for classification by MLD. The number of the feature for classification was determined from preliminary comparison (through 10-fold cross validation accuracy) with numbers of 2, 4, 6 and 8.

4. Results

4.1. Sensor–based ERD/ERS visualization

ERD/ERS visualizations for 4 subjects are included from MEG sensor data to demonstrate characteristic power changes located over motor cortical regions (Figure 2). Power changes were notable for a sustained decrease in the 8-30 Hz range beginning 1-1.5 second before S2 and continuing through the time of execution of movement. From the ERD images, it was observed that ERD signals were enhanced during the period of motor execution compared with the movement intention period.

4.2. SAM–based spatial visualization of ERD activation

Spatially filtered ERD activity was visualized using SAM. Figure 3 demonstrates SAM images from 4 subjects demonstrating activation of motor areas corresponding to the intention to move under the four different conditions. Virtual channels were derived from the areas of peak ERD activation for power analysis, feature extraction and classification.

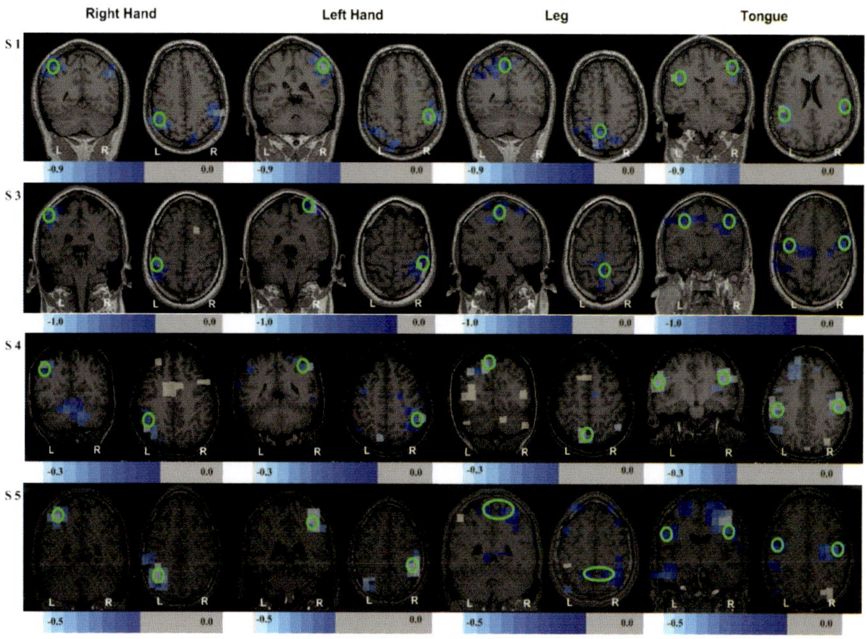

Figure 3. SAM image. Coronal and axial views of the head are shown for subjects S1, S3, S4 and S5. Virtual channels corresponding to the ERD (Blue) over areas of activation corresponding to movement intention were chosen from areas marked by the green circle for further classification.

4.3. Virtual channel power analysis

Time-frequency analysis was performed on single-trial MEG virtual sensor data. The time course of ERD/ERS changes from virtual channels demonstrates consistent patterns of desynchronization associated with the time period chosen for prediction (Figure 4).

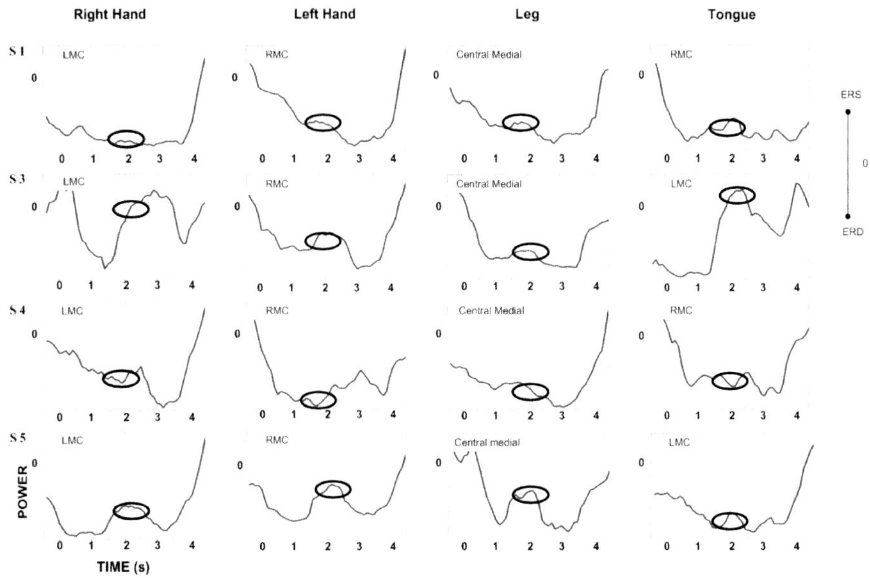

Figure 4. Time course of event-related power change for SAM-Virtual channel signal. Time-power maps for events Right hand, Left Hand, Leg and Tongue for the single-trial MEG data for subjects S1, S3, S4 and S5 are plotted for corresponding SAM-Virtual channels over regions of interest (LMC – left motor cortex, Central medial cortex, RMC – right motor cortex). The region of interest corresponding to the active state period for movement intention is marked by the black ellipse.

4.4. Classification

To compare the advantage of using SAM, results from virtual channel classification were compared with MEG sensor based classification. Classification of signals using 2 different classification methods (GA-MLD and DTC) were higher using MEG virtual sensors compared to raw sensors (Table 1). The virtual channel-based classification accuracy for four classes using GA-MLD was on average 88.90% with standard deviation of 7.74%. Similarly, virtual channel based classification using direct DTC was 73.34% with standard deviation of 16.71%.

Classification with MEG sensors was much less accurate. MEG sensor based classification accuracy using GA-MLD was 42.41% with standard deviation of 7.26%. Using direct DTC, accuracy was 30.13% with standard deviation 5.56%.

Subject	**SAM Virtual Sensor**		**MEG Sensor Domain**		**Total no. of**
	GA-MLD (%)	DTC (%)	GA-MLD (%)	DTC (%)	samples/trials
S 1	96 ± 0.44	85.19 ± 4.14	40.78 ± 2.11	30.44 ± 3.01	191
S 2	87.31 ± 1.32	61.75 ± 2.04	33.57 ± 2.32	26.14 ± 3.56	219

Subject	SAM Virtual Sensor		MEG Sensor Domain		Total no. of
	GA-MLD (%)	DTC (%)	GA-MLD (%)	DTC (%)	samples/trials
S 3	89.17 ± 1.62	85.75 ±1.86	44 ± 1.36	31.37 ± 2.97	181
S 4	84.25 ± 1.55	73.37 ±1.86	51.11 ± 2.16	29.5 ± 2.53	200
S 5	99.14 ± 0.19	97.16 ± 0.85	53.15 ± 1.66	41.90 ± 0.66	202
S 6	79.69 ± 2.36	42.68 ± 3.12	44.56 ± 1.57	32 ± 2.79	202
S7	96.58 ± 0.97	71.25 ± 3.61	38.18 ± 2.91	25.55 ± 3.33	177
S8	79.08 ± 2.06	69.58 ± 4.52	33.94 ± 2.07	24.17 ± 2.77	173

Table 1. SAM-Virtual channel signal vs. MEG-Sensor signal Classification

5. Discussion

In this study, a prediction based BCI was designed using spatially filtered MEG signals associated with four different movement intentions. Successful classification of discrete movement intentions was achieved with a high degree of accuracy. The results from this study demonstrate that the spatiotemporal activity associated with human movement intention is predictable and can be spatially separated and used for classification. These movement intentions can be potentially used as control mechanisms. Previously, we reported our results in [16] classifying movement based intentions from MEG using ERD/ERS patterns generated from right and left hand movement. The limitations of the previous paradigm are the reliance on the integrity of hand movement, which is often compromised in BCI user populations such as those with unilateral stroke or motor neuron disease. The ability to differentiate effector specific movement intentions from a range of body parts allows for a greater flexibility of our BCI approach.

All subjects demonstrated ERD before and during the movement, followed by ERS after the movement. ERD occurred in similar regions for the intention and movement execution period. As expected, desynchronization signals were stronger during actual movement than during movement intention. Distinct movement intentions led to distinctly different regions of activity in the brain, although some overlapping regions were also found. ERD activation was seen bilaterally suggesting coordination between both the hemispheres, although generally one side would dominate. For left hand movement, right motor cortex was predominantly activated whereas for right hand movement left motor cortex region showed greater activity. For leg movement, mesial motor cortex was activated. Tongue activity showed a great deal of variation across the subjects activating regions of both hemispheres. Global activation of motor networks have been reported for movements of the foot and tongue in [62], potentially making the distinction between classes more difficult due to overlap of activation. The tongue representation is relatively small and distributed across both hemispheres. The hand area also was activated during tongue movement. This may occur because the tongue is more difficult to move as compared to hand or foot, leading to a broader region of activation overlap as detailed in [62,63]

All subjects showed dynamic activity mostly in the beta band (15-30 Hz). This is consistent with previous studies demonstrating the important role of beta band activity in motor control [3]. All eight subjects showed different regions of activation for different movement intentions, but these regions varied from subject to subject. Each individual subject had particular pairs of movement intentions which produced better results than the rest, but the trends were not consistent across the subjects. This variability may be related to inherent differences in terms of individual motor learning and movement strategy. More research in this area may explain this trend. More generally, such research could lead to a better understanding of different neural activity involved in the learning of a motor task.

Previous studies have demonstrated the feasibility of using MEG signals for BCI purposes in [64-67]. In [65], a MEG study exploring the decoding of movement directions, a reasonable detection accuracy was achieved from signals associated with the motor execution of physical movement. Although it seems more intuitive for BCI users to control directional movement, practical application of BCI substitutes more reliable control for the intuitiveness of the approach. Comparing the premovement data to the results in that study, our BCI provided much better classification accuracy. The best detection accuracy was found to be after movement onset, which may not be useful in subject populations who can not physically move. Furthermore, the approach utilized in that study was performed on the sensor domain level. The conclusions from this study suggest that spatial filtering may lead to improved performance using their paradigm. Another study in [66] used MEG and sensorimotor mu rhythm control with successful results in 6 out of 8 patient, but their approach required extensive training over several weeks. In contrast, our BCI requires less extensive training and a faster response time due to the natural motor task performed.

Our method showed that MEG provides high resolution both spatially and temporally. If optimized techniques are used for source imaging, robust results can be obtained for suitable multi dimensional BCI control. By applying SAM filter, the classification accuracy was significantly improved with the average classification accuracy 91±12%. These results demonstrate that SAM spatial filter may effectively improve MEG signal spatial resolution to achieve an accurate classification of movement intentions. Four-class classification in this study using spatial filtering was highly accurate despite the visualized overlap of activation across different body parts. BCI results using this method may be further improved by replacing tongue movement with an alternative movement, such as the right foot. With better classification technique it may be possible to classify even finger movements, which may help in complex higher level control.

6. Conclusion

A high performance BCI was designed using spatially filtered MEG signals to decode movement intentions on a single trial basis. The combination of a natural motor task paradigm, SAM spatial filtering and event-related desynchronization analysis at the source level was able to discriminate four different movement intentions with a high level of accuracy. Although the computational analysis was performed offline, the robust performance suggests that online implementation using this paradigm would be effective in the setting of real-time feedback and user adaptation. Overall, this BCI has the following advantages over other BCIs: two-dimensional control, a more natural control scheme, less training time, high spatial resolution, and robust performance.

Due to the lack of portability and higher costs, MEG is less practical for BCI use compared with EEG. However, the advantages of MEG include high spatiotemporal resolution and robust spatial filtering methods facilitating reduced computational load and improved decoding and classification accuracy. The high level of multidimensional control attainable through the use of MEG signals as demonstrated in this study has great potential for future BCI applications. Such a MEG-based system could be used for patients to monitor and enhance ERD sensorimotor rhythms to facilitate motor rehabilitation or to practice in improving the efficiency of motor intention or imagery for BCI purposes using less costly technology such as EEG.

Author details

Peter T. Lin[1], Kartikeya Sharma[2], Tom Holroyd[3], Harsha Battapady[2], Ding-Yu Fei[2] and Ou Bai[2]

1 Department of Neurology, Santa Clara Valley Medical Center, Santa Clara, USA

2 Department of Biomedical Engineering, Virginia Commonwealth University, Richmond, USA

3 MEG Core Facility, National Institutes of Mental Health, Bethesda, USA

References

[1] Shibasaki H, Hallett M. What is the Bereitschaftspotential? Clinical Neurophysiology 2006;117 2341-56.

[2] Shibasaki H. Cortical activities associated with voluntary movements and involuntary movements. Clinical Neurophysiology 2012;123(2) 229-43.

[3] Stancak A Jr, Pfurtscheller G. Event-related desynchronisation of central beta-rhythms during brisk and slow self-paced finger movements of dominant and non-dominant hand. Brain Research Cognitive Brain Research 1996;4 171-83.

[4] Bai O, Mari Z, Vorbach S, Hallett M. Asymmetric spatiotemporal patterns of event-related desynchronization preceding voluntary sequential finger movements: a high-resolution EEG study. Clinical Neurophysiology 2005;116 1213-21.

[5] Pfurtscheller G, Pregenzer M, Neuper C. Visualization of sensorimotor areas involved in preparation for hand movement based on classification of mu and central beta rhythms in single EEG trials in man. Neuroscience Letters 1994;181 43-6.

[6] Pfurtscheller G, Neuper C, Andrew C, Edlinger G. Foot and hand area mu rhythms. International Journal of Psychophysiology 1997;26 121-35.

[7] Andersen RA, Hwang EJ, Mulliken GH. Cognitive neural prosthetics. Annual Review of Psychology 2010;61 169-90.

[8] Wolpaw JR, Birbaumer N, McFarland DJ, Pfurtscheller G, Vaughan TM. Brain-computer interfaces for communication and control. Clinical Neurophysiology 2002;113 767-91.

[9] Hochberg LR, Bacher D, Jarosiewicz B, Masse NY, Simeral JD, Vogel J, Haddadin S, Liu J, Cash SS, van der Smagt P, Donoghue JP. Reach and grasp by people with tetraplegia using a neurally controlled robotic arm. Nature 2012;485 372-5.

[10] Wessberg J, Stambaugh CR, Kralik JD, Beck PD, Laubach M, Chapin JK, Kim J, Biggs SJ, Srinivasan MA, Nicolelis MA. Real-time prediction of hand trajectory by ensembles of cortical neurons in primates. Nature 2000;408 361-5.

[11] Musallam S, Corneil BD, Greger B, Scherberger H, Andersen RA. Cognitive control signals for neural prosthetics. Science 2004;305 258-62.

[12] Laconte SM, Peltier SJ, Hu XP. Real-time fMRI using brain-state classification. Human Brain Mapping 2007;28(10) 1033-44.

[13] Hamalainen MS. Magnetoencephalography: a tool for functional brain imaging. Brain Topography 1992;5 95-102.

[14] Hinterberger T, Schmidt S, Neumann N, Mellinger J, Blankertz B, Curio G, Birbaumer N. Brain-computer communication and slow cortical potentials. IEEE Transactions on Biomedical Engineering 2004;51 1011-8.

[15] Wolpaw JR, McFarland DJ. Control of a two-dimensional movement signal by a non-invasive brain-computer interface in humans. Proceedings of the National Academy of Sciences USA 2004;101 17849-54.

[16] Krusienski DJ, Grosse-Wentrup M, Galan F, Coyle D, Miller KJ, Forney E, Anderson CW. Critical issues in state-of-the-art brain-computer interface signal processing. Journal of Neural Engineering 2011;8 025002.

[17] Blankertz B, Muller KR, Curio G, Vaughan TM, Schalk G, Wolpaw JR, Schlogl A, Neuper C, Pfurtscheller G, Hinterberger T, Schroder M, Birbaumer N. The BCI Com-

petition 2003: progress and perspectives in detection and discrimination of EEG single trials. IEEE Transactions in Biomedical Engineering 2004;51(6) 1044-51.

[18] Morash V, Bai O, Furlani S, Lin P, Hallett M. Classifying EEG signals preceding right hand, left hand, tongue, and right foot movements and motor imageries. Clinical Neurophysiology 2008;119 2570-8.

[19] Battapady H, Lin P, Holroyd T, Hallett M, Chen X, Fei DY, Bai O. Spatial detection of multiple movement intentions from SAM-filtered single-trial MEG signals. Clinical Neurophysiology 2009;120 1978-87.

[20] Graimann B, Pfurtscheller G. Quantification and visualization of event-related changes in oscillatory brain activity in the time-frequency domain. Progress in Brain Research 2006;159 79-97.

[21] Lotte F, Guan C. Regularizing common spatial patterns to improve BCI designs: unified theory and new algorithms. IEEE Transactions in Biomedical Engineering 2011;58(2) 355-62.

[22] Babiloni F, Cincotti F, Bianchi L, Pirri G, del R Millan J, Mourino J, Salinari S, Marciani MG. Recognition of imagined hand movements with low resolution surface Laplacian and linear classifiers. Medical Engineering Physics 2001;23(5) 323-8.

[23] Vallabhaneni A, He B. Motor imagery task classification for brain computer interface applications using spatiotemporal principle component analysis. Neurological Research 2004;26(3) 282-7.

[24] Mak JN, Arbel Y, Minett JW, McCane LM, Yuksel B, Ryan D, Thompson D, Bianchi L, Erdogmus D. Optimizing the P300-based brain-computer interface: current status, limitations and future directions. Journal of Neural Engineering 2011;8(2) 025003.

[25] Vialatte FB, Maurice M, Dauwels J, Cichocki A. Steady-state visually evoked potentials: focus on essential paradigms and future perspectives. Progress in Neurobiology 2010;90(4) 418-38.

[26] Dornhege G, Blankertz B, Kraudelat M, Losch F, Curio G, Muller KR. Combined optimization of spatial and temporal filters for improving brain-computer interfacing. IEEE Transactions in Biomedical Engineering 2006;53 2274-81.

[27] Bai O, Lin P, Vorbach S, Li J, Furlani S, Hallett M. Exploration of computational methods for classification of movement intention during human voluntary movement from single trial EEG. Clinical Neurophysiology 2007;118 2637-55.

[28] Adjamian P, Worthen SF, Hillebrand A, Furlong PL, Chizh BA, Hobson AR, Aziz Q, Barnes GR. Effective electromagnetic noise cancellation with beamformers and synthetic gradiometry in shielded and partly shielded environments. Journal of Neuroscience Methods 2009;178 120-7

[29] Gaetz W, Cheyne D. Localization of sensorimotor cortical rhythms induced by tactile stimulation using spatially filtered MEG. Neuroimage 2006;30 899-908.

[30] Taniguchi M, Kato A, Fujita N, Hirata M, Tanaka H, Kihara T, Ninomiya H, Hirabuki N, Nakamura H, Robinson SE, Cheyne D, Yoshimine T. Movement-related desynchronization of the cerebral cortex studied with spatially filtered magentoencephalography. Neuroimage 2000;12 298-306.

[31] Xiang J, Wilson D, Otsubo H, Ishii R, Chuang S. Neuromagnetic spectral distribution of implicit processing of words. Neuroreport 2001;12(18) 3923-7.

[32] Nagarajan S, Kirsch H, Lin P, Findlay A, Honma S, Berger MS. Preoperative localization of hand motor cortex by adaptive spatial filtering of magnetoencephalography data. Journal of Neurosurgery 2008;109(2) 228-37.

[33] Hirata M, Goto T, Barnes G, Umekawa Y, Yanagisawa T, Kato A, Oshino S, Kishima H, Hashimoto N, Saitoh Y, Tani N, Yorifuji S, Yoshimine T. Language dominance and mapping based on neuromagnetic oscillatory changes: comparison with invasive procedures. Journal of Neurosurgery 2010;112(3) 528-38.

[34] Oshino S, Kato A, Wakayama A, Taniguchi M, Hirata M, Yoshimine T. Magnetoencephalogrpahic analysis of cortical oscillatory activity in patients with brain tumors: Synthetic aperture magnetometry (SAM) functional imaging of delta band activity. Neuroimage 2007;34(3) 957-64.

[35] Kirsch HE, Robinson SE, Mantle M, Nagarajan S. Automated localization of magnetoencephalographic interictal spikes by adaptive spatial filtering. Clinical Neurophysiology 2006;117(10) 2264-71.

[36] Cincotti F, Mattia D, Aloise F, Bufalari S, Astolfi L, De Vico Fallani F, Tocci A, Bianchi L, Grazia Marciani M, Gao S, Millan J, Babiloni F. High-resolution EEG techniques for brain-computer interface applications. Journal of Neuroscience Methods 2008;167 31-42.

[37] Grosse-Wentrup M, Liefhold C, Gramann K, Buss M. Beamforming in noninvasive brain-computer interfaces. IEEE Transactions on Biomedical Engineering 2009;56 1209-19.

[38] Noirhomme Q, Kitney RI, Macq B. Single-Trial EEG Source Reconstruction for Brain-Computer Interface. IEEE Transactions on Biomedical Engineering 2008;55 1592-1601.

[39] Congedo M, Lotte F, Lecuyer A. Classification of movement intention by spatially filtered electromagnetic inverse solutions. Physics in Medicine and Biology 2006;51:1971-1989.

[40] Ahn M, Hong JH, Jun SC. Feasibility of approaches combining sensor and source features in brain-computer interface. Journal of Neuroscience Methods 2012;204 168-178.

[41] Barbati G, Sigismondi R, Zappasodi F, Porcaro C, Graziadio S, Valente G, Balsi M, Rossini PM, Tecchio F. Functional source separation from magnetoencephalographic signals. Human Brain Mapping 2006;27 925-34.

[42] Kauhanen L, Nykopp T, Sams M. Classification of single MEG trials related to left and right index finger movements. Clinical Neurophysiology 2006;117 430-9.

[43] Lee PL, Wu YT, Chen LF, Chen YS, Cheng CM, Yeh TC, Ho LT, Chang MS, Hsieh JC. ICA-based spatiotemporal approach for single-trial analysis of postmovement MEG beta synchronization. NeuroImage 2003;20 2010-30.

[44] Tecchio F, Porcaro C, Barbati G, Zappasodi F. Functional source separation and hand cortical representation for a brain-computer interface feature extraction. Journal of Physiology 2007;580 703-21.

[45] Oldfield RC. The assessment and analysis of handedness: the Edinburgh inventory. Neuropsychologia 1971;9 97-113.

[46] Vrba J, Robinson SE. Signal processing in magnetoencephalography. Methods 2001;25 249-71.

[47] Bai O, Lin P, Vorbach S, Floeter M K, Hattori N, Hallett M. A high performance sensorimotor beta rhythm-based brain-computer interface associated with human natural motor behavior. Journal of Neural Engineering 2008;5 24-35

[48] Toro C, Deuschl G, Thatcher R, Sato S, Kufta C, Hallett M. Movement-related desynchronization and movement-related cortical potentials on the ECoG and EEG. Electroencephalography and Clinical Neurophysiology 1994;93(5) 380-9.

[49] Muller-Gerking J, Pfurtscheller G, Flyvbjerg H. Designing optimal spatial filters for single-trial EEG classification in a movement task. Clinical Neurophysiology 1999;110 787-98.

[50] Pfurtscheller G, Berghold A. Patterns of Cortical Activation During Planning of Voluntary Movement. Electroencephalography and Clinical Neurophysiology 1989;72 250-8.

[51] Welch PD. The Use of Fast Fourier Transform for the Estimation of Power Spectra: A Method Based on Time Averaging Over Short, Modified Periodograms. IEEE Trans. Audio Electroacoust. AU-15;1967 70-3.

[52] Marques JP. Pattern recognition: concepts, methods and applications. Berlin: Springer-Verlag; 2001.

[53] Whitley D. A Genetic Algorithm Tutorial. Statistics and Computing 1994;4 65-85.

[54] Li Q, Doi K. Analysis and minimization of overtraining effect in rule-based classifiers for computer-aided diagnosis. Medical Physics 2006;33 320-8.

[55] Babiloni F, Babiloni C, Carducci F, Romani GL, Rossini PM, Angelone LM, Cincotti F. Multimodal integration of high-resolution EEG and functional magnetic resonance imaging data: a simulation study. Neuroimage 2003;19 1-15.

[56] Huang D, Lin P, Fei D Y, Chen X, Bai O. Decoding human motor activity from EEG single trials for a discrete two-dimensional cursor control. Journal of Neural Engineering 2009;6 046005.

[57] Babiloni F, Bianchi L, Semeraro F, Millan J, Mourinyo J. Mahalanobis distance-based classifiers are able to recognize EEG patterns by using few EEG electrodes. Conference Proceedings IEEE Engineering Med Biol Soc 2001;651-4

[58] Duda RO, Hart PE, Stork DG. Pattern Classification. New York: John Wiley; 2001.

[59] Jung P, Baumgartner U, Bauermann T, Magerl W, Gawehn J, Stoeter P, Treede RD. Asymmetry in the human primary somatosensory cortex and handedness. Neuroimage 2003;19 913-23.

[60] Kawashima R, Yamada K, Kinomura S, Yamaguchi T, Matsui H, Yoshioka S, Fukuda H. Regional cerebral blood flow changes of cortical motor areas and prefrontal areas in humans related to ipsilateral and contralateral hand movement. Brain Research 1993;623 33-40.

[61] Volkmann J, Schnitzler A, Witte OW, Freund H. Handedness and asymmetry of hand representation in human motor cortex. Journal of Neurophysiology 1998;79 2149-54.

[62] Stippich C, Blatow M, Durst A, Dreyhaupt J, Sartor K. Global activation of primary motor cortex during voluntary movements in man. Neuroimage 2007;34 1227-37.

[63] Loose R, Hamdy S, Enck P. Magnetoencephalographic response characteristics associated with tongue movement. Dysphagia 2001;16 183-5.

[64] Mellinger J, Schalk G, Braun C, Preissl H, Rosenstiel W, Birbaumer N, Kubler A. An MEG-based brain-computer interface (BCI) Neuroimage 2007;36 581-93.

[65] Waldert S, Preissl H, Demandt E, Braun C, Birbaumer N, Aertsen A, Mehring C. Hand movement direction decoded from MEG and EEG. Journal of Neuroscience 2008;28 1000-8.

[66] Buch E, Weber C, Cohen L G, Braun C, Dimyan M A, Ard T, Mellinger J, Caria A, Soekadar S, Fourkas A, Birbaumer N. Think to move: a neuromagnetic brain-computer interface (BCI) system for chronic stroke. Stroke 2008;39 910-7.

[67] Wang W, Sudre GP, Xu Y, Kass RE, Collinger JL, Degenhart AD, Bagic AI, Weber DJ. Decoding and cortical source localization for intended movement direction with MEG. Journal of Neurophysiology 2010;104:2451-2461.

Chapter 3

Brain Mapping of Developmental Coordination Disorder

Mitsuru Kashiwagi and Hiroshi Tamai

Additional information is available at the end of the chapter

http://dx.doi.org/10.5772/56496

1. Introduction

This chapter discusses the brain mapping of developmental coordination disorder (DCD). DCD is a neurological disorder characterised by impaired motor coordination and impaired performance of daily activities that require motor skills. In the Diagnostic and Statistical Manual of Mental Disorders, fourth edition (DSM-IV) [1], DCD is included in the *Learning Disorders* and the *Motor Skills Disorders* sections [1]. DCD is one of the most common disorders in childhood, and it affects 5% to 6% of school-age children.

DCD is a heterogeneous disorder, and its manifestations are varied and often complex. A meta-analysis of DCD literature that was published between 1974 and 1996 showed that the greatest deficiency in these patients was in visual-spatial processing [2]. The latest meta-analysis of 128 studies suggested that children with DCD show underlying problems in the visual-motor translation (namely inverse modelling) of movements that are directed within and outside peripersonal space, adaptive postural control, and the use of predictive control (namely forward modelling), which impacts their ability to adjust movement to changing constraints in real time [3]. The underlying cognitive mechanisms are still a matter of discussion.

Previous clinical and experimental studies have indicated that motor skill difficulties in DCD children may be related to dysfunction in the parietal lobe [4], the cerebellum (CB) [5], the basal ganglia (BG) [6], the hippocampus [7] and the corpus callosum [8]. However, because the motor system is highly complex, this is not a given conclusion.

Neuroimaging, including functional magnetic resonance imaging (fMRI), will create a new standard in the understanding of the complex cognitive functions in a child's brain. Therefore, it is useful to review the data from current DCD neuroimaging studies as the next critical step in enhancing our understanding of DCD. Clarifying DCD pathogenesis will be beneficial to clinicians as well as to children suffering from DCD.

2. Neuroimaging studies of DCD

We researched the Medline database with the terms 'neuroimaging' and 'DCD' for original research articles that were written in English. There were few DCD neuroimaging studies, and only 6 neuroimaging studies that involved the direct identification of the neural substrates responsible for DCD were available (Table 1).

No.	Citation	types of neuroimaging study	numbers (age)		object	task	results	remarks
1	Querne et al	fMRI	DCD, 9 control, 10	:7 boys 2 girls (9.9±1.8 years) :7 boys 3 girls (10.0±1.1years)	To assess the impact of DCD on effective connectivity applied to a putative model of inhibition.	go-nogo	[path coefficents] DCD<control, right hemisphere :striatum/parietal cortex DCD>control, left hemisphere :MFC/ACC/IPC	not motor task small sample size
2	Kashiwagi et al	fMRI	DCD, 12 control, 12	:12 boys (129.4±11.6 months) :12 boys (125.3±11.9 months)	To detect the mechanisms underlying clumsiness in DCD children.	visually guided tracking	[brain activity] tracking condition - watching condition DCD<control, left hemisphere :PPC(SPL,IPL)/postcentral gyrus [magnetic signal change for the DCD and control in IPL] negatively correlated with the task performace	The only study to reveal significant correlation of brain actication with task performance
3	Zwicker et al	fMRI	DCD, 7 control, 7	:6 boys 1 girl (10.8±1.5 years) :3 boys 4 girls (10.9±1.5years)	To determine whether patterns of brain activity differed between children with and without DCD.	trail-tracing	[brain activity] DCD<control, left hemisphere :percuneus/superior frontal, inferior frontal, postcentral (gyrus) right hemisphere :superior temporal gyrus/insula DCD>control, left hemisphere : IPL right hemisphere :middle frontal, supramarginal, lingual, parahippocampal posterior cingulate precentral, medial frontal, superior temporal (gyrus)/cerebellar lobule VI	small sample size
4	Zwicker et al	fMRI	DCD, 7 control, 7	:6 boys 1 girl (10.8±1.5 years) :3 boys 4 girls (10.9±1.5years)	To known whether DCD children employ a different set of brain regions than control children during skilled motor practice.	motor skill practice of trail-tracing	[brain activity] retention practice - early pracice DCD<control, left hemisphere :fusiform gyrus/cerebellar lobule VI IX /inferior parietal lobule right hemisphere :inferior parietal lobule/ lingual, middle frontal (gyrus)/cerebellar lobule I	motor learning paradigm small sample size
5	Maien et al	99m-ECD SPECT	DCD, 1 woman (19 years old)		To investigate the neural correlates of DCD.	-	[decrease of perfusion] left hemisphere :medial prefrontal right hemisphere :cerebellar/occipital region	Case report 19 years old
6	Zwicker et al	Diffusion Tensor Imaging	DCD, 7 control, 7	:6 boys 1 girl (10.8±1.5 years) :3 boys 4 girls (10.9±1.5years)	To explored the integrity of motor, sensory, and cerebellar pathways in children with and without DCD.	-	Fractional anisotropy of motor and sensory tracts and diffusion parameters in cerebellar peduncles did not differ. Mean diffusivity of the corticospinal tract and posterior thalamic radiation was lower in DCD children. Axial diffusivity was significantly correlated with motor impairment scores for both the corticospinal tract and posterior thalamic radiation.	not motor task small sample size

Table 1. DCD neuroimaging studies

2.1. Four fMRI studies

[No. 1] In 2008, Querne et al. [9] reported that DCD children exhibited abnormal brain hemispheric specialisation during development when performing a go/no-go task. Connectivity analyses in the middle frontal cortex-anterior cingulate cortex-inferior parietal cortex (IPC) network indicated that children with DCD are less able than healthy children to easily or promptly switch between go and no-go motor responses. This was the first fMRI study to clarify the attentional brain network of DCD children.

[No. 2] In 2009, Kashiwagi et al. [10] (our group) showed poor performance and less activation in the left superior parietal lobe (SPL), the left inferior parietal lobe (IPL), and the left postcentral gyrus in DCD children during visuomotor tasks. This was the first fMRI study to elucidate the neural underpinnings of DCD children by using a visuomotor task. Furthermore, a connection between the brain activity in the left IPL and task performance that represented clumsiness was suggested.

[No. 3] In 2010, Zwicker et al. [11] demonstrated that DCD children activate different brain regions compared to control children when performing the same trail-tracing task. They found that a correlation of the activation of the right middle frontal gyrus with the number of traces indicated cognitive effort in the children with DCD.

[No. 4] In 2011, Zwicker et al. [12] found that DCD children demonstrated decreased activation in cerebellar-parietal and cerebellar-prefrontal networks as well as in brain regions associated with visuospatial learning. This was the first study in DCD children to examine changes in the patterns of brain activation that were associated with skilled motor practice.

2.2. One single-photon emission computed tomography study

[No. 5] In 2010, Marien et al. [13] reported that the CB is crucially implicated in the pathophysiological mechanisms of DCD, and this reflects a disruption of the cerebello-cerebral network that is involved in executing planned actions, visuospatial cognition, and affective regulation. This was the first single-photon emission computed tomography study of children with DCD.

2.3. One diffusion tensor imaging (DTI) study

[No. 6] In 2012, Zwicker et al. [14] showed that the mean diffusivity of motor and sensory pathways is lower in DCD children. In addition, differences in the intrinsic characteristics of axons or in the extra-axonal/extracellular space may underlie some of the deficits that are observed in DCD children. This was the first DTI study in children with DCD.

3. Different patterns of activation of cerebral areas in DCD patients compared to controls in fMRI motor control tasks

In order to elucidate the main mechanisms underlying the impaired motor skills in DCD patients, we have to examine brain activities that are related to motor performances during motor control tasks. There were 3 fMRI studies (No. 2, 3, and 4) on motor control tasks in DCD patients. One study included a motor learning task. The cerebral areas listed below showed significant differences in activation between DCD children and control children during the motor control task and motor learning task and the functions of those areas.

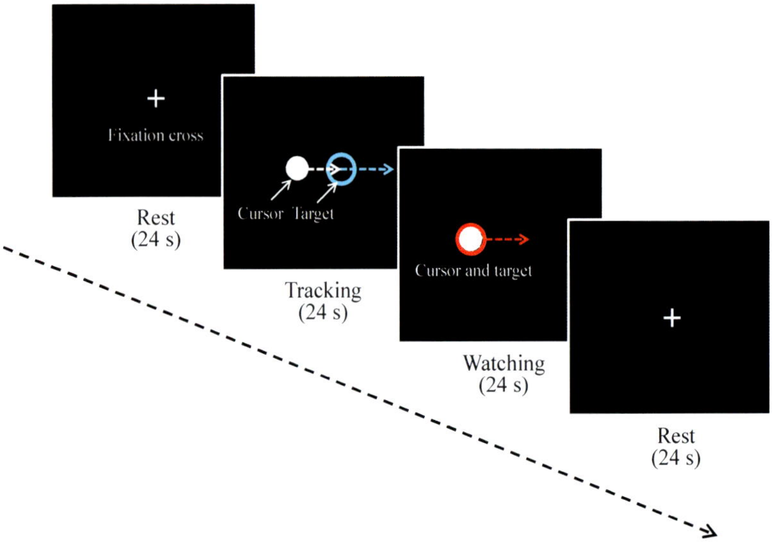

Figure 1. Our study (No. 2) design and conditions. The experiment was designed in a block manner and consisted of 3 conditions. Each condition lasted 24 s and was repeated 6 times in a pseudo-randomised order.

3.1. No. 2: Our study

3.1.1. Study design and conditions

The experiment was designed in a block manner and consisted of the following 3 conditions:

1) Tracking condition (TC): tracking the moving blue target by manipulating the joystick,

2) Watching condition (WC): watching the moving red target and white cursor without hand manipulation

and

3) Resting condition (RC): looking at a fixation cross.

Each condition lasted for 24 s and was repeated 6 times in a pseudo-randomised order (Figure 1). All of the participants were trained through 40 trials of tracking before scanning. The participants achieved their best performance after several trials. Task performance was represented by the distance (pixels) between the centre of the target and the cursor. We recorded 6 sets of data on the distance and the velocity changes for each participant, and the effects of the group and the participants (within group) on these data were analysed by a two-factor nested design analysis of variance. Furthermore, the effects of the trial numbers and the participants on the task performance during the final 6 training trials and 6 scanning trials were analysed with a factorial two-way analysis of variance.

3.1.2. Behavioural data

Figure 2. (a) shows the behavioural results for a DCD child and a control child. The DCD child showed much error at the return point and particularly at the beginning point compared to the control child.

The distance between the target and the cursor and the change in the velocity of the cursor were significantly greater in the DCD group than in the control group (mean distance, 22.8 vs. 19.5 pixels, $P = 0.001$; mean velocity change, 398.5 vs. 369.9 pixels/s/s, $P = 0.013$). The number of trials did not significantly affect task performance in either group over the final 6 training trials and 6 scanning trials [training trials: DCD group, $F(5,55) = 0.41$, $P = 0.839$ and $F(5,55) = 1.20$, $P = 0.322$; control group, $F(5,55) = 0.49$, $P = 0.784$] [scanning trials: DCD group, $F(5,55) = 0.41$, $P = 0.839$; control group, $F(5,55) = 0.49$, $P = 0.780$] (Figure 2. (b)).

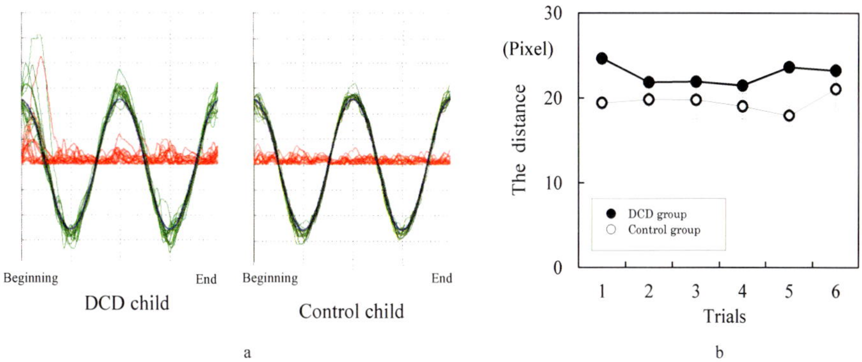

Figure 2. (a) The behavioural results of a child with DCD and a control child. The blue line shows the trajectory of the target, the green line shows the trajectory of the cursor and the red line shows the distance between the target and the cursor. (b) Mean task performances for the DCD and control groups during 6 scanning trials. The vertical bars indicate the standard errors of the means for each data point.

3.1.3. Imaging data

In the comparison of the watching condition versus the resting condition (WC - RC), both the DCD-greater-than-control and control-greater-than-DCD comparisons did not reveal significant differences in the activation maps between the groups. In the comparison of the tracking condition versus the watching condition [(TC - RC) - (WC - RC)], greater activation was not observed in the DCD-greater-than-control comparison. Inversely, the control-greater-than-DCD comparison showed differences in the activation in the left hemisphere.

Different brain activation in the comparison of the tracking condition versus the watching condition [(TC - RC) - (WC - RC)] in the visually guided tracking task between DCD patients and controls

(DCD < control only)

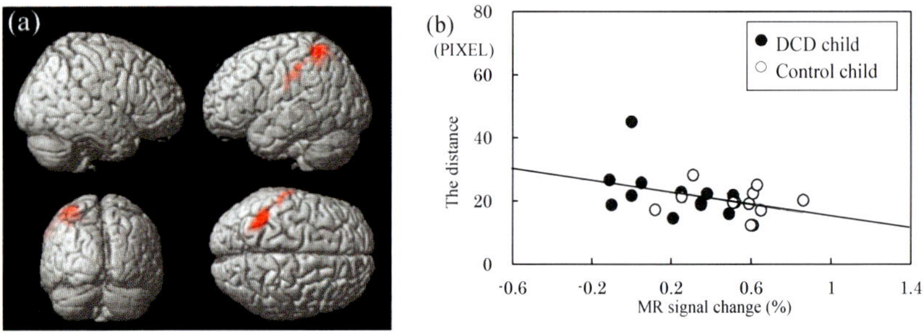

Figure 3. (a) Brain activity differences between the DCD and control groups. In the comparison of the tracking condition versus the watching condition, the control-greater-than-DCD comparison showed differences in left hemisphere activation in the left SPL and IPL and the left postcentral gyrus ($P < 0.001$ at the voxel level and $P < 0.05$ with a correction for multiple comparisons at the cluster level); (b). Mean task performances and magnetic resonance signal changes for the DCD and control groups in the IPC. The vertical bars indicate the standard errors of the means, and the horizontal bars indicate the 90% confidence intervals for each data point.

Left posterior parietal cortex (SPL and IPL): The main brain region involved in skilled motor functions, eye movements, multimodal encoding of locations near the head, reaching and pointing movements with the arm and finger, grasping movements that require preshaping of the hand [15], tool use and motor attention [16], internal representation of the dynamic body schema [17], hand movements [18] and motor imagery [19]. **Left postcentral gyrus**: proprioceptive control of movement [20]. (Table 2, Figure 3.(a).)

The correlations between task performance and the maximal magnetic resonance signal changes within a diameter of 8 mm of each local maximum were analysed. Only the magnetic resonance signal changes in the left IPL negatively correlated with task performance [r, -0.413; $P < 0.05$] (Figure 3(b)).

Region	Cluster				MNI coordinates (mm)		
	L/R	Size	$P_{corrected}$	Z	x	y	z
superior parietal lobe (BA7)	L	1024	0.001	4.02	-40	-48	66
postcentral gyrus (BA2)	L			3.89	-68	-20	34
inferior parietal lobe (BA40)	L			3.83	-36	-52	50

BA, Brodmann area; L, left; R, right

Table 2. Cluster size, Z-values, and coordinates

3.2. No. 3: Zwicker et al. study

Different brain activation in the trail-tracing task between DCD patients and controls

(DCD < control)

Left precuneus: visuospatial processing and initiation of movement programming [21, 22]. **Left superior frontal gyrus**: spatially oriented processing [23]. **Left inferior frontal gyrus**: inhibitory control over motor responses [24]. **Left postcentral gyrus**: motor control and motor learning [25, 26]. **Right insula**: motor control [27], motor learning [28] and error processing [29].

(DCD > control)

Left IPL: interpretation of sensory information [30, 31]. **Right supramarginal gyrus**: visuomotor/visuospatial processing [32, 33]. **Right posterior cingulate gyrus**: spatial attention [34]. **Right lingual gyrus**: visuospatial processing [35]. **Right precentral and parahippocampal gyri**: spatial memory [36-38]. **Right CB (lobule VI)**: spatial processing [39].

3.3. No. 4: Zwicker et al. study

Different brain activation of the retention condition versus the early condition in the trail-tracing task between DCD patients and controls

(DCD < control only)

Right cerebellar crus I: working memory and executive functions [40]. **Left cerebellar lobule VI**: part of the sensorimotor network of the CB [40], spatial processing [41], performance of a variety of tasks, including serial reaction time tasks [42], motor sequence learning [43], reaching tasks [44] and planned, discretely aimed arm movements [45] as well as the magnitude of motor correction during visuomotor learning [46]. **Left cerebellar lobule IX**: unclear [40]. **Right IPL**: spatial working memory [47]. **IPL**: the processing of sensory information and visual feedback [48]. **Right dorsolateral prefrontal cortex**: the initial stages of explicit motor learning [49], motor and visuomotor sequences [50, 51] and attentional control [52]. **Left fusiform gyrus**: higher level visual and visuospatial processing during the consolidation of visuomotor learning [53]. **Right lingual gyrus**: visuospatial processing [54].

4. Discussion

4.1. Previous studies of DCD (terminology, clumsiness, motor learning, and brain area)

4.1.1. What is DCD? Historical perspectives

At the beginning of the 20th century, an awareness of different levels of motor performance was clearly described in studies that identified the motor abilities of children as very clever, clever, medium, awkward or very awkward [55]. As early as 1926, Lippitt was concerned specifically with poor muscular coordination in children [56]. Orton's (1937) discussion of developmental apraxia or abnormal clumsiness was strongly influenced by ideas about adult apraxia and damage to the dominant hemisphere [57]. Since the early 1960s, many terms have been used to describe children whose motor difficulties interfere with daily living, and these include developmental apraxia and agnosia, minimal cerebral dysfunction (Wigglesworth,

1963) [58], minimal brain dysfunction (Clements, 1966) [59], minimal cerebral palsy (Kong, 1963) [60] and developmental dyspraxia [61].

At a 1994 consensus meeting in London, Ontario (Polatajko et al., 1995) [62], a multidisciplinary group of internationally recognised researchers who work with children with motor clumsiness agreed to use the term developmental coordination disorder as described by the American Psychiatric Association (APA) in the DSM-IIIR (APA, 1987) and revised in DSM-IV (APA, 1994).

4.1.2. What is clumsiness? What is dexterity?

Clumsiness is defined by Morris and Whiting as a maladaptive motor behaviour in relation to expected or required movement performance [63]. The antonym of clumsiness is dexterity.

Dexterity is the ability to find a motor solution for any external situation or to adequately solve any emerging motor problem correctly (adequately and accurately), quickly (with respect to both decision making and achieving a correct result), rationally (expediently and economically) and resourcefully (quick-wittedly and initiatively). In many movements and actions, there are no absolutely unpredictable events, but these movements nevertheless require quick and accurate movement adaptation to external events that cannot be predicted with certainty. This accurate movement adaptation is important for dexterity. The heart of the problem is to quickly and correctly find a solution in conditions of an unexpectedly changed environment. Dexterity apparently is not in the motor action itself but is revealed by its interaction with changing external conditions, including the uncontrolled and unpredicted influences from the environment. The established essential feature of dexterity is that it always refers to the external world. Moreover, dexterity is a complex activity. Real-life movements have an element of adaption to various, although perhaps minor, unexpected events [64].

Quick and correct motion is fundamental to dexterity performance. Quick motion means the rapid initiation of action and fleetness of the performance itself. Accurate motion implies spatially and temporally accurate performance. As we move more rapidly, we become more inaccurate in terms of the goal we are trying to achieve. The adage haste makes waste has been a long-standing viewpoint about motor skills.

Identifying optimal measurements of skill learning is not trivial [65]. Previous studies have typically defined skill acquisition in terms of a reduction in the speed of movement execution or reaction times, increases in accuracy or decreases in movement variability. Yet, these measurements are often interdependent, in that, faster movements can be performed at the cost of reduced accuracy and vice versa, which is a phenomenon which has often been referred to as the speed-accuracy trade-off. The principles of speed-accuracy trade-offs, which are known as Fitts' law, are specific to the goal and nature of the movement tasks [66]. One solution to this issue is through the assessment of changes in the speed-accuracy trade-off functions. Therefore, we should assess task performances with both speed and accuracy. The visually guided tracking task that we adopted in our fMRI study has been experimentally used for evaluating motor skills. We assessed task performance as the change in the velocity of the cursor for speed and the distance between the target and the cursor for accuracy.

4.1.3. What is motor learning?

Children with DCD have difficulties with motor performance and motor learning [67]. Most clinicians and researchers agree that difficulty with motor learning is a key feature of DCD.

Motor learning depends on maturation, experience, and active learning. Motor learning has been described as a set of processes that are associated with practice or experience and that lead to relatively permanent changes in the capabilities for producing skilled actions [68]. Motor skill learning means, in other words, dexterity learning. Therefore, as mentioned above, accurate movement adaptation is an important fact in motor skill learning.

For motor learning, 3 main theories apply. Fitts and Posner (1967) distinguished the following 3 phases of motor learning: cognitive, associative and autonomous [69].

Hikosaka and colleagues proposed a model of motor skill learning. According to this model, 2 parallel loop circuits operate in the learning of the spatial and motor features of sequences. Whereas the learning of spatial coordinates is supported by the frontoparietal associative BG-CB circuit, the learning of motor coordinates is supported by the primary motor cortex-sensorimotor BG-CB circuit. According to this model, transformations between the 2 coordinate systems rely on the contribution of the supplementary motor area (SMA), the pre-supplementary motor area (preSMA) and the pre-motor cortices. Importantly, it has been suggested that the learning of spatial coordinates is faster, yet requires additional attentional and executive resources that are putatively provided by prefrontal cortical regions [70] (Figure 4. (a)).

Similarly, on the basis of brain imaging studies, Doyon and Ungerleider (Doyon and Ungerleider's model of motor skill learning) [71] proposed that cerebral plasticity is important within the cortico-striatal and cortico-cerebellar systems during the course of learning a new sequence of movements (motor sequence learning) or the adaptation to environmental perturbations (motor adaptation).

This model proposes that, depending upon the nature of the cognitive processes that are required during learning, both motor sequence and motor adaptation tasks recruit the following similar cerebral structures early in the learning phase: the striatum, CB, motor cortical regions, in addition to prefrontal, parietal, and limbic areas. Dynamic interactions between these structures are likely to be crucial in establishing the motor routines that are necessary for the learning of the skilled motor behaviour. A shift of the motor representation from the associative to the sensorimotor striatal territory can be seen during sequence learning, whereas additional representation of the skill can be observed in the cerebellar nuclei after practice in a motor adaptation task. When consolidation has occurred, the subject has achieved asymptotic performance, and their performance has become automatic; however, the neural representation of a new motor skill at that stage is believed to be distributed in a network of structures that involves the cortico-striatal or cortico-cerebellar circuit, depending on the type of motor learning acquired. At this stage, the model suggests that the striatum is no longer necessary for the retention and execution of the acquired skill for motor adaptation; regions representing the skill at this stage include the CB and related cortical regions. In contrast, a reverse pattern of plasticity is thought to occur in motor sequence learning, such that the CB is no longer essential with extended practice, and the long-lasting retention of the skill is believed at this stage to involve representational changes in the striatum and the associated motor cortical regions (Figure 4. (b)).

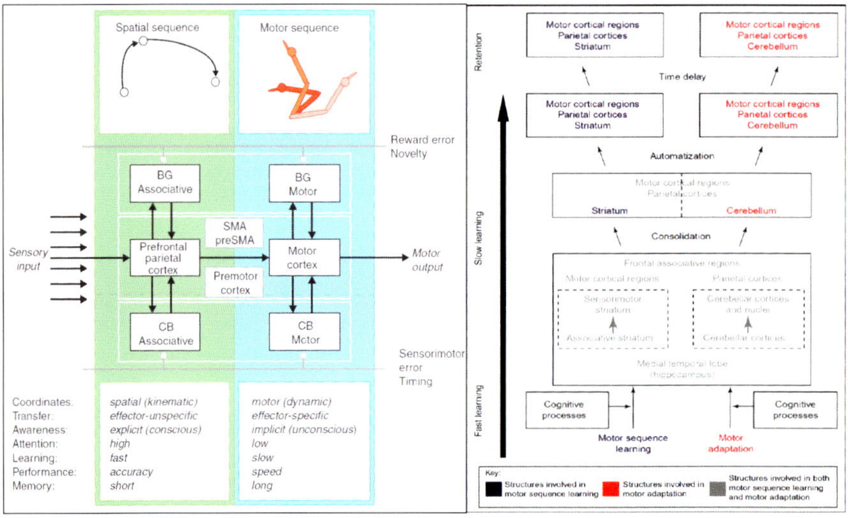

(a) (b)

Figure 4. (a). Hikosaka et al.'s scheme of motor skill learning. The figure is from Curr Opin Neurobiol 2002;12(2) 217-222.; (b). Doyon et al.'s model of skill learning. The figure is from Curr Opin Neurobiol 2005;15(2) 161-167.

Both models share the view that motor skill learning involves interactions between distinct cortical and subcortical circuits that are crucial for the unique cognitive and control demands that are associated with this stage of skill acquisition [65].

4.1.4. Where is brain area associated with DCD?

The parietal lobe

The parietal lobe plays a critical role in numerous cognitive functions, particularly in the sensory control of action [72]. As we know, lesions in the left posterior parietal cortex (PPC) are associated with apraxia, which is a higher order motor disorder, whereas lesions in the right PPC are associated with unilateral neglect, which is an attentional disorder [73].

The results of a meta-analysis of the information processing deficits that are associated with DCD children showed that DCD children have significantly poorer visual spatial processing than healthy controls [2, 3]. This evidence suggests that the parietal lobe may be implicated in DCD children because of its primary role in the processing of visual spatial information [74]. In addition, DCD children are less competent in their ability to recognise emotion [75], which has been linked to parietal lobe involvement [76]. Some clinical studies have supported the notion that the parietal lobe is associated with the mechanisms underlying the impaired motor skills in DCD children. Wilson et al. [77] conducted a study on procedural learning in DCD children and stated that the neurocognitive underpinnings of the disorder may be located in the parietal lobe and not in the BG. Another study involving mental rotation tasks indicated that DCD children might have dysfunction in the parietal lobe, which is involved in the internal representation of the movement [78]. In a recent study, Hyde et al. found that children with DCD show a similar response pattern as patients with lesions of the PPC on a number of paradigms that assess aspects of internal modelling. This has led to the hypothesis that DCD may be attributable to dysfunction at the level of the PPC [79].

Furthermore, a study on imagined motor sequences revealed that the performance of real and imagined tasks are dissociated in DCD children; this finding indicates that a disruption in the motor networks of the parietal lobe is associated with the generation of the internal representations of motor acts [80]. In addition, this group found that the ability of motor imagery in DCD children varied according to their level of motor impairment [81], and motor imagery training ameliorated the clumsiness in DCD children [82]. Recommendations of the definition, diagnosis, and intervention of DCD by the European Academy for Childhood Disability [3] only refer to the fact that Katschmarsky considered parietal dysfunction an underlying organic defect in DCD children from their study [4].

The cerebellum

The CB is related to motor skill learning. Given the CB's role in motor coordination and postural control, it may be involved in the neuropathology of DCD [74]. Geuze reported that the major characteristics of poor control in DCD are the inconsistent timing of muscle activation sequences, co-contraction, a lack of automation and the slowness of response. Converging evidence indicates that cerebellar dysfunction contributes to the motor problems of children with DCD [83]. Motor adaptation, which is also thought to reflect cerebellar function [71], has been demonstrated in children with DCD [84]. Waelvelde reported that the parameterization of movement execution in the Rhythmic Movement Test in children with DCD was significantly less accurate both in time and in space than the performance of same-aged typically developing children. The data of that study support the notion that some children with DCD manifest impairments in the generation of internal representations of motor actions and support the hypothesis that there is some form of cerebellar dysfunction in some children with DCD [85].

The basal ganglia

The BG is involved in motor control and motor skill learning. Clumsiness is a term that is associated in childhood with problems in the learning and execution of skilful movements, the neuronal basis of which is, however, poorly understood. Groenewegen reported that, as far as deficient motor programming is involved, the BG probably plays a role [86]. Wilson et al. did not identify any evidence that the BG is implicated in DCD [77].

The hippocampus

Hippocampal, cortico-cerebellar, and cortico-striatal structures are crucial for building the motor memory trace [71]. Neural structures, such as the hippocampus, parietal cortex, and CB, have been proposed to contribute to the process of learning new motor sequences. Gheysen et al. found that the sequence learning problems of DCD children might be located at the stage of motor planning rather than at sequence acquisition [87]. The fact that the hippocampus and CB could be involved in the neuropathology of DCD has been frequently proposed given their function in motor coordination and adaptation [71,88].

The corpus callosum

Sigmundsson reported that only DCD children showed significant performance differences in favour of the preferred hand in visual/proprioceptive or proprioceptive conditions. This finding was thought to suggest that the developmental lag that is exhibited by DCD children might have pathological overtones that are possibly related to the development of the corpus callosum [89].

4.2. Present studies of DCD (neuroimaging studies and current conclusion)

4.2.1. Recent neuroimaging studies

The parietal lobe and CB are key brain regions that have been highlighted in recent neuroimaging studies of the visuomotor performance of children with DCD. The brain functions of these 2 regions are known to involve the motor adaptation of motor learning in the past 2 models of motor skill learning. In addition, the parietal lobe and striatum are known to be involved in the motor sequence learning of motor learning. Accordingly, the parietal lobe is a region that is associated with sensory input, motor output, motor adaptation, and motor sequence learning.

In our results, parietal dysfunction reflected the difference in brain activities between DCD and control children during the phase of automation. The task in our study was easy to master, and, therefore, the performances of DCD patients and controls had already reached their plateau before the scanning trials. Thus, this study did not involve motor learning effects. In our fMRI task, the speed of the target was changed sinusoidally during its 12-s round trip. Consequently, we studied both motor sequence learning and motor adaptation in our fMRI task. We reported that DCD children showed poor performance and less activation in the left PPC and postcentral gyrus during the visuomotor task. Thus, a connection was suggested between brain activity of the left PPC and clumsiness.

In the results from other studies, dysfunction of the CB may reflect the different brain activities of consolidation conditions versus cognitive processes between DCD children and controls during the early–slow learning phases. In that study, tracing accuracy in control children improves from early practice to consolidation and shows increased activation in several brain regions. In contrast, the DCD children did not show any improvements in tracing accuracy. The authors noted that further work with a larger sample is needed to confirm the hypothesis that these areas of brain activation may contribute to improved motor performance. In this study design, the results mainly showed motor adaptation.

4.2.2. Current conclusion: Why are DCD children clumsy?

DCD is a disorder of impaired performances in daily activities that require motor skill. The movement parameters of daily activities appear to be encoded by delayed recall and require easy motor skills. Even though DCD children can learn easy motor skills, why they usually require more practice than healthy children and their quality of movement may be compromised is a pressing question.

From the viewpoints of the recent model of motor skill learning, previous studies, and the recent neuroimaging studies, DCD children have some difficulties with the cognitive processes in the fast learning phase, consolidation in the slow learning phase and automation in the retention phase during simple and easy motor skill learning (motor sequence learning and motor adaptation). Accordingly, it is not always easy for DCD children to perfectly acquire even simple motor skills. In fact, real-life movements that are required for daily simple and easy activities require an element of adaption to various, although perhaps minor, unexpected events. Therefore, we assumed that DCD children always seem to be required to adapt to the daily simple and easy activities as unexpected new motor learning every day because it is hard for DCD children to perfectly consolidate motor skills. In addition, DCD children show that the more a task demands the integration and adaptation of different information, the more vulnerable it is. Accordingly, we considered that motor adaptation is more important than motor sequence learning for DCD children.

Given that the main clinical finding in DCD children is motor adaptation, dysfunction in the parietal lobe and CB contributes to the mechanism underlying DCD. In addition, considering that DCD children have problems with sensory input and motor output, we conclude that the parietal lobe is the main neural substrate that is responsible for DCD.

4.3. Future studies of DCD (mirror neuron system, functional connectivity approaches, default mode network, intervention, and motor imagery training)

4.3.1. The mirror neuron system hypothesis

DCD includes impairments in motor skills, motor learning, and imitation. A better understanding of the neural correlates of the motor and imitation impairments in DCD children holds the potential for informing the development of treatment approaches that can address these impairments. In recent years, the discovery of a frontoparietal circuit, which is known as the mirror neuron system (MNS), has enabled researchers to better understand imitation, general motor functions, and aspects of social cognition. Given its involvement in imitation and other motor functions, they propose that dysfunction in the MNS may underlie the characteristic impairments of DCD [90].

4.3.2. Functional connectivity approaches

Most past studies of brain function have built on the concept of the localisation of function, in that different brain regions support different forms of information processing. Yet, no brain region exists in isolation. Information flows between the regions through the action potentials that are conducted by axons, which are bundled into large fibre tracts. For more than a century, neuroanatomists have mapped the anatomical connections between brain regions in an attempt to understand the structural connectivity of the brain. While much remains to be discovered, the study of the anatomical connections between brain regions has provided a cornerstone for neuroscience research.

Despite the value of this anatomical research, the knowledge of the structural connections between brain regions can only provide a limited picture of information flow in the brain. Descriptions of functional connectivity or of how the activity of one brain region influences activity in another brain region are also needed. Many researchers who are interested in functional connectivity have adopted fMRI techniques because of their utility for measuring changes in activation throughout the entire brain. This approach is useful for the brain mapping of DCD [91]

4.3.3. Default mode network

Functional brain imaging studies with fMRI in normal human subjects have consistently revealed expected task-induced increases in regional brain activity during goal-directed behaviours. These changes are detected when comparisons are made between a task state, which is designed to place demands on the brain, and a resting state with a set of demands that are uniquely different from those of the task state. Functional imaging studies should consider the need to obtain information about the baseline.

Researchers have also frequently encountered task-induced decreases in regional brain activity, even when the control state consists of the subject lying quietly with their eyes closed or passively viewing a stimulus. Whereas cortical increases in activity have been shown to be task specific and therefore to vary in location depending on the task demands, many decreases appear to be largely task independent and to vary little in their location across a wide range of tasks. This consistency with which certain areas of the brain participate in these decreases makes us wonder whether there might be an organised mode of brain function that is present as a baseline or default state [92]. Spatial patterns of spontaneous fluctuations in blood oxygenation level-dependent signals reflect the underlying neural architecture. The study of the brain networks that are based on these self-organised patterns is termed resting-state fMRI.

The notion of a default mode of brain function (DMN) has taken on certain relevance in human neuroimaging studies and in relation to a network of lateral parietal and midline cortical regions that show prominent activity fluctuations during the resting state [93]. The DMN is a prominent large-scale brain network that includes the ventral medial prefrontal cortex, the posterior cingulate/retrospenial cortex, the IPL, the lateral temporal cortex, dorsal medial prefrontal cortex, and hippocampal formation [94]. The parietal lobe is also an important area in the DMN. The DMN is unique in terms of its high resting metabolism, deactivation profile during cognitively demanding tasks and increased activity during the resting state and high-level social cognitive tasks. There is growing scientific interest in understanding the DMN underlying the resting state and higher-level cognition in humans. A recent study found that a goodness-of-fit analysis applied at the individual subject level suggested that the activity in the default-mode network might ultimately prove to be a sensitive and specific biomarker for incipient Alzheimer's disease [95].

The functional and structural maturation of networks that are comprised of discrete regions is an important aspect of brain development. The putative functions of the DMN, as well as the maturation of cognitive control mechanisms, develop relatively late in children, and they are often compromised in neurodevelopmental disorders, such as autism spectrum disorders and attention-deficit/hyperactivity disorder [96]. The relationship between DMN structure and function in DCD children is not known. Examining the developmental trajectory of the DMN is important not only for the understanding of how the structures of the brain change during development and impact the development of key functional brain circuits, but also for understanding the ontogeny of cognitive processes that are subserved by the DMN [97]. These multimodal imaging analyses will be important for a better understanding of how local and large-scale anatomical changes shape and constrain typical and atypical functional development. Future research should systematically explore the developmental trajectory of the DMN in a normal population and compare this with the maturation of the DMN in DCD children.

4.3.4. Intervention

Can dexterity be individually developed? Is it an exercisable capacity? The answer is positive and multifaceted. It is obvious that natural, inborn, and constitutional prerequisites for dexterity are and will be as different in different persons as their other psychophysical abilities. The attainable individual peaks of development, the degrees of difficulty, and the necessary amount of time for achieving a certain result will inevitably cause great individual variations. It is much more important to state that all natural prerequisites for dexterity can be developed. Both aspects of the structural complex that result in use dexterity can be exercised and developed.

In a systematic review of interventions on DCD children, Hillier generally concluded that an intervention for DCD is better than no intervention [98]. Independently, the guideline group performed a systematic literature search of studies that were published from 1995 to 2010. There is sufficient evidence that physiotherapy and/or occupational therapy intervention are better than no interventions for DCD children [3].

There are many different treatment approaches for DCD. The approaches to interventions are divided into the following 2 categories: process-oriented or bottom-up and task-oriented or top down [99]. Process oriented approaches include sensory integration therapy, kinaesthetic training, and perceptual motor therapy. Task-oriented approaches include Cognitive-Orientation to Occupational Performance, neuromotor task training, and motor imagery training [3]. In addition, studies have shown that process-oriented approaches may sometimes be effective but are less so than the task-oriented approaches, which are based on motor learning theories [100].

4.3.5. Motor imagery training

Motor imagery (MI) training is a cognitive approach that was developed by Wilson [101]. It uses the internal modelling of movements that facilitate the child in predicting the consequences for actions in the absence of overt movement. MI is a new intervention method for DCD children. The past literature has already described MI training as a method in stroke rehabilitation [102, 103]. MI training was investigated once in a randomised controlled trial, and it showed a positive effect if it was combined with active training [81].

In an fMRI study that investigated whether the neural substrates mediating MI differed among participants showing high or poor MI ability, intergroup comparisons revealed that good imagers exhibited more activation in the parietal and ventrolateral premotor regions, which are known to play a critical role in the generation of mental images [104]. Our data also indicated that dysfunction in the parietal lobe, such as that in motor imagery, might be a mechanism underlying the motor skill deficits in DCD children. Thus, from our data, MI training may be a helpful strategy for DCD children.

5. Conclusion

From clinical and neuroimaging studies and models of motor skill learning, we conclude that parietal lobe dysfunction is the main mechanism underlying DCD. In addition, the parietal lobe is a key area of the MNS and MI training. However, the parietal lobe is not the only neural correlate brain region in DCD. Dysfunctions in the CB, striatum, and hippocampus are also related to the neurobiology underlying DCD. In order to further elucidate the pathogenesis and interventions of DCD, additional neuroimaging studies that include DMN and DTI are needed that link the neural networks and the functional connectivity of brain regions during motor performance.

Author details

Mitsuru Kashiwagi[1,2] and Hiroshi Tamai[3]

1 Department of Pediatrics, Hirakata-City Hospital, Osaka, Japan

2 Department of Developmental Brain Science, Osaka Medical College, Osaka, Japan

3 Department of Pediatrics, Osaka Medical College, Osaka, Japan

References

[1] American Psychiatric Association. Diagnostic and statistical manual of mental disorders (4th ed). Washington DC: American Psychiatric Association; 1994.

[2] Wilson PH, McKenzie BE. Information processing deficits associated with developmental coordination disorder: a meta-analysis of research findings. J Child Psychol Psychiatry 1998;39(6) 829-840.

[3] Blank R, Smits-Engelsman B, Polatajko H, Wilson P. European Academy for Childhood Disability (EACD): recommendations on the definition, diagnosis and intervention of developmental coordination disorder (long version). Dev Med Child Neurol 2012;54(1) 54-93.

[4] Katschmarsky S, Cairney S, Maruff P, Wilson PH, Currie J. The ability to execute saccades on the basis of efference copy: impairments in double-step saccade performance in children with developmental co-ordination disorder. Exp Brain Res 2001;136(1) 73-78.

[5] Van Waelvelde H, De Weerdt W, De Cock P, Janssens L, Feys H, Smits Engelsman BC. Parameterization of movement execution in children with developmental coordination disorder. Brain Cogn 2006;60(1) 20–31.

[6] Groenewegen HJ. The basal ganglia and motor control. Neural Plast 2003;10(1-2) 107–120.

[7] Gheysen F, Van Waelvelde H, Fias W. Impaired visuo-motor sequence learning in Developmental Coordination Disorder. Res Dev Disabil 2011;32(2) 749-756.

[8] Sigmundsson H. Perceptual deficits in clumsy children: inter- and intra-modal matching approach-a window into clumsy behavior. Neural Plast 2003;10(1-2) 27-38.

[9] Querne L, Berquin P, Vernier-Hauvette MP, Fall S, Deltour L, Meyer ME, de Marco G. Dysfunction of the attentional brain network in children with developmental coordination disorder: A fMRI study. Brain Res 2008;1244 89–102.

[10] Kashiwagi M, Iwaki S, Narumi Y, Tamai H, Suzuki S. Parietal dysfunction in developmental coordination disorder: a functional MRI study. Neuroreport 2009;20(15) 1319-1324.

[11] Zwicker JG, Missiuna C, Harris SR, Boyd LA. Brain activation of children with developmental coordination disorder is different than peers. Pediatrics 2010;126(3) e678-686.

[12] Zwicker JG, Missiuna C, Harris SR, Boyd LA. Brain activation associated with motor skill practice in children with developmental coordination disorder: an fMRI study. Int J Dev Neurosci 2011;29(2) 145-152.

[13] Mariën P, Wackenier P, De Surgeloose D, De Deyn PP, Verhoeven J. Developmental coordination disorder: disruption of the cerebello-cerebral network evidenced by SPECT. Cerebellum 2010;9(3) 405-410.

[14] Zwicker JG, Missiuna C, Harris SR, Boyd LA. Developmental coordination disorder: a pilot diffusion tensor imaging study. Pediatr Neurol 2012;46(3) 162-167.

[15] Culham JC, Cavina-Pratesi C, Singhal A. The role of parietal cortex in visuomotor control: what have we learned from neuroimaging? Neuropsychologia 2006;44(13) 2668–2684.

[16] Iacoboni M. Visuo-motor integration and control in the human posterior parietal cortex: evidence from TMS and fMRI. Neuropsychologia 2006;44(13) 2691–2699.

[17] Ogawa K, Inui T. Lateralization of the posterior parietal cortex for internal monitoring of self-generated versus externally generated movements. J Cogn Neurosci 2007;19(11) 1827–1835.

[18] Taira M, Kawashima R, Inoue K, Fukuda H. A PET study of axis orientation discrimination. Neuroreport 1998;9(2) 283–288.

[19] Gerardin E, Sirigu A, Lehéricy S, Poline JB, Gaymard B, Marsault C, Agid Y, Le Bihan D. Partially overlapping neural networks for real and imagined hand movements. Cereb Cortex 2000;10(11) 1093–1104.

[20] Grefkes C, Ritzl A, Zilles K, Fink GR. Human medial intraparietal cortex subserves visuomotor coordinate transformation. Neuroimage 2004;23(4) 1494–1506.

[21] Cavanna AE, Trimble MR. The precuneus: a review of its functional anatomy and behavioural correlates. Brain 2006;129(pt 3) 564 –583.

[22] Treserras S, Boulanouar K, Conchou F, Simonetta-Moreau M, Berry I, Celsis P, Chollet F, Loubinoux I. Transition from rest to movement: brain correlates revealed by functional connectivity. Neuroimage 2009;48(1) 207–216.

[23] du Boisgueheneuc F, Levy R, Volle E, Seassau M, Duffau H, Kinkingnehun S, Samson Y, Zhang S, Dubois B. Functions of the left superior frontal gyrus in humans: a lesion study. Brain 2006;129(pt 12) 3315–3328.

[24] Swick D, Ashley V, Turken AU. Left inferior frontal gyrus is critical for response inhibition. BMC Neurosci 2008;9: 102.

[25] Cunnington R, Windischberger C, Deecke L, Moser E. The preparation and execution of self-initiated and externally-triggered movement: a study of event-related fMRI. Neuroimage 2002;15(2) 373—385.

[26] Frutiger SA, Strother SC, Anderson JR, Sidtis JJ, Arnold JB, Rottenberg DA. Multivariate predictive relationship between kinematic and functional activation patterns in a PET study of visuomotor learning. Neuroimage 2000;12(5) 515–527.

[27] Fink GR, Frackowiak RS, Pietrzyk U, Passingham RE. Multiple nonprimary motor areas in the human cortex. J Neurophysiol 1997;77(4) 2164 –2174.

[28] Mutschler I, Schulze-Bonhage A, Glauche V, Demandt E, Speck O, Ball T. A rapid sound-action association effect in human insular cortex. PLoS One 2007;2(2) e259.

[29] Ullsperger M, von Cramon DY. Neuroimaging of performance monitoring: error detection and beyond. Cortex 2004;40(4 –5) 593– 604.

[30] Clower DM, West RA, Lynch JC, Strick PL. The inferior parietal lobule is the target of output from the superior colliculus, hippocampus,and cerebellum. J Neurosci 2001;21(16) 6283– 6291.

[31] Halsband U, Lange RK. Motor learning in man: a review of functional and clinical studies. J Physiol Paris 2006;99(4 – 6) 414–424.

[32] Bjoertomt O, Cowey A, Walsh V. Near space functioning of the human angular and supramarginal gyri. J Neuropsychol 2009;3(pt1) 31– 43.

[33] Medina J, Kannan V, Pawlak MA, Kleinman JT, Newhart M, Davis C, Heidler-Gary JE, Herskovits EH, Hillis AE. Neural substrates of visuospatial processing in distinct reference frames: evidence from unilateral spatial neglect. J Cogn Neurosci 2009;21(11) 2073–2084.

[34] Small DM, Gitelman DR, Gregory MD, Nobre AC, Parrish TB, Mesulam MM. The posteriorcingulate and medial prefrontal cortex mediate the anticipatory allocation of spatial attention. Neuroimage 2003;18(3) 633– 641.

[35] Clements-Stephens AM, Rimrodt SL, Cutting LE. Developmental sex differences in basic visuospatial processing: differences in strategy use? Neurosci Lett 2009;449(3) 155–160.

[36] Leung HC, Oh H, Ferri J, Yi Y. Load response functions in the human spatial working memory circuit during location memory updating. Neuroimage 2007;35(1) 368 – 377.

[37] Eichenbaum H, Lipton PA. Towards a functional organization of the medial temporal lobe memory system: role of the parahippocampal and medial entorhinal cortical areas. Hippocampus 2008;18(12) 1314–1324.

[38] Okudzhava VM, Natishvili TA, Gurashvili TA, Gogeshvili KSh, Chipashvili SA, Bagashvili TI, Andronikashvili GT, Kvernadze GG, Okudzhava NV. Spatial recognition in cats: effects of parahippocampal lesions. Neurosci Behav Physiol 2009;39(7) 613–618.

[39] Stoodley CJ, Schmahmann JD. Functional topography in the human cerebellum: a meta-analysis of neuroimaging studies. Neuroimage 2009;44(2) 489 –501.

[40] Habas C, Kamdar N, Nguyen D, Prater K, Beckmann CF, Menon V, Greicius MD. Distinct cerebellar contributions to intrinsic connectivity networks. Journal of Neuroscience 2009;29(26) 8586–8594.

[41] Stoodley CJ, Schmahmann JD. Functional topography in the human cerebellum: a meta-analysis of neuroimaging studies. Neuroimage 2009;44(2) 489–501.

[42] Seidler RD, Purushotham A, Kim SG, Uğurbil K, Willingham D, Ashe J. Cerebellum activation associated with performance change but not motor learning. Science 2002;296(5575) 2043–2046.

[43] Orban P, Peigneux P, Lungu O, Albouy G, Breton E, Laberenne F, Benali H, Maquet P, Doyon J. The multifaceted nature of the relationship between performance and brain activity in motor sequence learning. Neuroimage 2010;49(1) 694–702.

[44] Diedrichsen J, Hashambhoy Y, Rane T, Shadmehr R. Neural correlates of reach errors. Journal of Neuroscience 2005;25(43) 9919–9931.

[45] Boyd LA, Vidoni ED, Siengsukon CF, Wessel BD. Manipulating time-to- plan alters patterns of brain activation during the Fitts' task. Experimental Brain Research 2009;194(4) 527–539.

[46] Grafton ST, Schmitt P, Van Horn J, Diedrichsen J. Neural substrates of visuomotor learning based on improved feedback control and prediction. Neuroimage 2008;39(3)1383–1395.

[47] Anguera JA, Reuter-Lorenz PA, Willingham DT, Seidler RD. Contributions of spatial working memory to visuomotor learning. J Cogn Neurosci 2010;22(9) 1917-1930.

[48] Clower DM, West RA, Lynch JC, Strick PL. The inferior parietal lobule is the target of output from the superior colliculus, hippocampus, and cerebellum. J Neurosci 2001;21(16) 6283-6291.

[49] Halsband U, Lange RK. Motor learning in man: a review of functional and clinical studies.J Physiol Paris. 2006 ;99(4-6) 414-424.

[50] Jenkins IH, Brooks DJ, Nixon PD, Frackowiak RS, Passingham RE. Motor sequence learning: a study with positron emission tomography. J Neurosci. 1994 Jun;14(6): 3775-90.

[51] Sakai K, Hikosaka O, Miyauchi S, Takino R, Sasaki Y, Pütz B. Transition of brain activation from frontal to parietal areas in visuomotor sequence learning.J Neurosci 1998 Mar 1;18(5):1827-40.

[52] Fassbender C, Murphy K, Foxe JJ, Wylie GR, Javitt DC, Robertson IH, Garavan H. A topography of executive functions and their interactions revealed by functional magnetic resonance imaging.Brain Res Cogn Brain Res 2004;20(2) 132-143.

[53] Graydon FX, Friston KJ, Thomas CG, Brooks VB, Menon RS. Learning-related fMRI activation associated with a rotational visuo-motor transformation. Brain Res Cogn Brain Res 2005;22(3) 373-383.

[54] Clements-Stephens AM, Rimrodt SL, Cutting LE. Developmental sex differences in basic visuospatial processing: differences in strategy use?Neurosci Lett 2009;449(3) 155-160.

[55] Bagley, W. C. On the correlation of mental and motor ability in school children. The American Journal of Psychology 1901;12(2) 193-205.

[56] Lippitt, L. C. A manual of corrective gymnastics. New York: Macmillan; 1926

[57] Orton, S.T. Reading, writing and speech problems in children. New York: Norton; 1937.

[58] Wigglesworth, R. The importance of recognising minimal cerebral dysfunction in paediatric practice. In: Bax M, MacKeith R. (ed.) Minimal cerebral dysfunction. Little Club Clinics in Developmental Medicine No. 10. London: Heinemann Medical; 1963. p.34-38.

[59] Clements, SD. Minimal brain dysfunction in children; Terminology and identification. Phase I of a Three-Phase Project, NINBD Monograph 3. Washington, DC: U. S. Government; 1966.

[60] Kong, E. Minimal cerebral palsy: The importance of its recognition. In: Bax M, MacKeith R. (ed.) Minimal cerebral dysfunction. Little Club Clinics in Developmental Medicine No. 10. London: Heinemann Medical;1963. p.29-31.

[61] Cermak, S. Developmental dyspraxia. In Roy EA. (ed.), Neuropsychological studies of apraxia and related disorders. Amsterdam: North-HoUand; 1985. p.225-248.

[62] Polatajko, H. J., Fox, A. M., & Missiuna, C. An international consensus on children with developmental coordination disorder. Canadian Journal of Occupational Therapy 1995;62(1) 3-6.

[63] Morris PR, Whiting HTA. Motor impairment and compensatory education. Philadelphia: G. Bell and Sons; 1971.

[64] Bernstein NA., Latash ML, Latash MT. Dexterity and Its Development. NY: Psyhology Press;1996.

[65] Dayan E, Cohen LG. Neuroplasticity subserving motor skill learning. Neuron 2011;72(3) 443-454.

[66] Fitts PM. The information capacity of the human motor system in controlling the amplitude of movement. Journal of Experimental Psychology 1954;47 381-391.

[67] Cermak S. A., Larkin, D.Developmental coordination disorder. Albany, NY: Delmar/ Thompson Learning; 2002

[68] Shumway-Cook A. Woollacott MH. Motor Control: Translating Research into Clinical Practice. Philadelphia: Lippincott Williams & Wilkins; 2011.

[69] Fitts PM, Posner MI. Human performance. Belmont, CA: Brooks/Cole;1967.

[70] Hikosaka O, Nakamura K, Sakai K, Nakahara H. Central mechanisms of motor skill learning. Curr Opin Neurobiol 2002 ;12(2) 217-222.

[71] Doyon J, Benali H. Reorganization and plasticity in the adult brain during learning of motor skills. Curr Opin Neurobiol 2005;15(2) 161-167.

[72] Culham JC, Cavina-Pratesi C, Singhal A. The role of parietal cortex in visuomotor control: what have we learned from neuroimaging? Neuropsychologia 2006; 44(13) 2668–2684.

[73] Heilman, K. M., & Valenstein, E. Clinical neuropsychology (4th ed.).New York, NY: Oxford University Press; 2003.

[74] Zwicker JG, Missiuna C, Boyd LA. Neural correlates of developmental coordination disorder: a review of hypotheses. J Child Neurol 2009;24(10) 1273-1281.

[75] Cummins A, Piek JP, Dyck MJ. Motor coordination, empathy, and social behaviour in school-aged children. Dev Med Child Neurol 2005;47(7) 437-442.

[76] Adolphs R, Damasio H, Tranel D, Damasio AR. Cortical systems for the recognition of emotion in facial expressions. J Neurosci 1996;16(23) 7678-7687.

[77] Wilson PH, Maruff P, Lum J. Procedural learning in children with developmental coordination disorder. Hum Mov Sci 2003;22(4-5) 515–526.

[78] Wilson PH, Maruff P, Butson M, Williams J, Lum J, Thomas PR. Internal representation of movement in children with developmental coordination disorder: a mental rotation task. Dev Med Child Neurol 2004; 46(11) 754–759.

[79] Hyde C, Wilson P. Online motor control in children with developmental coordination disorder: chronometric analysis of double-step reaching performance. Child Care Health Dev 2011;37(1) 111-122.

[80] Maruff P,Wilson PH, Trebilcock M, Currie J. Abnormalities of imaged motor sequences in children with developmental coordination disorder. Neuropsychologia 1999;37(11) 1317–1324.

[81] Williams J, Thomas PR, Maruff P, Wilson PH. The link between motor impairment level and motor imagery ability in children with developmental coordination disorder. Hum Mov Sci 2008; 27(2) 270–285.

[82] Wilson PH, Thomas PR, Maruff P. Motor imagery training ameliorates motor clumsiness in children. J Child Neurol 2002; 17(7) 491–498.

[83] Geuze RH. Postural control in children with developmental coordination disorder. Neural Plast 2005;12(2-3) 183-196; discussion 263-272.

[84] Kagerer FA, Contreras-Vidal JL, Bo J, Clark JE. Abrupt, but not gradual visuomotor distortion facilitates adaptation in children with developmental coordination disorder. Hum Mov Sci 2006;25(4-5) 622-633.

[85] Van Waelvelde H, De Weerdt W, De Cock P, Janssens L, Feys H, Smits Engelsman BC. Parameterization of movement execution in children with developmental coordination disorder. Brain Cogn 2006;60(1) 20-31.

[86] Groenewegen HJ. The basal ganglia and motor control. Neural Plast 2003;10(1-2) 107-120.

[87] Gheysen F, Van Waelvelde H, Fias W. Impaired visuo-motor sequence learning in Developmental Coordination Disorder.Res Dev Disabil 2011;32(2) 749-756.

[88] Gheysen F, Van Opstal F, Roggeman C, Van Waelvelde H, Fias W. Hippocampal contribution to early and later stages of implicit motor sequence learning. Exp Brain Res 2010;202(4) 795-807.

[89] Sigmundsson H, Ingvaldsen RP, Whiting HT. Inter- and intrasensory modality matching in children with hand-eye coordination problems: exploring the developmental lag hypothesis. Dev Med Child Neurol 1997;39(12) 790-796.

[90] Werner JM, Cermak SA., Aziz-Zadeh L. Neural Correlates of Developmental Coordination Disorder: The Mirror Neuron System Hypothesis. Journal of Behavioral and Brain Science 2012;2,:258-268 doi:10.4236/jbbs.2012.22029 (accessed May 2007)

[91] Scott A. Huettel, Allen W. Song, Gregory McCarthy. Functional Magnetic Resonance Imaging. Massachusetts: Sinauer Associates Inc.; 2009

[92] Raichle ME, MacLeod AM, Snyder AZ, Powers WJ, Gusnard DA, Shulman GL. A default mode of brain function. Proc Natl Acad Sci U S A 2001;98(2) 676-682.

[93] Harrison BJ, Pujol J, López-Solà M, Hernández-Ribas R, Deus J, Ortiz H, Soriano-Mas C, Yücel M, Pantelis C, Cardoner N. Consistency and functional specialization in the default mode brain network. Proc Natl Acad Sci U S A 2008;105(28) 9781-9886.

[94] Buckner RL, Andrews-Hanna JR, Schacter DL. The brain's default network: anatomy, function, and relevance to disease. Ann N Y Acad Sci 2008;1124 1-38.

[95] Greicius MD, Srivastava G, Reiss AL, Menon V. Default-mode network activity distinguishes Alzheimer's disease from healthy aging: evidence from functional MRI. Proc Natl Acad Sci U S A. 2004;101(13) 4637-46742.

[96] Broyd SJ, Demanuele C, Debener S, Helps SK, James CJ, Sonuga Barke EJ. Default-mode brain dysfunction in mental disorders: a systematic review. Neurosci Biobehav Rev 2009;33(3) 279-296.

[97] Supekar K, Uddin LQ, Prater K, Amin H, Greicius MD, Menon V. Development of functional and structural connectivity within the default mode network in young children. Neuroimage 2010;52(1) 290-301.

[98] Hillier, S. Intervention for children with developmental coordination disorder: A systematic review. The Internet Journal of Allied Health Sciences and Practice 2007;5(3) http://ijahsp.nova.edu

[99] Sugden D. Current approaches to intervention in children with developmental coordination disorder. Dev Med Child Neurol 2007;49(6) 467-471.

[100] Pless M, Carlsson M. Effects of motor skill intervention on developmental coordination disorder: a meta-analysis. Adapt Phys Activ Q 2000;17(4) 381–401.

[101] Wilson PH. Practitioner review: approaches to assessment and treatment of children with DCD: an evaluative review. J Child Psychol Psychiatry 2005; 46(8) 806–823.

[102] Braun SM, Beurskens AJ, Borm PJ, Schack T, Wade DT. The effects of mental practice in stroke rehabilitation: a systematic review. Arch Phys Med Rehabil 2006;87(6) 842-852.

[103] Langhorne P, Coupar F, Pollock A.. Motor recovery after stroke: a systematic review. Lancet Neurol. 2009;8(8) 741-754.

[104] Guillot A, Collet C, Nguyen VA, Malouin F, Richards C, Doyon J. Functional neuroanatomical networks associated with expertise in motor imagery. Neuroimage 2008;41(4) 1471-1483.

Chapter 4

Shared Neural Correlates for Speech and Gesture

Meghan L. Healey and Allen R. Braun

Additional information is available at the end of the chapter

http://dx.doi.org/10.5772/56493

1. Introduction

Humans are inherently social creatures: we spend a remarkable portion of our waking hours communicating with one another. We share our thoughts, goals, and desires, tell stories about what happened at lunch and make plans for the weekend. Although messages can be written, signed, or typed, the majority of this communication occurs through spoken language and face-to-face dialogue. These interactions demand that message recipients attend not only to words and sentences, but also to numerous nonverbal cues that include body language, facial expressions, and gestures, among others.

Hand gestures have been the focus of a substantial body of research in recent decades. While the body as a whole can be used to signify general emotional state, hand gestures tend to represent more precise semantic content. These spontaneous movements can be used independently or in conjunction with speech. For example, a "thumbs up" sign in the absence of any speech may indicate "I'm okay" after a bad fall, while wiggling index and middle fingers accompanying the statement "I went to the store earlier" may indicate the subject walked rather than drove. These and other examples suggest that gestures convey semantic and/or pragmatic information much in the same way that speech does. In light of this, some researchers have suggested that gesture, which is still relied upon by our primate ancestors for communication, may constitute the evolutionary basis of spoken language [1]. The following chapter will offer a comprehensive look at this intimate relationship between gesture and language, as well as a critique of the so-called "gestural origins theory." More specifically, we will address the following questions: (1) Are gesture and speech fundamentally linked, representing two parts of a single system that underlies human communication? (2) Did language initially emerge as a purely manual system?

2. Overview of gesture

While we may fail to recognize it, we use gestures constantly to convey and extract meaning. The variety of gestures we use on a daily basis also goes somewhat unnoticed. Some gestures are idiosyncratic, while others are more conventionalized. Some require the co-presence of speech to be interpretable, while others can stand alone. Although researchers have begun to focus on the characteristics of different gesture types, the field still lacks a consistent nomenclature system. Types of gestures overlap, sub-groups are combined, and definitions vary slightly, all depending on who is doing the labeling. Of course, this makes it difficult to formally conceptualize the nature of gestural communication and to compare findings across studies conducted by different research groups. Figure 1 below illustrates the wide range of gestures that have been individually defined.

Efforts have been made to develop a more systematic method for categorizing gesture types. The simplest of these schemes may be the one McNeill [2] termed "Kendon's continuum." According to this scheme, hand movements progress in the following linear sequence:

gesticulations → speech-framed gestures → pantomimes → emblems → sign languages

Moving from left to right along the continuum, the necessity for concurrent speech disappears and the presence of language-like properties increases. At the left extreme of the spectrum, gesticulations are defined as spontaneous and idiosyncratic movements of the hands and arms that rarely occur independent of speech (in fact, these gestures are temporally synchronized with the speech they accompany ninety percent of the time). Within this category, McNeill distinguishes between iconics, metaphorics, deictics, and beats. He explains that each gesture type performs a different function within discourse: iconic gestures refer to concrete events or features of a scene, metaphoric gestures to abstract concepts or relationships, deictic gestures to locations and orientations, and beat gestures to thematic highlights (see [2] for more information). The majority of research, including the next sections of this chapter, focuses on these subcategories of gesticulations. See Figure 1 below for definitions and examples of speech-framed gestures, pantomimes, emblems, and sign languages.

Regardless of type, gesture production can be defined in three stages: preparation, stroke, and retraction. The stroke of the gesture contains the content of the message. Gestures are generally performed in the front of the body; McNeill writes that "the gesture space can be visualized as a shallow disk in front of the speaker, the bottom half flattened when the speaker is seated" ([2], p.86).

3. Competing theories

While there is a general consensus that gestures are used to communicate, the exact nature of the relationship between gesture and speech is still a matter of some controversy. David McNeill [2] was first to propose that, at their core, gesture and speech reflect the same cognitive process: only the modality of expression differs. Others, like Robert Krauss [3] for example,

http://dx.doi.org/10.5772/56493

Gesture Type	Definition	Example
Gesticulations	Spontaneous and idiosyncratic movements of the hands and arms. Rarely occur in absence of speech/ require speech for full comprehension.	Any iconic, metaphoric, deictic, or beat gestures.
Iconic Gestures	Visually represents the co-expressive speech content.	While describing a car accident, hands form a T-shape, representing how the two collided.
Metaphoric Gestures	Represent abstract concepts or relationships.	Using the hands to form a spherical shape, representing the idea of "wholeness"
Deictic Gestures	Also known as pointing gestures. Locate objects and actions in space. Can be concrete or abstract.	Classical deictic gesture is an extended index finger.
Beat Gestures	Also known as "baton" gestures. Provide temporal highlighting to speech. Signal the speaker feels part of the message is particularly important.	Generally a rhythmic waving of the hands or arms.
Speech-framed gestures	Fill a grammatical slot in a sentence. Do not overlap with speech, but require speech to set up the context.	"The ball went [gesture indicates ball bounced up and down repeatedly]."
Pantomimes	Hands are used to imitate objects or actions. Speech is not obligatory. Can combine multiple gestures to demonstrate a sequence. ** The term transitive gesture is also used to represent those gestures imitating use of everyday tools. Intransitive gestures, on the contrary, do not involve tools.	Hands assume the shape of a camera and index finger moves downward, imitating taking a photograph.
Emblems	Arbitrary but conventionalized representations of linguistic meaning. Can function independently. Emblems are culturally specific. *Instrumental gestures (gestures intended to influence the behavior of another, e.g. "come here") generally fall into this category.	Thumbs up sign means "I'm okay" or "Everything is good" One finger to the lips means "be quiet"
Instrumental Gestures	Meant to influence or direct the behavior of another. Generally these gestures can also be classified as emblems.	"Come here" sign with one finger extending and then forming a hook back to the speaker.
Expressive Gestures	Express inner feeling states. May also be classified as emblems.	Hands turned up and to the sides to indicate "I don't know"
Sign Language	Full-fledged language system with syntactic structure and a community of users.	American Sign Language, Nicaraguan Sign Language

Figure 1. Names, definitions, and examples of commonly-referred to gesture types.

take an alternate view, arguing that gesture and speech are separate and independent systems, only loosely related. According to this second camp, gesture is merely used as an auxiliary support when speech processing is unusually difficult.

Evidence is accumulating in favor of the first proposal that gesture and speech are intimately connected and combine to form a single system of meaning. While they are undoubtedly used to bolster communication under adverse conditions (e.g. loud environments), gestures are used far more widely than this hypothesis would suggest. Instead, McNeill explains that gestures are able to convey ideas that cannot always be captured with conventional spoken language (e.g. information about spatial relationships). While speech is highly structured and arbitrary, gesture provides information in a more holistic and imagistic fashion [4]. Gesture and speech serve distinct, but complementary functions in this regard: a speaker's message cannot always be expressed, nor understood in its entirety without this composite signal. The movement of the hands is not just a "bonus" feature; it is fundamental to successful transmission of the message.

There are several lines of evidence that support McNeill's claim of an intimate relationship between speech and gesture: 1) gesture and speech are temporally synchronized, 2) speech and gesture co-develop in children, 3) there is a correlation between handedness and the cerebral lateralization of language, 4) people readily incorporate gestural information into the retelling of speech-only content, and 5) the use of gesture does not disappear when people are physically removed from their audience [5-19]. Each of these arguments will be explored in more detail below.

4. Temporal synchronization of speech and gesture

When we produce gestures, we instinctively produce them so they overlap with their co-expressive speech. Consider an example cited by McNeill [2]: while describing a scene from a comic in which a character bends a tree towards the ground, the speaker grips an imaginary branch and pulls it inwards and down (from the upper gesture space to the body). The gesture stroke concludes as the subject finishes the utterance "he grabs a big oak tree and he bends it way back" [2, p.25]. Here, the gesture and speech are carefully synchronized so the hand movement can be linked to the content it both depends and elaborates upon. In general, the gesture stroke generally precedes speech onset, within a certain restricted time window. The gesture stroke is rarely, if ever, initiated after the speech it is meant to represent or supplement.

Several researchers have examined the sensitive nature of temporal relationship between speech and gesture. For example, Rauscher, Krauss, and Chen [5] manipulated participants' ability to gesture while they described a cartoon to a listener. In those conditions where hand movement was restricted, subjects spoke less fluently and produced more unfilled pauses. Based on these findings, the authors argue that gestures facilitate the speech production process itself (in particular access to the mental lexicon), rather than serving as a backup mechanism for communication once speech has failed.

Mayberry and Jaques [6] reach a similar conclusion in their work on persons who stutter. When these individuals narrate cartoons, gestures are only produced alongside fluent speech. In the cases when gestures have been initiated prior to a stuttering event, the gesture stroke is frozen until speech is resumed and the two can continue to co-occur. Again, the results directly contradict the independent systems theory: if gesture and speech were separate processes, persons who stutter would be expected to continue gesturing even when speech is temporarily interrupted. In fact, these people would likely gesture more in order r to compensate for the breakdown in speech. This bidirectional relationship—the fact that the gesture stroke is halted in time with the stuttering events-- suggests speech and gesture must be linked at a deep, neural level. Mayberry and Jaques [6] exclude the possibility that it is simply a "manual-motor shutdown" that prevents gesturing during stuttering events by showing that only speech-related hand movements (and not simultaneous button-pressing, finger-tapping, etc.) are suspended during dysfluencies. Instead, the two must be connected at a planning stage, prior to motor execution.

5. Co-development of speech and gesture

Speech and gesture are known to show similar developmental trajectories in children. Bates and Dick [7] provide a comprehensive review of these parallel milestones, starting with the co-emergence of rhythmic hand movements and babbling in six to eight month olds. The same trends continue as children age and language abilities expand rapidly. Between twelve and eighteen months, gesture and naming are positively correlated (children who gesture earlier also name objects earlier). By18 months of age, toddlers begin to form both gesture-word and gesture-gesture combinations, and at 24 months, the ability to reproduce arbitrary sequences of manual actions is correlated with grammatical competence [7,8].This tight developmental link between speech and gesture can be easily understood if we believe speech and gesture are supported by a common and amodal system of communication.

Interestingly, hand banging is significantly correlated with onset of babbling and single word production even in infants with Williams Syndrome (WS), a rare genetic disorder causing broad developmental delays. More importantly, these manual movements in infants with WS are *not* correlated with other motor milestones; the link is specific to these early precursors of spoken language and gesture [9]. Also interesting is the observation that in congenitally deaf children, the emergence of manual babbling is developmentally appropriate, coinciding with the emergence of vocal babbling in typical hearing children [10]. This suggests that infants are innately disposed to acquire language, but that the system is flexible in terms of the input (e.g. visual or auditory) it will accept and later imitate.

Relatedly, studies have also shown that language and handedness both emerge early in development. The left hemisphere has long been known to support language function, and the majority of the global population develops a right handed bias for motor activity (motor activity on the right side of the body is also controlled by the left hemisphere of the brain). Interestingly, this handedness effect is stronger when producing symbolic rather than non-communicative hand movements [11]. These results suggest that that there is a common network within the left hemisphere that may support any type of communicative act, whether it is achieved through spoken language or manual movements.

6. Incorporation of gesture into speech retell

Numerous studies have demonstrated that people incorporate gestural information into the retelling of stories [12-15,among others]. For example, Church, Garber, and Rogalski [12] compared subject recall for ambiguous statements (e.g. "My brother went to the gym") alone versus when accompanied by a complementary gesture (e.g. shooting a basketball). At testing, researchers found a significant memory enhancement effect when both speech and gesture were available to subjects. Moreover, when asked to recall the speech items, 75% of the subjects added pieces of information based on the accompanying gestures. This pattern of results suggests that the brain does not "tag" the incoming information as originating in separate channels, but immediately integrates the two sources and processes them together.

Subjects may also add new content to a narrative in order to resolve potential mismatches between speech and gesture. For example, a conflict is introduced if a subject hears the phrase "and then Granny gives him a penny" but sees a gesture suggesting that Granny was actually on the *receiving* end of the interaction. In this case, the subject might insert additional information in their retelling: "and she threw him a penny, so he picked up the penny." Now, the gesture towards the body is aligned with "he picked up the penny," which is more logical than the mismatch that was originally presented [13]. Importantly, the subject does not ignore the gestural information in favor the speech. Instead, the two are seen as equally viable sources of information that must be linked in some fashion.

7. Gesture in self-only conditions

An additional line of evidence verifying the intimate relationship for speech and gestures comes from the repeated observation that the presence of gesture does not disappear entirely when a speaker's audience is removed (i.e. separated by a partition, on the phone, etc.). While the rate of gesturing is always higher in conditions where the receiver of the message is visible to the speaker), we do not stop gesturing in monologue or non face-to-face conditions. Why gesture if it cannot ease the comprehension load of our listener? Some researchers hypothesize that in these instances, gestures are used to benefit the speaker by facilitating word retrieval and lexical access, while others suggest that it is simply the result of habit. However, in the context of other research, it seems most likely that because gesture and speech are so tightly and inextricably linked, it becomes challenging to produce the speech without simultaneously producing the gesture [16-18]

Similarly, there is evidence that congenitally blind individuals gesture as well, suggesting that – since they have never observed it—their use of gesture and its association with speech is innate rather than learned. Moreover, they gesture at a rate that is comparable to sighted individuals [19]. This behavior persists even when they are talking to individuals whom they know to be blind and could not benefit from the visual input.

8. Evidence from neuroimaging

While the behavioral studies described above are somewhat convincing, neuroimaging techniques may provide more compelling evidence that speech and gesture are best described as two example of a singular process. Functional magnetic resonance imaging (fMRI) and electroencephalography /event-related potentials (EEG/ERP) provide useful methods to explore what the brain is doing as it processes speech and gesture, either separately or together. Results of imaging studies have demonstrated that 1) gestures influence the earliest stages of speech processing, 2) gestures are subject to the same semantic processing as speech, and 3) speech and gesture activate a common neural network.

9. Early sensory processing

A handful of studies have indicated that gestures can affect the earliest stages of language processing [20-25]. In an ERP experiment, Kelly, Kravitz, and Hopkins [21] showed a modulatory effect of gesture on the sensory P1-N1 and P2 components elicited at frontal sites. Since these early components are generally reflective of low level and automatic sensory processing, this suggests that the interaction between speech and gesture occurs obligatorily and prior to any conscious semantic processing. Such a finding directly contradicts the view that gesture is an "add-on" or "bonus" feature, only used post-hoc in cases when speech fails. Similarly, in an fMRI experiment, Hubbard et al. [23] presented subjects with videos of speech accompanied by spontaneous production of beat gestures (i.e. rapid movements of the hands which provide 'temporal highlighting' to accompanying speech; [1]), nonsense hand movements, or no hand movements. Analysis revealed higher BOLD signal in brain regions relevant to speech perception, including the left superior temporal gyrus and the right planum temporale, in the beat gesture condition.

Gestures do not only affect how we process speech; they also affect how we produce it. Bernardis and Gentilucci [24] compared the properties of speech and gesture emitted in multimodal (speech + gesture) conditions versus unimodal (speech only or gesture only) conditions. The authors found increased F2 and pitch in vocal spectra when words were accompanied by meaningful gestures, but no effect when words were accompanied by aimless arm movements. Similarly, speaking a word, but not a pseudoword, aloud reduced the maximal height reached by the hands and duration of meaningful gestures. These findings offer clear evidence that there is a bi-directional relationship between speech and gesture: producing one automatically and reflexively influences how we produce the other. Krahmer and Swerts [25] confirm that producing a gesture (in this case, a beat gesture) influences how a speaker generates co-occuring speech in terms of its acoustic features (emphasis, duration, frequency, etc). The reverse is also true: when participants can see a speaker's gesture, they rate the accompanying word as more "prominent."

10. Semantic processing of speech and gesture

A series of ERP experiments has shown that speech and gesture reflect the same semantic and cognitive processing. These experiments focus on the N400 component, which is thought to be an index of semantic integration and is commonly elicited by both words and gestures that are incongruent with the ongoing discourse. While the N400 was initially reported as generated by incongruent or unexpected words [26], the N400 to incongruent gestures is an incredibly robust finding [21, 27-29, among others]. For example, Kelly, Kravitz, and Hopkins [21] showed participants video clips in which an actor gestured to one of two objects (a short, wide dish or a tall, thin glass) and then described the same object aloud. The N400 was smallest when the gesture and verbal descriptor referred to the same object and largest when they referred to different objects. Similarly, Holle and Gunter [27] used homonyms to investigate the ability of gesture to disambiguate speech. An N400 effect to the homonym was found when the ongoing discourse failed to support the meaning that was previously indicated via gesture.

11. Shared neural networks

A smaller body of research has examined the processing of autonomous gestures, like emblems and pantomimes. Studying these gesture types, rather than the gesticulations dependent on speech for context, allows researchers to contrast the brain's response to each form of communication separately. For example, a recent fMRI study [30] demonstrated that language and symbolic gestures both activate a common, left-lateralized network of inferior frontal and posterior temporal regions, including the inferior frontal gyrus/Broca's Area (IFG), posterior middle temporal gyrus (pMTG), and superior temporal sulcus (STS) (see Figure 2 for illustration).The authors suggest that these regions are not language-specific but rather function more broadly to link symbols with their meaning. This is true regardless of the modality or form the symbol adopts: sounds, words, gestures, pictures, etc.

12. The gestural origins theory

The findings that speech and gesture are tightly integrated at multiple stages of processing and that they appear to activate a common neural system have significant implications for the question of how language evolved. The Gestural Origins Theory, made popular by Michael Arbib, Michael Tomasello, and Michael Corballis, proposes that spoken language emerged

http://dx.doi.org/10.5772/56493

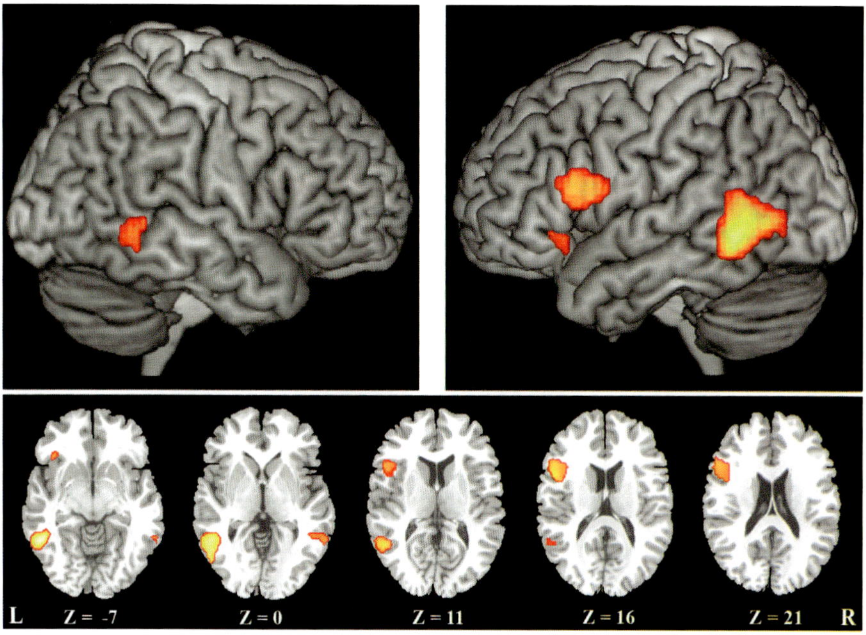

Figure 2. Common areas of activation for processing symbolic gestures and spoken language minus their respective baselines, identified using a random effects conjunction analysis. The resultant t map is rendered on a single subject T1 image: 3D surface rendering above, axial slices with associated z axis coordinates, below. See [30] for more details.

from the system of gestural communication we still see today in non-human primates (see [31] for review). In humans, a growth in brain size and the development of the vocal tract permitted a gradual transition to a more complex language system based upon vocalizations. Subsequently, and although we still use gestures to express ourselves, spoken language became the dominant mode of communication because it freed the hands for simultaneous tool use, was less demanding of energy resources, and did not require the speaker and addressee to be in the same physical (not to mention well-lit) location.

13. Gesture in our primate ancestors

Renowned primatologist Jane Goodall, as well as many other scientists, cites our sophisticated spoken language system as the crucial difference between humans and chimpanzees. Our primate relatives do produce sounds in order to communicate, but these vocalizations are limited in their scope and function and are used mainly to direct attention. Instead, it is their gesticulations that serve a more "language-like" function. These gestures are numerous: pointing, shaking, begging, and offering are all common [32]. These manual gestures can also be used intentionally, flexibly, and across many contexts, unlike facial and vocal gestures which are more automatic and ritualized [33].

So, the question is now what is unique about humans that supports spoken language ability? Spoken language requires the same careful coordination of motor systems as manual gestures, only the same fine motor control of the hands gradually transitioned to similar movements of the vocal tract. This transition was only possible due to skeletal changes: the lowering of the larynx, lengthening of the tongue and neck, etc. A popular theory claims that a genetic mutation in the FOXP2 gene located on chromosome 7 may be responsible for the development of fine motor skills necessary for articulation and vocalization [34].

14. Gesture and the mirror neuron system

The discovery of the mirror neuron system lent added credence to the gestural origins theory. Mirror neurons were first identified in area F5 of the monkey ventral premotor cortex and fire whether an animal executes or observes an action (for review, see [35]). A similar system is thought to exist in humans, and the areas of the human MNS, activated both by speech and by gesture, overlap largely with the classical language areas (i.e. Brodmann Area 44/Broca's Area). In terms of the Gestural Origins Theory, the mirror neuron system accounts for what Michael Arbib terms parity: the fact that what a listener hears and understands is the message that the speaker intended to send [36]. However, the role of the MNS has been hotly debated in recent years, with some researchers suggesting that it cannot account for the complex semantic features of our language system [37] and suggesting its role in action understanding may be overstated [38-39].

15. Gesture as a universal language

The existence of a communication system is a feature of every human culture. However, spoken language is not a unitary phenomenon: depending on geographic location and the community we belong to, we speak one or two (or in some circumstances, maybe three or four) out of hundreds of modern languages. When an English speaker travels to China for the first time, for example, it is highly unlikely he will understand even simple words or phrases if he has not spent extensive time memorizing vocabulary and practicing with fluent speakers first. In these situations, we turn to gestures. Unlike speech, gestures, such as pointing, is relatively consistent across cultures (emblems, of course, are culturally bound and the exception to this rule). For example, Liszkowski et al. [40] showed that infants and caregivers from seven different cultures all pointed with the same general frequency and under the same circumstances, suggesting a universal and prelinguistic basis for communication.

Many studies have examined the frequency of gesture usage in situations where no common language exists between speakers or when an individual is speaking in his non-native language. In general, speakers rely more upon gesture when communicating in their second language (L2) [41-42]; gesture under these circumstances likely function to decrease the production burden for the speaker and increase the likelihood of comprehension for the listener. Another line of research has been study the role of gesture in L2 vocabulary acquisition. This work has demonstrated that learning novel words paired with meaningful gestures helps learners retain the material over time [43-45].

Similarly, it seems that it is easier for members of deaf communities to develop a common gesture or sign-based language than it is for members of separate speech communities to develop a new spoken language. The most notable example is perhaps Nicaraguan Sign Language, which emerged in the 1970s after the opening of a special education school that brought deaf children in the community together for the first time [46]. In sum, the fact that 1) we rely upon gesture as a common platform for communication when we lack a common language and 2) signed (but not spoken) languages still arise spontaneously, suggest that gestures may indeed form the core of our communication system.

16. Conclusions

Evidence overwhelmingly favors the view that speech and gesture are tightly integrated with one another, at both the behavioral and neural levels, suggesting that forms of verbal and nonverbal communication are parts of one amodal system that enables complex human communication.

Considered broadly, evidence also seems to support a view of language evolution rooted in manual gesture. The mechanisms that underlie this, however, are still somewhat unclear. The mirror neuron system may be the center of the "language-ready brain," but this theory is not free from controversy. Equally viable (and not mutually exclusive) is the proposal we advocate here: the system that supported nonverbal communication was co-opted over the course of evolution to support spoken language.

Nevertheless, David McNeill, whose work we see as central to both of these hypotheses, is actually a critic of the "gesture-first" view, instead claiming that speech and gesture emerged alongside one another and in response to the same environmental pressures. Challenging this view, however, is the literature on comparative biology, primate vocalizations and gesture, molecular, and the developmental trajectories of gesture and speech in children, all of which all suggest that speech lags behind gesture in our evolutionary history.

In the end, the question of how language evolved and whether or not it emerged from a system built on manual gestures is not as important as what the relationship is between speech and gesture, now that they both exist. The intimate relationship between the two, which is now well established, has important implications for education, acquisition of second languages, effective public speaking, treatment of patients with communication disorders, and much, much more.

Author details

Meghan L. Healey and Allen R. Braun

Language Section, Voice, Speech, and Language Branch, National Institutes on Deafness and Other Communication Disorders, Bethesda, MD, USA

References

[1] Call, J., & Tomasello, M. (2007). The gestural communication of apes and monkeys. New York: Lawrence Erlbaum Associates.

[2] McNeill, D. (1992). Hand and mind: What gestures reveal about thought. Chicago: University of Chicago Press.

[3] Krauss, R. M. (1998). Why do we gesture when we speak? Current Directions in Psychological Science, 7, 54–59.

[4] McNeill, D., Cassell, J., & McCullough, K. (1994). Communicative effects of speech-mismatched gestures. Research on Language and Social Interaction, 27(3), 223-237.

[5] Rauscher, F. H., Krauss, R. M., & Chen, Y. (1996). Gesture, speech, and lexical access: The role of lexical movements in speech production. Psychological Science, 7, 226–231.

[6] Mayberry, R. & Jaques, J. (2000). Gesture production during stuttered speech: insights into the nature of gesture-speech integration. In D. McNeill (ed.). Language and gesture, pp. 199-214. Cambridge: Cambridge University Press.

[7] Bates, Elizabeth & Dick, Frederic. (2002). Language, gesture and the developing brain. In B. J. Casey & Y. Munakata (eds.), Special issue: Converging Method Approach to the Study of Developmental Science. Developmental Psychobiology 40: 293- 310.

[8] Bauer, P.J., Herstgaard, L.A., Dropik, P., & Daly, B.P. (1998). When even arbitrary order becomes important: Developments in reliable temporal sequencing of arbitrarily ordered events. Memory, 6, 165-198.

[9] Masataka, N. (2001). Why early linguistic milestones are delayed in children with Williams syndrome: Late onset of hand banging as a possible rate-limiting constraint on the emergence of canonical babbling. Developmental Science, 4, 158-164.

[10] Petitto, L.A. & Marentette, P.F. (1991). Babbling in the manual mode: evidence for the ontogeny of language. Science, 251(5000), 1493-6.

[11] Bates, E., O'Connell, B., Vaid, J., Sledge, P. & Oakes, L. (1986). Language and hand preference in early development. Developmental Neuropsychology, 2(1), 1-15.

[12] Church, R. B., Garber, P., & Rogalski, K. (2007). The role of gesture in memory and social communication. Gesture, 7(2), 137-158.

[13] Cassell, J., McNeill, D., & McCullough, K. (1999). Speech–gesture mismatches: Evidence for one underlying representation of linguistic and nonlinguistic information. Pragmatics & Cognition, 7(1), 1-34.

[14] Kelly, S. D. (2001). Broadening the units of analysis in communication: Speech and nonverbal behaviours in pragmatic comprehension. Journal of Child Language, 28(2), 325-349.

[15] Kelly, S. D., Barr, D. J., Church, R. B., & Lynch, K. (1999). Offering a hand to pragmatic understanding: The role of speech and gesture in comprehension and memory. Journal of Memory and Language, 40(4), 577-592.

[16] Bavelas, J. B., Gerwing, J., Sutton, C., & Prevost, D. (2008). Gesturing on the telephone: Independent effects of dialogue and visibility. Journal of Memory and Language 58, 495-520.

[17] Alibali, M. W., Heath, D. C., & Myers, H. J. (2001). Effects of visibility between speaker and listener on gesture production: Some gestures are meant to be seen. Journal of Memory and Language, 44(2), 169-188.

[18] Clark, H. H. (1996). Using language. Cambridge: Cambridge University Press.

[19] Iverson, J.M. & Goldin-Meadow, S. (1997). What's communication got to do with it? Gesture in children blind from birth. Developmental Psychology, 33(3), 453-67.

[20] Wu, Y. C., & Coulson, S. (2010). Gestures modulate speech processing early in utterances. Neuroreport, 21(7), 522-526.

[21] Kelly, S. D., Kravitz, C., & Hopkins, M. (2004). Neural correlates of bimodal speech and gesture comprehension. Brain and Language, 89(1), 253-260.

[22] Skipper, J. I., Goldin-Meadow, S., Nusbaum, H. C., & Small, S. L. (2007). Speech-associated gestures, broca's area, and the human mirror system. Brain and Language, 101(3), 260-277.

[23] Hubbard, A. L., Wilson, S. M., Callan, D. E., & Dapretto, M. (2009). Giving speech a hand: Gesture modulates activity in auditory cortex during speech perception. Human Brain Mapping, 30(3), 1028-1037.

[24] Bernardis, P. & Gentilucci, M. (2006). Speech and gesture share the same communication system. Neuropsychologia, 44, 178–190.

[25] Krahmer, E. and M. Swerts (2007). "The effects of visual beats on prosodic prominence: acoustic analyses, auditory perception and visual perception." Journal of Memory and Language, 57, 396-414.

[26] Kutas, M., & Hillyard, S. A. (1980). Reading senseless sentences: Brain potentials reflect semantic incongruity. Science, 207, 203–204.

[27] Holle, H., & Gunter, T. C. (2007). The role of iconic gestures in speech disambiguation: ERP evidence. Journal of Cognitive Neuroscience, 19(7), 1175-1192.

[28] Ozyurek, A., Willems, R. M., Kita, S., & Hagoort, P. (2007). On-line integration of semantic information from speech and gesture: Insights from event-related brain potentials. Journal of Cognitive Neuroscience, 19(4), 605-616.

[29] Bernardis, P., Salillas, E., & Caramelli, N. (2008). Behavioural and neurophysiological evidence of semantic interaction between iconic gestures and words. Cognitive Neuropsychology, 25(7-8), 1114-1128.

[30] Xu, J., Gannon, P.J., Emmorey, K., Smith, J.F., & Braun, A.R. (2009). Symbolic gestures and spoken language are processed by a common neural system. Proceedings of the National Academy of Sciences, 106(49), 20664-20669.

[31] Gentilucci, M., & Corballis, M.C. (2006). From manual gesture to speech: A gradual transition. Neuroscience & Biobehavioral Reviews, 30(7), 949-960.

[32] Tomasello, M., Call, J., and Gluckman, A. (1997). Comprehension of novel communicative signs by apes and human children. Child Development, 68(6), 1067-80.

[33] Pollick, A.S. & de Waal, F.B.M. (2007) Ape gestures and language evolution. Proceedings of the National Academy of Sciences, 104(19): 8184-8189.

[34] Corballis, M.C. (2004). FoxP2 and the mirror neuron system. TRENDS in Cognitive Science. 8(3), 95-6.

[35] Rizzolatti, G., & Craighero,L. (2004). The mirror-neuron system. Annual Review of Neuroscience, 27, 169-192.

[36] Arbib, M.A. (2008). From grasp to language: embodied concepts and the challenge of abstract. Journal of Physiology, 102(1-3), 4-20.

[37] Tettamanti, M. & Moro, A. (2012). Can syntax appear in a mirror system? Cortex, 48(7), 923-35.

[38] Hickok, G. (2009). Eight problems for the mirror neuron theory of action understanding in monkeys and humans. Journal of Cognitive Neuroscience, 21(7), 1229-43.

[39] Lingnau, A., Gesierich, B., & Caramazza, A. (2009). Asymmetric fMRI adaptation reveals no evidence for mirror neurons in humans. Proceedings of the National Academy of Sciences, 106(24), 9925-30.

[40] Liszkowski, U., Brown, P., Callaghan, T., Takada, A., & de Vos, C. (2012). A prelinguistic gestural universal of human communication. Cognitive Science. 36(4), 698-713.

[41] Gullberg, M. (1998). Gesture as a Communication Strategy in Second Language Discourse: A Study of Learners of French and Swedish. Lund, Sweden: Lund University Press.

[42] Hadar, U., Dar, R., & Teitelman, A. (2001). Gesture during Speech in First and Second Language: Implications for Lexical Retrieval. Gesture, 1(2),151-165.

[43] Kelly, S. D., McDevitt, T., & Esch, M. (2009). Brief training with co-speech gesture lends a hand to word learning in a foreign language. Language and Cognitive Processes, 24, 313-334.

[44] Macedonia, M. & Knosche, T. (2011). Body in mind: how gestures empower foreign language learning. Mind, Brain, and Education, 35(4),196-211.

[45] Macedonia, M., Muller, K., & Friederici, A.D. (2011). The impact of iconic gestures on foreign language word learning and its neural substrate. Human Brain Mapping, 31(6), 982-98.

[46] Senghas, A., Kitas, S., & Ozyurek, A. (2004). Children creating core properties of language: evidence from an emerging sign language in Nicaragua. Science, 305(5691): 1779-82.

Chapter 5

Brain Mapping of Language Processing Using Functional MRI Connectivity and Diffusion Tensor Imaging

Todd L. Richards and Virginia W. Berninger

Additional information is available at the end of the chapter

http://dx.doi.org/10.5772/56501

1. Introduction

Because the brain's language systems have no end organs for interacting directly with the external world, language systems work with sensory (ears or eyes) and motor (mouth and hands) systems, which are the only brain systems with direct links to external environment. Liberman contributed to understanding of how the language by ear (listening) and language by mouth (reading) systems work together at the behavioral level and also become integrated to support acquisition of language by eye (reading) [1]. Berninger and colleagues extended the work of Liberman and colleagues at the Haskins Laboratory to language by hand (writing), which is not just a motor skill as many assume [2]. This University of Washington research team also showed that Language by Ear, Language by Mouth, Language by Eye, and Language by Hand are separate, but interacting functional language systems, which draw on common as well as unique processes at the behavioral [3] and brain levels of analysis [4]. Moreover, each of the functional language systems has different levels of organization, ranging from subword, to word, to syntax, to text, and has connections with other brain systems such as working memory, attention and executive functions, and cognitive.

The emerging work on the complex functional language systems that connect with other brain systems illustrates the need for brain imaging methods that not only assess localized brain areas or functions but also their structural and functional connections. First, we discuss how the modern imaging techniques have confirmed knowledge of localized structures and functions first acquired in autopsy studies with patients. Second, we discuss how advances in imaging techniques are adding knowledge about the structural and functional connections among specific functional language systems.

1.1. Localized structures and functions

In early work in neurolinguistics researchers studied people with brain lesions and discovered relationships between the patient's specific language deficit and the location of the lesion. In this way, they discovered that two areas in the brain are involved in language processing: Wernicke's area located in the posterior section of the superior temporal gyrus in the dominant cerebral hemisphere. People with a lesion in this area of the brain develop receptive aphasia, a condition in which there is a major language comprehension impairment, but the capability for speech production remains intact. The other area is Broca's area located in the posterior inferior frontal gyrus of the dominant hemisphere. Patients with a lesion to this area develop expressive aphasia and are unable to produce speech even though they are able to understand other's that they hear [4].

Neurolinguist researchers have adopted non-invasive brain imaging techniques such as functional magnetic resonance imaging and electrophysiology to study language processing in individuals without impairments [5]. For example, in the study of phonological processing, the receptive processing of phonemes in heard words has been localized to Wernicke's area (posterior Brodmann's Area [BA] 22) and BA 40 [6] [7-11], and expressive production of phonemes during speech has been localized to the posterior Broca's area (BAs 44 and 6) [11-15]. Thus, research using these newly developed brain imaging techniques has confirmed what was was classically thought based on patient studies for right-handed individuals: The two major language areas are Broca's area for production of language by mouth [16] and Wernicke's area for comprehension of language by ear [17], which receives input from the ear through the auditory cortex. The arcuate fasciculus, a fiber pathway that originates in the temporal lobe and curves in an anterior/posterior direction to project to the frontal lobe [18], was thought to connect these 2 areas.

Figure 1 that follows shows these important language processing areas of the brain superimposed on a side/surface view of the brain based on more recent non-invasive brain imaging methods. These areas may also play a role in production of language by hand (writing) and comprehension of language by eye (reading), via related processing in angular gyrus and supramarginal gyrus [4].

2. Brain's structural and functional connectivity

In 2010 the US National Institute of Health (NIH) announced the Human Connectome Project:

"Knowledge of human brain connectivity will transform human neuroscience by providing not only a qualitatively novel class of data, but also by providing the basic framework necessary to synthesize diverse data and, ultimately, elucidate how our brains work in health, illness, youth, and old age." Included in this connectome is the study of language-related neural connections which enable the brain to perform written and oral language.

Mullen [19] has on online manual that defines several important terms used in research about structural and functional networks.

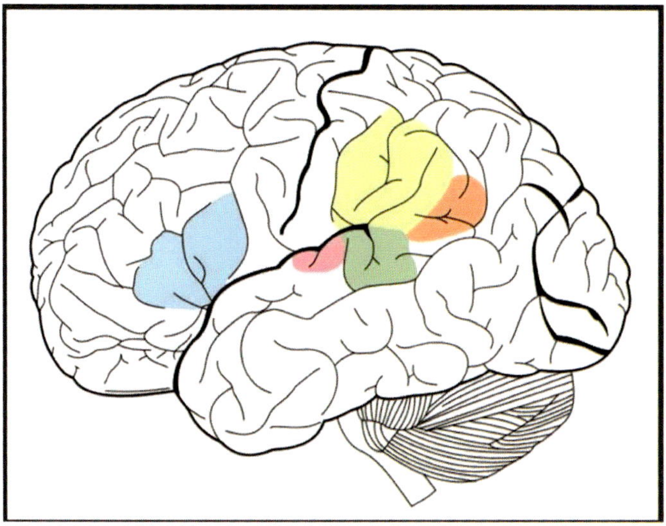

Figure 1. Brain regions important for language. Broca's area (blue), auditory cortex (pink), Wernicke's area (green), Supramarginal gyrus (yellow), angular gyus (orange). (Figure from the wikipedia website http://en.wikipedia.org/wiki/File:Brain_Surface_Gyri.SVG).

The study of human brain connectivity generally falls under one or more of three categories: structural, functional, and effective [20].

2.1. DTI structural connectivity studies of brain

Structural connectivity denotes networks of anatomical (e.g., axonal) links) for which the primary goal is to understand what brain structures are capable of influencing each other via direct or indirect axonal connections. Structural connectivity might be studied in vivo using invasive axonal labeling techniques or noninvasive MRI-based diffusion weighted imaging (DWI/DTI) methods. These methods cannot measure individual axons but can measure the water diffusion signal from a group of axons that have parallel geometric properties within a fiber bundle. DTI connectivity is influenced by the number of axons and the amount of myelination within the fiber bundle.

Diffusion Tensor Imaging (DTI) tractography is a neuroimaging technique that allows for the virtual dissection of fiber tracts in the living brain based on the directionally biased diffusion of water in white matter [21]. DTI analysis provides several parameters that quantify the properties of the fiber bundle: fractional anisotropy (a measure of the amount of anisotropy of water diffusion between the primary fiber direction and the perpendicular to the primary fiber direction); axial water diffusion diffusivity (the amount of water diffusion along the primary direction of the fiber bundle); radial diffusivity (the amount the water diffusion perpendicular to the primary direction of the fiber bundle); mean diffusivity (characterizes the overall mean-squared displacement of water molecules); relative anisotropy; and volume ratio. These parameters can be calculated on a voxel by voxel basis within the DTI image The exact equations used to calculate these DTI parameters have been published by LeBihan et al [22]. Other important parameters that characterize the fiber bundle are the tractography analysis which is a procedure to demonstrate the neural tracts[23]. These neural tracts have properties such as mean fiber length, fiber volume, and mean FA within the fiber tract. This tractography analysis can be used to measure connectivity between specific regions of the brain such as between Broca's area and Wernicke's area or other language-related brain regions. The figures that follow (Figures 2 A, 2B, and 2C) show an example of fibers tract4s connected to Broca's area in the left hemisphere.

DTI [24-27] has been used to study language connections. For example, DTI studies have identified association between variation in white matter microstructure and differences in reading skill [28] [29] [30]. Klingberg et al [30] found that white matter diffusion anisotropy in the temporo-parietal region of the left hemisphere was significantly correlated with reading scores within the reading-impaired adults and within the control group. Nioqi et al [28] found strong correlation between fractional anisotropy (FA) values in a left temporo-parietal white matter region and standardized reading scores of typically developing children. Deutsch et al [29] found that white matter structure (as measured by fractional anisotropy) and coherence index (CI) significantly correlated with behavioral measurements of reading, spelling, and rapid naming performance in children. Glasser et al used Diffusion Tensor Imaging (DTI) tractography to detect leftward asymmetries in the arcuate fasciculus [31]. The arcuate fasciclus is a pathway that links temporal and inferior frontal language cortices and is divided into 2 segments with different hypothesized functions, one terminating in the posterior superior temporal gyrus (STG) and another terminating in the middle temporal gyrus (MTG). STG terminations were strongly left lateralized and overlapped with phonological activations in the left but not the right hemisphere, suggesting that only the left hemisphere phonological cortex is directly connected with the frontal lobe via the arcuate fasciculus. MTG terminations were also strongly left lateralized, overlapping with left lateralized lexical--semantic activations. Smaller right hemisphere MTG terminations overlapped with right lateralized prosodic activations. They used a recent model of brain language processing to explain 6 aphasia syndromes [31].These studies demonstrate the potential for using DTI to measure white matter structural changes in dyslexia.

2.2. Brain studies of functional and effective connectivity

Functional connectivity denotes symmetrical correlations in activity between brain regions during information processing. Here the primary goal is to understand which regions are functionally related through correlations in their activity, as measured by some imaging technique. Functional connectivity is a powerful noninvasive technique used to investigate the distribution of neural networks in healthy participants and affected subjects, which can be characterized by low-frequency fluctuations in the BOLD signal when the subject is performing a task [32, 33]. The BOLD response of a continuous task leads to coherent signal changes in anatomically different, but functionally connected, brain structures and thus implies the

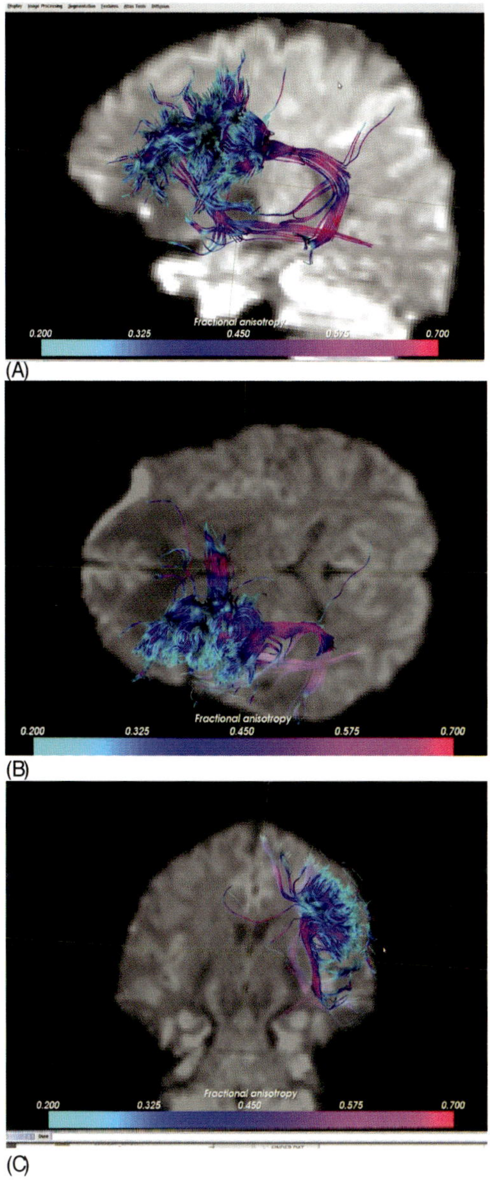

Figure 2. DTI fiber tracts connected to Broca's area. Sagittal view (part A), axial view (part B), and coronal view (part C) showing fibers in the frontal and temporal lobe. The color coding of the fibers is related to the amplitude of the fractional anisotropy within the fiber. A color scale bar is shown at the bottom.

existence of neuronal connections between these regions. Coherent signal changes in anatomically different brain structures imply the existence of neuronal connections between these regions. Exploratory data analysis methods have the attractive feature of being model free and thus allowing unbiased studies of brain signal responses.

Examples in fMRI/PET include principal component analysis (PCA), independent component analysis (ICA), and cluster analysis. There are also model-free analyses of interregional connectivity [34-41]. A popular form of functional connectivity analysis using functional magnetic resonance imaging (fMRI) has been to compute the pairwise correlation (or partial correlation) in BOLD activity for a large number of voxels or regions of interest within the brain volume. The figure 3 below shows an example pair of BOLD signals that have a high degree of correlation. For example functional MRI connectivity can be used to study the functional signal correlations between Broca's area and Wernicke's area.

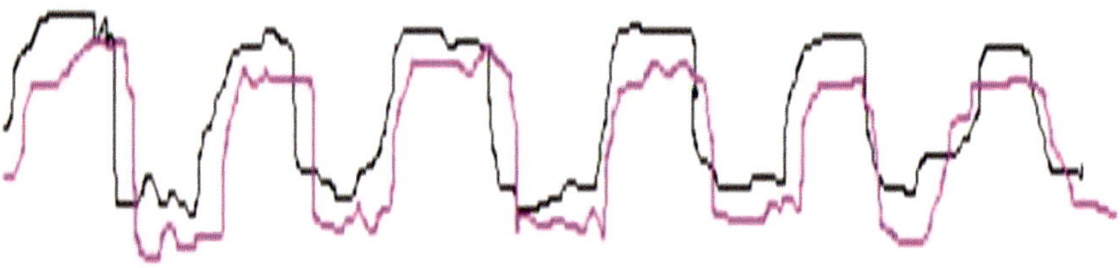

Figure 3. Example of the time course of fMRI signals from two different brain regions which are functionally connected. Notice that the two signals (black and red lines) are closely correlated but not exactly the same.

In contrast to the symmetric nature of functional connectivity, effective connectivity denotes asymmetric or causal dependencies between brain regions. Here the primary goal is to identify which brain structures in a functional network are causally influencing other elements of the network during some stage or form of information processing. Often the term "information flow" is used to indicate directionally specific (although not necessarily causal) effective connectivity between neuronal structures. Popular effective connectivity methods, applied to fMRI and/or electrophysiological (EEG, iEEG, MEG) imaging data, include dynamic causal modeling, structural equation modeling, transfer entropy, and Granger-causal methods. An example of fMRI connectivity using Broca's area as a seed region is shown below in Figure 4.

3. Connectivity imaging studies of specific learning disabilities

3.1. Functional connectivity studies

Currently, imaging research studies of dyslexia are moving away from simply localizing task-related activation to regions of interest (ROI) to analyzing functional connectivity among different brain regions in specific task environments [42] or resting states [43]. Previous functional connectivity studies of dyslexia were mostly focused on the angular gyrus. Asyn-

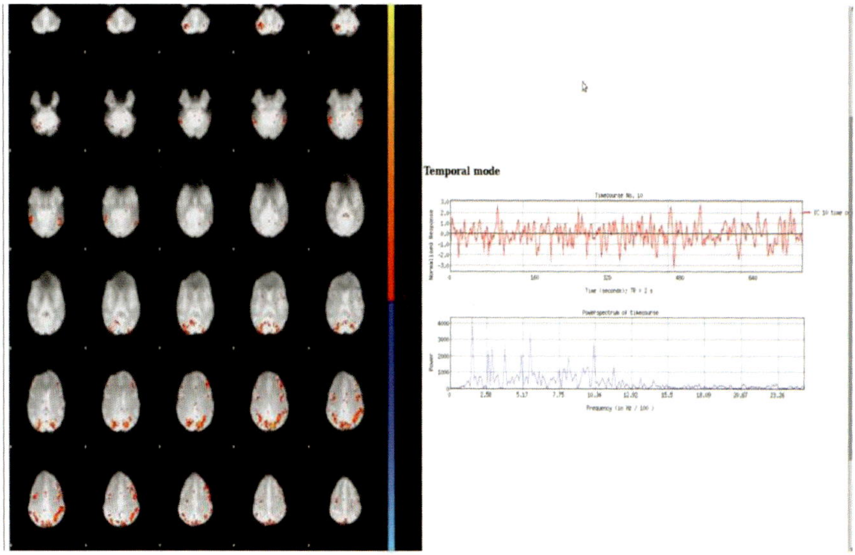

Figure 4. FMRI connectivity analysis related to left-sided Broca's area using FSL's Independent Component Analysis software Melodic combined with UW software. The red plot shows the time course of this ICA component and the plot in blue shows the frequency spectrum. Notice that there are several anatomical regions of the brain that are involved in this component including the left frontal lobe (which includes Broca's area), left and right parietal lobe, left and right temporal lobe.

chrony of regional cerebral blood flow changes in the angular gyrus and extrastriate occipital/temporal lobe regions suggested functional disconnection during single word reading [44]. Pugh et al [45] showed functional disconnections between the angular gyrus and temporal and occipital areas (namely, lateral extrastriate, medial extrastriate, and primary visual cortex) in the left hemisphere specific to the phonological processing. Shaywitz et al. [46] found functional connections between the occipitotemporal region and inferior frontal gyrus in the left hemisphere in normal readers under a real-word reading condition. Poor readers, in contrast, exhibited more functional connections between the left occipitotemporal region and right middle and inferior frontal gyri [46].

Shaywitz et al documented that the important difference between compensated young adults with a history of dyslexia and young adults who are good readers without a history of dyslexia lies in connectivity among regions rather than in regions of activation per se [46]. Milne et al. [47] reported that an individual with developmental dyslexia showed increased activation, as the phonological processing demands increased, in the left inferior frontal gyrus, right parietal cortex, right occipital cortex, and cerebellum. Both the Shaywitz et al. [46] and Milne et al. [47] studies had shown the importance of connectivity between posterior and anterior language systems in supporting the reading process. Betan et al, [48] have recently used fMRI connectivity to examine task-specific modulations of effective connectivity within a left-hemisphere

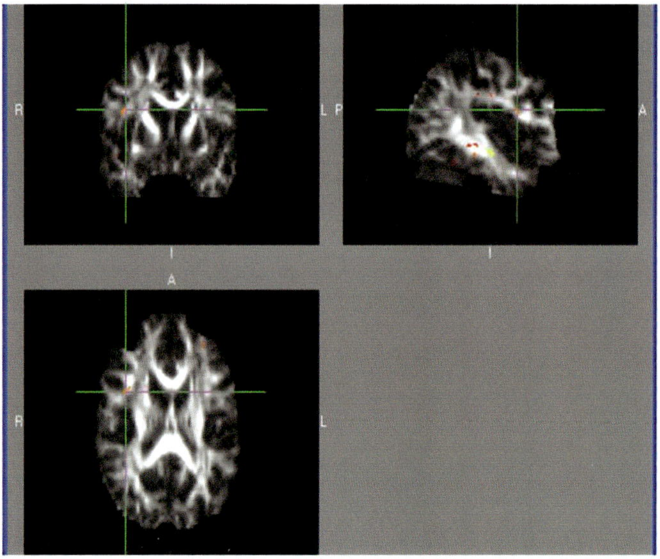

Figure 5. Group differences for controls > dyslexics in analysis of fractional anisotropy with FSL-based TBSS software. Crosshair on a significant cluster near R inf. frontal gyrus.

language network during spelling and rhyming judgments on visually presented words. They used dynamic causal modeling to show that each task preferentially strengthened modulatory influences converging on its task-specific site (LTC for rhyming, IPS for spelling). Their findings also showed that switching tasks led to changes in the target area influenced by the IFG, suggesting that the IFG may play a pivotal role in setting the cognitive context for each task [48].

3.2. Converging fMRI and DTI Imaging findings

Our first DTI Study [49] identified differences between adults with and without dyslexia (which is also a writing disorder, [50]) in the right inferior gyrus (See Figure 5). This is one of the same regions where structural differences were found between dyslexics and good readers in an MRI structural study (Eckert et al., 2003) [51] and the same region where functional differences were found in an fMRI orthographic task contrast before but not after orthographic treatment (Richards et al., 2006a) [52]. Trends towards less activation in right inferior frontal gyrus were associated with improved phonological decoding following treatment (Richards et al., 2006b) [53].

Trends towards less activation in right inferior frontal gyrus were associated with improved phonological decoding following treatment [53]. These findings suggest that right inferior frontal gyrus plays a role in orthographic coding, a process which our behavioral studies for nearly two decades have shown contributes uniquely to handwriting, spelling, and composi-

http://dx.doi.org/10.5772/56501

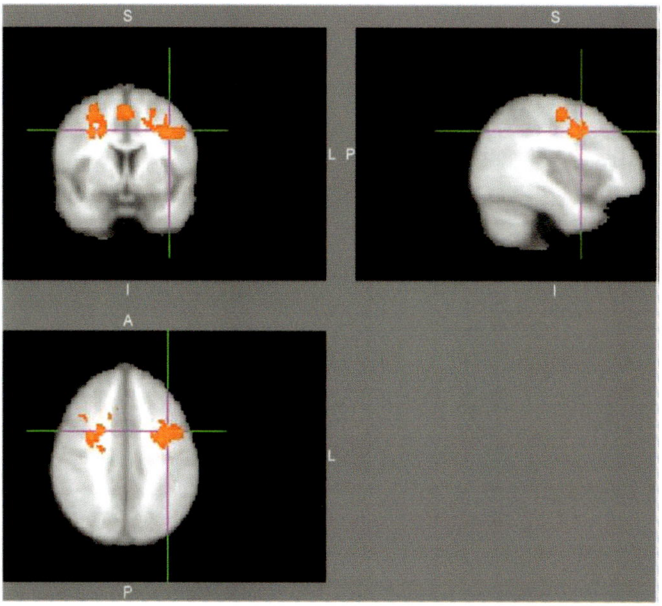

Figure 6. Group difference map for dyslexics greater than controls. The individual maps used in this analysis were correlation maps created when the seed ROI in the left inferior frontal gyrus was compared to the rest of the brain voxels.

tion[54]. Thus, we predict that in studies in progress children with handwriting disabilities will differ from good writers in the right inferior frontal gyrus.

Differences in functional connectivity were also found between children with and without dyslexia before but not after treatment on a phonological spelling task (phoneme mapping—deciding whether letter(s) in pair of pronounceable nonwords could stand for the same sound[55]. These data were analyzed with a seed point correlational method for functional connectivity from four seed points based on prior studies: inferior frontal gyrus, middle frontal gyrus, the occipital region, and cerebellum. Before treatment, there was a significant difference in fMRI connectivity between children with dyslexia and normal reading controls in the degree of connectivity between left inferior frontal gyrus and the following regions: right and left middle frontal gyrus, right and left supplemental motor area, left precentral gyrus, and right superior frontal gyrus. There were no significant differences when seed regions were placed in the middle frontal gyrus, occipital gyrus or cerebellum. Children with dyslexia had greater functional connectivity from the left inferior frontal gyrus seed point to the right inferior frontal gyrus than did the children without dyslexia as shown in Figure 6.

The children with dyslexia then participated in a 3-week instructional program that provided explicit instruction in linguistic awareness, alphabetic principle (taught in a way to maximize temporal contiguity of grapheme–phoneme associations and to train both phonological and orthographic loops), decoding and spelling. At Time2, the treated children with did not differ from the children without dyslexia in any of the clusters in the group. The main result was that children with dyslexia had greater functional connectivity from the left inferior frontal gyrus seed point to the right inferior frontal gyrus than did the children without dyslexia before but not after treatment [55]. Thus, the structural and functional connectivity studies provided converging evidence for abnormalities related to inferior frontal gyrus (on right or left) in children with dyslexia.

3.3. Stanberry model of fMRI connectivity in dyslexia

Stanberry et al [35] developed a model of fMRI connectivity based on earlier results that predicts that for normal readers there will be functional connectivity among 5 major reading-related brain regions: (a) frontal lobe (including the inferior frontal gyrus and middle frontal gyrus); (b) parietal lobe (including the angular gyrus); (c) visual processing areas (including occipitotemporal region); (d) fusiform/lingual word form region; and (e) the cerebellum. This model is generally consistent with that reported by other research groups for normal reading [46]; it is also consistent with phonological loop in verbal working memory as a deficit in dyslexia [56, 57]. We predicted that individual dyslexics may have impaired connectivity in any one or a combination of these major circuits. In our first fMRI connectivity study, we investigated differences in cortical networks used by adult controls compared to adult dyslexics during the previously described Phoneme Mapping. By definition, functional connectivity refers to a correlation or synchronization between the time courses of activation of two brain regions. We hypothesized that two brain regions that work together have similar temporal response profiles [58]. A model-independent method was used to analyze the time-synchronized activations induced by the phoneme mapping paradigm (adapted from [59]) presented during a continuous task presentation. A standard fMRI acquisition and analysis of the on-off block design was also performed using Phoneme Mapping. Native English speakers ranging in age from 30 to 45 years participated in the connectivity study: 10 healthy right-handed control males (fathers from the family genetics study who did not meet research criteria for dyslexia on tests and also did not have a history of reading problems) and 13 right-handed, otherwise healthy, adult males who did meet the research criteria for dyslexia and had a history of reading and writing problems. The two groups did not differ significantly in mean Verbal IQ [dyslexics, M=113.8 (SD = 10.3); controls, M=107.7 (SD=11.1), but the dyslexics were significantly lower than the control fathers on each of the reading, spelling, and RAN measures.

Structural and functional MR images were collected in accordance with institutional regulations (IRB approval) on a commercial 1.5T MR scanner (General Electric, Waukesha, WI) equipped with echo-speed gradients and a standard birdcage head coil. Functional images were acquired using an echo-planar sequence with imaging parameters set as follows:
"On-Off" task: 20 axial slices, FOV 24cm x 24cm, BW +/- 62.5 kHz, TR 2000ms, TE 40ms, Flip 82 deg, slice thickness 6mm, gap 1mm, resolution 64x64, 162 time points; Continuous task: 20 axial slices, FOV 24cm x 24cm, BW +/- 62.5 kHz, TR 2000ms, TE 40 ms, Flip 82 deg, slice thickness 6mm, gap 1mm, resolution 64x64, 483 time points.

Cardiac and respiratory rates were digitally recorded with a pulse oximeter and a flexible belt, respectively, using a sampling frequency of 100Hz. Three different seed regions were used for connectivity analysis – right and left inferior frontal gyrus and cerebellum.

For the standard block fMRI acquisition and analysis of controls, fMRI brain activation was detected in the following brain regions: for the right side - inferior frontal gyrus, middle frontal gyrus, cerebellum crus I, cerebellum crus II, occipital gyrus, superior parietal gyrus, inferior parietal gyrus, angular gyrus, lingual gyrus, and fusiform gyrus; for the left side – superior parietal gyrus, angular, occipital gyrus, cerebellum crus I, cerebellum crus II, lingual.

For the fMRI connectivity analysis of the continuous phoneme mapping paradigm, we narrowed the five region model above to a focus on three regions based on structural MRI differences in dyslexics from a family genetics study [51]. Results showed that (a) when the right IFG was chosen as the seed region, significant differences ($p<.05$) were found between dyslexics and controls in right inferior frontal triangularis, bilateral fusiform, bilateral middle and inferior occipital gyri, right angular gyrus, bilateral ITG and cerebellum; (b) when the left IFG was chosen as the seed region, significant differences ($p<.05$) were found between dyslexics and controls in the following brain regions: right inferior frontal triangularis, right middle occipital gyrus, right inferior occipital gyrus, and right cerebellum (VI); and (c) when the cerebellum was chosen as the seed region, significant differences ($p<.05$) were found between dyslexics and controls in the following brain regions: bilateral superior frontal gyrus, left middle frontal gyrus, right angular gyrus, and right middle occipital gyrus. Adult dyslexics, when compared to controls, had impaired cortical connections in brain regions important for phonological processing. The abnormality in functional connectivity from cerebellum in dyslexics may be related to Klingberg et al.'s [30] finding, based on DTI, that white matter diffusion anisotropy in the temporo-parietal region of the left hemisphere is significantly correlated with reading in normal and dyslexic readers. Insufficient myelination of the axonal pathways is one possible explanation for the low anisotropy index values observed in poor readers [60]. Structural abnormalities in white matter pathways could interfere with neuronal transmission, which will directly affect the synchrony of the BOLD signal. Of most importance, functional disconnections were also observed when seed regions were set in bilateral IFG. Bilateral IFG and right cerebellum were found to be abnormal in child dyslexics compared to normal controls ascertained using the same research criteria in our structural MRI studies [51]. Also see Berninger, Raskind, Richards et al. [50].

4. Future perspectives

One of the great potential techniques in this area of language connectivity analysis is the integration of both functional and structural connectivity as shown by Morgan et al [61]. They measured connections between Wernicke's (WA), Broca's (BA) and supplementary motor area (SMA). Along the path between BA and SMA, they showed that fibers tracked measured from DTI generally formed a single bundle and the mean radius of the bundle was positively correlated with functional connectivity. They concluded that the insights gained from this work offers a useful guidance for non-invasive means to evaluate brain network integrity in vivo for use in diagnosing and determining disease progression and recovery [61]. The concept of integrating information across brain imaging modalities will allow the study of human language network as a systems approach. Another futuristic concept has been described by Rota et al [62] where they discuss the mechanisms of cortical reorganization underlying the enhancement of speech. They were able to measure changes in functional and effective connectivity induced in subjects who learned to deliberately increase activation in the right inferior frontal gyrus [62]. Also, see [63] for a model of the four multi-leveled functional language systems, which provides the conceptual framework for testing a model that differentiates among typical oral and written language learners (OWLs), dysgraphia, dyslexia, and OWL LD at the behavioral (phenotype and response to instruction) and brain levels of analysis.

5. Conclusions

The language connectivity findings discussed in this chapter suggest that structural and functional connectivity are adding and will continue to add to our understanding of language and language learning. There are specific language pathways and connections that are crucial for language acquisition and function. The integrity of these connections can be tested using structural DTI and functional MRI connectivity imaging. Individuals with learning and language disabilities have been reported to have different fMRI and DTI measurable connections than those with normal language functions. Once the techniques have been fully tested and developed, the application of language connectivity techniques to the individual assessment, treatment design, and response to treatment would also have enormous practical applications in the clinic and schools.

Acknowledgements

This project received support from the NIH/NICHD Grant 1P50HD071764 (overall PI Virginia Berninger, PI of project 3 Todd Richards).

Author details

Todd L. Richards[1*] and Virginia W. Berninger[2]

*Address all correspondence to: toddr@u.washington.edu

1 Department of Radiology, University of Washington Medical Center, Seattle, WA, USA

2 Department of Educational Psychology, University of Washington, Seattle, WA, USA

References

[1] Liberman A. The reading researcher and the reading teacher need the right theory of speech. Scientific Studies of Reading 1999;3:95-111.

[2] Berninger V, Graham S. Language by hand: A synthesis of a decade of research on handwriting. Handwriting Review 1998;12:11-25.

[3] Berninger V. Development of language by hand and its connections to language by ear, mouth, and eye. Topics in Language Disorders, 20, 65-84 2000;20:65-84.

[4] Trask RL. Language: The Basics. New York: Routledge; 1999.

[5] Lesser R. Language in the Brain: Neurolinguistics, An Encyclopedia of Language. New York: Routledge; 1989.

[6] Binder JR, Frost JA, Hammeke TA, Cox RW, Rao SM, Prieto T. Human brain language areas identified by functional magnetic resonance imaging. J Neurosci 1997;17:353-362.

[7] Binder JR, Frost JA, Hammeke TA, Bellgowan PS, Springer JA, Kaufman JN, et al. Human temporal lobe activation by speech and nonspeech sounds. Cereb Cortex 2000;10(5):512-28.

[8] Cannestra AF, Bookheimer SY, Pouratian N, O'Farrell A, Sicotte N, Martin NA, et al. Temporal and topographical characterization of language cortices using intraoperative optical intrinsic signals. Neuroimage 2000;12(1):41-54.

[9] Castillo EM, Simos PG, Davis RN, Breier J, Fitzgerald ME, Papanicolaou AC. Levels of word processing and incidental memory: dissociable mechanisms in the temporal lobe. Neuroreport 2001;12(16):3561-6.

[10] Jancke L, Wustenberg T, Scheich H, Heinze HJ. Phonetic perception and the temporal cortex. Neuroimage 2002;15(4):733-46.

[11] McDermott KB, Petersen SE, Watson JM, Ojemann JG. A procedure for identifying regions preferentially activated by attention to semantic and phonological relations using functional magnetic resonance imaging. Neuropsychologia 2003;41(3):293-303.

[12] Bookheimer S. Functional MRI of language: new approaches to understanding the cortical organization of semantic processing. Annu Rev Neurosci 2002;25:151-88.

[13] Hickok G, Poeppel D. Dorsal and ventral streams: a framework for understanding aspects of the functional anatomy of language. Cognition 2004;92(1-2):67-99.

[14] Price CJ, Mummery CJ, Moore CJ, Frakowiak RS, Friston KJ. Delineating necessary and sufficient neural systems with functional imaging studies of neuropsychological patients. J Cogn Neurosci 1999;11(4):371-82.

[15] Paulesu E, Goldacre B, Scifo P, Cappa SF, Gilardi MC, Castiglioni I, et al. Functional heterogeneity of left inferior frontal cortex as revealed by fMRI. Neuroreport 1997;8(8):2011-7.

[16] Broca P. Nouvelle observation d'aphemie produite par une lesion de la troisieme circonvolution frontale. Bulletins de la Societe anatomie (Paris), 2e serie 1861;6:398-407.

[17] Wernicke C. The symptom complex of aphasia (1874). Reprinted in English in Proc. Boston Colloq. Philos. Sci. 1874;4:34-97.

[18] Dejerine J. Anatomy of central nervous system. Paris: Masson; 1895.

[19] Mullen T. SIFT Online Handbook and User Manual. http://sccn.ucsd.edu/wiki/SIFT 2010.

[20] Bullmore E, Sporns O. Complex brain networks: graph theoretical analysis of structural and functional systems. Nat Rev Neurosci 2009;10(3):186-98.

[21] Beaulieu C. The basis of anisotropic water diffusion in the nervous system - a technical review. NMR Biomed 2002;15(7-8):435-55.

[22] Le Bihan D, Mangin JF, Poupon C, Clark CA, Pappata S, Molko N, et al. Diffusion tensor imaging: concepts and applications. Journal of magnetic resonance imaging: JMRI 2001;13(4):534-546.

[23] Filler AI. The History, Development and Impact of Computed Imaging in Neurological Diagnosis and Neurosurgery: CT, MRI, and DTI. Internet Journal of Neurosurgery 2010;7(1).

[24] Catani M, Mesulam M. The arcuate fasciculus and the disconnection theme in language and aphasia: history and current state. Cortex 2008;44(8):953-61.

[25] Nucifora PG, Verma R, Melhem ER, Gur RE, Gur RC. Leftward asymmetry in relative fiber density of the arcuate fasciculus. Neuroreport 2005;16(8):791-4.

[26] Parker GJ, Luzzi S, Alexander DC, Wheeler-Kingshott CA, Ciccarelli O, Lambon Ralph MA. Lateralization of ventral and dorsal auditory-language pathways in the human brain. Neuroimage 2005;24(3):656-66.

[27] Powell HW, Parker GJ, Alexander DC, Symms MR, Boulby PA, Wheeler-Kingshott CA, et al. Hemispheric asymmetries in language-related pathways: a combined functional MRI and tractography study. Neuroimage 2006;32(1):388-99.

[28] Niogi SN, McCandliss BD. Left lateralized white matter microstructure accounts for individual differences in reading ability and disability. Neuropsychologia 2006;44: 2178-2188.

[29] Deutsch GK, Dougherty RF, Bammer R, Siok WT, Gabrieli JD, Wandell B. Children's reading performance is correlated with white matter structure measured by diffusion tensor imaging. Cortex 2005;41:354-363.

[30] Klingberg T, Hedehus M, Temple E, Salz T, Gabrieli JD, Moseley ME, et al. Microstructure of temporo-parietal white matter as a basis for reading ability: evidence from diffusion tensor magnetic resonance imaging [see comments]. Neuron 2000;25(2):493-500.

[31] Glasser MF, Rilling JK. DTI tractography of the human brain's language pathways. Cereb Cortex 2008;18(11):2471-82.

[32] Hampson M, Peterson B, Skudlarski P., Gatenby J, Gore J. Detection of functional connectivity using temporal correlations in MR images. Human Brain Mapping 2002;15:247-262.

[33] Lowe M, Mock B, Sorenson J. Functional connectivity in single and multislice echoplanar imaging using resting-state fluctuations. Neuroimage 1998;7:119-132.

[34] Stanberry L, Nandy R, Cordes D. Cluster analysis of fMRI Data using Dendrogram Sharpening. Human Brain Mapping 2003;20:201-219.

[35] Stanberry LI, Richards T, Berninger VW, Stock P, Nandy RR, Aylward E, et al. Low Frequency Signal Changes Reflect Differences in Functional Connectivity between Good Readers and Dyslexics during Continuous Phoneme Mapping. Magnetic Resonance Imaging 2006;24:217-229.

[36] Nandy R, Cordes D. Improving the spatial specificity of canonical correlation analysis in fMRI. Magn Reson Med 2004;52(4):947-52.

[37] Nandy RR, Cordes D. Novel nonparametric approach to canonical correlation analysis with applications to low CNR functional MRI data. Magn Reson Med 2003;50(2): 354-65.

[38] Nandy RR, Cordes D. Novel ROC-type method for testing the efficiency of multivariate statistical methods in fMRI. Magn Reson Med 2003;49(6):1152-62.

[39] Cordes D, Haughton V, Carew JD, Arfanakis K, Maravilla K. Hierarchical clustering to measure connectivity in fMRI resting-state data. Magn Reson Imaging 2002;20(4): 305-17.

[40] Cordes D, Haughton VM, Arfanakis K, Carew JD, Turski PA, Moritz CH, et al. Frequencies contributing to functional connectivity in the cerebral cortex in "resting-state" data. AJNR Am J Neuroradiol 2001;22(7):1326-33.

[41] Cordes D, Haughton VM, Arfanakis K, Wendt GJ, Turski PA, Moritz CH, et al. Mapping functionally related regions of brain with functional connectivity MR imaging [In Process Citation]. AJNR Am J Neuroradiol 2000;21(9):1636-44.

[42] Büchel C, Coull, J., Friston, K. The predictive value of changes in effective connectivity for human learning. Science 1999;283:1538-1540.

[43] Cordes D, Haughton VM, Arfanakis K, Wendt GJ, Turski PA, Moritz CH, et al. Mapping functionally related regions of brain with functional connectivity MR imaging. AJNR Am J Neuroradiol 2000;21(9):1636-44.

[44] Horwitz B, Rumsey JM, Donohue BC. Functional connectivity of the angular gyrus in normal reading and dyslexia. Proc Natl Acad Sci U S A 1998;95(15):8939-44.

[45] Pugh K, Mencl, W., Shaywitz, B., Shaywitz, S., Fulbright, R., Constable, R., Skudlarski, P., Marchione, K., Jenner, A., Fletcher, J., Liberman, A., Shankweiler, D., Katz, L., Lacadie, C., Gore,J. The angular gyrus in developmental dyslexia: Task-specific differences in functional connectivity within posterior cortex. Psychological Science 2000;11:51-56.

[46] Shaywitz SE, Shaywitz BA, Fulbright RK, Skudlarski P, Mencl WE, Constable RT, et al. Neural systems for compensation and persistence: young adult outcome of childhood reading disability. Biol Psychiatry 2003;54(1):25-33.

[47] Milne D, Syngeniotis A, Jackson G, Corballis M. Mixed lateralization of phonological assembly in developmental dyslexia. Neurocase 2002;8:205-209.

[48] Bitan T, Booth JR, Choy J, Burman DD, Gitelman DR, Mesulam MM. Shifts of effective connectivity within a language network during rhyming and spelling. J Neurosci 2005;25(22):5397-403.

[49] Richards T, Stevenson J, Crouch J, Johnson LC, Maravilla K, Stock P, et al. Tract-based spatial statistics of diffusion tensor imaging in adults with dyslexia. AJNR Am J Neuroradiol 2008;29(6):1134-9.

[50] Berninger VW, Raskind W, Richards T, Abbott R, Stock P. A multidisciplinary approach to understanding developmental dyslexia within working-memory architecture: genotypes, phenotypes, brain, and instruction. Dev Neuropsychol 2008;33(6): 707-44.

[51] Eckert MA, Leonard CM, Richards TL, Aylward EH, Thomson J, Berninger VW. Anatomical correlates of dyslexia: frontal and cerebellar findings. Brain 2003;126(Pt 2): 482-494.

[52] Richards T, Aylward E, Berninger V, Field K, Parsons A, Richards A, et al. Individual fMRI activation in orthographic mapping and morpheme mapping after orthographic or morphological spelling treatment in child dyslexics. Journal of Neurolinguistics 2006;19:56-86.

[53] Richards T, Aylward E, Raskind W, Abbott R, Field K, Parsons A, et al. Converging evidence for triple word form theory in child dyslexia. Special Issue on Brain Imaging in Developmental Neuropsychology 2006;in press.

[54] Berninger V, Richards T. Inter-relationships among behavioral markers, genes, brain and treatment in dyslexia and dysgraphia. Future Neurol 2011;5(4):597-617.

[55] Richards TL, Berninger VW. Abnormal fMRI Connectivity in Children with Dyslexia During a Phoneme Task: Before But Not After Treatment. J Neurolinguistics 2008;21(4):294-304.

[56] Heilman KM, Voeller K, Alexander AW. Developmental dyslexia: a motor-articulatory feedback hypothesis. Ann Neurol 1996;39(3):407-12.

[57] Chen SH, Desmond JE. Cerebrocerebellar networks during articulatory rehearsal and verbal working memory tasks. Neuroimage 2005;24:332-338.

[58] Koshino H, Carpenter PA, Minshew NJ, Cherkassky VL, Keller TA, Just MA. Functional connectivity in an fMRI working memory task in high-functioning autism. Neuroimage 2005;24(3):810-21.

[59] Aylward EH, Richards TL, Berninger VW, Nagy WE, Field KM, Grimme AC, et al. Instructional treatment associated with changes in brain activation in children with dyslexia. Neurology 2003;61(2):212-9.

[60] Wimberger DM, Roberts TP, Barkovich AJ, Prayer LM, Moseley ME, Kucharczyk J. Identification of 'premyelination" by diffusion-weighted MRI. J Comput Assist Tomogr 1995;19:28-33.

[61] Morgan VL, Mishra A, Newton AT, Gore JC, Ding Z. Integrating functional and diffusion magnetic resonance imaging for analysis of structure-function relationship in the human language network. PLoS One 2009;4(8):e6660.

[62] Rota G, Handjaras G, Sitaram R, Birbaumer N, Dogil G. Reorganization of functional and effective connectivity during real-time fMRI-BCI modulation of prosody processing. Brain Lang 2011;117(3):123-32.

[63] Berninger V, Niedo J. Individualizing instruction for students with oral and written language difficulties. In: Mascolo J, Flanagan D, Alfonso V, editors. Essentials of planning, selecting and tailoring intervention: Addressing the needs of unique learners. New York: Wiley; 2013. In Press

Chapter 6

Pre-Attentive Processing of Mandarin Tone and Intonation: Evidence from Event-Related Potentials

Gui-Qin Ren, Yi-Yuan Tang, Xiao-Qing Li and Xue Sui

Additional information is available at the end of the chapter

http://dx.doi.org/10.5772/56503

1. Introduction

In tonal languages (e.g., Chinese and Thai), the meaning of a word cannot be defined solely by consonants and vowels without a lexical tone, which varies in pitch patterns. The pitch patterns associated with Mandarin lexical tones are used to distinguish lexical meaning. Mandarin Chinese has four lexical tones and tones 1-4 can be described phonetically as high level, high rising, low rising, and high falling pitch patterns respectively. The syllable /ma/ in Chinese, for example, can stand for "mother" [tone1], "hemp" [tone2], "horse" [tone3], or "scold" [tone4]. Previous studies have shown that the native speakers of tone languages are highly sensitive to changes in lexical tones regardless of whether the subjects focus their attention on the stimuli or not (Tsang et al., 2011; Ren et al., 2009). The pitch patterns associated with Mandarin intonation, however, may serve a variety of linguistic functions such as attitudinal meanings, discoursal meanings, or grammatical meanings (Cruttenden, 1997; Pell, 2006). A cross-linguistic (Chinese and English) study showed that whereas pitch contours associated with intonation are processed predominantly in the right hemisphere whereas the pitch contours associated with tones are processed in the left hemisphere by Chinese listeners only (Gandour et al., 2003).

The neurophysiological study of the processing of tone and intonation can provide valuable insight into the nature of pitch patterns perception. Other than non-tone languages such as English, lexical tone and intonation in Chinese are both signaled primarily by changes in fundamental frequency (*F*0) while their linguistic functions are different. Furthermore, most models on Mandarin intonation suggest that lexical tone affects intonation (Chao, 1968; Shen, 1992; Yuan, 2004). Chao (1968) has pointed that intonation is realized by changing pitch range and interacts with lexical tone by addition. In Chinese, interrogative intonation has a higher pitch contour than that of its declarative counterpart (Yuan, 2004). Among the four Mandarin tones, tone 2 in isolation is rising in its' phonological representation (Xu, 2005) and the average F0 contour of tone2 resembles that of interrogative intonation. The questions arise as to whether the cortical processing of pitch patterns associated with lexical tone is distinguishable from that associated with intonation, and whether the interrogative intonation associated with tone 2 can be identified when native speakers' attention is withdrawn from stimuli input.

The issue of whether or not attention is needed during speech perception has provoked a large amount of researches such as the influence of attention in audiovisual speech perception (Astheimer & Sanders, 2009; Navarra et al., 2010) and role of selective attention in speech perception (Astheimer & Sanders, 2009; 2012). There exists evidences either supports for the view that the audiovisual integration of speech is an attention modulated process, or for the view that audiovisual integration of speech is an automatic process (Navarra et al., 2010; Astheimer & Sanders, 2009; Jones & Munhall, 1997). Concerning the role of attention in speech comprehension, Andersen et al. (2009) demonstrated that temporally selective attention may serve a function that allows preferential processing of highly relevant acoustic information such as word-initial segments during normal speech perception. In subsequently study, Andersen et al. (2012) examined the use of temporally selective attention in 3-to 5-year –old children and found that, like adults, preschool aged children modulate temporally selective attention to preferentially process the initial portions of words in continuous speech. By directly comparing the effects of attention on different speech stimuli, Hugdahl et al. (2003) revealed that attention to speech sounds may act to recruit stronger neuronal activation compared to when the same stimulus is processed in the absence of attention. Although previous results showed that cognitive processing of many aspects of language such as semantic, syntactic, and pitch information take place indexed by MMN regardless of whether subjects focus their attention on linguistic stimuli, the size of the MMN can be modulated by the level of attention (Pulvermüller & Shtyrov, 2003; 2006). The MMN is larger when subjects attend to the stimuli, as compared with that of subjects are involved in a distraction task.

Tone languages are advantageous for examining the nature of pitch patterns processing. In recent years, the functional asymmetry of two human cerebral hemispheres in the processing prosody information has received a considerable attention. The left hemisphere has been thought to be dominant for language-related behaviours (Gandour et al., 2002; Klein, Zatorre, Milner, & Zhao, 2001) and the right hemisphere to be dominant for pitch-related behaviours (Warrier & Zatorre, 2004; Zatorre & Belin, 2001). However, what cues are used by the brain to determine the labor division is still a matter of debate. The functional hypothesis (Pell & Baum, 1997; Wong, 2002) states that the psychological functions of sounds determine which neural mechanisms are engaged during speech processing. Those sounds that carry a greater linguistic load (e.g., lexical tone) are preferentially processed in the left hemisphere, while those that carry a less linguistic load (e.g., intonation) are preferentially processed in the right hemisphere. However, the acoustic hypothesis (Zatorre & Belin, 2001; Zatorre, Belin, & Penhune, 2002) states that all pitch patterns are lateralized to the right hemisphere regardless of psychological functions.

http://dx.doi.org/10.5772/56503

More recently, the dynamic models such as two-stage model and a more comprehensive model have been put forward, which integrate the acoustic hypothesis and functional hypothesis. The two-stage model (Luo et al., 2006) states that speech is initially processed as a general acoustic signal with lateralized to the right hemisphere at a pre-attentive stage, and then mapped into a semantic representation with lateralized to the left hemisphere at an attentive stage. This point of view is compatible with the notion put forward by Zatorre et al (2002) that the left hemisphere lateralization effect in linguistic functions may arise from a slight initial advantage in decoding speech sounds. According to the more comprehensive model proposed by Gandour and his colleagues (Gandour et al., 2004; Tong et al., 2005), speech prosody perception is mediated primarily by the right hemisphere for complex sound analysis while left hemisphere is dominant when language processing is required. What is more, both the left and right hemispheres were found to contribute to pitch patterns perception (Pell, 2006; Xi, Zhang, Shu, Zhang, & Li, 2010). The prosodic speech information can be processed on either hemisphere depending on whether the speech information is emotional or the linguistic prosodic cues (Pell, 2006). The acoustic and linguistic information is processed in parallel at an early stage of speech perception (Xi et al., 2010).

The left hemisphere lateralization in the perception of lexical tones is supported by evidence from a number of studies including dichotic-listening (Wang, Jongman, & Sereno, 2001) and functional imaging studies (Gandour et al., 2002; Klein, Zatorre, Milner, & Zhao, 2001). For example, when Thai and Chinese subjects were required to perform discrimination judgments of Thai tone, only Thai subjects displayed an increased activation in the left inferior prefrontal cortex (Gandour et al., 2002). Similar hemispheric dominance was obtained in Chinese speakers when Chinese and English speakers were required to discriminate the pitch patterns in Chinese words (Klein, Zatorre, Milner, & Zhao, 2001). Nevertheless, those studies mentioned above likely reveal the temporally aggregated brain activity of auditory processing due to the coarse temporal resolution of fMRI or PET.

The specific aims of this study are to further investigate the neural mechanisms underlying the perception of linguistic pitch patterns by comparing the early pre-attentive processing of Mandarin tone and intonation, and examine whether the pitch changes of the intonation associated with Mandarin tone 2 can be detected by native speaker of Chinese at the early pre-attentive stage. Here a method of combining event-related potentials and a source estimation technique Low-resolution electromagnetic tomography (LORETA) was used. The ERP component of interest is the mismatch negativity (MMN), which peaks at about 100-250 ms after stimulus onset and is present by any discriminable changes in auditory processing irrespective of subjects' attention or task (Näätänen & Escera, 2000; Näätänen, Paavilainen, Rinne, & Alho, 2007; Näätänen, Tervaniemi, Sussman, Paavilainen, & Winkler, 2001). A new MMN paradigm was applied in this study, which allows one to obtain different MMNs in a short time (Näätänen, Pakarinen, Rinne, & Takegata, 2004). The sources of the MMNs were estimated by LORETA, an approach that has been successfully used in the studies on auditory processing to locate the sources of the neural activities (Liu & Perfetti, 2003; Marco-Pallarés, Grau, & Ruffini, 2005).

2. Materials and methods

Subjects:

Thirteen graduate students (age rang 21-25; six male, seven female) participated in this study as paid volunteers. All subjects were native speakers of Mandarin Chinese and right-handed, with no history of neurological or psychiatric impairment. Informed consent was obtained from all subjects.

Stimuli and procedure:

Stimuli consisted of two meaningful auditory Chinese words that have the same consonant and vowel (/lai/) but different lexical tone, pronounced in high rising tone (tone 2) and high falling tone (tone 4) respectively. The syllable /lai4/ was pronounced in a declarative intonation, and the syllable /lai2/ was pronounced in a declarative intonation or an interrogative intonation respectively. The standard stimulus was the syllable /lai2/ pronounced in a declarative intonation. Deviant stimuli differed from the standard in either intonation (/lai2/, intonation deviant) or lexical tone (/lai4/, lexical tone deviant).

A new passive auditory odd-ball paradigm (Näätänen, Pakarinen, Rinne, & Takegata, 2004) was applied to present the stimuli. In order to control the effect of physical stimulus features to obtain the relatively pure contribution of the memory network indexed by MMN (Pulvermüller & Shtyrov, 2006; Pulvermüller, Shtyrov, Ilmoniemi, & Marslen-Wilson, 2006), we created three sequences including one oddball sequence and two control sequences to calculate the identity MMN. The oddball sequence preceded by 15 standard was a pseudorandom block of 1015 stimuli which included standard ($P = 0.8$) and two deviants ($P = 0.1$ for each). The two control sequences for each deviant comprised 400 trials respectively and each deviant stimulus was presented alone ($P = 1$). The subjects were instructed to ignore the sounds from the headphone and watch a silent movie during the course of experiment. The order of the presentation of the three sequences was randomized across the subjects.

The auditory stimuli were pronounced in isolation by a trained female speaker and digitized at a sampling rate of 22, 050 Hz. The stimuli were modified with Praat software (doing phonetics by computer version 4.4.13, download from www.praat.org) and normalized to 450 ms in duration, including 5 ms rise and fall times. The stimuli were presented binaurally at an intensity of 70 dB through headphones in a soundproof room with a stimulus onset asynchrony of 700 ms. The maximum fundamental frequency between the two deviants was comparable. Fig. 1 shows the acoustic features of the experimental stimuli.

Recording:

The EEG was recorded using the 64 electrodes secured in an elastic cap (Neuroscan Inc.) with a sampling rate of 500 Hz, and a band-pass from 0.05 to 40 Hz. The bilateral mastoids serve as the reference and the GND electrode on the cap serve as the ground. The vertical and horizontal electrooculograms were monitored by electrodes placed at the outer canthus of each eye and the electrodes above and below the left eye respectively. All impedances were kept below 5 kΩ.

Data analysis:

http://dx.doi.org/10.5772/56503

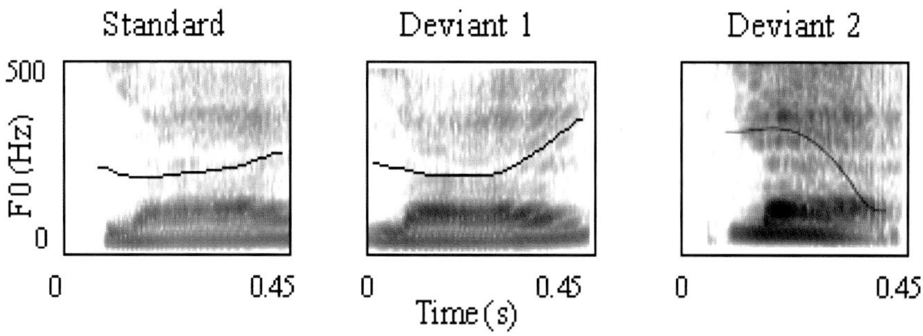

Figure 1. Acoustic features of the stimuli. The data set consists of spectrograms with voice fundamental frequency contours superimposed as a black line. The standard, the pronunciation of syllable /lai2/ in a declarative intonation; Deviant 1, same syllable as the standard but in an interrogative intonation; Deviant 2, syllable /lai4/ in a declarative intonation.

The raw EEG data were first corrected for eye-blink artifacts and filtered with a band-pass filter 0.1-30 Hz. Trials with artifacts exceeding ±75μV in any channel were excluded from the averaging. Epochs were 600 ms including a 100 ms pre-stimulus baseline. ERPs elicited by deviants in the oddball sequence and the identical stimulus in the control sequences were averaged separately across subjects and electrodes.

Although the MMN is generally obtained by subtracting the responses to standard from that to deviant stimulus, it is possible that the physical differences between standard and deviant stimuli influence the responses. In order to control the physical stimulus properties in a more stringent manner (Pulvermüller & Shtyrov, 2006; Pulvermüller, Shtyrov, Ilmoniemi, & Marslen-Wilson, 2006), we calculated the MMN (identity MMN) by subtracting from the ERP to a deviant stimulus presented in the oddball sequence, the ERP to the identical stimulus in the control sequence.

The grand ERP wave shapes were first analyzed by visual inspection and the time window of MMN was defined 110-240 ms. The MMN amplitudes were measured as mean voltages using a 40 ms time-window centered at the peak latency from the electrode Cz, since the largest response was observed at Cz in the grand average waveform. Two different analyses of variance (AVOVA) were done on the mean amplitudes. A original ANOVA for the original mean amplitudes was performed to estimate the two MMNs (one for the lexical tone and the other for the intonation) with condition (lexical tone, intonation), type (deviant, the identical stimulus presented alone), and electrode (F3, F4, Fz, C3, C4, Cz, P3, P4, Pz) as independent factors. To compared the MMN elicited by lexical tone condition with the MMN elicited by the intonation condition, a difference ANOVA was conducted for the difference waveforms with condition (lexical tone, intonation), lobe (frontal, central, parietal), and hemisphere (left, right) as within subject factors. The Greenhouse-Geisser adjustment was applied when the variance sphericity assumption was not satisfied.

Low resolution electromagnetic tomography (LORETA) was used to estimate the sources of the MMN elicited in the experiment. LORETA is a tomographic technique that can help find the best possible solution of all possible solutions consistent with the scalp distribution (Pascual-Marqui, Michel, & Lehmann, 1994). The LORETA-KEY (http://www.unizh.ch/keyinst/NewLORETA/LORETA01.htm) (Pascual-Marqui, Esslen, Kochi, & Lehmann, 2002) was used and the results are illustrated in Talairach space (Talairach & Tournoux, 1988). We computed the LORETA solutions on each time point covered the MMN. The input for LORETA was the grand averaged ERP, sampled over the MMN window. The outputs were 3D maps of activity value for each of 2,394 cortex pixels, based on the scalp distribution of each time point, with a subtraction of the averaged scalp distribution during the 100 ms prior to stimulus onset which corresponding to the baseline. Those pixels among the top 5% in activation value of each 3D map were treated as "active" pixels to allow focusing on a reduced set of highly activated brain regions (Liu & Perfetti, 2003; Ren, Liu, & Han, 2009 a; Ren, Yang, & Li, 2009 b).

3. Results

Fig. 2 shows the grand average waveforms to the deviant stimuli in the oddball sequence (P=0.1) and to the identical stimuli in the control sequences (P=1). The deviant-minus-control difference waveforms are shown in Fig. 3.

The original three-way [condition×type×electrode] ANOVA revealed a significant main effect of condition (F (1, 12) = 34.132, p = 0.000) indicating a larger negative-going deflection for lexical tone than intonation (effect magnitude: -1.328 uV), a main effect of type (F (1, 12) = 15.263, p = 0.002) due to a larger negative-going deflection for the deviant in the oddball sequence than the identical stimulus in the control sequence (effect magnitude: -1.065 uV), and a main effect of electrode (F (8, 96) = 9.096, p = 0.001). In addition, there was a significant interaction effect between condition and type (F (1, 12) = 7.211, p = 0.02), and between electrode and type (F (8, 96) = 6.923, p = 0.002). Subsequently simple effect analyses showed that the ERPs to the deviant were significantly more negative than to the identical controls only in the lexical tone condition (F (1, 12) = 17.45, p = 0.001), and the same differences patterns of types was observed at Fz, F4, Cz, C3, C4, and P4 electrode sites (F (1, 12) = 7.99, p = 0.015; F (1, 12) = 8.09, p = 0.015; F (1, 12) = 12.36, p = 0.004; F (1, 12) = 7.29, p = 0.019; F (1, 12) = 29.52, p = 0.000; F (1, 12) = 19.42, p = 0.001).

A difference three-way [condition×lobe×hemisphere] ANOVA revealed a main effect of condition (F (1, 12) = 23.924, p = 0.000) indicating that the lexical tone evoked a larger negative deflection than the intonation (effect magnitude: -1.879 uV), a main effect of lobe (F (2, 24) = 7.677, p = 0.013) due to the fact that a larger negative deflection existed at frontal and central than parietal sites (effect magnitude: -0.929 uV, -0.893 uV, respectively), and a main effect of hemisphere (F (1, 12) = 5.691, p = 0.034) due to the fact that a larger negative deflection existed for right than left hemisphere (effect magnitude: -0.296 uV). In addition, there was a significant interaction between condition and lobe (F (2, 24) = 8.459, p = 0.002). Subsequently simple effect analyses showed that a larger negative deflection existed over frontal and central than parietal sites only in the tone condition (F (2, 24) = 11.71, p = 0.000). However, the difference ANOVA with peak latency as dependent variable found no significant effect.

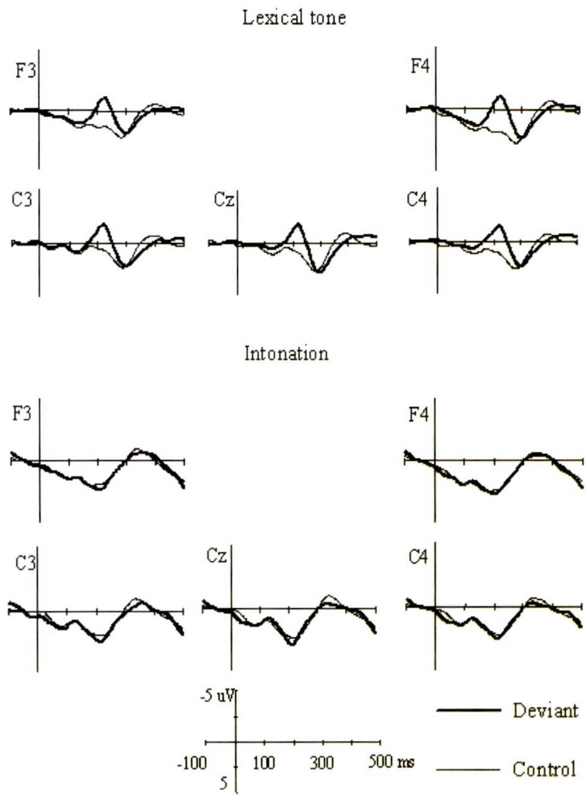

Figure 2. Grand average waveforms to the deviant stimuli in the oddball sequence (thick line) and to the identical stimuli in the control sequence (thin line).

Given the latency and topography of the difference negative deflection (see fig.1 and fig. 2), we classified it as MMN (Rinne et al., 2006). Since no MMN was elicited for the intonation, only the source of the MMN for the lexical tone was analyzed. The local maximum of the MMN was located in the right middle temporal gyrus (BA 21, Talairach coordinates of the maximum: x = 53; y = 3; z = -13).

4. Disscussion

The present study examined the early cortical processing of linguistic pitch patterns by comparing the ERP responses to Mandarin tone and intonation. The results demonstrated that MMN was elicited only by the lexical tone contrast and no MMN was obtained to the intonation

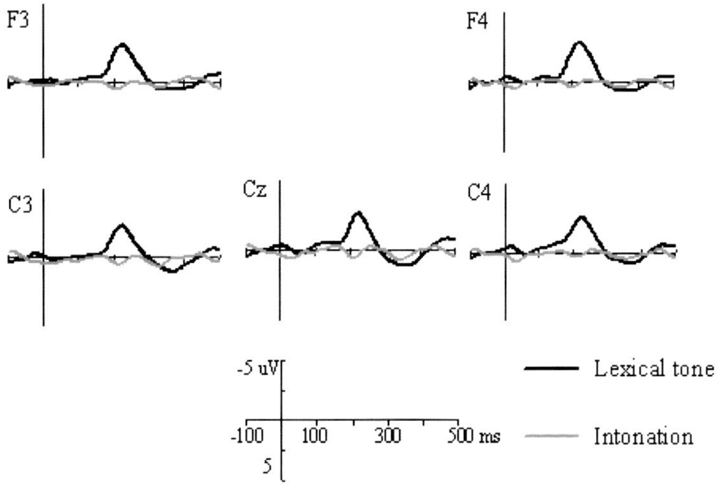

Figure 3. Grand difference waveforms (deviant —control ERPs) in the tone and intonation conditions

contrast which associated with a Mandarin tone 2. Source estimation of the MMN showed that the highest activation of brain areas underlying lexical tone processing was located into the right hemisphere, the right middle temporal gyrus (BA 21).

A clear MMN was observed for the lexical tone contrast and the highest activation of the MMN was located into the right temporal gyrus. The result of right hemisphere dominance for lexical tone in the early pre-attentive processing is converging with previous studies (Luo et al., 2006; Ren et al., 2009 b). Ren et al. (2009 b) demonstrated that both the sources of the MMNs to Mandarin lexical tone and its hummed version were located in the right hemisphere in the early pre-attentive processing. By comparing the early pre-attentive processing of Mandarin tones and consonants, Luo et al (2006) found that Mandarin tones evoked a stronger pre-attentive response in the right hemisphere than in the left hemisphere. Those results above presumably reflect the role of right hemisphere in acoustic processing and compatible with the acoustic hypothesis (Zatorre & Belin, 2001) and the dynamic models (Zatorre et al., 2002; Gandour et al., 2004; Tong et al., 2005 ; Luo et al., 2006), but cannot be explained by the functional hypothesis which predicts lexical tones are preferentially processed in the left hemisphere (Pell & Baum, 1997; Wong, 2002). However, the functional hypothesis was supported by the data from fMRI or PET studies (Hsieh et al., 2001; Klein et al., 2001; Gandour et al., 2002; 2003) which revealed the left hemisphere dominance of native speakers in the perception of lexical tones and suggest that hemispheric lateralization is sensitive to linguistic functions of pitch patterns and language experience. Taken together, these findings seem to reflect the dynamic interaction between the two hemispheres and are compatible with the dynamic models of speech perception (Gandour et al., 2004; Luo et al., 2006; Zatorre, Belin, & Penhune, 2002). Just as proposed by Gandour et al (2004) that both acoustics and linguistics are all necessary ingredients for developing a neurobiological model of speech prosody. High-level linguistic processing might initially have developed from low-level acoustic processing (Zatorre et al., 2002; Luo et al., 2006).

LORETA analysis for the MMN to lexical tone was located into the right middle temporal gyrus (BA 21), one major source of the MMN (Luo et al., 2006; Näätänen et al., 2001). Besides the temporal lobe, there are other sources contribute to the MMN generators, such as frontal lobe (Molholm, Martinez, Ritter, Javitt, & Foxe, 2005) and parietal lobe (Levänen, Ahonen, Hari, McEvoy, & Sams, 1996; Marco-Pallarés, Grau, & Ruffini, 2005). It appears that the change of MMN generators is associated with the time points of the current sources and is feature dependent (Levänen et al., 1996; Molholm et al., 2005). In this study, the cortical locus reported as the MMN generator was the highest level of activation region covering the time window of the MMN. It can be seen that although the solution of LORETA produces a "blurred-localized" image of a point source, it conserves the location of maximal activity and allows at least the discussion of asymmetric hemispheric involvement in pitch perception (Liu & Perfetti, 2003; Mulert et al., 2007; Ren et al., 2009a; 2009b).

The result that no MMN was elicited by the intonation contrast (declarative vs. interrogative) demonstrated the perceptual difficulties when the intonation is combined with the Mandarin tone 2. The MMN, an index of change-detection of brain response to any change in auditory stimuli, can enable one to determine discrimination accuracy which usually with a good correspondence with behavioural discrimination (Näätänen et al., 2007; 2012). It suggested in the study that the listeners cannot tease part the two types of intonation at the pre-attentive processing stage. For the four Mandarin tones, the average fundamental frequency contours produced in isolation reflect directly the canonical forms of the tones (Xu, 1997). The F0 contour of tone 2 in isolation is rising in its' phonological representation (Xu, 2005; Yuan, 2004) and resembles that of interrogative intonation. When tone 2 is at the end of sentences, it is more difficult for native speakers of Chinese to identify the interrogative intonation (Ren et al., 2011; Yuan, 2004). Three mechanisms were proposed by Yuan (2004) to explain the perception of interrogative intonation, such as the phrase curve mechanism, the strength mechanism, and the tone-dependent mechanism. Among the mechanisms, the strength mechanism may conflict with the tone-dependent mechanism on the Mandarin tone 2. This conflict likely leads to the perceptual difficulties of interrogative intonation for tone 2.

The perceptual difficulties of intonation contrast showed in the present study also suggested the interaction between lexical tone and intonation. Gandour et al. (1997) demonstrated the interaction between lexical tone and intonation in Thai by analyzing intonational characteristics of the Thai sentences which produced by normal and brain-damaged speakers at a conversational speaking rate. Most models on Mandarin intonation are in terms of contour interaction (Chao, 1968; Shen, 1992; Yuan, 2004). For example, Chao (1968) likened syllabic tone and sentence intonation to small ripples riding on large waves in the ocean and stated that they interact by addition. Based on perceptual and acoustic studies, Yuan (2004) proposed a tone-dependent mechanism for intonation perception, which flattens the falling slope of the falling tone (such as Mandarin tone 4) and steepens the rising slope of the rising tone (such as Mandarin tone 2). It can be reasoned that the contrast of declarative and interrogative intonation might be detected more difficult or easier for certain tone. In a prior experiment, we found a clear MMN to intonation contrast for Mandarin tone 4 (Ren et al., 2009 b).

In summary, the present study demonstrated the right hemispheric dominance of lexical tone in the early pre-attentive processing, which is compatible with the acoustic hypothesis (Zatorre & Belin, 2001) and the dynamic models (Gandour et al., 2004; Tong et al., 2005 ; Luo et al., 2006), but cannot be counted by the functional hypothesis (Pell & Baum, 1997, Wong, 2002). Moreover, the current results provide clearly evidence that listeners can not tease apart the declarative and interrogative intonation when the target was Mandarin tone 2 at the early stage of pre-attentive processing. However, how tone and intonation interact and how intonation is perceived remain to be determined, and we will focus on them in the further experiments.

Acknowledgements

This research was supported by Grants from the National Natural Science Foundation of China (31100732 and 31271091) and Specialized Research Fund for the Doctoral Program of Higher Education (20112136120003).

Author details

Gui-Qin Ren[1], Yi-Yuan Tang[2], Xiao-Qing Li[3] and Xue Sui[1]

*Address all correspondence to: renguiqin@126.com

1 School of Psychology, Liaoning Normal University, Dalian, China

2 Institute of Neuroinformatics and Laboratory for Body and Mind, Dalian University of Technology, Dalian, China

3 State Key Laboratory of Brain and Cognitive Science, Institute of Psychology, Chinese Academy of Sciences, Beijing, China

References

[1] Andersen, T, Tiippana, S, Laarni, K, Kojo, J, & Sams, I. M. ((2009). The role of visual spatial attention in audiovisual speech perception. *Speech Communication*, , 51, 184-193.

[2] Astheimer, L, & Sanders, L. (2009). Listeners modulate temporally selective attention during natural speech processing. *Biological. Psychology*, 80 (1), 23-34.

[3] Astheimer, L, & Sanders, L. (2012). Temporally selective attention supports speech processing in 3- to 5-year-old children. *Developmental Cognitive Neuroscience, ,* 2, 120-128.

[4] Chao, Y. R. (1968). *A Grammar of Spoken Chinese,* Berkeley: University of California Press, Berkeley, CA.

[5] Cruttenden, A. (1997). *Intonation.* (2nd ed.). Cambridge, England: Cambridge University Press.

[6] Gandour, J, Dzemidzic, M, Wong, D, Lowe, M, Tong, Y. X, Hsieh, L, et al. (2003). Temporal integration of speech prosody is shaped by language experience: An fMRI study. *Brain and Language, ,* 84, 318-336.

[7] Gandour, J, Ponglorpisit, S, Potisuk, S, Khunadorn, F, Boongird, P, & Dechongkit, S. (1997). Interaction between tone and intonation in Thai after unilateral brain damage. *Brain and Language, ,* 58, 174-196.

[8] Gandour, J, Tong, Y, Wong, D, Talavage, T, Dzemidzic, M, Xu, Y, et al. (2004). Hemispheric roles in the perception of speech prosody. *NeuroImage, ,* 23, 344-357.

[9] Gandour, J, Wong, D, Lowe, M, Dzemidzic, M, Satthamnuwong, N, Long, Y, et al. (2002). Neural circuitry underlying perception of duration depends on language experience. *Brain and Language, ,* 83, 268-290.

[10] Hugdahl, K, Thomsen, T, Ersland, L, Rimol, L, & Niemi, M. J. ((2003). The effects of attention on speech perception: an fMRI study. *Brain and Language, ,* 85, 37-48.

[11] Jones, J. A, & Munhall, K. G. (1997). The effects of separating auditory and visual sources on audiovisual integration of speech. *Canadian Acoustics, ,* 25, 13-19.

[12] Klein, D, Zatorre, R, Milner, B, & Zhao, V. PET study of tone perception in Mandarin Chinese and English speakers. *NeuroImage, ,* 13, 646-653.

[13] Levänen, S, Ahonen, A, Hari, R, Mcevoy, L, & Sams, M. (1996). Deviant auditory stimuli activate human left and right auditory cortex differently. *Cerebral Cortex, 6,* 288-296.

[14] Liu, Y, & Perfetti, C. A. (2003). The time course of brain activity in reading English and Chinese: An ERP study of Chinese bilinguals. *Human Brain Mapping, ,* 18, 167-175.

[15] Luo, H, Ni, J. T, Li, Z. H, Li, X. O, Zhang, D. R, Zeng, F. G, et al. (2006). Opposite patterns of hemisphere dominance for early auditory processing of lexical tones and consonants. *Proceedings of the National Academy of Sciences of the United States of America, ,* 103, 19558-19563.

[16] Marco-pallarés, L, Grau, C, & Ruffini, G. (2005). Combined ICA-LORETA analysis of mismatch negativity. *NeuroImage, ,* 25, 471-477.

[17] Molholm, S, Martinez, A, Ritter, W, Javitt, D. C, & Foxe, J. J. (2005). The neural circuitry of pre-attentive auditory change-detection: An fMRI study of pitch and duration mismatch negativity generators. *Cerebral Cortex, 15*, 545-551.

[18] Mulert, C, Leicht, G, Pogarell, O, Mergl, R, Karch, S, Juckel, G, et al. (2007). Auditory cortex and anterior cingulated cortex sources of the early evoked gamma-band response: relationship to task difficulty and mental effort, *Neuropsychologia,* , 45, 2294-2306.

[19] Navarra, J, Alsius, A, Soto-faraco, S, & Spence, C. (2010). Assessing the role of attention in the audiovisual integration of speech. *Information Fusion,* , 11, 4-11.

[20] Näätänen, R, & Escera, C. (2000). Mismatch negativity: clinical and other applications. *Audiol Neurootol,* , 5, 105-110.

[21] Näätänen, R, Kujala, T, Escera, C, Baldeweg, T, Kreegipuu, K, Carlson, S, et al. (2012). The mismatch negativity (MMN)- A unique window to disturbed central auditory processing in ageing and different clinical conditions. *Clinical Neurophysiology,* , 123, 424-458.

[22] Näätänen, R, Paavilainen, P, Rinne, T, & Alho, K. (2007). The mismatch negativity (MMN) in basic research of central auditory processing: A review. *Clinical Neurophysiology, 118*, 2544-2590.

[23] Näätänen, R, Pakarinen, S, Rinne, T, & Takegata, R. (2004). The mismatch negativity (MMN): towards the optimal paradigm. *Clinical Neurophysiology, 115*, 140-144.

[24] Näätänen, R, Tervaniemi, M, Sussman, E, Paavilainen, P, & Winkler, I. (2001). Primitive intelligence' in the auditory cortex. *Trends in Neurosciences,* , 24, 283-288.

[25] Pascual-marqui, R. D, Esslen, M, Kochi, K, & Lehmann, D. (2002). Functional imaging with low resolution brain electromagnetic tomography (LORETA): review, new comparisons, and new validation. *Japanese Journal of Clinical Neurophysiology, 30*, 81-94.

[26] Pascual-marqui, R. D, Michel, C. M, & Lehmann, D. (1994). Low resolution electromagnetic tomography: a new method for localizing electrical activity in the brain. *International Journal of Psychophysiology, 18*, 49-65.

[27] Pell, M. D. (2006). Cerebral mechanisms for understanding emotional prosody in speech. *Brain and Language,* , 96, 221-234.

[28] Pell, M, & Baum, S. (1997). Unilateral brain damage and the acoustic cues to prosody: Are prosodic comprehension deficits perceptually based? *Brain and Language,* , 57, 195-214.

[29] Pulvermüller, F, & Shtyrov, Y. (2006). Language outside the focus of attention: the mismatch negativity as a tool for studying higher cognitive processes. *Progress in Neurobiology, 79*, 49-71.

[30] Pulvermüller, F, & Shtyrov, Y. (2003). Automatic processing of grammar in the human brain as revealedbythemismatchnegativity. *Neuroimage, 20*, 159-172.

[31] Pulvermüller, F, Shtyrov, Y, Ilmoniemi, R. J, & Marslen-wilson, W. D. (2006). Tracking speech comprehension in space and time. *NeuroImage*, , 31, 1297-1305.

[32] Ren, G. Q, Han, Y. C, Zou, Y. L, & Ren, Y. T. (2011). Early cortical processing of Mandarin intonation, *Acta Psychologica Sinica (in Chinese)*, , 43, 241-248.

[33] Ren, G. Q, Liu, Y, & Han, Y. C. (2009 a). Phonological activation in Chinese reading: an event-related potential study using low-resolution electromagnetic tomography. *Neuroscience*, , 164, 1623-1631.

[34] Ren, G. Q, Yang, Y, & Li, X. (2009 b). Early cortical processing of linguistic pitch patterns as revealed by the mismatch negativity. *Neuroscience*, , 162, 87-95.

[35] Shen, J. (1992). Hanyu yudiao moxing chuyi [On Chinese intonation model]. *Yuwen Yanjiu, 45*, 16-24.

[36] Talairach, J, & Tournoux, P. (1988). *Co-planar sereotaxc atlas of the human brain*. (Rayport, M., Translator.), New York: Thieme Medical Publishers.

[37] Tong, Y, Gandour, J, Talavage, T, Wong, D, Dzemidzic, M, Xu, Y, Li, X, et al. (2005). Neural circuitry underlying sentence-level linguistic prosody. *NeuroImage*, , 28, 417-428.

[38] Tsang, Y-K, Jia, S, Huang, J, & Chen, H-C. (2011). ERP correlates of pre-attentive processing of Cantonese lexical tones: the effects of pitch contour and pitch height. *Neuroscience Letters*, , 487, 268-272.

[39] Warrier, C. M, & Zatorre, R. J. (2004). Right temporal cortex is critical for utilization of melodic contextual cues in a pitch constancy task. *Brain, 127*, 1616-1625.

[40] Wong, P. C. M. (2002). Hemispheric specialization of linguistic pitch patterns. *Brain Research Bulletin*, , 59, 83-95.

[41] Wang, Y, Jongman, A, & Sereno, J. A. (2001). Dichotic perception of Mandarin tones by Chinese and American listeners. *Brain and Language*, , 78, 332-348.

[42] Xi, J, Zhang, L. J, Shu, H, Zhang, Y, & Li, P. (2010). Categorical perception of lexical tones in Chinese revealed by mismatch negativity. *Neuroscience*, , 170, 223-231.

[43] Xu, Y. (2005). Speech melody as articulatorily implemented communicative functions. *Speech Communication*, , 46, 220-251.

[44] Xu, Y. (1997). Contextual tonal variations in Mandarin. *Journal of Phonetics, 25*, 61-83.

[45] Yuan, J. (2004). Intonation in Mandarin Chinese: acoustics, perception, and computation modeling, *Cornell University*, dissertation.

[46] Zatorre, R. J, & Belin, P. (2001). Spectral and temporal processing in human auditory cortex. *Cerebral Cortex, 11*, 946-953.

[47] Zatorre, R. J, Belin, P, & Penhune, V. B. (2002). Structure and function of auditory cortex: music and speech. *Trends in Cognitive Science,* , 6, 37-46.

Chapter 7

Exploring the Effect of Verbal Emotional Words Through Event-Related Brain Potentials

Andrés Antonio González-Garrido,
Fabiola Reveca Gómez-Velázquez and
Julieta Ramos-Loyo

Additional information is available at the end of the chapter

http://dx.doi.org/10.5772/56494

1. Introduction

For centuries, philosophers and neuroscientists have questioned whether the use of language and the ability to solve complex problems are related and, if so, what the nature of the relationship between language and thought is. Most of the attention – and controversy – have been focused on the claim that the structure of language shapes non-linguistic thinking; so-called *linguistic relativity.*

Human intelligence directly derives from brain activity and it is closely linked to the natural languages that humans speak [1]. The Language, this complex system of sound-meaning connections, not only provides a comprehensive description of the world, but its acquisition is one of the most fundamental human traits, and it is obviously the brain that undergoes the developmental changes.

Brain development seems to be non-linear, with sensitive periods of time in which the characteristics of experiences determine different possible outcomes [2]. In fact, during development, the brain not only stores linguistic information but also adapts to the grammatical regularities of language.

Language acquisition might be oversimplified as the way in which the brain learns, perceives, represents and integrates complex sequences of verbal events. The temporal nature of sounds, structural integration, expectations, and cognitive sequencing allows the brain to construct progressively intricate representations of the environment, and with progressive maturity, even aspects of emotion or cognition not readily verbalized may be influenced by linguistically based thought processes.

No matter whether it is verbal or not the new material we have to deal with, once it appears it is processed through a group of co-acting neural specific subsystems which allow us to detect, encode, temporarily hold and compare incoming stimuli with previous material, along with the decision making on what to do next. In this context, it is crucial to understand that certain characteristics of the stimulus might influence its processing and, if so, how these characteristics interact with cognitive processing.

1.1. Evaluating incoming information

Presently, it is generally accepted that incoming information is initially processed in the working memory (WM), which is a theoretical construct used to refer to the system or mechanism underlying the maintenance of task-relevant information during the performance of a cognitive task. WM is crucial for a wide range of complex cognitive activities but has a limited capacity [3-5]. Enough empirical evidence supports that WM plays an important role in recognition, encoding and manipulation of task-related and concurrent distractor stimuli, while WM load influences attention modulation. In fact, the working memory central executive system [6,7], concept based on the "Supervisory Attentional System" proposed by Shallice [8, 9], is critical for systematizing a continuous "background monitoring" that searches for new relevant information, even though the information may be irrelevant to the ongoing act [10,11]. These "background-monitoring" mechanisms seem to be designed to eventually interrupt the current action and trigger an updating of working memory [12]; thus, WM provides goal-directed control of visual selective attention and allows the minimization of interference caused by goal irrelevant distractors [13].

The interaction between attention and working memory is bidirectional. It has been postulated that the maintenance of information in working memory is accomplished by directing attention to the neural representations of the information itself [14], whereas attentional orienting within working memory can retroactively influence maintenance-related activity in functionally specialized posterior areas by engaging selective retrieval functions [see reference 15 for a review]. Even while flexible switching between goals may require maintaining higher sensitivity to possibly relevant information, distracting stimuli must be continuously evaluated and suppressed. Therefore, behavioral performance could be sensitive to the "on-line" appearance of environmental distractors; especially when they could be "relevant" to the subject.

1.2. Processing information with affective valence

Several theories posit that emotionally salient stimuli have privileged access during information processing [16,17] which implies that affective stimuli have the capacity to transcend task boundaries, disrupting ongoing processing regardless of whether they are relevant to the current task-set or not.

Numerous studies have addressed the effects of affective stimuli on cognitive processes such as attention, memory and executive functions [18-27]. Actually, it seems that the appearance of an emotional stimulus might interfere with the processing of other stimuli emerging in the temporal vicinity, basically due to the fact that stimuli with emotional content attract attentional resources because of their adaptive relevance [28-31].

The acceptance of the assumption that affective stimuli disrupt subsequent cognitive processing raises the question whether there is an asymmetry between emotional and cognitive processing (i.e., emotional distractors disrupt cognitive processing, but not vice versa). Recently, Reeck and Egner [32] studied this issue using a face-word Stroop protocol adapted to independently manipulate (a) the congruency between target and distractor stimulus features, (b) the affective salience of distractor features, and (c) the task-relevance of emotional compared to non-emotional target features. As a result of this study, the authors concluded that task-irrelevant emotional distractors resulted in equivalent performance costs as task-relevant non-emotional distracters, whereas task-irrelevant non-emotional distractors did not produce performance costs comparable to those generated by task-relevant emotional distractors. In other words, this study documented the abovementioned asymmetry between affective and cognitive processing, supporting the notion that affective stimuli are prioritized in human information processing.

On the other hand, an increased arousal of the stimulus has been associated with a more intense defensive response when compared to appetitive motivational systems [33-35]. Accordingly, the arousal of unpleasant stimuli is comparatively higher, leading to what has been termed as *emotional negativity bias* [36-38]. In addition, it has been postulated an *emotional positivity offset* when lower arousal stimuli are processed, as is possible to infer from the enhanced processing of pleasant compared to unpleasant stimuli, when they both are lower arousal ones [33,39,40].

Emotional words are consistently acknowledged as low arousal stimuli [41-44], particularly in comparison with emotional scenes or faces [45-47]. This effect has been explained as a result that words depict emotional events less vividly [42]. Interestingly, it has been proposed that verbal material is less capable of disrupting cognitive performance than pictures, particularly when using negative words, what reinforces the notion that emotional verbal stimuli associate with lower brain responsivity. However, it seems that arousing verbal stimuli can lead to amygdala activation similar to that induced by emotional faces, pictures, or conditioned stimuli [48].

1.3. Neural basis of emotional processing

Recent advances in neuroimaging techniques have demonstrated that the amygdala, ventromedial prefrontal cortex (VMPFC), anterior cingulate, insula, nucleus accumbens and basal ganglia are all involved in emotion processing and executive control in some capacity [49-53]. In fact, it has been found that left and right interior frontal gyrus (IFG) regions differentiate between interference and noninterference trials across neutral and emotional stimuli; a region of the left anterior insula and right orbital frontal cortex (OFC) is capable to differentiate between interference and non-interference trials for emotional stimuli, regardless of valence, whereas the insula, OFC and ventral anterior cingulate cortex (ACC) seem to be sensitive to interference resolution for a select valence and that the left amygdala differentiated emotional and neutral stimuli at encoding and response [54]. Furthermore, the behavioral patterns observed in patients with either left temporal lesion or right OFC lesion suggest that the left amygdala and right OFC are both critical to the emotion facilitation effect [55].

In the last few years, the temporal course of the brain processing of emotional words has been studied through event-related brain potentials (ERPs) techniques, showing that earlier components as P120, N170 and P200 (including a variant closely related to N170 and termed as vertex-positive potential: VPP) could be sensitive to the emotional content of the word and the subsequent attentional allocation process [42,45,56], while later ERP changes as Early Posterior Negativity, N400 and Late Positive Components could reflect semantic stages of processing [40,57,58].

Even though there is a general consensus that emotionally arousing faces or scenes capture a substantial amount of visual processing resources even if they appear as distractors for a concurrent cognitive task, scarce data is available on the effect due to task-irrelevant emotional words.

A recent study evaluated the effect of written emotional words sharing the scene in which subjects had to perform a simultaneous visual perceptual task [59]. The authors reported emotion effects of task-irrelevant words on the ERPs before 300 ms, but not any interference with the visual foreground task was evidenced by task-related steady-state visual evoked potential amplitudes or behavioral data. The results were interpreted as suggesting a specificity of emotion effects on sensory processing that might depend on the information channel from which emotional significance is derived. However, these effects appeared when distractors and task-relevant stimuli shared the same sensory modality –visual-, along with a similar temporal appearance. Therefore, one could speculate if there is any effect of emotional irrelevant words when equating the nature of both relevant and task-irrelevant stimuli, while delivering distractors through a different sensory modality, but immediately preceding the task onset.

1.4. Evaluating the cross-modal influence of verbal affective stimuli on subsequent cognitive processing

Following the previous idea, we studied the effect of auditory emotional words on the ERPs and behavioral performance of a subsequent highly demanding visual verbal working memory task, with the general hypothesis that the enhanced capture of lexico-semantic processing resources by emotional distractor words could last long enough as to interfere verbal subsequent processing, particularly in high cognitive demand situations.

Next, various methodological considerations and results from the abovementioned study are detailed, as well as how they could be interpreted in the context of the previously discussed related literature.

2. Methods

Subjects. In order to explore our hypothesis, 18 healthy, right-handed, university female subjects were recruited to voluntarily participate in the experiment (mean age= 26.1 years; SD= 4.1).

Experimental task. Behavioral data and ERPs were obtained during task performance. Subjects performed a dual working memory task. The first part of the task consisted in the serial presentation of two-syllable, four-letter words during 500 ms. Participants were given explicit instructions to first read the word silently and then, as soon as possible, pronounce aloud an arrangement of letters made up of the second syllable of the word followed by the inverted letters of the first syllable (e.g. BOTE – TEOB). Pronunciation times (RT) and the number of correct responses were measured for all trials. In the second part of the task, subjects were asked to decide, by pressing a key, if a string of four letters (which appear during 500 ms) represented – or not – the inverted order of the first word that was presented [e.g. BOTE – ETOB (inverse; 50% of the stimuli) or OTEB (not inverse: 50% of the stimuli)]. The time interval between the visual appearance of the word and the string of letters was 1000 ms. One hundred and fifty different high frequency words [60] were used as stimuli. Figure 1 shows the experimental flow chart.

Participants were seated comfortably in a quiet, dimly lit room. Visual stimuli were presented on an SVGA monitor (refresh rate: 100 Hz). Words were written in white capital letters (Arial) against a black background displaying a visual angle of 0.80°. Preceding each one of the trials of the task, a context was presented to the subjects. Five blocks of 50 trials each – a total of two hundred and fifty trials – were configured by combining three randomly-distributed main conditions. After each block, subjects had a brief rest period. The presentation order of the blocks was counterbalanced. The two conditions that constituted the trial blocks were:

A (reference trials): Fifty trials in which the WM trial was free from preceding stimuli.

B (auditory preceding stimuli) 200 trials in which the WM trials were preceded by words – delivered binaurally- showing different emotional content:

Ba - positive (50 trials)

Bb - negative (50 trials)

Bc - neutral (50 trials)

C - control (50 trials)

Auditory stimuli. Auditory stimuli were designed based on the results of a verbal production paradigm performed by 50 female voluntary subjects with similar ages and educational level with the participants in the ensuing electrophysiological experiment. They were instructed to write words freely with three different emotional contents: positive, negative and neutral. Subsequently, the most common 50 words in each category were selected and randomly presented to another group of 50 subjects –similar ages and educational level than participants-with the instruction to classified them in a continuum from very negative (0) to very positive (10) with 5 as the neutral emotional content.

Later, twenty-five words with averaged scores below 1.5 were selected and labeled as "negative" (i.e. "TONTA"; "SILLY"). Other twenty-five exemplars with averaged scores above 8.5 were selected and labeled as "positive" (i.e. "BONITA", "PRETTY"), while further twenty-five words with scores ranging from 4 to 6 points were selected and labeled as "neutral" (i.e. "LADO", "SIDE"). Both positive and negative words were female adjectives. The 75 resultant words were tape-recorded in a professional facility studio by a professional broadcaster. The length of the audio files was digitally restricted to 500 ms each. Besides, other 75 audio-files were created to be used as controls, by inverting the 75 files containing the spoken words, with the aim to keep similar physical characteristics but avoiding semantic bias.

Using the selected audio-files, three semi-randomized lists with different emotional content -50 words each- were created (each word was presented twice in its corresponding list). In addition, another list of 50 inverted audio-files was created to act as control (C), including 16 inverted positive, 16 inverted negative and 18 inverted neutral spoken words.

All the auditory stimuli were delivered binaurally via COBY (CV-200) headphones (COBY Electronics, Corp., U.S.A) controlled by the software MindTracer (Neuronic S.A., Cuba), at 85 dB SPL. Previous pilot studies were done to guarantee that the sound level used were not only audible but comfortable.

ERP Acquisition. ERPs were obtained, in all conditions, time-window starting 500 ms after auditory stimuli onset, which corresponded to 300 ms before dual WM task onset, until 750 ms after it. ERPs were recorded from the Fp1, Fp2, F7, F8, F3, F4, C3, C4, P3, P4, O1, O2, T3, T4, T5, T6, Fz, Cz, and Pz scalp electrode sites, according to the International 10-20 system. The electrooculogram (EOG) was recorded from the outer canthus and infraocular orbital ridge of the right eye.

Electrophysiological recordings were made using 10 mm diameter gold disk electrodes (Grass Type E5GH) and Grass electrode cream. All recording sites were referred to linked mastoids. Interelectrode impedances were below 5 kΩ. EEG and EOG signals were amplified at a bandpass of 0.5–30 Hz (3-dB cutoff points of 6 dB/octave rolloff curves) with a sampling period of 4 ms on the MEDICID-04 system. Single trial data were examined off-line for averaging and analysis.

ERP Scoring. Prior to scoring, EEG data was visually corrected for artifacts due to eye movement. Epochs of data on all channels were excluded from averages when voltage in a given recording epoch exceeded 100 μV on any EEG or EOG channel. In general, 3 to 7 epochs had to be rejected in each condition per subject. Thirty free-artifact correct trials were considered to obtain the individual ERP in each condition, reaching a signal-noise ratio higher than 1.5 in all cases. Amplitude and latency for the ERP components of focal interest were measured according to a 100-ms pre-stimulus baseline. All scoring was conducted baseline-to-peak through visual inspection.

Data Analysis. Repeated Measure Analyses of Variance (RM-ANOVAs) were used to study behavioral responses and reaction times. Electrophysiological data was analyzed using

http://dx.doi.org/10.5772/56494

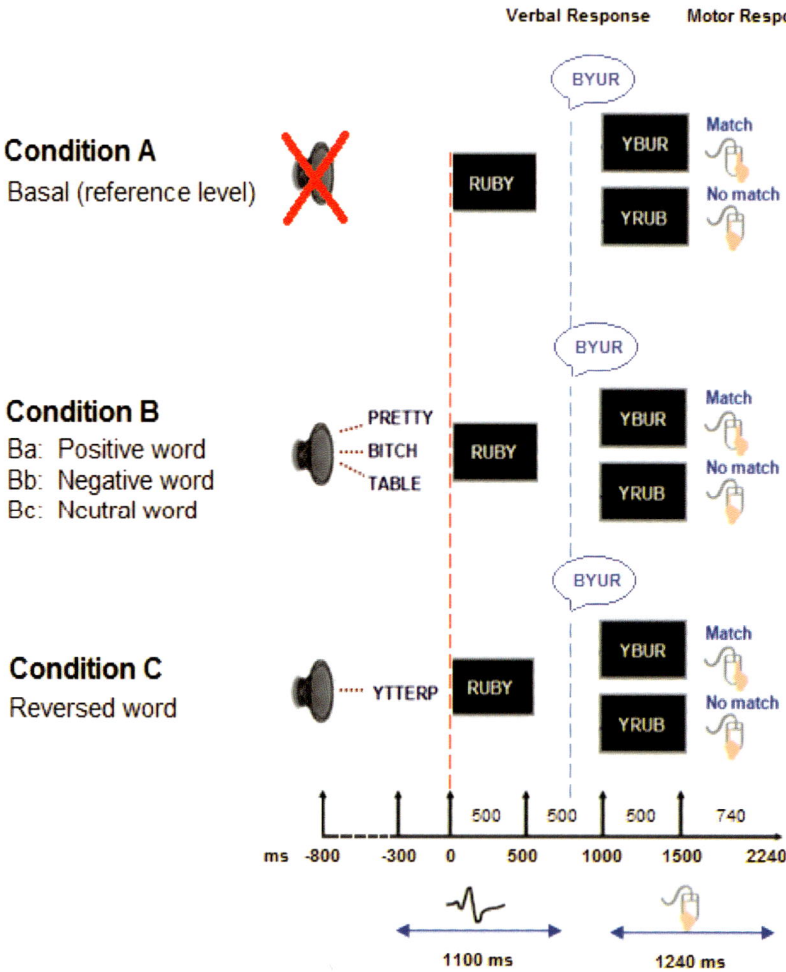

Figure 1. Experimental design and flow chart.

Randomized-block Analysis of Variance [Conditions x Recording Sites; see reference 61] with average voltage across each time window as the dependent variable. The latency and amplitude of each ERP component were quantified by the highest peak within each respective latency window. Considering the appearance of the task-relevant stimuli as the initial time instant (t_0), several time windows were used to examine averaged ERP-waveforms. In addition, post-hoc Tukey's HSD tests were carried out to explore the trend of the differences found.

3. Results

Behavioral results. The analysis of the correct responses showed significant differences between the experimental conditions ($F_{(4,60)}$= 4.65, p<0.05). Post-hoc comparisons showed that when the WM task onset was preceded by positive words, the number of correct responses significantly decreased, as compared to negative (Bb) or control (C) auditory stimuli (p<0.05), and when compared to neutral (Bc) or none (A) precedent stimuli (p<0.01) as well. Although the comparison between negative and control stimuli did not reached statistical significance, when negative stimuli preceded the task the amount of correct responses tended to decreased. The Table 1 shows the behavioral performances in the experimental task.

Experimental Task Performance	No Auditory Stimuli		**Auditory words with emotional content**						**Auditory Control stimuli**	
	Mean	**SD**	**Mean**	**SD**	**Mean**	**SD**	**Mean**	**SD**	**Mean**	**SD**
			Neutral		**Positive**		**Negative**			
Correct Responses	42.3	6.6	42.3	6.1	38.6	6.4	39.8	4.3	41.4	5.3
Reaction Times	868.3	88.0	908.4	112.6	986.4	104.2	896.7	76.4	896.7	76.4

SD: standard deviations. Reaction times are expressed in milliseconds.

Table 1. Behavioral performances.

The pronunciation times - the time it took the subject to give the verbal response – were also significantly different across conditions ($F_{(4,60)}$= 6.18, p<0.05). Post hoc analyses showed that the WM task performance preceded by positive words was significantly slower than that associated to control auditory stimuli or the lack of any precedent one (p<0.01). In addition, performances preceded by positive words were also slower than those preceded by neutral or negative words (p<0.05). See Table 1.

Electrophysiological results. Regarding the visual inspection of the resultant ERPs waveforms, three main components were discernible over the fronto-central region, when there was not any auditory stimulus preceding the WM task; an early negativity peaking over 80 ms subsequent to the instant in which the first visual stimuli (word) appeared, followed by a prominent P2 component (VPP) reaching its maximum at 170 ms, and a slow negativity with maximum about 400 ms at vertex. Probably due to the fact that the WM task involved mental manipulation of visual words, a left-lateralized N170 was discernible over the posterior regions. Figure 2 shows the grand-averaged ERPs that correspond to three experimental conditions: none auditory stimuli (A), neutral words (Bc) and reversed-words (C: control) preceding the beginning of the WM dual task.

http://dx.doi.org/10.5772/56494

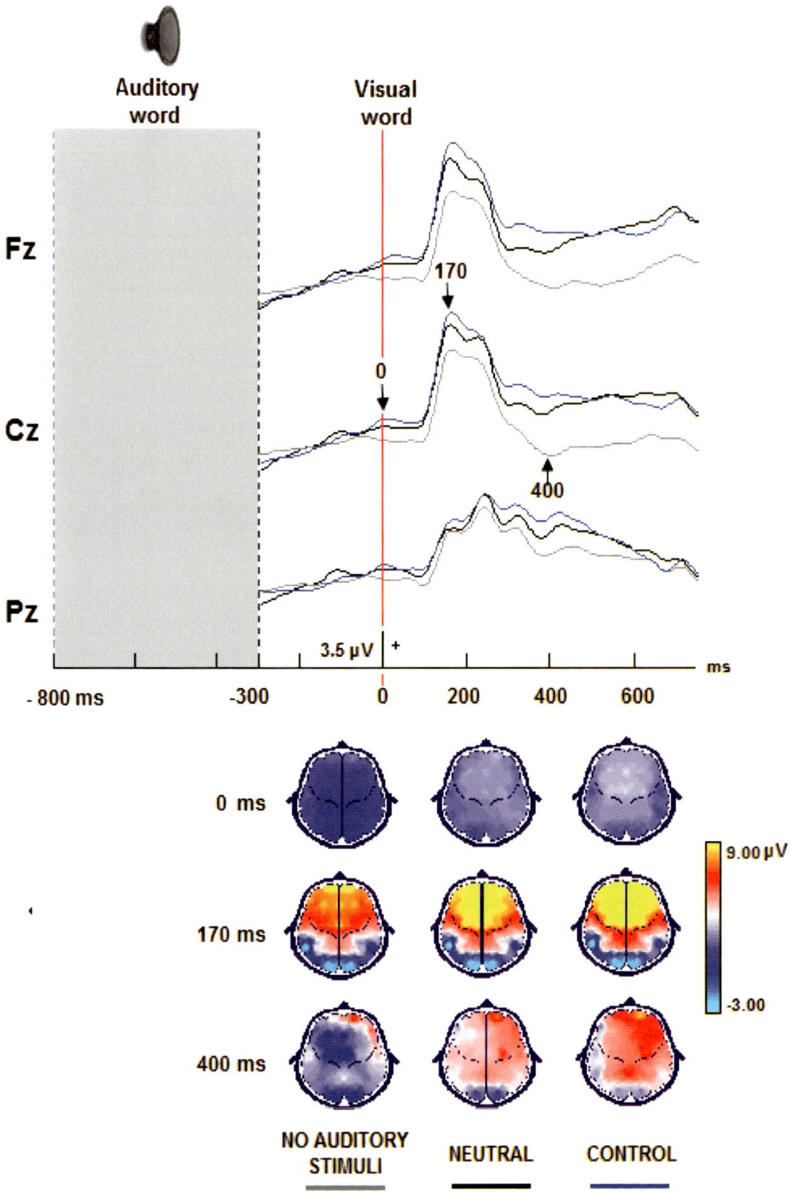

Figure 2. Grand-averaged ERPs in three experimental conditions: without auditory stimuli (A), neutral words (Bc), and reversed-words (C: control), preceding the beginning of the WM dual task.

One first ERP analysis was performed with the aim to elucidate the effect of any auditory stimuli preceding the beginning of the WM task on task-related visual ERP waveforms. With this goal, the three time windows which best represented the main ERPs changes were analyzed in the locations where they mainly occurred (-300-0, 0-300, and 300-750 ms, respectively). The presentation of the first task-relevant stimuli was taken as the initial time instant (t_0).

Randomized-block ANOVAs using two factors [Condition (3: A, Bc and C); Recording Sites (8: Fp1, Fp2, F3, F4, C3, C4, Fz, and Cz)] were performed, showing significant differences for both factors (Condition: $F_{(2,322)}$=17.94, p<0.0001, and recording sites: $F_{(2,322)}$=5.10, p<0.0001), in the time window that preceded the beginning of the experimental task. No relevant interaction was found. This finding is compatible with the decrease observed in the slight early negative shift during conditions in which auditory stimulus were delivered.

The analysis of the time window in which N80 and P170 occurred, showed significant differences between conditions [(F(2,322)= 39.65, p<0.0001)], recording sites [(F(7,322)= 41.11, p<0.0001)], and their interaction [(F(14,322)= 2.99, p<0.001)]. Post-hoc analysis demonstrated that at fronto-central locations, ERPs reached significantly minor voltage amplitude when there was no preceding auditory stimuli (A), in comparison with the conditions in which they were presented (Bc and Bd; p<0.01).

Finally, the analysis of the N400 component also showed significant differences between conditions [(F(2,322)= 26.74, p<0.0001)], recording sites [(F(7,322)= 2.78, p<0.001)] and their interaction [(F(14,322)= 2.66, p<0.01)]. In this case, post-hoc tests showed that N400 was widely located, while showing significantly greater amplitude when no auditory stimuli were present, in comparison to the conditions in which they were (p<0.01).

Following an analog procedure, randomized-block ANOVAs were performed to clarify the effect of the emotional content of the preceding auditory stimuli on task performance. Therefore, two factors were analyzed [Condition: positive (Ba), negative (Bb) and neutral words (Bc); and Recording sites (Pz, P3, P4, O1, O2, T5 and T6)] in the time-windows which corresponded to the main ERP changes: -300-0 ms, 0-250 ms, 250-500, and 500-750 ms. Figure 3 shows the grand-averaged ERPs that correspond to three experimental conditions preceded by the following auditory stimuli: positive words (Ba), negative words (Bb) and neutral words (Bc).

The ERP analysis of the time elapsed from the auditory stimuli to the task onset (-300-0 ms) showed significant differences between conditions [(F(2,238)= 8.64, p<0.001)] and recording sites [(F(6,238)= 6.55, p<0.0001)] without any relevant interaction. In this case, the experimental conditions preceded by positive and negative words showed significantly minor voltages than that preceded by neutral words. This result suggests that visual ERP are capable of depicting a cross-modal effect of the emotional content of the auditory stimuli even earlier than the beginning of the task-related cognitive effort.

Similarly, the analysis of the time-window between the task-onset and the subsequent 250 ms showed significant differences only between conditions [(F(2,238)= 9.03, p<0.001)] and

http://dx.doi.org/10.5772/56494

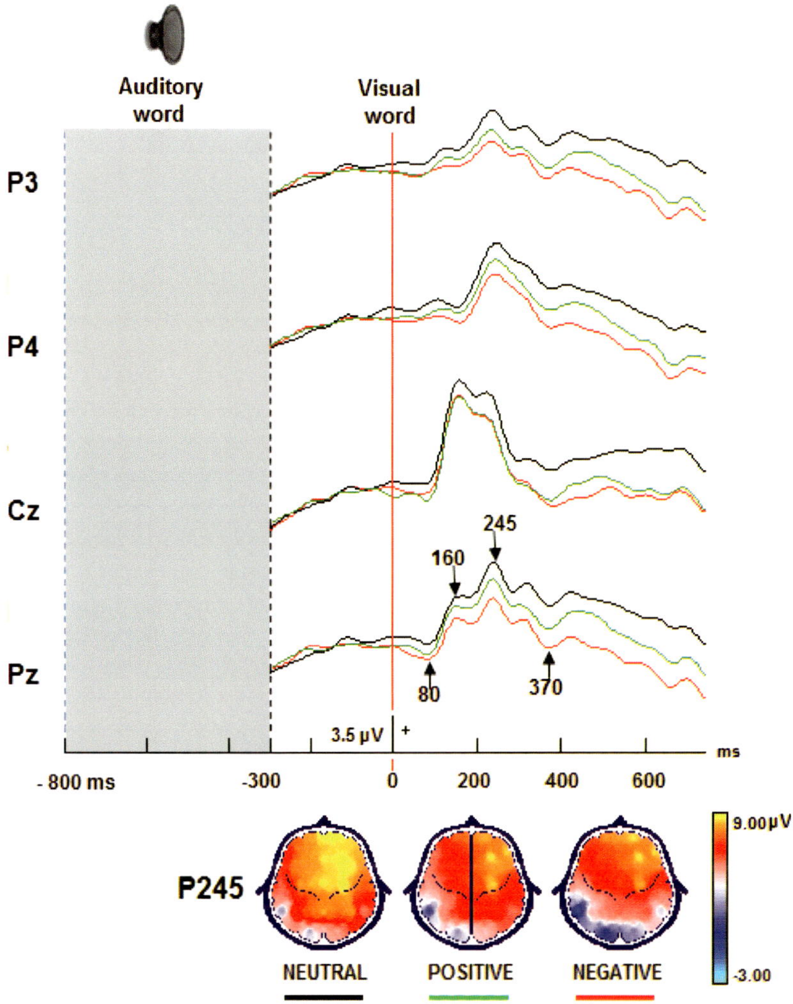

Figure 3. Grand-averaged ERPs in three experimental conditions: positive words (Ba), negative words (Bb) and neutral words (Bc), preceding the beginning of the WM dual task.

recording sites [(F(6,238)= 43.83, p<0.0001)]. In this time window the conditions preceded by positive and negative words also showed significantly minor voltages than the neutral ones.

The analysis of the time period between 250 and 500 ms subsequent to the task-onset demonstrated significant differences between conditions [(F(2,238)= 14.43, p<0.0001)] and recording sites [(F(6,238)= 13.68, p<0.0001)] without relevant interactions. As it occurred in the previous time-windows, minor voltages corresponded to trials preceded by positive and negative words, what reinforces the notion that neural effects caused by distracting affective stimuli might last longer than expected.

Finally, the analysis of the later period of time showed that conditions [(F(2,238)= 15.55, p<0.0001)] and recording sites [(F(6,238)= 3.95, p<0.01)] reached statistical significance, also without any significant interaction. In this case, there were also higher voltages in trials preceded by neutral words.

4. Discussion

4.1. Unraveling behavioral results

The analysis of the correct responses achieved while performing the experimental task showed that when the onset of the WM task was preceded by positive words, the number of correct responses significantly decreased, as compared to the alternative conditions, while negative words tended to show the same effect without attaining statistical significance. In addition, the pronunciation times were significantly different across conditions, being particularly longer when positive words preceded the task onset.

Therefore, one possible first conclusion might be that auditory emotional words evoked a sustained interfering effect on task performance, even though they were task-irrelevant. This finding coincides with the report from Sakaki and colleagues [62] who recently studied the effect of emotional events on the cognitive processing of subsequent stimuli. Despite the fact that not all types of later cognitive processes are impaired by preceding negative events, they found that the presentation of negative pictures interferes with subsequent semantic processing. In our experiment, the use of female adjectives might have enhanced the arousal elicited by the auditory verbal stimuli with emotional content, particularly considering that the participants in the experiment were female subjects.

It has been reported that when the subjects are instructed to perform a semantic categorization using emotional words as distractors, affective mismatches are detected automatically and modulate a binding of irrelevant information with responses [63]. Furthermore, the notion that the effect of emotional words could be narrowed to certain aspects of cognitive processing is reinforced by recent findings pointing out that negative words interfere with the allocation of dimensional attention to different features of an attended object, but they do not capture spatial or object-based mechanisms of visual attention [64].

Whatever the effect of emotional stimuli might be, it should depend on their distinctive characteristics. In this regard, it has been reiteratively demonstrated that the arousal associated to the stimulus definitely influences its subsequent processing. Despite the low arousal attributed to verbal stimuli, emotional words might be more arousing than neutral ones, probably due to their intrinsic relevance to individual social suitability. In fact, these differences in the word-arousal level could explain distinct processing outcomes as it occurred when Guillet and Arndt [65] demonstrated that while examining memory for peripheral information, memory for peripheral words was enhanced when it was encoded in the presence of emotionally arousing taboo words but not when it was encoded in the presence of words that were only negative in valence.

The effects of the emotional valence of the stimuli have been profusely discussed in the literature. However, beyond the different neural subsystems underlying emotional recognition, the exact effect of emotional words on cognitive processing remains far from being elucidated. During the previous paragraphs, some empirical evidence supporting the notion that negative stimuli interfere with subsequent cognitive processing has been documented. This could portray the tendency observed for some behavioral responses in the present study, but do not elucidate the predominant effect of positive distractors preceding the experimental task.

4.2. Emotional positivity bias

In order to clarify the effect of preceding positive words on later cognitive processing at least two variables must be considered: a) positive emotional valence and b) dissimilarities in sensory activation when distractors are auditory stimuli while task-relevant targets are visually displayed.

Abundant empirical evidence supports the idea that stimuli with positive valence influence subsequent processing. Visual scenes such as smiling and attractive faces, appetizing foods and beautiful pictures can evoke strong emotions. People routinely employ such emotional imagery in the media and even during ordinary social interactions to attempt to bias the decisions of others. However, not all positive stimuli are equally influential. In fact, human smiling facial expressions and images of cute animals bias decisions more than food [66, 67]. Furthermore, there is a recognition bias for information consistent with the physical attractiveness stereotype [68].

Recent evidence from brain damaged patients has been interpreted as suggesting that the proper recognition of both negative and positive facial expressions relies on the right hemisphere, and that the left hemisphere produces a default state resulting in a bias towards evaluating expressions as happy [69]. The recent report commenting that the activation of the left dorso-lateral prefrontal cortex favors the memory retrieval of positive emotional information [70] additionally supports this hemispheric disquisition. These findings lead to the conclusion that the positive bias not only includes the recognition process but also the memory and its retrieval, functionally involving several brain neural structures.

With respect to the latter topic to consider -the possible cross-modal effect that time-related auditory and visual stimuli have on cognitive processing- recent studies have found, using different auditory-visual distraction paradigms, that task-irrelevant novel sounds preceding visual targets cause behavioral distraction in adults as reflected by increased reaction times to the visual target preceded by novel sounds when compared to those preceded by standard sounds [71].

Regarding this issue, San Miguel and colleagues [72] have proposed that (together with other factors) attention task demands and the temporal position of the novel relative to the encoding or retrieval of the task-related visual information influences whether a novel stimulus causes distraction or facilitation. In fact, they reported a reduced distraction under high memory load [73]. On the other hand, Muller-Gass & Schröger [74] studied whether the distraction effect is modulated by the difficulty of the auditory task. They found that the distraction effect increased while rising memory load task demands, but not while increasing its perceptual difficulty. Interpreting these results together it could be possible to assume that channel separation between task-relevant information and task-irrelevant distracting information has an interactive effect with task demands in determining the magnitude of auditory distraction. Therefore, when channel separation is possible distraction increases, as it occurred in the experiment conducted by San Miguel and colleagues [73], and distraction decreases when processing information in both auditory and visual channels concur. In the present study, we used auditory irrelevant stimuli preceding the performance of a highly cognitive demanding WM visual task, thus it could strengthen the potential impact of the attentional capture elicited by the significant sounds and its consequences on subsequent behavioral task-performance.

4.3. Event-related brain potentials

Two main effects can be inferred from the ERP data; 1) visual ERP components reach significantly minor voltage amplitude when there are none preceding auditory stimuli in comparison with conditions in which they are present, 2) When the auditory irrelevant stimuli had an emotional content, there is a discernible decrease in the voltage amplitude of the ERP components which appears very early in the processing stream.

Voltage increases are usually interpreted as signs of greater neural recruitment, which is commonly seen in more novel tasks or ones that are more difficult [75]. Other possible explanations for the amplifying effect that task-preceding irrelevant distractors impinge on the ERP voltage magnitudes was postulated by Nataanen and colleagues in 1982 [76]. These authors proposed that deviant stimulus elicit two overlapping sequences of brain events: exogenous and endogenous. They described the former as an earlier automatic and inflexible set of brain processes that might provide a central-level stimulus to the latter. In addition, they suggest that there is a subsequent endogenous set of brain waves regarded as a sign of stimulus deviance.

In the same logic, we expected to obtain the overlapped effects of the neural state triggered by the auditory stimuli and that necessary to fulfill task demands. Accordingly, the auditory stimuli processing could either distract neural resources from task performance leading to poorer achievements or deploy additional resources thus improving task performance. The present results favored the latter conjecture.

On the other hand, one important point to elucidate resides on the time in which auditory distracting stimuli influence the visual ERP. The simplest assumption might be that any stimulus preceding the task onset should only influence the ERP corresponding to the beginning of the task due to an earlier processing closure related to the task irrelevance of the former stimulus. However, the present results might suggest that the processing closure of the auditory relevant stimuli could take longer than expected, probably due to the different sensory modality in which task-irrelevant and task-relevant stimuli are delivered.

4.3.1. N170

In general, the N170 component has been interpreted as a hallmark of visual orthographic specialization [77, 78] that may reflect increased visual processing expertise [79], most likely in pre-lexical orthographic processing [80]. The present results seem to correspond well to previously reported findings on the N170 component, where source localization and imaging studies have shown that this early stage of perception processing occurs in the fusiform gyrus and is lateralized depending upon the nature of the stimuli (left side for words; right side for pictures; 81,82]. Accordingly, the component N170 was lateralized at the left side, suggesting that experimental manipulations with the visual words might be performed in a sub-lexical perceptual processing level.

4.3.2. VPP component

The vertex-positive potential is an ERP waveform that has been described as a positive counterpart at centro-frontal sites of the N170 component. The entire N170/VPP complex has been accounted for by two dipolar sources located in the lateral inferior occipital cortex/ posterior fusiform gyrus [82]. These authors postulated that early processes in object recognition respond to category-specific visual information, and are associated with strong lateralization and orientation bias. In addition, it is very probably that differences between N170 and VPP effects observed in ERP studies could be accounted for by differences in reference methodology [83].

In the present experiment the VPP waveform showed greater amplitude at fronto-central regions in the trials preceded by auditory stimuli, whereas its amplitude decreased when the distractors had an emotional content. Despite this component is usually related with configurational information processing more than with emotional processing, the voltage decrement observed in trials preceded by emotional words might depict the amount of resources engaged in the processing of irrelevant stimuli but needed for the concurrent task performance.

4.3.3. Slow negativity

A component named N2b, one that exhibits peaks later than 250 ms in adults, has been reported during performance of category comparison tasks [84, 85]. Experimental evidence suggests that while the N400 component is a specific marker of semantic incongruity, N2b represents a general correlate of inconsistencies in the detection process, or "conflicts" [85] between representations of task-relevant stimuli features [84]. Both components could fit the explanation for the slight negativity subsequent to the P2 like component observed in the present experiment. However, due to its latency, N400 waveform seems to be more likely to occur in the present conditions.

In our experiment the visual word had to be read and further manipulated in working memory to fulfill the task requirements. The N400 like component observed might be depicting the link between the steps in which visual descriptive information of words is first encoded in semantic memory and subsequently visualized via the network for object working memory [86]. Alternatively, it could depict the timing of the effect resemble brain responses linked to engagement of working memory resources, as it was interpreted recently by Wlotko and Federmeier [87] while evaluating the influence of contextual information on semantic processing. The differences between conditions preceded by auditory stimuli -emotional versus neutral- seem to additionally address the contextual influence on working memory processing.

5. Conclusions and final statements

Conjunctively, behavioral and electrophysiological results suggest that when verbal distractors precede the beginning of a high demanding verbal WM task, its performance is influenced by the characteristics of the distractors, irrespective of whether they appear in different sensory modalities.

In the present study, a "positivity offset" was confirmed, where positive irrelevant stimuli interfered with task performance. It occurred despite the temporal shift between the appearance of distractors and task-relevant stimuli, as well as, the different sensory modality in which they were both delivered. This could be probably explained as part of the competing effect between irrelevant and relevant stimuli for processing cross-modal common resources.

Even though the topic concerning environmental influences on cognitive processing remains incompletely elucidated, we hope that this work could contribute to the understanding of these important relationships. In fact, increasing experimental evidence on the topic suggest that more attention will be paid in the future to the interaction between contextual environment and cognitive processing demands, due to the general idea that verbal positive material could help to process concurrent information, when it seems that exactly the opposite occurs.

In a more general context, the present results should be interpreted within the extensive framework of emotion-cognitive processing relationships. The multisensory continuous assessment of the environment carried on by the central executive systems is constantly challenged by environmental demands, while its response capacity is limited by the amount of available processing resources. Fortunately, this neurofunctional dynamic seems to run asymmetric, in which the intrinsic relevance of certain stimuli (e.g. faces, words, and emotional stimuli) benefit from a special cognitive treatment.

Acknowledgements

The authors are grateful to Psic. Vanessa Ruiz-Stovel for her revision of the text and useful comments.

http://dx.doi.org/10.5772/56494

Author details

Andrés Antonio González-Garrido[1,2*], Fabiola Reveca Gómez-Velázquez[1] and Julieta Ramos-Loyo[1]

*Address all correspondence to: gonzalezgarrido@gmail.com

1 Instituto de Neurociencias. Universidad de Guadalajara, Guadalajara, Mexico

2 O.P.D. Hospital Civil de Guadalajara, Mexico

References

[1] Borzenko A. Language processing in human brain. In Proceedings of the First AGI Conference "Frontiers in Artificial Intelligence and Applications", Wang, P, Goertzel, B and Franklin, S. Eds. IOS Press, 171, 2008. pp. 232-239.

[2] Dawson G, Ashman SB, Carver LJ. The role of early experience in shaping behavioral and brain development and its implications for social policy. Development and Psychopathology 2000; 12 695–712.

[3] Baddeley AD, Hitch GJ. Working memory. In: Bower, G.H. (Ed.), The Psychology of Learning and Motivation. Advances in Research and Theory, vol. 8. Academic Press, New York, 1974. pp. 47–89.

[4] Carpenter PA, Just MA, Reichle ED. Working memory and executive function: evidence from neuroimaging. Current Opinion in Neurobiology 2000; 10(2), 195–199.

[5] Just MA, Carpenter PA. A capacity theory of comprehension: individual differences in working memory. Psychological Review 1992; 99(1) 122–149.

[6] Baddeley A. The episodic buffer: a new component of working memory? Trends in Cognitive Science 2000; 4(11) 417–423.

[7] Repovs G, Baddeley A. The multi-component model of working memory: explorations in experimental cognitive psychology. Neuroscience 2006; 139(1) 5–21.

[8] Norman DA, Shallice T. Attention to action. Willed and automatic control of behavior. In: Davidson RJ, Schwartz GE, Shapiro D, editors. Consciousness and self-regulation. Advances in research and theory, Vol. 4. New York: Plenum Press; 1986. p. 1–18.

[9] Shallice T. From neuropsychology to mental structure. Cambridge: Cambridge University Press; 1988.

[10] Carter CS, Braver TS, Barch DM, Botvinick MM, Noll DC, Cohen JD. Anterior cingulate cortex, error detection, and the online monitoring of performance. Science 1998; 280 747–749.

[11] Dreisbach G. How positive affect modulates cognitive control: the costs and benefits of reduced maintenance capability. Brain and Cognition 2006; 60(1) 11–19.

[12] Braver TS, Cohen JD. On the control of control: the role of dopamine in regulating prefrontal function and working memory. In: Monsell, S., Driver, J. (Eds.), Control of cognitive processes: Attention and performance XVIII, MA. MIT Press, Cambridge, 2000. pp. 711–737.

[13] Lavie N, de Fockert J. The role of working memory in attentional capture. Psychonomic Bulletin and Review 2005; 12(4) 669–674.

[14] Curtis CE, D'Esposito M. Persistent activity in the prefrontal cortex during working memory. Trends in Cognitive Sciences 2003; 7(9) 415–423.

[15] Lepsien J, Nobre AC. Cognitive control of attention in the human brain: insights from orienting attention to mental representations. Brain Research 2006; 1105, 20–31.

[16] LeDoux JE. Review Emotion circuits in the brain. Annual Review of Neuroscience 2000; 23 155–184. doi: 10.1146/annurev.neuro.23.1.155.

[17] Vuilleumier P, Huang YM. Emotional attention: uncovering the mechanisms of affective biases in perception. Current Directions in Psychological Science 2009; 18 148–152. doi: 10.1111/j.1467-8721.2009.01626.x.

[18] Banich MT, Mackiewicz KL, Depue BE, Whitmer AJ, Miller GA, Heller W. Cognitive control mechanisms, emotion and memory: A neural perspective with implications for psychopathology. Neuroscience & Biobehavioral Reviews 2009; 33 613–630.

[19] Delplanque S, Lavoie ME, Hot P, Silvert L, Sequeira H. Modulation of cognitive processing by emotional valence studied through event-related potentials in humans. Neuroscience Letters 2004; 356 1-4.

[20] Fenske MJ, Eastwood JD. Modulation of focused attention by faces expressing emotion: evidence from flanker tasks. Emotion 2003; 3(4) 327–343.

[21] Hoffstetter Ch, Achaibou C, Vuilleumier P. Reactivation of visual cortex during memory retrieval: content specificity and emotional modulation. Neuroimage 2012; 60 1734-1745.

[22] Lindström BR, Bohlin G. Threat-relevance impairs executive functions: Negative impact on working memory and response inhibition. Emotion 2012; 12(2) 384-93.

[23] Pessoa L. Emotion and attention effects: is it all a matter of timing? Not yet. Frontiers in human Neuroscience 2010; 4.pii: 172.

[24] Pessoa L. Beyond brain regions: Network perspective of cognition-emotion interactions. The Behavioral and Brain Sciences 2012; 35(3)158-9.

[25] Pessoa L, Padmala S, Kenzerm A, Bauer A. Interactions between cognition and emotion during response inhibition. Emotion 2012; 12(1) 192-7.

[26] Phelps E. Emotion and cognition: Insights from studies of the human amygdala. Annual Reviews of Psychology 2006; 57 27–53.

[27] Pourtois G, Schettino A, Vuilleumier P. Brain mechanisms for emotional influences on perception and attention: What is magic and what is not. Biological Psychology 2012. In press.

[28] LeDoux JE. The Emotional Brain. New York. Simon & Schuster; 1996.

[29] González-Garrido AA, Ramos-Loyo J, Gómez-Velázquez F, Alvelais-Alarcón M., de la Serna Tuya J.M. Visual verbal working memory processing may be interfered by previously seen faces. International Journal of Psychophysiology 2007; 65(2) 141–151.

[30] González-Garrido AA, Ramos-Loyo J, López-Franco AL, Gómez-Velázquez F. (2009). Visual processing in a facial emotional context: An ERP study. International Journal of Psychophysiology 2009; 71(1) 25–30.

[31] Vuilleumier P, Armony JL, Driver J, Dolan RJ. Effects of attention and emotion on face processing in the human brain: an event-related fMRI study. Neuron 2001; 30 829–841.

[32] Reeck C, Egner T. Affective privilege: asymmetric interference by emotional distracters. Frontiers in Psychology 2011; 2232.

[33] Cacioppo JT, Gardner WL. Emotion. Annual Review of Psychology. 1999; 191-214.

[34] Peeters G, Czapinski J. Positive-negative asymmetry in evaluations: The distinction between affective and informational negativity effects. European review of social psychology 1990; 1 33-60.

[35] Taylor SE. Asymmetrical effects of positive and negative events: the mobilization-minimization hypothesis. Psychological bulletin 1991; 110 67.

[36] Hansen CH, Hansen RD. Finding the face in the crowd: an anger superiority effec

[37] Carretié L, Mercado F, Tapia M, Hinojosa JA (2001) Emotion, attention, and the negativity bias', studied through event-related potentials. International journal of psychophysiology 2001; 41(1)

[38] Huang YX, Luo YJ. Temporal course of emotional negativity bias: An ERP study. Neuroscience Letters 2006; 398 91-96.

[39] Cacioppo JT, Berntson GG. Relationship between attitudes and evaluative space: A critical review, with emphasis on the separability of positive and negative substrates. Psychological bulletin 1994; 115 401.

[40] Kanske P, Plitschka J, Kotz S.A. Attentional orienting towards emotion: P2 and N400 ERP effects. Neuropsychologia 2011; 49(11) 3121-9.

[41] Ito T, Cacioppo J. Variations on a human universal: Individual differences in positivity offset and negativity bias. Cognition & Emotion 2005; 19 1-26.

[42] Liu B, Jin Z, Wang Z, Hu Y. The interaction between pictures and words: evidence from positivity offset and negativity bias. Experimental Brain Research 2009; 201 141-153.

[43] Carretié L, Hinojosa JA, Albert J, López-Martín S, de La Gándara BS, Igoa JM, Sotillo M. Modulation of ongoing cognitive processes by emotionally intense words. Psychophysiology 2008; 45 188-196.

[44] Hinojosa JA, Carretié L, Valcarcel MA, Mendez-Bertolo C, Pozo MA. Electrophysiological differences in the processing of affective information in words and pictures. Cognitive, Affective, & Behavioral Neuroscience 2009; 9 173-189.

[45] Kissler J, Assadollahi R, Herbert C. Emotional and semantic networks in visual word processing: insights from ERP studies. Progress in brain research 2006; 156 147-183.

[46] Keil A, Ihssen N, Heim S. Early cortical facilitation for emotionally arousing targets during the attentional blink. BMC biology 2006; 4 23.

[47] Mogg K, Bradley BP. A cognitive-motivational analysis of anxiety. Behaviour research and therapy 1998; 36 809-848.

[48] Baas D, Aleman A, Kahn RS. Lateralization of amygdala activation: a systematic review of functional neuroimaging studies. Brain Research Brain Research Reviews 2004; 45(2) 96-103.

[49] Hikosaka O, Nakamura K, Nakahara H. Basal Ganglia orient eyes to reward. Journal of Neurophysiology. 2006; 95567–584.

[50] Kringelbach ML. The human orbital frontal cortex: linking reward to hedonic experience. Nature Reviews Neuroscience 2005; 6691–702.

[51] Luu P, Collins P, Tucker DM. Mood, personality, and self-monitoring: negative affect and emotionality in relation to frontal lobe mechanisms of error monitoring. Journal Experimental Psychology: General 2000; 129(1) 43–60.

[52] Pessoa L. How do emotion and motivation direct executive control? Trends in Cognitive Science 2009; 13(4)160–166.

[53] Phelps EA, LaBar KS, Anderson AK, O'Connor KJ, Fulbright RK, Spencer DS. Specifying the contributions of the human amygdala to emotional memory: A case study. Neurocase 1998; 4527–540.

[54] Levens SM, Phelps EA. Insula and orbital frontal cortex activity underlying emotion interference resolution in working memory. Journal of Cognitive Neuroscience 2010; 22(12) 2790-803.

[55] Levens SM, Devinsky O, Phelps EA. Role of the left amygdala and right orbital frontal cortex in emotional interference resolution facilitation in working memory. Neuropsychologia 2011; 49(12) 3201–3212. doi:10.1016/j.neuropsychologia.2011.07.021.

[56] Landis T. Emotional words: what's so different from just words? Cortex 2006; 42(6) 823–830.

[57] Méndez-Bértolo C, Pozo MA, Hinojosa JA. Early effects of emotion on word immediate repetition priming: electrophysiological and source localization evidence. Cognitive, affective and behavioral neuroscience 2011; 11(4)652-65.

[58] Palazova M, Mantwill K, Sommer W, Schacht A. Are effects of emotion in single words non-lexical? Evidence from event-related brain potentials. Neuropsychologia 2011; 49(9) 2766-2775.

[59] Trauer SM, Andersen SK, Kotz SA, Müller MM. Capture of lexical but not visual resources by task-irrelevant emotional words: a combined ERP and steady-state visual evoked potential study. Neuroimage 2012; 60(1) 130-8.

[60] Alameda JR, Cuetos F. Diccionario de frecuencias de las unidades linguísticas del castellano. Universidad de Oviedo, Oviedo; 1995.

[61] Kirk RE. Experimental design: procedures for the behavioral sciences, 3rd. ed. Brooks/Cole Publishing Company, Belmont. 1995.

[62] Sakaki M, Gorlick MA, Mather M. Differential interference effects of negative emotional states on subsequent semantic and perceptual processing. Emotion 2011; 11(6) 1263-78.

[63] Giesen C, Rothermund K. Affective matching moderates S-R binding. Cognition & Emotion 2011; 25(2) 342-350.

[64] Frings C, Wühr P. Don't be afraid of irrelevant words: The emotional Stroop effect is confined to attended words. Cognition & Emotion 2012; 26(6)1056-68.

[65] Guillet R, Arndt J. Taboo words: the effect of emotion on memory for peripheral information. Memory and Cognition 2009; 37(6) 866-879.

[66] Furl N, Gallagher S, Averbeck BB. A selective emotional decision-making bias elicited by facial expressions. PLoS One 2012; 7(3) e33461.

[67] Sherman GD, Haidt J, Coan JA. Viewing cute images increases behavioral carefulness. Emotion 2009; 9(2) 282–286.

[68] Rohner JC, Rasmussen A. Recognition bias and the physical attractiveness stereotype. Scandinavian Journal of Psychology 2012; 53(3) 239-46. doi: 10.1111/j.1467-9450.2012.00939.x.

[69] Nijboer TC, Jellema T. Unequal impairment in the recognition of positive and negative emotions after right hemisphere lesions: a left hemisphere bias for happy faces. Journal of Neuropsychology 2012; 6(1) 79-93. doi: 10.1111/j.1748-6653.2011.02007.x.

[70] Balconi M, Ferrari C. RTMS stimulation on left DLPFC affects emotional cue retrieval as a function of anxiety level and gender. Depression and Anxiety 2012; doi: 10.1002/da.21968.

[71] Ruhnau P, Wetzel N, Widmann A, Schröger E. The modulation of auditory novelty processing by working memory load in school age children and adults: a combined behavioral and event-related potential study. BMC Neuroscience 2010; 11 126.

[72] San Miguel I, Linden D, Escera C. Attention capture by novel sounds: Distraction vs. facilitation. European Journal of Cognitive Psychology 2010; 22 481–515. doi: 10.1080/09541440902930994.

[73] San Miguel I, Corral MJ, Escera C. When loading working memory reduces distraction: behavioral and electrophysiological evidence from an auditory-visual distraction paradigm. Journal of Cognitive Neuroscience 2008; 20(7) 1131-45.

[74] Muller-Gass A, Schröger E. Perceptual and cognitive task difficulty has differential effects on auditory distraction. Brain Research 2007; 1136(1) 169-77.

[75] Ciesielski KT, Harris RJ, Cofer LF. Posterior brain ERP patterns related to the go/no-go task in children. Psychophysiology 2004; 41(6) 882-892.

[76] Näätänen R, Simpson M, Loveless NE. Stimulus deviance and evoked potentials. Biological Psychology 1982; 14(1-2) 53-98.

[77] Bentin S, Mouchetant-Rostaing Y, Giard MH, Echallier JF, Pernier J: ERP manifestations of processing printed words at different psycholinguistic levels: time course and scalp distribution. Journal of Cognitive Neuroscience 1999; 11 235-260.

[78] Brem S, Lang-Dullenkopf A, Maurer U, Halder P, Bucher K, Brandeis D. Neurophysiological signs of rapidly emerging visual expertise for symbol strings. NeuroReport 2005; 16 45-48.

[79] Cao X, Li S, Zhao J, Lin S, Weng X: Left-lateralized early neurophysiological response for Chinese characters in young primary school children. Neuroscience Letters 2011; 492 165-169.

[80] Simon G, Petit L, Bernard C, Rebaï M. N170 ERPs could represent a logographic processing strategy in visual word recognition. Behavioral brain functions 2007; 321.

[81] Maillard L, Barbeau EJ, Baumann C, Koessler L, Bénar C, Chauvel P, Liégeois-Chauvel C: From perception to recognition memory: time course and lateralization of neu-

ral substrates of word and abstract picture processing. Journal of Cognitive Neuroscience 2011; 23 782-800.

[82] Rossion B, Joyce CA, Cottrell GW, Tarr MJ: Early lateralization and orientation tuning for face, word, and object processing in the visual cortex. Neuroimage 2003, 20: 1609-1624.

[83] Joyce C, Rossion B. The face-sensitive N170 and VPP components manifest the same brain processes: the effect of reference electrode site. Clinical Neurophysiology 2005; 116(11) 2613-2631.

[84] Szucs D, Soltesz F, Czigler I, Csepe V. Electroencephalography effects to semantic and non-semantic mismatch in properties of visually presented single-characters: the N2b and the N400. Neuroscience Letters 2007; 412(1) 18-23.

[85] Zhang X, Wang Y, Li S, Wang L. Event-related potential N270, a negative component to identification of conflicting information following memory retrieval. Clinical Neurophysiology 2003; 114(12) 2461- 2468.

[86] vanSchie HT, Wijers AA, Mars RB, Benjamins JS, Stowe LA. Processing of visual semantic information to concrete words: temporal dynamics and neural mechanisms indicated by event-related brain potentials. Cognitive Neuropsychology 2005; 22(3) 364-86.

[87] Wlotko EW, Federmeier KD. So that's what you meant! Event-related potentials reveal multiple aspects of context use during construction of message-level meaning. Neuroimage 2012; 62(1) 356-366.

Section 2

Functional Neuroimaging in Vision, Mood and Cognition

Chapter 8

Genetic Marker Mice and Their Use in Understanding Learning and Memory

Mark Murphy, Yvette M. Wilson and
Christopher Butler

Additional information is available at the end of the chapter

http://dx.doi.org/10.5772/56498

1. Introduction

The advent of genetically encoded marker proteins to follow functional and structural change in neurons has been a major technical advance in neuroscience. These proteins have been used to image cellular changes *in vitro* and *in vivo* and have enabled the identification of activated neurons which are involved in a diverse array of functions in the brain. Particular marker proteins have also been employed to trace the changes in neuronal activation following different functional stimuli both *in vitro* and *in vivo*. Another major advance in utilising genetically encoded marker proteins has been the development of techniques which allow the specific stimulation or inhibition of neuronal function of specified subsets of neurons which express these proteins. This has allowed the precise targeting of subpopulations of neurons within sub-nuclei within the brain to determine their function. In this article, we will summarise the major types of genetically encoded marker proteins and their uses in studies of neuronal function, predominantly in the mouse. We will give examples where they have been used in behavioural studies, with a particular emphasis on learning and memory.

2. Transgenic marker mice

In contrast to traditional staining or dye-injection techniques, labelling cells using a genetic approach enables the identification of specific cell types, sub-types, as well as the temporal and spatial aspects of genetic expression [1]. One of the most widely used reporter proteins is the bacterial β-galactosidase (βgal) enzyme, encoded by the *E. coli* gene *LacZ* [2]. Inserting the *LacZ* gene into a cell under the control of a given set of transcriptional elements enables the biochemical labelling of cells in which expression of the gene of interest has taken place. One of the first such studies in learning and memory utilized a transgenic mouse containing the *LacZ* gene regulated by six cAMP response elements (CREs) upstream of a minimal promoter [3, 4]. The CRE system and CRE binding protein (CREB) are important transcription elements involved in learning and memory. CRE-mediated *LacZ* expression was induced by long term potentiation (LTP) in area CA1 of the hippocampus and was also induced in CA1 and CA3 and amygdala following different forms of fear conditioning [3, 4], which is consistent with neurons in these areas of the brain being involved in contextual and fear memory.

This *CRE-LacZ* mouse was also used to examine neuronal activation in the barrel fields of the somatosensory cortex, which receive and map sensory information from the facial whiskers. Removal of all but one facial whisker resulted in highly specific *LacZ* expression in layer IV of the spared whisker barrel, and was accompanied by an increase in responsiveness of neurons in layer II/III of the same barrel. These findings suggested that CRE expression in layer IV was in neurons presynaptic to the altered neurons in layer II/III [5].

Given that βgal diffusion into the processes of a *LacZ* expressing neuron is minimal, this traditional method of *LacZ* reporting can only provide limited information in studies of the nervous system, where data on the morphology, structure, and connections between neurons is often required [1]. Neurons and their processes can thus be visualised by the use of *LacZ*-fusion genes, whereby the *LacZ* gene is fused to a gene encoding a separate, neuronal protein that is known to be trafficked throughout the cell [2]. For example in *Drosophila*, the entire neuron has been labelled by fusing *LacZ* with the gene for the microtubule-binding protein tau [2].

The *Fos-Tau-LacZ* (*FTL*) transgenic mouse was created to enable the identification of functionally activated neurons in the mouse brain following a given behavioural task [6]. The mouse expresses a transgene that encodes the tau-βgal fusion protein, driven by the promoter for the immediate early gene c-*fos*. This immediate-early gene is expressed in neurons following functional stimulation, with expression shown to occur following a range of stimuli including stress, ischemia, sensory stimulation, endocrine hormones and various pharmacological agents [6]. The *FTL* transgene is thus rapidly expressed in neurons following functional stimulation, and trafficked throughout the cell body, dendrites and axon. This labelling enables the localisation of functionally activated neurons, the identification of their cellular morphologies and the connections they make with other neurons in the brain [6]. Labelling experiments that utilise the *FTL* mouse include the identification of the neuronal nuclei involved in osmoregulation [6], as well as the identification of light activated pathways in the visual system [7]. However, the findings most pertinent to this review occur from the analysis of *FTL* mouse brains following context fear conditioning.

Context fear conditioning is a model for learning, and training *FTL* mice to associate the context of a shock chamber with the aversive stimulus of a foot-shock enables the identification of the neurons that are functionally activated by this association. Initially, a discrete population of glutamatergic neurons were identified along the lateral edge of the lateral amygdala [8]. These FTL^+ neurons only appeared in those *FTL* mice that had learned to associate the context with shock, indicating that these cells may be involved in the circuits responsible for this learning process [8]. A further study was able to identify other nuclei of labelled neurons, in the medial amygdala, the amygdalo-striatal transition region, and the ventromedial hypothalamus [9]. It was also shown that these regions were not activated following the recall of memory or following fear expression, but specifically by the association of context to shock, suggesting that these neurons were involved in this learning event [9]. These anatomically restricted populations were hypothesised to be nodes within a circuit for fear conditioning [9]. In this way, a modified version of the βgal marker protein has contributed to our understanding of the circuitry that underlies the formation of fear memories in mammals.

Perhaps the most widely studied cellular marker protein is the Green Fluorescent Protein (GFP). First isolated from *Aequorea* jellyfish, GFP was found to produce bright green fluorescence in the presence of ultraviolet light [10]. The GFP gene was first used as a marker of genetic expression [11], with the finding that both prokaryotic and eukaryotic cells were capable of expressing the protein and that this expression was non-toxic to the cell. In a similar fashion to βgal, GFP is thus capable of acting as a marker of genetic expression as well as enabling the labelling of specific populations of cells.

Fos-GFP mice have been generated and used to study plasticity in the barrel cortex in a series of studies following on from those using the *CRE-LacZ* mice [5, 12-15]. Similar to the results from the *CRE-LacZ* mice, expression of GFP in the *fos-GFP* mice was specific to the barrel field of the spared whisker in mice where all whiskers bar one were removed. The use of GFP as a marker also permitted electrophysiological recordings of these neurons, and it was found that both the GFP^+ and GFP^- neurons within the same region of the spared barrel had altered action potentials and spike frequencies compared to neurons in non-spared barrels. Subsequent experiments with *fos-GFP* mice identified increased amplitudes of the AMPA glutamate receptor in the spared barrel column [13]. This was due to the specific delivery of AMPA receptors at the inputs to the spared, but not deprived, barrels. These findings suggested that delivery of AMPA receptors is a normal feature of synaptic strengthening underlying experience dependent plasticity [13]. Further experiments studied the effects of ongoing stimulation of the spared whisker [12]. *N*-methyl-D-aspartate (NMDA) receptors were required to initiate synaptic strengthening at the layer IV-II/III synapse. However with additional sensory activity, strengthening was dependent on activation of metabotropic glutamate receptors, which suggests a mechanism whereby continued experience can result in synaptic strengthening over time [12].

Recently, the Barth group studied the properties of GFP^+ neurons in the cortex of unstimulated *fos-GFP* mice as a method to study neurons which were recently active in cortex [16]. GFP^+ neurons had higher firing rates compared to GFP^- neurons, which was due to increased excitatory and decreased inhibitory drive of the GFP^+ neurons. Paired cell recordings indicated that the GFP^+ neurons had a greater likelihood of being connected to each other. These results suggested that the GFP^+ neurons represented interconnected neuronal ensembles in neocortex, possibly involved in coding of sensory information [16].

Since its initial discovery, a number of GFP variants have been created, improving the efficiency and stability of the protein as well as altering its spectral properties [17]. In this way, different colours of emitted light can be produced. Red, yellow and cyan fluorescent proteins (RFP, YFP, and CFP, or XFPs collectively) have each been created, enabling experiments that label multiple cell types or expression profiles within the same biological sample [18]. The use of multiple XFPs is perhaps exemplified by the creation of the 'Brainbow' mouse, whereby individual neurons in the mouse brain express different ratios of the XFPs, enabling the distinctive tagging of individual neurons with at least 90 different fluorescent colours [19]. The Brainbow mouse enables the visualisation of the precise morphology of closely juxtaposed neurons, and has had major contributions to the study of neural connections in the brain [20].

Specifically targeting the expression of XFPs to neurons is typically achieved by driving expression of the XFPs by the promoter for the thymocyte antigen protein Thy-1, a cell surface protein. Thy-1 is a known marker of axonal processes in mature neurons, thus Thy1-XFP transgenes specifically label neurons in the brain [21]. A large number of learning and memory studies that utilise the various XFPs have also used the Thy-1-XFP fusion transgene to fluorescently tag neurons and their processes. These neurons can then be visualised *in vitro* using fluorescence confocal microscopy, as well as visualising *in vivo* using two-photon microscopy.

2.1. Conditional transgenic marker mice

In addition to the marker mice described above, it is also possible to conditionally regulate the gene which controls marker expression. Some of the conditional expression systems include Cre recombinase/lox site insertions, excisions and other modifications, and the tetracycline (tet) systems based on the tet-controlled transactivator (tTa) and reverse tet-on transactivator (rtTA) that allow downregulation or induction of gene expression [22]. A conditional transgenic mouse employing the tet system has been developed and used in studies of learning and memory [23]. This *TetTag* mouse has two transgenes: 1. containing the c-*fos* promoter regulating expression of tTa, which will bind to 2. the *TetO* promoter regulating expression of *tau-LacZ*. Binding to the *TetO* promoter is inhibited by doxycycline, and thus by maintaining the mice on doxycycline, this system is blocked. However, the second transgene also contains a doxycycline insensitive tTa, and once this transgene is activated, a feedback loop is established which will maintain expression of the doxycycline insensitive tTa and consequently also *tau-LacZ*. This allows for the long term tagging of neurons which express c-*fos* during the window when the mice were taken off doxycycline [23]. Using this *TetTag* mouse, a small number of neurons in the basolateral amygdala, which were activated and tagged during fear conditioning learning, were found to be subsequently reactivated during recall of fear conditioning [23]. It was thus suggested that these neurons were a stable neural correlate of fear memory.

A variant of this experiment involved the c-*fos*-tTa transgene in combination with a *TetO*-GFP-GluR1 transgene [24]. GluR1 is a major subunit of the AMPA glutamate receptor and using this conditional marker mouse, the location of newly synthesised AMPA receptors could be followed using GFP fluorescence. Following fear conditioning, newly synthesised GluR1 receptors were found to be selectively associated with mushroom-type dendritic spines on hippocampal CA1 neurons [24]. These results were argued to be consistent with a synaptic tagging model whereby activated synapses capture new AMPA receptors as part the learning and memory process.

2.2. Viral-mediated gene delivery

Genetic manipulation of the neurons involved in learning and memory has also been achieved using viral methods of transgene delivery, enabling targeting of specific brain regions. In one series of studies, the question of how neurons become involved in memory was addressed and if the transcriptional status of the neuron at the time of learning was important in this process. For this, the function of CREB was manipulated via delivery of a series of different CREB containing viruses to the lateral amygdala [25, 26]. Increasing CREB function in any lateral amygdala neuron appeared to increase the probability that this neuron was recruited into the fear memory trace, suggesting that CREB status is important in determining which neurons are involved in memory [25]. Further, ablation of these overexpressing CREB neurons after learning blocked the expression of the specific fear memory in which they were involved, establishing that these neurons were functionally required for that specific fear memory [26]. Broadly consistent results were found when the CREB viruses were targeted to the auditory thalamus [27].

3. Two-photon imaging using transgenic marker mice

Transgenic marker mice have been used very successfully to follow changes in neuron structure over time. In initial studies of this kind, individual neurons were imaged in developing hippocampus of rat brains expressing enhanced GFP, via infection with GFP encoding Sindbis virus [28]. Imaging of the neurons was done using two-photon laser scanning microscopy, which has the advantage of detecting the fluorescence signal with very low levels of photobleaching and phototoxicity. This allows for repeated high resolution imaging deep into living neural tissue with little effect on the imaged neurons. These studies demonstrated change in dendritic structure driven by high frequency synaptic stimulation, suggesting that synaptic activation during development could contribute to development of neural circuitry [28].

Subsequent studies have undertaken imaging of dendritic spines over time. Dendritic spines are protrusions from dendrites and are the postsynaptic sites of excitatory synapses. Thus imaging changes in dendritic spines over time is a very good approach to studying structural synaptic plasticity. Synaptic plasticity is thought to be a prime candidate mechanism underlying the processes involved in learning and memory. Two-photon imaging of dendritic spines was undertaken in hippocampal slices [29] using one of the lines of thy1-GFP expressing mice (line M) generated by Feng et al. [18]. Induction of LTP in these slices resulted in a transient increase in spine area of a small fraction of spines. Similar to LTP, this increase was dependent on NMDA receptor activation which is hypothesised to contribute to the synapse remodelling that occurs in LTP [29]. Similar results were obtained in experiments using hippocampal slices from non-transgenic rats [30].

In further experiments using the thy1-GFP-M mice [18], two-photon microscopy was used to study relationships between spines following LTP [31]. Following induction of LTP at individual synapses of hippocampal pyramidal neurons, the response thresholds at closely neighbouring synapses on the same dendrite were found to be altered [31]. Thus, presentation of low level stimuli, which were normally too weak to induce LTP, resulted in robust LTP and spine enlargement at these neighbouring synapses. The reduction in this threshold for LTP was short lived (~10 minutes) and extended over 10 micron of dendrite length. It was proposed that these interactions between neighbouring synapses were consistent with clustered models of plasticity in memory storage as well as providing a mechanism for binding of behaviourally linked information within a small region of a dendrite [31].

3.1. Two-photon imaging *in vivo*

The two-photon imaging approach has been extended to studies of living animals to great effect. This is done by removing a small area of skull from the mice, which allows for repeated imaging of the exposed cortex using two-photon microscopy. The major advance in this approach is that single neurons can be studied in living mice over extended periods of time, up to many months. This allows for the mapping of spines on a particular dendrite and the tracking of the changes in spine number, morphology and lifetime of individual spines over this time. Thus, one can examine the effects of learning on spines, and accompanying studies can ask if the observed spine changes result in synaptic changes.

The first studies to use this approach undertook imaging of spines in individual pyramidal neurons in visual cortex and barrel cortex over periods of a month to over a year [32, 33]. Using thy1-GFP-line H mice [18], they found that dendritic structure was essentially stable, and that spines appear and disappear. In barrel cortex, 50% of spines were stable for at least a month, with the other spines present for days or less [32]. These spine changes were shown to correlate with synaptic change. Further, sensory experience of the facial whiskers (the principle input for the barrel cortex) resulted in increased spine turnover [32]. In adult visual cortex, the great majority of spines were stable for at least one month [33]. However, in visual cortex of young mice during the critical period of visual cortical development, about 70% of spines were stable for at least one month, with most changes due to spine elimination [33]. These findings thus demonstrated spine turnover in cortex, and that developmental stage and sensory experience can alter that turnover. Further studies in different regions of the mouse cortex also confirmed that spine turnover varies across the cortex [34].

Most synapses which occur on dendritic spines are excitatory, and most of the changes described above probably represent changes in excitatory synapses. There is no obvious morphological hallmark for inhibitory synapses. Recently, genetic markers have been developed to allow the visualisation of both inhibitory synapses and dendritic spines on pyramidal neuron dendrites. The markers were a) teal fluorescent protein fused to gephyrin, a postsynaptic protein only expressed in inhibitory synapses, and b) YFP to label neuronal morphology [35]. Plasmids expressing these markers were inserted into the embryonic cortices of mice via electroporation. Using this combination of markers, it was found that inhibitory synapses and dendritic spines (as proxy for excitatory synapses) differed in their distribution pattern across the dendritic arbor [35]. However, remodelling of both inhibitory synapses and dendritic spines occurred within the same spatially clustered regions on the dendritic arbor and this clustering was influenced by sensory input. These findings suggested that both excitatory and inhibitory synapse rearrangement occurs and may be coordinated at the dendritic level [35].

Whereas dendritic structure is stable in pyramidal neurons, other classes of neurons in the cortex show dynamic changes in dendritic structure over time. Imaging of thy1-GFP-S mice [18] showed that GABA+ inhibitory interneurons extend and retract dendritic branches over periods of months and in a small proportion of neurons, new branch tips emerge [36]. In the visual cortex, visual deprivation stimulates this structural remodelling, affecting up to 16% of branch tips [37]. Visual deprivation induces branch retractions, which is accompanied by loss of inhibitory inputs to neighbouring pyramidal neurons and results in a decrease in inhibitory tone [37]. Further studies show that interneuron remodelling occurs across the major primary sensory cortex regions, but may differ in degree between primary and higher order sensory cortical areas [38]. These studies show that the dendritic arbor of inhibitory neurons changes over time, is influenced by sensory input, and that these changes correlate with functional changes in sensory cortex.

3.2. Two-photon imaging in learning and memory

The effects of learning have been directly studied using *in vivo* imaging of dendritic spines. In two such studies, young (1 month) and adult thy1-GFP-H mice [18] were trained specific motor skills and the effects of that training on motor cortex were followed [39, 40]. Training in a forelimb reaching task resulted in formation of dendritic spines within one hour in the pyramidal neurons in contralateral motor cortex [39]. Training on a rotarod also increased production of new spines in motor cortex [40]. These new spines were stabilised by subsequent training and persisted long after training stopped and into adulthood [39, 40]. However, spines present before training were selectively eliminated and thus overall spine density returned to its original level. Other motor skills resulted in production of different sets of spines [39]. These findings suggested that specific motor skills are encoded by particular sets of newly generated and long lasting synaptic connections [39, 40].

Subsequent studies using the motor learning model showed that a third of the new spines formed during learning emerged as clusters, generally as pairs of spines [41]. These clustered spines were more likely to persist than newly formed single spines. The clusters were formed in succession, with later spines in the cluster formed during repetition of the motor task [41]. Thus, these new clusters are formed by repetitive activation of particular cortical circuits and correspond to the strength of the motor memory.

Other studies in learning and memory using two-photon imaging of YFP+ dendritic spines have provided somewhat counter-intuitive findings. Studies of fear conditioning by pairing an auditory cue with a foot-shock provide evidence that this results in an increase in the rate of spine elimination in frontal association cortex [42]. In contrast, extinguishing the fear memory by presenting the auditory cue without foot-shock, increased the rate of spine formation. Both of these changes in spine number were observed on the same dendrites and within the same region of the dendrite. Further reconditioning of the mice tended to result in elimination of the spines which were formed by extinction [42]. These findings suggest both that the fear memory trace is partly generated through reduction of particular synaptic contacts and that this is eliminated through opposing actions of extinction on these synapses.

4. Genetically engineered calcium indicators

Ca^{2+} is one of the master second messengers for the cell, being involved in a vast array of cellular processes. Many studies have employed various chemical Ca^{2+} indicators to study Ca^{2+} flux in the cell. These chemical Ca^{2+} indicators are generally based on the Ca^{2+} chelator BAPTA (1,2-bis(o-aminophenoxy)ethane-N,N,N',N'-tetraacetic acid). A particular advantage of the Ca^{2+} indicators is the very high temporal resolution (millisecond scale) as these indicators are changing their fluorescence essentially in time with Ca^{2+} flux in the cell. In recent years, a new class of Ca^{2+} indicators has been developed; the genetically engineered Ca^{2+} indicators (GECI; 43-45). These indicators are formed by the fusion of genetically engineered fluorescent proteins with proteins which bind Ca^{2+}. Upon binding of Ca^{2+} the confirmation of the GECI changes, which results in a change in its fluorescence properties. The principal advantages of the GECIs over the chemical Ca^{2+} indicators is that they can be targeted to specific functional subpopulations of neurons by the use of cell specific gene promoters to control their expression, they can be delivered to particular brain regions using viral injection, and expression is relatively stable for several months.

The first GECIs were the Cameleons, which were fusions of blue- or cyan- variants of GFP with calmodulin, the calmodulin-binding peptide M13, and an enhanced green- or yellow-emitting GFP [45]. Binding of Ca^{2+} results in consequent binding of M13 with calmodulin and an increase in fluorescent resonance energy transfer between the two GFPs in the protein [45]. Another form of GECI is the GCaMP (GFP–Calmodulin–M13 Protein), which uses a circularly permuted GFP where the N- and C- termini of GFP are fused [46, 47]. Calmodulin and M13 are fused to this circularly permuted GFP, and on binding of Ca^{2+}, the conformation of the fusion protein is altered which results in increased fluorescence of GFP [46, 47]. Other forms of GECIs use Troponin C instead of Calmodulin and M13 to induce binding of Ca^{2+} and conformational change in the fusion protein [48]. The different types of GECIs have different properties and particular advantages in Ca^{2+} imaging studies [43].

Ca^{2+} influx and regulation of signalling plays a fundamental role in the molecular mechanisms underlying learning and memory. For example, the NMDA glutamate receptor is regarded as one of the most important neurotransmitter receptors in the initial acquisition process of learning and memory [49-51]. The NMDA receptors are highly permeable to Ca^{2+} ions, but this permeability only occurs during both membrane depolarisation and glutamate binding [52]. Such conditions are regarded as a requirement for memory acquisition. Inside the neuron, Ca^{2+} regulates many intracellular signalling processes involved in memory formation [50, 51, 53]. Thus the use of GECIs may be useful in learning and memory studies; for example in identifying neuronal populations undergoing changes in Ca^{2+} concentrations during learning and memory and in studying the temporal progression of such changes. However, there have been few studies to date which have used this approach in learning and memory research.

http://dx.doi.org/10.5772/56498

Recent studies have developed methods for the cellular imaging of neural activity in awake behaving mice and which can be suitable for analysis of cellular responses during learning and memory. For example, one study describes a method to visualise cellular imaging of neural activity in the visual cortex of awake head restrained mice during visual discrimination learning as well as passive viewing of visual stimuli [54]. Neural activity was measured using the yellow Cameleon 3.6 GECI, virally transfected into visual cortex. Another approach has been developed which enables imaging the activity of neurons in head restrained mice which can still perform spatial behaviours within a virtual reality system [55]. In the example given, the activity of neurons in the CA1 region of the hippocampus was imaged through the expression of the GCaMP3 GECI. Populations of place cells were thus identified based on their place specific activity within the virtual environment and correlated with their location within the local hippocampal circuit [55].

An extension of the use of GECIs is the development of indicators which detect the Ca^{2+} activation of Ca^{2+}/calmodulin-dependent protein kinase (CaMKII; 56). These are GECIs using CaMKII as the Ca^{2+} binding protein and thus are specific for CaMKII activation. This indicator has been used to detect changes in CaMKII activity in individual spines of particular regions of cortex before and after visual deprivation [56]. Visual deprivation is a model of experience dependent plasticity and thus this approach could be used in the analysis of spine changes occurring during learning and memory formation.

5. Optogenetics and learning and memory

Optogenetics is a technology currently sweeping through many areas of neuroscience. It relies on the targeted expression of light activated ion channels within any neuronal population one wishes to study [57-59]. The light activated channels belong to the family of microbial opsins. Two classes of these opsins are currently used: 1. Positive ion channels which upon light activation result in depolarisation and activation of the neuron (such as channelrhodopsins ChR1, ChR2, and VChR1), and 2. negative ion channels which upon light stimulation result in hyperpolarisation and inhibition of the neuron (such as *Natronomonas pharaonis* halorhodopsins, NpHR, enhanced halorhodopsins, eNpHR2 and eNpHR3, *Archaerhodopsin, Leptosphaeria maculans* fungal opsin, and enhanced bacteriorhodopsin). The channels are activated very quickly by light, allowing for the precise temporal control of neuronal activation. The light can be delivered by optic fibres to a small volume of brain tissue allowing for good spatial definition of activation and expression of the opsins can be genetically targeted to subpopulations of neurons within the brain region of interest. This combination thus permits the examination of the consequences of either activation or inhibition of neuronal function at a fine temporal, spatial and neuron-type level [58, 59].

5.1. Optogenetics in reward learning

Optogenetic technology has been used to study a number of different types of learning and memory. These include classical conditioning to both rewarding and aversive stimuli, and spatial learning and the role of the hippocampus. Most of these studies have been done in mice, with one study undertaken in *Drosophila* to date [60]. In studies of conditioning to a reward, one of the most important classes of neuron studied is the dopaminergic neuron in the ventral tegmental area (VTA), postulated to be involved in mediating the reward stimulus [61, 62]. However, it was unclear if firing of these neurons alone could result in reward conditioning. To test the role of these neurons, the Cre-inducible adeno-associated virus vector carrying the ChR2 gene fused to enhanced YFP (EYFP) was used [63]. Injection of this vector into the VTA of *Tyrosine hydroxylase – Cre* transgenic mice results in specific expression of ChR2-EYFP in the dopamine neurons. They then tested the effects of optogenetic stimulation of these dopamine neurons on conditioned place preference. The mice received phasic (50 Hz) optical stimulation in one chamber and 1 Hz stimulation in the other chamber of the place preference apparatus. The mice developed a clear place preference to the chamber in which they received the phasic stimulation [63]. These findings demonstrate that phasic firing of the dopamine neurons alone (in the absence of reward) is sufficient for reward conditioning.

These experiments involved conditioned place preference, which is passive behavioural conditioning. To look at the role of the dopaminergic neurons in operant conditioning, these neurons were optogenetically stimulated during an active food seeking operant task [64]. Phasic activation of the dopaminergic neurons enhanced the positive reinforcing actions (pressing a specific lever for a food reward) in this task. This enhancing effect was dependent on the presence of the food reward, in contrast to that seen in the passive conditioning task [64]. However, activation of the dopaminergic neurons alone was sufficient to reactivate a previously extinguished food seeking behaviour. These findings together suggested that activation of the dopaminergic neurons facilitates development of positive reinforcement during active reward seeking [64].

Within the dopamine system, the firing rate of the dopamine neurons is increased for only a very short time following reward events (200 milliseconds) and it was unclear if this was sufficient to be involved in reward learning. To test for this, mice with expression of ChR2-EYFP targeted to the dopamine neurons of the VTA were placed in testing chambers with a port, which when investigated with a nose-poke, triggered a 200 millisecond optogenetic stimulation. This resulted in the mice rapidly learning to nose-poke the port and receive the brief optical stimulations [65]. This demonstrated that the brief time of dopamine neuron firing was sufficient to drive reward learning. Optogenetics has also been used to study the role of GABA neurons in the VTA and shown that these neurons negatively regulate consummatory behaviour and dopamine release from the VTA [66].

Further experiments have looked at the role of other neurons in the putative reward circuit. The nucleus accumbens is strongly implicated in the reward pathway and its input from the basolateral amygdala (BLA) is thought to be involved in cue-triggered motivated behaviours. In order to investigate the function of the BLA to nucleus accumbens pathway during behaviour, the ChR2-EYFP virus was injected into the BLA, and the pathway to the accumbens was targeted for optogenetic stimulation [67]. Mice were then placed in the testing chambers which triggered optogenetic stimulation with a nose-poke. The mice rapidly learnt to receive optical stimulations [67]. To inhibit this pathway, the BLA was injected with a NpHR-EYFP virus, which results in hyperpolarisation upon light stimulation. Optically induced inhibition of the pathway reduced co-evoked intake of sucrose, demonstrating that this pathway controls naturally occurring reward related behaviour. These findings together show that the pathway from BLA to the nucleus accumbens promotes motivated behavioural responding in conjunction with the dopamine pathway from VTA [67].

The striatum is another part of the reward circuit and has been implicated both in positive learning reinforcement as well as negative reinforcement. The striatum contains two populations of projection neurons, characterised by their expression of either dopamine receptor 1 (D1) or 2 (D2). To determine possible roles of these two populations of neurons, they were selectively targeted for optogenetic stimulation [68]. Optical stimulation of the D1 receptor–expressing neurons induced persistent reinforcement, whereas stimulating D2 receptor–expressing neurons induced transient negative reinforcement, indicating that activation of these different populations of neurons has opposite behavioural effects and can result in distinctly different learning outcomes.

5.2. Optogenetics in classical fear conditioning

The amygdala is heavily implicated not only in reward but also in classical conditioning to aversive stimuli that occurs in fear conditioning paradigms. In particular the lateral amygdala is considered to be a site of plasticity underlying fear memory. In order to determine if stimulation of the principle neurons of the lateral amygdala could directly contribute to fear conditioning, mice were infected with the ChR2-EYFP virus to target these neurons [69]. The mice then received an auditory stimulus paired with optical stimulation of the LA neurons instead of being paired with a conventional aversive stimulus. It was found that pairing resulted in successful fear conditioning of the mice. These findings provided direct evidence that fear learning can be a consequence of a stimulus induced activation of the principle neurons of the lateral amygdala [69].

The central amygdala is thought to be involved in transmitting the behavioural response signal to other parts of the brain. Recent information also implicates the central amygdala in fear learning. To investigate this possibility, a series of different approaches, including optogenetically targeted activation of subpopulations of neurons in central amygdala were employed [70]. Neuronal activity in the lateral division of the central amygdala was found to be required for fear memory formation, whereas optogenetic stimulation of neurons in the medial division of the central amygdala indicated that these neurons were involved in fear related (freezing) behavioural expression [70]. These findings suggested that a part of the fear memory is acquired in inhibitory neurons of the medial division, which project to the lateral division of the central amygdala to control their output fear signalling.

Contextual fear conditioning is a form of fear conditioning which is dependent on the hippocampus. It was unclear if the hippocampal neurons which are activated during context fear learning contain enough information to drive fear behaviour when they are specifically re-activated. To test this, neurons which were activated during fear learning in the dentate gyrus of mice were targeted to express ChR2 [71], using a modified *TetTag* mouse described above [23]. Optical stimulation of dentate gyrus alone resulted in freezing, indicating light induced fear memory recall. Further, activation of cells targeted in a context not associated with fear did not result in freezing, suggesting that light-induced fear memory recall is context specific [71]. Essentially similar findings were obtained using non-optogenetic techniques [72]. Together these findings indicate that activation of a sparse and specific population of neurons in dentate gyrus, which were activated during learning, is sufficient for recall of that memory.

Another important issue on the role of the hippocampus in learning and memory is the observation that contextual and explicit memories are first dependent on hippocampus but loss of hippocampus some period of time after acquisition of these memories does not result in loss of these memories [73]. Based on these observations, it has been thought that memories somehow transfer from hippocampus to the cortex over time. Optogenetic approaches were employed to examine the contribution of the hippocampus to long term memories in real-time [74]. Excitatory neurons in dorsal CA1 hippocampus were virally targeted to express the chloride channel, eNpHR3.1. Rapid optical stimulation to inhibit these neurons resulted in reversible abolition of short and long term context fear memory (up to 9 weeks old), indicating hippocampal involvement throughout the period of memory retention [74]. However, when inhibition was extended significantly, the context fear memory became hippocampal independent; suggesting long term memory normally involves hippocampus but can shift to alternate structures. The anterior cingulate cortex had previously been implicated in storage of long term memories, and optogenetically induced inhibition of this region of the cortex resulted in inhibition of long term but not recent context fear memories [74]. These findings thus indicate a permanent role for hippocampus in context memory, with additional roles for anterior cingulate cortex in long term memory.

Another form of fear conditioning involves pairing the aversive stimulus to an auditory stimulus. This auditory fear conditioning is independent of hippocampus and probably involves auditory regions of the brain. Recent experiments indicate that auditory fear conditioning depends on recruitment of a disinhibitory microcircuit in the auditory cortex [75]. Disinhibition in auditory cortex is driven by foot-shock-mediated cholinergic activation of layer I interneurons, which generates inhibition of layer II/III parvalbumin-positive interneurons and subsequently leads to disinhibition of the layer II/III cortical pyramidal neurons. Importantly, optogenetic block of pyramidal neuron disinhibition abolishes fear learning [75]. These findings thus show the involvement of auditory cortex in associative fear learning, but also suggest that layer 1 disinhibition may be an important mechanism underlying different types of learning throughout the cortex.

5.3. Hippocampus and spatial learning

Where many studies have looked at the role of excitatory granule cells of the dentate gyrus in spatial learning, the function of the GABA-ergic inhibitory interneurons, which control the granule neuron activity, is unclear. To investigate the role of these neurons, their activity was inhibited via expression of targeted expression of eNpHR3.0 [76]. Optogenetic inhibition of these GABA-ergic interneurons impaired spatial learning and memory retrieval, without affecting memory retention, as determined in the Morris water maze, thus establishing a role for these neurons in spatial learning and retention [76].

5.4. Other studies in learning and memory

Sleep has been implicated in memory consolidation for many years. Sleep disruption results in memory deficits, which raises the question of whether the continuity of sleep is important for memory consolidation. However, it is difficult to disrupt one feature of sleep (i.e. sleep continuity) without disrupting other sleep features (such as duration and intensity). To introduce a precise way of disrupting sleep continuity, optogenetics was used to target hypocretin/orexin neurons, which play a key role in arousal [77]. Optogenetic activation of these neurons could fragment sleep without affecting total amount or intensity of sleep [77]. Fragmenting sleep this way disrupted performance of the mice in an object recognition task once the duration of sleep episodes decreased below 66% normal. These findings indicated that a minimum of uninterrupted sleep is required for memory consolidation [77].

6. Conclusion

The employment of genetically encoded markers both in transgenic mice and in viral constructs has been a major technical advance for neuroscience and for whole animal biology generally. In studies of learning and memory, the use of this technology is leading to improved understanding in many aspects of this large and varied field of knowledge. The use of this approach is aiding in the identification of the neurons which are involved in learning and memory, in identifying the changes within those neurons which may underlie different parts of the learning process, in understanding potential mechanisms which specify which neurons are involved in learning and memory, and in describing ensembles of neurons which together code the contextual memory in the hippocampus. Two photon imaging using genetic markers in living animals is producing remarkable findings of what synaptic changes occur in learning and memory and how synaptic homeostasis is achieved. The use of Genetically engineered Calcium indicators is at an early stage in learning and memory, but it promises to inform us of real time changes in neuronal activation during learning and memory events.

Optogenetics, which relies on the ability to specifically activate or inhibit specific markers, is rapidly becoming a critical technique throughout neuroscience. Overall, optogenetics is delivering in its promise to enhance our understanding of learning and memory, through its ability to target specific populations of neurons and activate or inhibit them very rapidly and reversibly. This has helped to define the role of these neurons in behaviours associated with the learning and memory process, to ask if these neurons are involved in learning or memory *per se*, and to determine directly the role of these neurons - without the complexity of relatively slow lesioning studies and attendant compensation which the brain undertakes to circumvent the lesion.

Author details

Mark Murphy*, Yvette M. Wilson and Christopher Butler

*Address all correspondence to: m.murphy@unimelb.edu.au

Department of Anatomy and Neuroscience, University of Melbourne, Melbourne, Victoria, Australia

References

[1] Callahan CA, Yoshikawa S, Thomas JB. Tracing axons. Curr Opin Neurobiol. 1998;8(5):582-6. Epub 1998/11/13.

[2] Callahan CA, Thomas JB. Tau-beta-galactosidase, an axon-targeted fusion protein. Proc Natl Acad Sci U S A. 1994;91(13):5972-6.

[3] Impey S, Mark M, Villacres EC, Poser S, Chavkin C, Storm DR. Induction of CRE-mediated gene expression by stimuli that generate long-lasting LTP in area CA1 of the hippocampus. Neuron. 1996;16(5):973-82. Epub 1996/05/01.

[4] Impey S, Smith DM, Obrietan K, Donahue R, Wade C, Storm DR. Stimulation of cAMP response element (CRE)-mediated transcription during contextual learning. Nat Neurosci. 1998;1(7):595-601.

[5] Barth AL, McKenna M, Glazewski S, Hill P, Impey S, Storm D, et al. Upregulation of cAMP response element-mediated gene expression during experience-dependent plasticity in adult neocortex. J Neurosci. 2000;20(11):4206-16.

[6] Wilson Y, Nag N, Davern P, Oldfield BJ, McKinley MJ, Greferath U, et al. Visualization of functionally activated circuitry in the brain. Proc Natl Acad Sci U S A. 2002;99(5):3252-7.

[7] Greferath U, Nag N, Zele AJ, Bui BV, Wilson Y, Vingrys AJ, et al. Fos-tau-LacZ mice expose light-activated pathways in the visual system. Neuroimage. 2004;23(3): 1027-38.

[8] Wilson YM, Murphy M. A discrete population of neurons in the lateral amygdala is specifically activated by contextual fear conditioning. Learn Mem. 2009;16(6):357-61.

[9] Trogrlic L, Wilson YM, Newman AG, Murphy M. Context fear learning specifically activates distinct populations of neurons in amygdala and hypothalamus. Learn Mem. 2011;18(10):678-87. Epub 2011/10/05.

[10] Shimomura O, Johnson FH, Saiga Y. Extraction, purification and properties of aequorin, a bioluminescent protein from the luminous hydromedusan, Aequorea. Journal of cellular and comparative physiology. 1962;59:223-39. Epub 1962/06/01.

[11] Chalfie M, Tu Y, Euskirchen G, Ward WW, Prasher DC. Green fluorescent protein as a marker for gene expression. Science. 1994;263(5148):802-5. Epub 1994/02/11.

[12] Clem RL, Celikel T, Barth AL. Ongoing in vivo experience triggers synaptic metaplasticity in the neocortex. Science. 2008;319(5859):101-4.

[13] Clem RL, Barth A. Pathway-specific trafficking of native AMPARs by in vivo experience. Neuron. 2006;49(5):663-70.

[14] Barth AL, Gerkin RC, Dean KL. Alteration of neuronal firing properties after in vivo experience in a FosGFP transgenic mouse. J Neurosci. 2004;24(29):6466-75.

[15] Benedetti BL, Glazewski S, Barth AL. Reliable and precise neuronal firing during sensory plasticity in superficial layers of primary somatosensory cortex. J Neurosci. 2009;29(38):11817-27. Epub 2009/09/25.

[16] Yassin L, Benedetti BL, Jouhanneau JS, Wen JA, Poulet JF, Barth AL. An embedded subnetwork of highly active neurons in the neocortex. Neuron. 2010;68(6):1043-50. Epub 2010/12/22.

[17] Tsien RY. The green fluorescent protein. Annual review of biochemistry. 1998;67:509-44. Epub 1998/10/06.

[18] Feng G, Mellor RH, Bernstein M, Keller-Peck C, Nguyen QT, Wallace M, et al. Imaging neuronal subsets in transgenic mice expressing multiple spectral variants of GFP. Neuron. 2000;28(1):41-51.

[19] Livet J, Weissman TA, Kang H, Draft RW, Lu J, Bennis RA, et al. Transgenic strategies for combinatorial expression of fluorescent proteins in the nervous system. Nature. 2007;450(7166):56-62. Epub 2007/11/02.

[20] Lichtman JW, Livet J, Sanes JR. A technicolour approach to the connectome. Nat Rev Neurosci. 2008;9(6):417-22. Epub 2008/05/01.

[21] Andra K, Abramowski D, Duke M, Probst A, Wiederhold KH, Burki K, et al. Expression of APP in transgenic mice: a comparison of neuron-specific promoters. Neurobiology of aging. 1996;17(2):183-90. Epub 1996/03/01.

[22] Bockamp E, Sprengel R, Eshkind L, Lehmann T, Braun JM, Emmrich F, et al. Conditional transgenic mouse models: from the basics to genome-wide sets of knockouts and current studies of tissue regeneration. Regenerative medicine. 2008;3(2):217-35. Epub 2008/03/01.

[23] Reijmers LG, Perkins BL, Matsuo N, Mayford M. Localization of a stable neural correlate of associative memory. Science. 2007;317(5842):1230-3.

[24] Matsuo N, Reijmers L, Mayford M. Spine-type-specific recruitment of newly synthesized AMPA receptors with learning. Science. 2008;319(5866):1104-7.

[25] Han JH, Kushner SA, Yiu AP, Cole CJ, Matynia A, Brown RA, et al. Neuronal competition and selection during memory formation. Science. 2007;316(5823):457-60.

[26] Han JH, Kushner SA, Yiu AP, Hsiang HL, Buch T, Waisman A, et al. Selective erasure of a fear memory. Science. 2009;323(5920):1492-6.

[27] Han JH, Yiu AP, Cole CJ, Hsiang HL, Neve RL, Josselyn SA. Increasing CREB in the auditory thalamus enhances memory and generalization of auditory conditioned fear. Learn Mem. 2008;15(6):443-53.

[28] Maletic-Savatic M, Malinow R, Svoboda K. Rapid dendritic morphogenesis in CA1 hippocampal dendrites induced by synaptic activity. Science. 1999;283(5409):1923-7. Epub 1999/03/19.

[29] Lang C, Barco A, Zablow L, Kandel ER, Siegelbaum SA, Zakharenko SS. Transient expansion of synaptically connected dendritic spines upon induction of hippocampal long-term potentiation. Proc Natl Acad Sci U S A. 2004;101(47):16665-70. Epub 2004/11/16.

[30] Matsuzaki M, Honkura N, Ellis-Davies GC, Kasai H. Structural basis of long-term potentiation in single dendritic spines. Nature. 2004;429(6993):761-6. Epub 2004/06/11.

[31] Harvey CD, Svoboda K. Locally dynamic synaptic learning rules in pyramidal neuron dendrites. Nature. 2007;450(7173):1195-200. Epub 2007/12/22.

[32] Trachtenberg JT, Chen BE, Knott GW, Feng G, Sanes JR, Welker E, et al. Long-term in vivo imaging of experience-dependent synaptic plasticity in adult cortex. Nature. 2002;420(6917):788-94. Epub 2002/12/20.

[33] Grutzendler J, Kasthuri N, Gan WB. Long-term dendritic spine stability in the adult cortex. Nature. 2002;420(6917):812-6.

[34] Majewska AK, Newton JR, Sur M. Remodeling of synaptic structure in sensory cortical areas in vivo. J Neurosci. 2006;26(11):3021-9. Epub 2006/03/17.

[35] Chen JL, Villa KL, Cha JW, So PT, Kubota Y, Nedivi E. Clustered dynamics of inhibitory synapses and dendritic spines in the adult neocortex. Neuron. 2012;74(2):361-73. Epub 2012/05/01.

[36] Lee WC, Huang H, Feng G, Sanes JR, Brown EN, So PT, et al. Dynamic remodeling of dendritic arbors in GABAergic interneurons of adult visual cortex. PLoS biology. 2006;4(2):e29. Epub 2005/12/22.

[37] Chen JL, Lin WC, Cha JW, So PT, Kubota Y, Nedivi E. Structural basis for the role of inhibition in facilitating adult brain plasticity. Nat Neurosci. 2011;14(5):587-94. Epub 2011/04/12.

[38] Chen JL, Flanders GH, Lee WC, Lin WC, Nedivi E. Inhibitory dendrite dynamics as a general feature of the adult cortical microcircuit. J Neurosci. 2011;31(35):12437-43. Epub 2011/09/02.

[39] Xu T, Yu X, Perlik AJ, Tobin WF, Zweig JA, Tennant K, et al. Rapid formation and selective stabilization of synapses for enduring motor memories. Nature. 2009;462(7275):915-9. Epub 2009/12/01.

[40] Yang G, Pan F, Gan WB. Stably maintained dendritic spines are associated with lifelong memories. Nature. 2009;462(7275):920-4. Epub 2009/12/01.

[41] Fu M, Yu X, Lu J, Zuo Y. Repetitive motor learning induces coordinated formation of clustered dendritic spines in vivo. Nature. 2012;483(7387):92-5. Epub 2012/02/22.

[42] Lai CS, Franke TF, Gan WB. Opposite effects of fear conditioning and extinction on dendritic spine remodelling. Nature. 2012;483(7387):87-91. Epub 2012/02/22.

[43] Tian L, Akerboom J, Schreiter ER, Looger LL. Neural activity imaging with genetically encoded calcium indicators. Prog Brain Res. 2012;196:79-94. Epub 2012/02/22.

[44] Tian L, Hires SA, Looger LL. Imaging neuronal activity with genetically encoded calcium indicators. Cold Spring Harbor protocols. 2012;2012 Jun(6):647-56. Epub 2012/06/05.

[45] Miyawaki A, Llopis J, Heim R, McCaffery JM, Adams JA, Ikura M, et al. Fluorescent indicators for Ca2+ based on green fluorescent proteins and calmodulin. Nature. 1997;388(6645):882-7. Epub 1997/08/28.

[46] Nakai J, Ohkura M, Imoto K. A high signal-to-noise Ca(2+) probe composed of a single green fluorescent protein. Nature biotechnology. 2001;19(2):137-41. Epub 2001/02/15.

[47] Tian L, Hires SA, Mao T, Huber D, Chiappe ME, Chalasani SH, et al. Imaging neural activity in worms, flies and mice with improved GCaMP calcium indicators. Nature methods. 2009;6(12):875-81. Epub 2009/11/10.

[48] Mank M, Santos AF, Direnberger S, Mrsic-Flogel TD, Hofer SB, Stein V, et al. A genetically encoded calcium indicator for chronic in vivo two-photon imaging. Nature methods. 2008;5(9):805-11. Epub 2009/01/23.

[49] Nicoll RA, Malenka RC. Expression mechanisms underlying NMDA receptor-dependent long-term potentiation. Ann N Y Acad Sci. 1999;868:515-25.

[50] Dunning J, During MJ. Molecular mechanisms of learning and memory. Expert reviews in molecular medicine. 2003;5(25):1-11. Epub 2004/02/28.

[51] Johansen JP, Cain CK, Ostroff LE, LeDoux JE. Molecular mechanisms of fear learning and memory. Cell. 2011;147(3):509-24. Epub 2011/11/01.

[52] Seeburg PH, Burnashev N, Kohr G, Kuner T, Sprengel R, Monyer H. The NMDA receptor channel: molecular design of a coincidence detector. Recent progress in hormone research. 1995;50:19-34. Epub 1995/01/01.

[53] Soderling TR. Calcium-dependent protein kinases in learning and memory. Advances in second messenger and phosphoprotein research. 1995;30:175-89. Epub 1995/01/01.

[54] Andermann ML, Kerlin AM, Reid RC. Chronic cellular imaging of mouse visual cortex during operant behavior and passive viewing. Frontiers in cellular neuroscience. 2010;4:3. Epub 2010/04/22.

[55] Dombeck DA, Harvey CD, Tian L, Looger LL, Tank DW. Functional imaging of hippocampal place cells at cellular resolution during virtual navigation. Nat Neurosci. 2010;13(11):1433-40. Epub 2010/10/05.

[56] Mower AF, Kwok S, Yu H, Majewska AK, Okamoto K, Hayashi Y, et al. Experience-dependent regulation of CaMKII activity within single visual cortex synapses in vivo. Proc Natl Acad Sci U S A. 2011;108(52):21241-6. Epub 2011/12/14.

[57] Boyden ES, Zhang F, Bamberg E, Nagel G, Deisseroth K. Millisecond-timescale, genetically targeted optical control of neural activity. Nat Neurosci. 2005;8(9):1263-8. Epub 2005/08/24.

[58] Tye KM, Deisseroth K. Optogenetic investigation of neural circuits underlying brain disease in animal models. Nat Rev Neurosci. 2012;13(4):251-66. Epub 2012/03/21.

[59] Fenno L, Yizhar O, Deisseroth K. The development and application of optogenetics. Annu Rev Neurosci. 2011;34:389-412. Epub 2011/06/23.

[60] Keene AC, Masek P. Optogenetic induction of aversive taste memory. Neuroscience. 2012;222:173-80. Epub 2012/07/24.

[61] Wise RA. Dopamine, learning and motivation. Nat Rev Neurosci. 2004;5(6):483-94. Epub 2004/05/21.

[62] Everitt BJ, Robbins TW. Neural systems of reinforcement for drug addiction: from actions to habits to compulsion. Nat Neurosci. 2005;8(11):1481-9. Epub 2005/10/28.

[63] Tsai HC, Zhang F, Adamantidis A, Stuber GD, Bonci A, de Lecea L, et al. Phasic firing in dopaminergic neurons is sufficient for behavioral conditioning. Science. 2009;324(5930):1080-4. Epub 2009/04/25.

[64] Adamantidis AR, Tsai HC, Boutrel B, Zhang F, Stuber GD, Budygin EA, et al. Optogenetic interrogation of dopaminergic modulation of the multiple phases of reward-seeking behavior. J Neurosci. 2011;31(30):10829-35. Epub 2011/07/29.

[65] Kim KM, Baratta MV, Yang A, Lee D, Boyden ES, Fiorillo CD. Optogenetic mimicry of the transient activation of dopamine neurons by natural reward is sufficient for operant reinforcement. PLoS One. 2012;7(4):e33612. Epub 2012/04/17.

[66] van Zessen R, Phillips JL, Budygin EA, Stuber GD. Activation of VTA GABA neurons disrupts reward consumption. Neuron. 2012;73(6):1184-94. Epub 2012/03/27.

[67] Stuber GD, Sparta DR, Stamatakis AM, van Leeuwen WA, Hardjoprajitno JE, Cho S, et al. Excitatory transmission from the amygdala to nucleus accumbens facilitates reward seeking. Nature. 2011;475(7356):377-80. Epub 2011/07/01.

[68] Kravitz AV, Tye LD, Kreitzer AC. Distinct roles for direct and indirect pathway striatal neurons in reinforcement. Nat Neurosci. 2012;15(6):816-8. Epub 2012/05/01.

[69] Johansen JP, Hamanaka H, Monfils MH, Behnia R, Deisseroth K, Blair HT, et al. Optical activation of lateral amygdala pyramidal cells instructs associative fear learning. Proc Natl Acad Sci U S A. 2010;107(28):12692-7. Epub 2010/07/10.

[70] Ciocchi S, Herry C, Grenier F, Wolff SB, Letzkus JJ, Vlachos I, et al. Encoding of conditioned fear in central amygdala inhibitory circuits. Nature. 2010;468(7321):277-82. Epub 2010/11/12.

[71] Liu X, Ramirez S, Pang PT, Puryear CB, Govindarajan A, Deisseroth K, et al. Optogenetic stimulation of a hippocampal engram activates fear memory recall. Nature. 2012;484(7394):381-5. Epub 2012/03/24.

[72] Garner AR, Rowland DC, Hwang SY, Baumgaertel K, Roth BL, Kentros C, et al. Generation of a synthetic memory trace. Science. 2012;335(6075):1513-6. Epub 2012/03/24.

[73] Milner B, Squire LR, Kandel ER. Cognitive neuroscience and the study of memory. Neuron. 1998;20(3):445-68.

[74] Goshen I, Brodsky M, Prakash R, Wallace J, Gradinaru V, Ramakrishnan C, et al. Dynamics of retrieval strategies for remote memories. Cell. 2011;147(3):678-89. Epub 2011/10/25.

[75] Letzkus JJ, Wolff SB, Meyer EM, Tovote P, Courtin J, Herry C, et al. A disinhibitory microcircuit for associative fear learning in the auditory cortex. Nature. 2011;480(7377):331-5. Epub 2011/12/14.

[76] Andrews-Zwilling Y, Gillespie AK, Kravitz AV, Nelson AB, Devidze N, Lo I, et al. Hilar GABAergic interneuron activity controls spatial learning and memory retrieval. PLoS One. 2012;7(7):e40555. Epub 2012/07/14.

[77] Rolls A, Colas D, Adamantidis A, Carter M, Lanre-Amos T, Heller HC, et al. Optogenetic disruption of sleep continuity impairs memory consolidation. Proc Natl Acad Sci U S A. 2011;108(32):13305-10. Epub 2011/07/27.

Chapter 9

Attractor Hypothesis of Associative Cortex: Insights from a Biophysically Detailed Network Model

Mikael Lundqvist, Pawel Herman and
Anders Lansner

Additional information is available at the end of the chapter

http://dx.doi.org/10.5772/56229

1. Introduction

Ever since Hebb proposed that cells that fire together wire together, the idea that memories are formed by distributed cell assemblies capable of self-sustained activity [1] has been one of the main hypothesis regarding memory formation and recall. It has laid the foundation for a theory of attractor memory extensively exploited in computational neuroscience. Memory representations, manifested as the selective activations of these cell assemblies, serve as attractors in simulated neural networks and can be retrieved as a result of external stimulation or intrinsic system dynamics.

Despite major efforts in neuroscience to investigate the attractor hypothesis experimentally, which have produced some supporting evidence, no conclusive result to prove or reject it has been provided. This current status can largely be attributed to the limitations in data collection and the distributed nature of Hebbian cell assemblies. For the attractor hypothesis of associative cortex to be validated, simultaneous spiking data from a vast number of cells over a large spatial scale should be recorded. In slices [2] and cell cultures [3], more accessible for such recordings, evidence for cell assemblies capable of self-sustained activity has been provided. In vivo however the task is more challenging since the use of intrusive techniques is limited. In addition, activity related to attractor dynamics can be obscured by spiking contributions reflecting other, parallel processes in behaving animals. In consequence, we must at this point rely on indirect evidence. Simulations in biophysically detailed attractor networks can provide useful insights in this regard and help to address questions relevant to a hypothesis of attractor computations in cortical circuits, for example:

- Is the known cortical connectivity with relatively sparse cell-to-cell connectivity sufficient to support the globally coherent phase-transitions and sustained activity states associated with attractor networks?
- Likewise, is the observed sparse and low rate cortical activity consistent with the activation of recurrently connected cell assemblies?
- What features of the neural activity in vivo could be linked to and interpreted in light of the simulated attractor dynamics?
- In what capacity can additional phenomena, such as oscillations in various frequency bands and cross-frequency coupling effects, be explained by the presence of attractors in the biological system?

In addition, models compliant with known biological data can then make several testable predictions and guide further experimental work. The last few decades, attractor networks have been used extensively as models for cortical memory in various paradigms [4-15]. The major distinguishing feature of the model presented here is that it operates in an oscillatory regime and has a modular structure [16-20]. Throughout this chapter we demonstrate evidence for biological relevance of these features and motivate functional advantages of oscillations in our attractor network.

2. Basic hypothesis

The ad hoc hypothesis adopted here is that layers 2/3 of associative cortex provide the neural substrate for attractor memory network. In the light of attractor hypothesis, cortical memory representations correspond to attractor states supported by recurrent excitatory connections. Attractor networks have several dynamical attractors, to which similar activity patterns in terms of a combination of specific active and inactive units are attracted. These attractors can be stored by means of synaptic learning. The attractor dynamics lends the memory system several attractive features. First of all, such memory networks are noise resistant and fault tolerant in the sense that a noisy, corrupted or incomplete stimulus can still activate a full corresponding memory pattern – the effect known as pattern completion. Furthermore, when conflicting stimuli are provided the phenomenon of pattern rivalry occurs. In addition, the use of local, synaptic learning rules are sufficient to form global memory patterns using highly parallel processing. Despite this locality, an attractor network trained with a Bayesian-Hebbian learning rule [21] retrieves the pattern provided with the stronger evidence based on the statistics of the input and previous learning examples. In addition, storage capacity in large-scale attractor networks appears to meet biological needs [22].

Despite a high degree of compatibility between the functionality of attractor networks and that of cortical memory, it is relevant to study the actual anatomical substrate of attractor dynamics in cortex. As mentioned in the beginning, we hypothetically designate layer 2/3 to be the main driver of such dynamics; mostly due to the predominant presence of dense recurrent connections, necessary to support attractor function. From a neurodynamical perspective, these layers

http://dx.doi.org/10.5772/56229

seem to be the main source of excitatory drive in the cortical circuitry [23, 24]. In addition, the phylogenetically oldest parts of the cerebral cortex only contain the superficial layers so if the attractor functionality is central to cortical processing, it should be harbored there. The deeper layers, which emerged later in evolution, could still be directly involved in or supporting attractor function. Then however they would be likely to rather address the needs arising from the expanding cortex size such as readout and output to subcortical structures [25, 26], or participate in the selection and modulation of both task-relevant and task-irrelevant cortical modalities. The latter notion is bolstered by the fact that layer 5 seems critical in the regulation of cortical up and down states [27, 28], i.e. in the regulation of global excitability of entire cortical areas.

In further support of attractor dynamics in the superficial layers, stimulus evoked neural activity exhibited in layers 2/3 is also sparser with lower average firing rate and is more selective to input statistics compared to the deeper layers [29, 30]. These characteristics are congruent with sparse and distributed memory patterns stored in attractor networks. However, a consequence of this relatively sparse activity is that it is likely to be obscured by deep layer activity when large quantities of spiking data is collected, which hinders the acquisition of direct neural evidence for attractor-like dynamics. It is not surprising therefore that the most direct in vivo evidence of attractor dynamics comes from olfactory cortex ([31, 32] and references found therein), and hippocampus [12, 33, 34], i.e. cortical structures that lack the deeper layers. There is also evidence for self-sustained and input specific activity from inferotemporal [35, 36] and prefrontal cortex [37-39], which are late in the processing stream and therefore should be more strongly influenced by the intrinsic connectivity. In addition, two-photon calcium imaging studies have produced relevant insights into the attractor hypothesis since the imaging method can reveal calcium current traces with good temporal resolution in tens to hundreds of neurons simultaneously within a small cortical volume of the superficial layers in vivo [40-43]. This technique was recently used to demonstrate non-linear attractor-like activity in auditory cortex [42]. In particular, spatially organized neuronal sub-groups were shown to respond discretely in time to specific auditory cortex input [42]. Here, groups of stimuli evoked all-or-nothing responses in distinct neural sub-groups. These discrete activities were however partly obscured by a large trial-to-trial variability.

Finally, there is evidence for attractor dynamics sustained by the recurrent connectivity in striate cortex [44, 45]. Using voltage-sensitive dye imaging, Kenet et al. [45] found that the superficial layers switched spontaneously and in a coordinated fashion between re-occurring states spanning several cortical columns. These spontaneous states showed strong correlation to visually evoked patterns of activity and have later also been reported to match the structured, horizontal long-range connections in layer 2/3 [46]. It thus seem likely that visually evoked states are strongly related to self-sustained attractor states supported by recurrent connectivity in superficial layers.

However, it is not clear whether such switches between stable activity patterns are indeed compatible with the dynamics of computational networks as for such models, unlike biology, full connectivity between units is often used. Further, single units in attractor networks display very high firing rates with low variability while superficial activity in vivo has low rate and is highly variable. From the modeling perspective, the implications of the questionable assumption about all-to-all cortical connectivity adopted in theoretical studies (mathematically it ensures convergence to stable states) have hardly been investigated in the context of biological plausibility of attractor dynamics and function. Nor have the very low firing rates reported in vivo been reproduced. Our approach relying on a biophysically detailed attractor network model of cortex with a spatial scale spanning several hypercolumns [16], which draws from known anatomy and connectivity, allows for addressing some of these questions.

3. The network model

The network contains two types of neurons, excitatory pyramidal and inhibitory basket cells, composed of several compartments modeled by Hodgkin-Huxley equations. The basic functional units of the network are however minicolumns, each containing 30 recurrently connected pyramidal cells (Figure 1), inspired by the columnar structure of sensory cortex [41, 47-49]. These should not necessarily be seen as anatomical columns but rather functional columns consisting of subgroups of more tightly connected neurons, as found throughout cortex [40, 42, 43, 50-55].

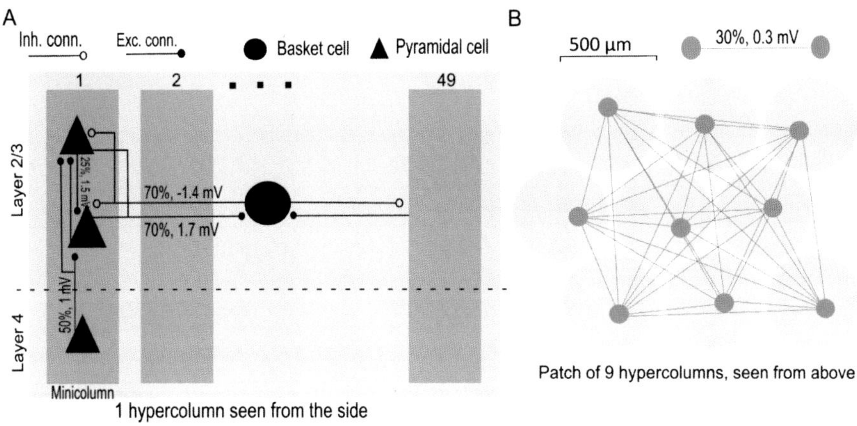

Figure 1. Network setup and connectivity.A: A detailed connectivity of a single hypercolumn, containing 49 minicolumns. B: A sketch of the long-range connectivity within a cortical patch, consisting of several hypercolumns (9 in a full patch). The numbers on the arrows give the connectivity and post synaptic potential (PSP) size at resting potential of the post-synaptic cell.

A cluster of minicolumns, spanning a few hundred microns, constitutes a hypercolumn in the network. Since the minicolumns within each cluster are coupled through a pool of basket cells, a hypercolumn can be defined by the extent of non-specific feedback inhibition [52] (Figure 1). In earlier studies [16] we used down-scaled hypercolumns containing 8 minicolumns, but in the subsequent work hypercolumns contained at least 49 minicolumns [17-20]. The feedback

http://dx.doi.org/10.5772/56229

from the basket cells has several functions. It normalizes activity in the network, provides the means for mutual competition that implements winner-take-all (WTA) dynamics within a hypercolumn and finally produce oscillations, which in turn add several interesting dynamical features to the network. Similar local WTA dynamics, on the scale of ~200 microns, was recently observed in auditory cortex in vivo [42].

We have typically modeled a cortical patch of about 1.5x1.5 mm using a 9-hypercolumn network. Distributed, retrievable and sparse patterns of activity are stored as attractors in this network. This is achieved by long-range interactions between pyramidal cells in minicolumns across different hypercolumns (Figure 1). Such structured, horizontal connections had originally been adopted in the model as an assumption but later on they received increased experimental support from studies of layer 2/3 connectivity [46, 56, 57]. In the work presented here, only orthogonal attractor patterns are stored, i.e. each minicolumn only participates in one global pattern. Although overlapping patterns, where each minicolumn participates in several patterns, increase memory storage capacity, they lead to similar results [58]. Data from in vivo paired recordings are used to bring connectivity and synaptic weights as close to biology as possible [59], but assumptions regarding long-rage connectivity have to be made.

4. Attractor properties, low firing rates and nested oscillations

We have found that stable attractor activity can indeed be maintained for plausible synaptic weights and very low firing rates, if the network is operating in an oscillatory regime (Figure 2). These oscillations, in the range of 25-40 Hz, correspond to upper beta [60] and gamma-like [61] oscillations in vivo, which have been correlated with active stimulus processing and memory recall [60-68]. In our network, the oscillations are generated by the strong feedback inhibition from basket cells (pyramidal interneuron gamma (PING) network; [69, 70]). This feedback inhibition also effectively underlies the selection of a winning population in the WTA circuit within a hypercolumn and controls firing rates in this winning cell assembly.

The oscillatory regime is also interesting for other computational reasons. Due to the gamma-cycle dynamics, an attractor cell assembly could maintain its activity and suppress the activity of competing assemblies already at an average firing rate of 3 s^{-1} per pyramidal cell [17]. This can be explained by the dynamics of the gamma cycle, which has a phase dominated by excitation where pyramidal cells have an opportunity to fire, and followed by a phase where the innervated basket cells shut down the activity in the network. As this inhibitions wears off, there is a race between populations of pyramidal cells to reach the firing threshold before recruited basket cells shut down the activity again [65]. As a result, only a small bias (low firing rates) to one of the competing populations is needed to activate or maintain a given attractor.

Since the network is highly dependent on the activity in the distant recurrently connected hypercolumns an intrinsic bias is mediated by long-range excitation, which arrives out of phase with respect to local excitatory inputs (Figure 2A), often in the inhibition-dominated part of the local gamma rhythm. This reflects an integration of global evidence for a given memory pattern on the gamma time-scale and implies that the resulting decision to either maintain current activity pattern in the network or not is made within a short temporal window in each gamma cycle, serving as a discrete time unit. Consequently, transitions from and to active attractor states are globally sharp. The inter-hypercolumnar connections underlying these computations in a modular network help to stabilize the oscillatory regime since the global excitation arrives out of phase with respect to the local firing [17].

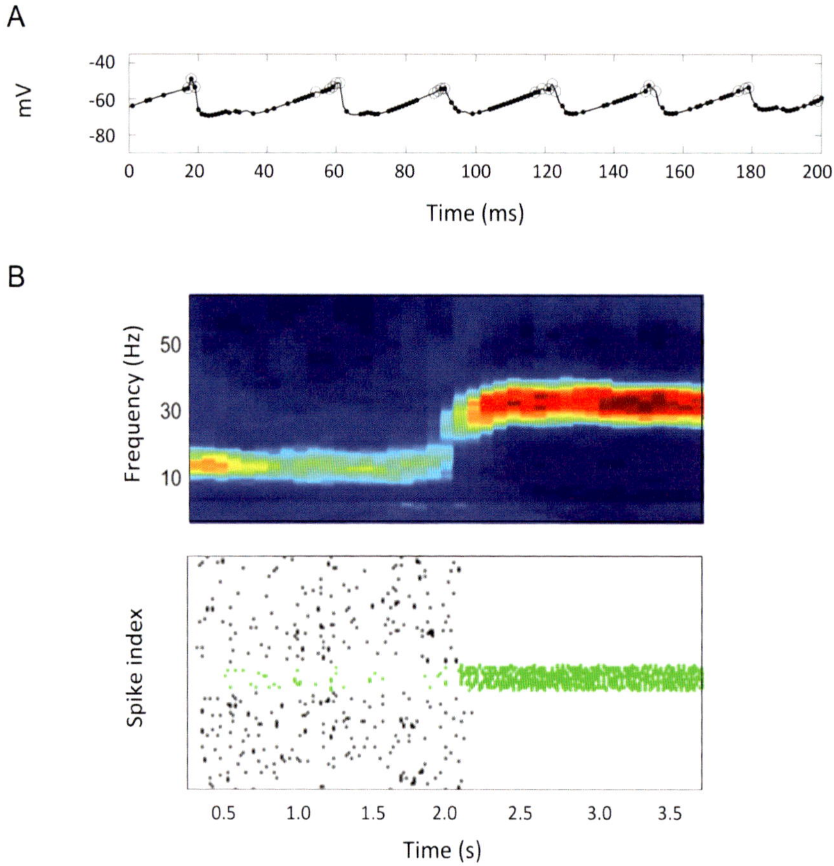

Figure 2. Oscillatory activity in the various network states. A: During attractor retrieval each minicolumn in the active assembly oscillates at gamma frequency (25-40 Hz). All pyramidal spiking within a minicolumn is concentrated to the peak of each oscillation (circles) while the incoming spikes from distant minicolumns are evenly distributed across the whole oscillatory cycle, stabilizing activity within the assembly. B: Bistable network receiving stimulation of one of its coding attractors at t = 2s. This time point marks a transition from alpha like (ground state) to gamma like (attractor state) oscillations (top) and a simultaneous transition from diffuse low rate firing to the concentrated higher rate spiking (bottom) in a specific cell assembly. Spiking from pyramidal cells in this assembly is shown as green dots while all other spikes are depicted as black dots.

The fast state transitions in the network can also be understood from the perspective of balanced excitation and inhibition [11, 71, 72]. Since spiking of individual neurons in balanced networks is driven by input fluctuations rather than average net excitation, with membrane potential close to the firing threshold, rapid state transitions can occur [71, 72]. The balance, which also results in highly irregular firing on the single cell level [72], is roughly preserved in a large parametric region of the oscillatory regime [17, 69]. The model can therefore operate in this regime without a need for fine-tuning or plasticity-induced synaptic changes, which are otherwise necessary in memory networks [9, 73]. The oscillatory regime thus results in fast transitions and irregular firing [17, 69] with a CV_2 close to one (during attractor activation), as often reported in vivo during delay match-to-sample tasks [39, 74, 75].

Classical attractor networks remain in an attractor state once they fall into one as long as there is no external input forcing a transition. One of the biological mechanisms that can cause such global transitions out of active attractor states is neural fatigue, implemented in our modeling work by the inclusion of cellular adaptation and synaptic depression in the model [76]. Together they render the attractor lifetime finite and the level of adaptation has a direct effect on the attractor duration (Figure 3A). The dynamics of activation and deactivation of attractors with finite life-times result in an increase in theta/delta-band power of the synthesized local field potentials (LFPs) (Figure 4A). The peak frequency of this rhythm corresponds roughly to the inverse of the attractor's dwell time. In consequence, the co-emerging gamma and theta/delta rhythms are coupled, i.e. the phase of slower theta/delta wave modulates the amplitude of faster gamma activity (Figure 4B). Such nested oscillations have been widely reported as a neural correlate of various memory paradigms [62, 77-81]. Theta oscillations by themselves have also been connected to both encoding, learning and retrieval of memory objects [68, 82-87]. In addition, theta phase modulations of firing rates observed in vivo [85] can also be found in the model (Figure 4C).

From the functional perspective, the network is capable of memory completion and pattern rivalry (Figure 5). Memory completion was tested by providing the network with partial stimuli of the stored patterns and examining whether full activation of the stored activity pattern was achieved via the lateral long-range connections. This occurs when roughly one third of the minicolumns in a pattern receives brief stimulation (Figure 5A, B). Pattern rivalry reflects the network's ability to resolve ambiguities in the input. When two patterns are simultaneously stimulated and their relative strengths vary, it turns out that small differences between stimuli can have a decisive impact on which pattern is activated and which one is extinguished [16]. Lundqvist et al. [16] demonstrated that relative differences in input strength of 25% consistently selected the more strongly stimulated assembly. This is by no means the lower limit though and here we used 10% differences (Figure 5B). Once the activity of the winning pattern is terminated due to adaptation and the same conflicting stimuli is applied again, the weakly stimulated pattern typically gets activated (Figure 5B).

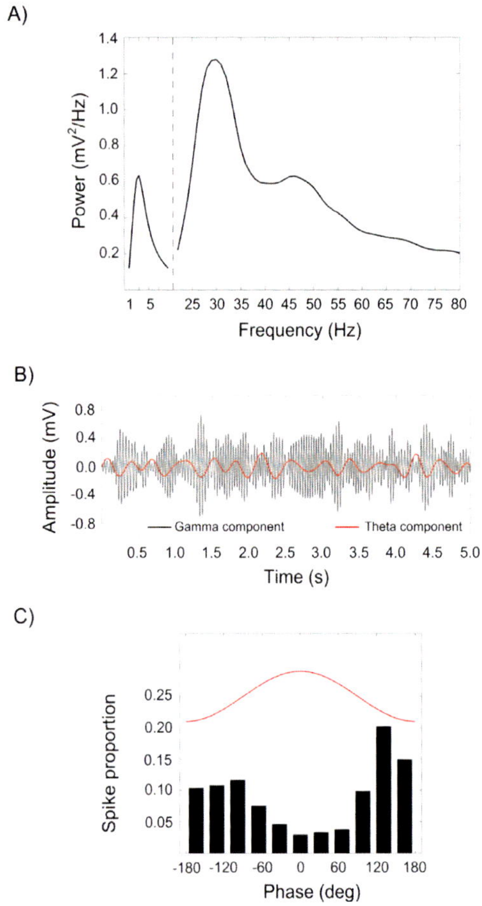

Figure 3. Cartoon of energy landscapes in various regimes. Solid lines depict the energy of various states at time t=0, and broken lines at a later time point (specified in A-C). The ball indicates what state the network is likely to be in, i.e. one of the states with the lowest energy. A: Network with attractors of limited life-time, t_{lt} (200-800 ms depending on parameters). The network will quickly end up in one of its attractor states at the onset of each simulation. At $t = t_{lt}$ (broken lines) neural fatigue and synaptic depression has increased the energy of this attractor such that noise will bump it to another attractor state. If there is no neural fatigue the attractor states will be persistently active until the network is deterred into a new state by external stimulation. B: Bistable network with one default state and several coding attractors. This bistability is achieved by either scaling up the network or increasing mutal inhibition between cell assemblies. At the onset of simulation we have here stimulated a specific coding attractor. At $t=t_{lt}$ (broken line) the network will again exit this state but now jump into the ground state. The network will remain in this state until one of the coding attractors are stimulated. C: Bistable network with added synaptic augmentation. Solid lines show the network state just after the stimulated attractor has terminated due to neural fatigue, and the network has retreated to its ground state. After some time t, larger than the fast decay of neural fatigue but smaller than the decay of the more long-lasting synaptic augmentation, the energy landscape is altered (broken lines). During this time window the network is likely to jump back in to the previously active attractor spontaneously.

http://dx.doi.org/10.5772/56229

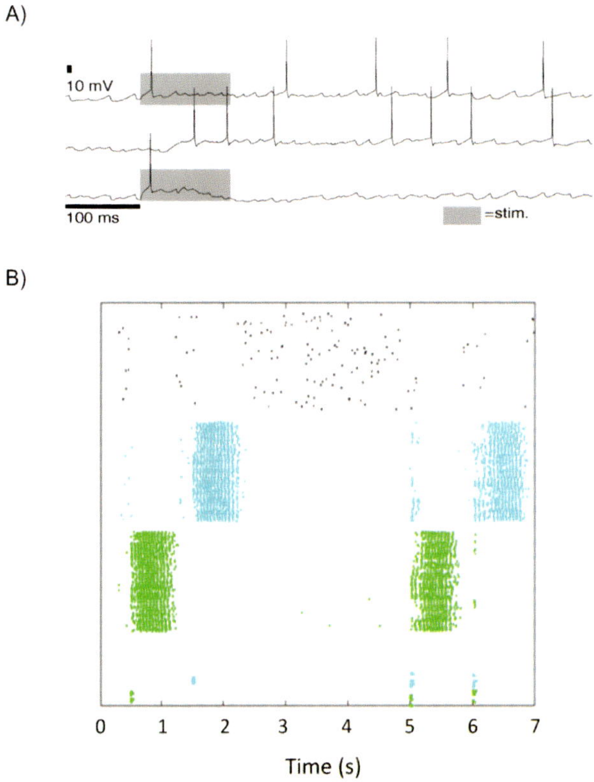

Figure 4. Gamma and theta phase locking. Gamma and theta power (A) and gamma-filtered (black) and theta-filtered (red) components during active sequential retrieval of attractors (B). C: Histogram of spike events in relation to the theta phase.

Conceptually, we consider minicolumns, rather than single cells, as the basic functional units of the network. This means that information processing does not rely on single cells but on recurrently connected neuronal populations. This perspective recently obtained additional experimental support [42] and has several important implications. Firstly, the connectivity within the network on the unit level can be increased without affecting the biologically realistic connectivity on the single cell level [22]. Since a pyramidal cell receives roughly 10 000 synapses, full cell-to-cell connectivity is not possible, even within a small cortical volume. With minicolumns acting as computational units, a closer approximation of the full connectivity, assumed in theoretical studies of attractor networks, can be obtained (another factor that reduces the need for full cell-to-cell connectivity is the dense local inhibition implementing di-synaptic connections between a vast number of pyramidal cells). Secondly, since the average output of each minicolumn rather than that of a single cell reflects the activation of a distributed memory pattern, memory retrieval is more robust to cellular variability or synaptic failures. In this light, irregular and rare firing of individual pyramidal cells does not undermine the stability of the retrieval process. On the contrary, this irregular firing is instead the manifestation of a dynamically regulated network state where the population activity does not depend on spike timing and firing rates of individual cells. In consequence, the network function is robust to cell death and synaptic loss [88]. Without adjusting the synaptic weights, more than 50% of cells could be removed with no detrimental effects to the attractor retrieval dynamics (Figure 6). As regards the removal of synapses, it can be performed in two different ways. First, if connections are removed from one cell at a time, a similar effect can be obtained by simply removing cells. Second, in the scenario where individual connections are removed at random the network becomes slightly more sensitive, but still tolerates a synaptic loss of roughly 40%. This number can be increased to 60% if the loss is compensated by increasing the conductance of the remaining synapses [88].

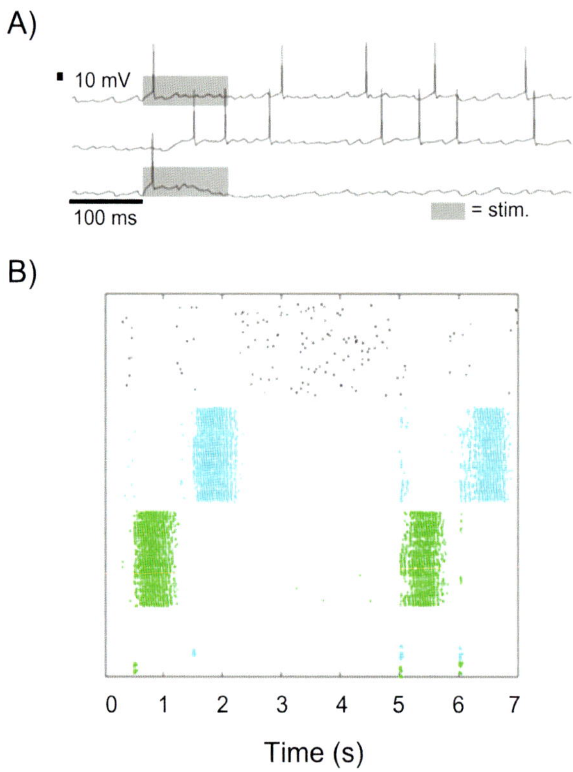

Figure 5. Pattern rivalry and completion. A: Single cell dynamics during pattern rivalry and completion. Two cells (top and bottom respectively), part of two distinct assemblies, receive input. The cell at the top is part of an assembly that

receives slightly stronger excitation and will sustain its activity while the cell at the bottom will be suppressed (pattern rivalry). The cell in the middle didn´t receive any stimulation but belonged to the winning assembly and becomes active (pattern completion). B: Global spiking dynamics demonstrating completion and rivalry. Two assemblies receive brief, partial input to 1/3 of their pyramidal cells at t=0.5 s (green) and t= 1.5 s (cyan). These inputs quickly spreads so that the full patterns are activated (pattern completion). At t=5 s both patterns receive stimulation simultaneously, but the green pattern receives 10% stronger input. This pattern quickly activates at the cost of the cyan pattern. At t=6 s the green pattern again receives 10% stronger input but due to the recent activation it is partly fatigued and the cyan pattern prevails.

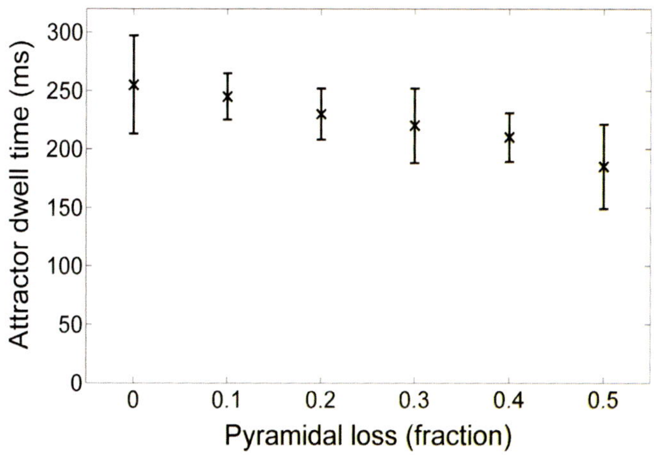

Figure 6. Tolerance to cellular death. The stability of attractor dynamics, measured as the dwell time (y-axis) of stimulated cell assemblies receiving brief stimulation. Cells are removed at random from the network (x-axis) without adjusting connectivity or synaptic weights.

5. Scaling the network and the emergence of bistability and alpha oscillations

Since the scale of the original model was small relative to a cortical area in terms of the number of hypercolumns and minicolumns (while the number of cells within each minicolumn was consistent with biological evidence), it becomes relevant to investigate whether biologically plausible neural dynamics and attractor function can be maintained at much larger simulated scales. For instance, the question as to whether a large distribution of axonal delays can coexist with stable and coherent activations of cell assemblies should be addressed. In addition, it is important to show that the relatively few connections that each pyramidal cell can form are sufficient for stable memory retrieval even at cortical scales. In order to handle these questions, we scaled the network considerably, up to the size of mouse cortex containing 22 million neurons and spanning 16 cm^2 [20].

Due to the modular structure of the network, and arguably cortex, it is indeed scalable with largely preserved dynamics. Once hypercolumns are scaled to realistic size, only the density in the connections across them has to be re-scaled in order to maintain the dynamical regime as the network grows. As the number of hypercolumns in the network was increased, we kept the number of long-range (cross-hypercolumnar) connections terminating on each pyramidal cell constant, progressively diluting the probability that two distant neurons connect. Since biological neurons have limited physical space to make connections on their dendrites, an equivalent process seems likely as in vivo systems are scaled up. As a result, a single cell sees roughly the same amount of excitatory and inhibitory input once an attractor state is entered regardless of network size. Dynamics and function during attractor retrieval were maintained even for the largest simulations without any parameter changes [20]. The transitions to and from attractor states turned out surprisingly coherent, even though the slowest time delays within each assembly were 50-60 ms. This effect was again, as described above, obtained due to the interdependence of minicolumns in each pattern mediated by the gamma cycle dynamics and the network operating in a balanced regime, where only small changes in excitation are needed for state transitions to occur.

Despite largely preserved attractor retrieval dynamics there are functional and dynamical consequences of scaling up the network. Most importantly, another dynamical state of the network emerges [11, 20] in addition to the aforementioned active attractor coding state (Figure 2B) once each hypercolumn has more than 25 minicolumns. Since this new state becomes the default condition of the bistable (Figure 3B) network in the absence of any external stimulation, it is referred to as the ground state. It is in our network manifested by global alpha-band (~10-20 Hz) oscillations (Figure 2B) and is characterized by very low levels of activity in all minicolumns without a dominance of any patterns. This state is facilitated by the mutual competition between attractor patterns [11], stabilized by feed-back inhibition growing with the network size. In the smaller network, noise fluctuations quickly activated one pattern at the expense of the others leading to a sequential recall of the patterns in a random order. In the larger network, on the other hand, it is possible to maintain the state of competition between attractor patterns as long as there is no sufficient bias to one of them, thus the emergence of a new stable state. This bias could be either in the form of external stimulation of a specific pattern or internal mechanisms such as synaptic facilitation, which we used to store a subset of patterns in working memory ([18, 19]; see section *Multi-item working memory*).

In the scaled-up bistable network, successful pattern activation by an external cue is coupled to a transition in the oscillatory dynamics from the alpha to gamma rhythm (Figure 2B). Similar stimulus induced transitions have been reported in layer 2/3 of the visual cortex in vivo [66, 89]. In the context of extensive experimental work on neural oscillations, our two distinct network states correspond with a general view that alpha reflects idling or pre-stimulus readiness (for a review see [90, 91]) and gamma is a correlate of active processing ([61]; for review see [64, 65]).

What are the mechanisms underlying these rhythms, and, more importantly, the transition between them in our network? In balanced networks with oscillatory population activity and irregular firing, the oscillatory frequency is dependent, among other factors, on the level of overall excitation in the network [92]. Comparing spiking populations in the two stable network states, the excitation level and firing rates are higher during active memory retrieval, thereby increasing the oscillatory frequency relative to the ground state. At the limit where the recurrent excitation within cell assemblies is just strong enough to promote stable attractor states, the switch from the ground state to one of the coding attractors is associated with a minimal increase in excitation and oscillatory frequency. Although the total amount of spikes elicited from the pyramidal cell population as a whole remains the same, after stimulation all spikes are elicited from the active cell assembly, i.e. the combination of single minicolumns across all the hypercolumns, instead of being spread out between all pyramidal cells as in the ground state [17]. This effect occurs since cells in the active assembly climb slightly faster to firing threshold in each oscillatory cycle, thereby shutting down competitors before they get a chance to spike and influence the network dynamics. It illustrates how a very small bias can have a strong impact on the spiking in oscillatory, balanced networks. As recurrent excitation is increased, the gap between the oscillatory frequencies in the two states also widens towards a clear distinction between alpha and gamma rhythms, hence reflecting the gradual stabilization of the active state. To maintain attractor-coding activity, a cell assembly has to oscillate faster than the ground state frequency. Towards the end of the attractor's lifetime the oscillatory frequency drops due to adaptation and the network consequently falls back into the ground state.

As with the balanced regime, the bistable regime with two simultaneously stable states exists also in non-oscillatory networks [11]. However, the advantage of oscillatory networks amounts to the fact that the parametric range of the bistable regime becomes much wider and less sensitive to perturbations in excitation [17]. The strong feedback inhibition needed for a stable ground state does not destabilize the active attractor states. On the contrary, it has relevant functional and dynamical implications for the network during memory retrieval, as discussed in the previous section.

In general, neural oscillations as a population phenomenon occur due to strong feedback inhibition that periodically shuts down activity in a network, and therefore typically destabilizes persistent activity in a cell assembly [93]. However, if this cell subset is biased in any way, in our case by the long-range excitation out of phase with respect to the local oscillations, the persistent activity in the oscillatory regime becomes extremely stable instead. Once the network can tolerate periodic hyperpolarization without terminating the activity permanently, strong feedback inhibition can be used to dynamically balance fast changes in excitation. Then, as long as the inhibition is strong enough to periodically shut down the network, it remains roughly balanced.

6. Multi-item working memory

Attractor networks have been proposed as a modeling framework for a working memory system, which temporarily maintains a small subset of memory items. Models of spatial working memory have for instance used persistent activity in bump-attractor networks to preserve a trace of a specific direction [8, 93]. We can obtain a similar effect in our network when the adaptation mechanisms are subdued. Then a stimulated attractor will remain persistently active as a cued memory over several seconds [17]. The persistent activity approach is limited however since only one item or direction can be stored at any given time due to the mutual inhibition between attractors, whereas working memory is reported to contain up to seven items simultaneously [94, 95]. In this section we discuss an alternative approach to working memory maintenance known as periodic replay [10, 14, 18, 19, 84, 96], which allows for storing multiple items.

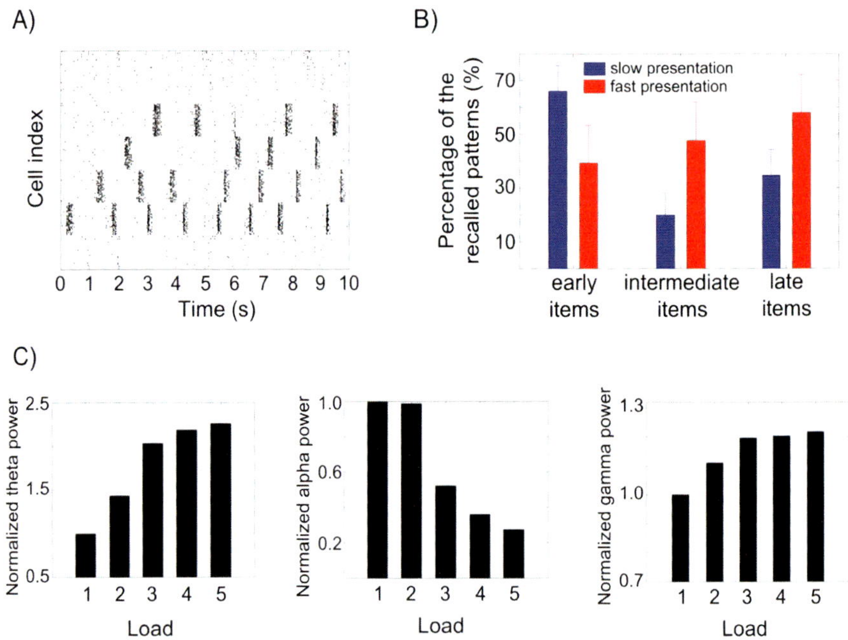

Figure 7. Multi-item working memory through synaptic augmentation. Synaptic augmentation causes attractors to spontaneously reactive some time after they have been terminated. This augmentation is then refreshed upon each reactivation, and the attractor is held in working memory in a cyclic fashion. A: Here four items are stimulated (at 0.2, 1.2, 2.2, and 3.2 sec), and the space between active recall is filled by ground state activity. The items presented early start their re-activations already during the presentation period (0-3.5 s). This can explain the bias for items presented early in the list to be remembered as seen in (B). Here 10 items are presented followed by a recall phase where we test which items that are replayed. Early (1, 2) and late (9, 10) items have a higher probability to be remembered than intermediate (4-6) items (blue bars). If the list is presented at the rate of 2 s^{-1} (red bars), the tendency for early items to be remembered is removed. C: Frequency modulations by memory load. Bars show integrated power in the three different power bands (2–6, 10–18, and 28–40 Hz) and five different load conditions. Bars are normalized relative to the power in Load 1 condition (one memory item), such that power in Load 1 is 1.

Although in both working memory models only one attractor can be active at any given time, in the periodic replay paradigm it has a brief lifetime instead of being persistently active. The encoded items are then retrieved in a sequence one after another and get periodically reactivated. In computational networks this effect can be achieved by incorporating either cellular [96] or synaptic [10, 14, 18, 19] mechanisms that adjust the excitability of activated neurons dynamically. In the latter case, it can be achieved by adding synaptic augmentation, observed in prefrontal neuronal subgroups [97], on top of faster synaptic depression in a bistable attractor network. On the single synapse level, this makes the conductance vary dynamically over time. During a brief pre-synaptic spike train the amplitude of excitatory post-synaptic potentials (EPSPs) remains static or slightly decreases over time due to the combined effect of synaptic augmentation and synaptic depression. However, due to the slower decay of the augmentation, a new spike arriving roughly one second after the initial burst elicits a significantly magnified EPSP. On the cell assembly level, this implies that an attractor that has been activated by stimulation is temporarily more excitable than the ground state some time after its termination (Figure 3C). During this window it has a high chance to spontaneously reactivate and in the process refresh the synaptic augmentation. This way, a pattern stimulated initially becomes periodically reactivated. During silent periods there is an opportunity for other assemblies to be replayed (Figure 7a). Due to the decay of augmentation, the subset of memory patterns selected for replay need to be reactivated within the decay time window following their last deactivation in order to maintain their elevated excitability. As a consequence, a limited number of items can be stored. In particular, up to ~6 attractor memories can be simultaneously augmented and hence periodically reactivated [18, 19] for biologically realistic levels of synaptic augmentation.

The notion that individual memory objects are replayed at a theta time-scale during working memory maintenance has support from human MEG recordings [84]. The model can also explain the widely reported finding that alpha-band power decreases [98, 99] while gamma- and theta-band power increase [67, 98-100] with working memory load. We obtain this effect (Figure 7C) since for each additional memory item encoded in working memory, the network spends on average shorter time in the alpha-dominated ground state and longer time in its active retrieval state, correlated with nested theta-gamma oscillations [18]. The effect saturates at the full memory capacity of the network.

The notion of theta-coupled replay of memory items with accompanying theta-gamma phase-amplitude coupling is also consistent with single-cell spike statistics obtained from recordings in prefrontal areas and superficial layers of cortex, where a relative abundance of cells displaying clumpy-bursty behavior with Lv [101] and CV_2 [102] well above 1 was observed [103, 104]. This clumpy-bursty behavior can be reproduced when single cells burst in specific theta periods and are silent in the other ones as is seen in the periodic replay paradigm [19]. Although the estimated variability during the active theta periods results in Lv close to 1, the inclusion of long inter-spike intervals (ISIs) introduced by the silent theta periods boosts Lv to 1.5 (Figure 8), as reported for clumpy-bursty cells in vivo. This effect occurs for firing rates within a certain range, overlapping with the ones observed in our network model [19].

Finally, we would also like to present unpublished results from a study aimed at reproducing the phenomenon of recency and primacy effects [105] in list-learning paradigms. When a list of items exceeding the capacity of working memory is to be remembered by a subject, there is a marked tendency for objects from the beginning (primacy) and the end (recency) of the list to be recalled with a greater likelihood. To simulate this, the network is presented with 10 memory items at the rate of 1 s^{-1} followed by a 10 s period corresponding to a free recall phase. On average in 100 trials, 5.0±0.7 (mean ± standard deviation) items are maintained such that they are replayed in the recall phase. In addition, memory items in the beginning and at the end of the list are more frequently encoded than those presented in the middle (Figure 7B). The simulated recency effect can be explained by the fact that augmentation in the assemblies activated towards the end of the presentation period is relatively high when the free recall period starts. The primacy effect, on the other hand, can be explained by the fact that the network has time in between presentations to replay these items already in the presentation phase, and thus re-enforce their increased excitability. If the network is largely denied this opportunity by presenting the list of items in quicker succession (at the rate of 2s^{-1}), around five items are again maintained in working memory (4.9±0.8), but the first items now have the smallest chance of being remembered (Figure 7B). At their cost, the last items instead have an even elevated chance of being replayed during the free recall period.

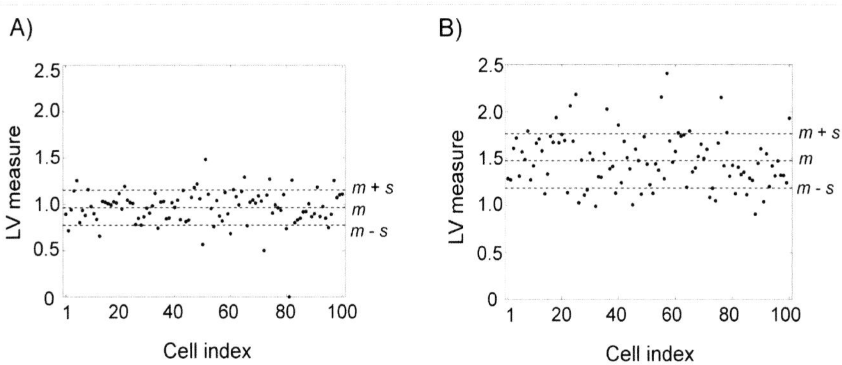

Figure 8. Scatter plot of Lv for 100 cells drawn from the persistently active network (A) and the replay network (B). The dotted lines mark the range of Lv values within one standard deviation from the mean.

7. Attentional blink

Attractor networks also allow us to study attentional mechanisms and their functional consequences. Attentional effects can be incorporated into such models in several different ways. For instance, it has been studied how top-down activity can bias certain attractors at the cost of others and thus serve as a model for top-down attention [13, 106]. Generally, in our work we rather focus on the potential neural manifestations of attention and examine how they correlate with the network's capability to retrieve weakly stimulated memory pattern. In that vein, we are currently studying the effects of both phase and power modulations of ongoing alpha oscillations on the network's performance. Here, however, we want to discuss results related to the attentional blink phenomenon [107-110]. It is concerned with an inability to detect and process two relevant stimuli presented in quick succession by humans; the first item masks the perception of the second one even if they are presented equally long. This masking effect is not maximal when the visual targets are shown immediately one after another, but instead when the relative delay is around 300 ms [108, 109]. The attentional blink phenomenon was correlated with the P300 component [108] and evoked gamma oscillations in the electroencephalography signals [109].

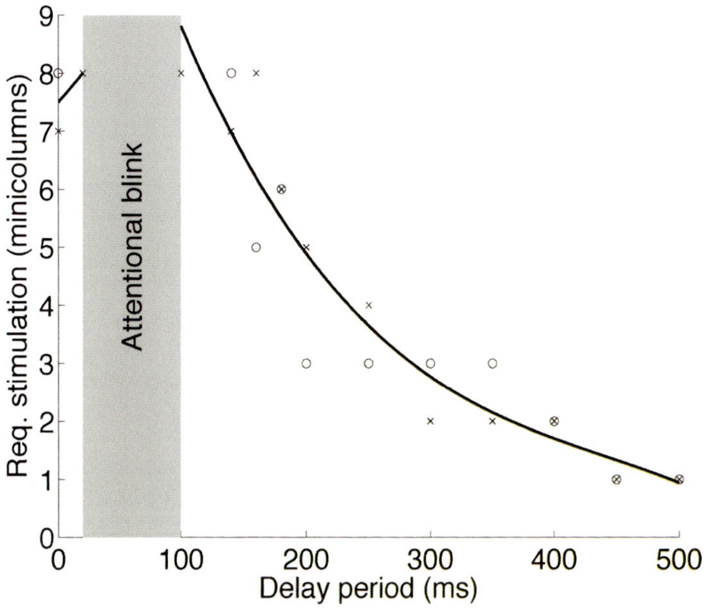

Figure 9. Attentional blink. In the period of time closely after activation of one stored pattern in the network, triggering another pattern requires more stimulation than otherwise. Here, one pattern was first activated at t = 0. After some delay, a second stimulus was applied to a different pattern, attempting to trigger its activation. Two data series (rings and crosses) are shown, corresponding to separate experiments (random seeds). Each data point shows the minimum number of minicolums in a pattern that have to be stimulated in order to activate the second pattern after a given delay. Third degree polynomia have been fitted to the data points.

In the network, we obtain qualitatively similar time-dependent attentional blink effect [16] related to evoked gamma oscillations. This is due to the fact that an activated cell assembly attains a peak in firing rates after some delay relative to the stimulation. The delay corresponds to the time needed for the recurrent network to build up activity before the adaptation causes the reduction in rates again. Other competing assemblies are maximally suppressed and thus harder to activate at this peak of activity. We associate this effect with the impaired ability to detect the subsequent stimuli in consistence with psychophysical data ([108, 109], Figure 9). This phenomenon was recently studied in more detail using the same network model [58].

8. Summary and conclusions

We have reviewed evidence that the neural activity of superficial cortical layers is to a large extent compatible with the non-linear dynamics displayed in recurrent attractor networks. Research in the field of computational neuroscience has touched upon various aspects of the attractor theory with emphasis on its biological relevance and functional implications. In our modeling work, where we have used a biophysically detailed attractor network inspired by cortical connectivity, we have demonstrated how novel features such as modular structure and oscillatory dynamics render the model more robust and consistent with biological findings. In addition, we have shown how our mesoscopic network model can be utilized to link lower-level neural substrate with higher-order cognitive or behavioral phenomena. In particular, we have conceptually replicated recency, primacy and attentional blink effects. In the light of the network's dynamics we have also motivated the limited capacity of working memory. The model can be perceived as a crude model of the superficial layers of associative cortex taking the form of a large distributed network of attractor networks. Future work is intended to follow the direction of diverging individual cortical areas with respect to connectivity and function. We envisage that this work will be accelerated by the concerted effort in computational neuroscience to study cortical function from a bottom-up perspective.

Author details

Mikael Lundqvist*, Pawel Herman and Anders Lansner

KTH and Stockholm University, Stockholm, Sweden

References

[1] Hebb DO (1949) The Organization of Behaviour. New York: Wiley.

[2] Cossart R, Aronov D, Yuste R (2003) Attractor dynamics of network UP states in the neocortex. Nature 423: 283-288.

[3] Plenz D, Thiagarajan (2007) The organizing principles of neural avalanches: cell assemblies in the cortex? TINS (30): 101-110.

[4] Hopfield JJ (1982) Neural networks and physical systems with emergent collective computational properties. PNAS 81:3088–3092.

[5] Palm G (1982) Neural assemblies. An alternative approach to artificial intelligence. Berlin: Springer.

[6] Lansner A, Fransén E (1992) Modeling Hebbian cell assemblies comprised of cortical neurons. Network: Comput Neural Systems 3: 105–119.

[7] Fransén E, Lansner A (1998) A model of cortical associative memory based on a horizontal network of connected columns. Network: computations in neural systems 9(2): 235-264.

[8] Compte A, Brunel N, Goldman-Rakic PS, Wang XJ (2000) Synaptic mechanisms and network dynamics underlaying spatial working memory in a cortical network model. Cereb Cortex 10: 910–23.

[9] Barbieri F, Brunel N (2008) Can attractor network models account for the statistics of firing during persistent activity in prefrontal cortex? Front Neurosci 2: 114-122.

[10] Sandberg A, Tegnér J, Lansner A (2003) A working memory model based on fast Hebbian learning. Network 14: 789-802.

[11] Amit DJ, Brunel N (1997) Model of global spontaneous activity and local structured activity during delay periods in cerebral cortex. Cereb Cortex 7 (3): 237-252.

[12] Treves A, Rolls ET (1994) Computational Analysis of the Role of the Hippocampus in Memory. Hippocampus 4: 374–391.

[13] Deco G, Thiele A (2009) Attention - oscillations and neuropharmacology. Eur J Neurosci 30: 347-354.

[14] Mongillo G, Barak O, Tsodyks M (2008) Synaptic theory of working memory. Science 319: 1543-1546.

[15] Lansner A (2009) Associative memory models: from the cell-assembly theory to biophysically detailed cortex simulations. Trends Neurosci 32: 178–186.

[16] Lundqvist M, Rehn M, Djurfeldt M, Lansner A (2006) Attractor dynamics in a modular network model of neocortex. Network 17: 253-276.

[17] Lundqvist M, Compte A, Lansner A (2010) Bistable, Irregular Firing and Population Oscillations in a Modular Attractor Memory Network. PLoS Comput Biol 6(6): e1000803. doi:10.1371/journal.pcbi.1000803.

[18] Lundqvist M, Herman P, Lansner A (2011) Theta and gamma power increases and alpha/beta power decreases with memory load in an attractor network model. J Cog Neurosci 23: 3008–3020.

[19] Lundqvist M, Herman P, Lansner A (2012) Variability of spike firing during theta-coupled replay of memories in a simulated attractor network. Brain Res 1434: 152–161.

[20] Djurfeldt M, Lundqvist M, Johansson C, Rehn M, Ekeberg Ö, Lansner A (2008) Brain-scale simulation of the neocortex on the IBM Blue Gene/L supercomputer. IBM Journal of Research and Development 52: 31-41.

[21] Sandberg A, Lansner A, Petersson KM, Ekeberg Ö (2002) A bayesian attractor network wth incremental learning. Network, 13: 179-184.

[22] Johansson C, Lansner A (2007) Imposing Biological Constraints onto an Abstract Neocortical Attractor Network Model. Neural Comput 19(7): 1871–1896.

[23] Weiler N, Wood L, Yu J, Solla SA, Shepherd GMG (2008) Top-down laminar organization of the excitatory network in motor cortex. Nat Neurosci. 11 (3): 360-366.

[24] Binzegger T, Douglas RJ, Martin KAC (2009) Topology and dynamics of the canonical circuit of cat V1. Neural Networks 22: 1071-1078.

[25] Wise SP, Jones EG (1977) Cells of origin and terminal distribution of descending projections of the rat somatic sensory cortex. J Comp Neurol 175: 129–157.

[26] Deschenes M, Bourassa J, Pinault D (1994) Corticothalamic projections from layer V cells in rat are collaterals of long-range corticofugal axons. Brain Res 664: 215–219.

[27] Shu Y, Hasenstaub A, McCormick DA (2003) Turning on and off recurrent balanced cortical activity. Nature 423: 288–293.

[28] Wester JC, Contreras D (2012) Columnar Interactions Determine Horizontal Propagation of Recurrent Network Activity in Neocortex. J Neurosci. 32 (16): 5454-5471.

[29] Sakata S, Harris KD (2009) Laminar Structure of Spontaneous and Sensory-Evoked Population Activity in auditory cortex. Neuron 64: 404-418.

[30] de Kock CPJ, Sakmann B (2009) Spiking in primary somatosensory cortex during natural whisking in awake head-restrained rats is cell-type specific. PNAS 106 (38): 16446-16450.

[31] Haberly LB, Bower, JM (1989) Olfactory Cortex: Model Circuit for Study of Associative Memory? Trends Neurosci. 12: 258–264.

[32] Wilson DA, Sullivan RM (2011) Cortical processing of odor objects. Neuron 72: 506-519.

[33] Wills TJ, Lever C, Cacucci F, Burgess N, O'Keefe J (2005) Attractor dynamics in the hippocampal representation of the local environment. Science 308: 873–876 .

[34] Niessing J, Friedrich RW (2010) Olfactory pattern classification by discrete neuronal network states. Nature 465, 47–52.

[35] Rolls ET, Tovee MJ (1994) Processing speed in the cerebral cortex and the neurophysiology of visual masking. Proceedings of the Royal Society, 257: 9-15.

[36] Desimone R (1996) Neural mechanisms for visual memory and their role in attention. PNAS 93(24): 13494-13499.

[37] Fuster JM, Alexander GE (1971) Neuron activity related to short-term memory. Science 173: 652–4.

[38] Goldman-Rakic PS (1995) Cellular basis of working memory. Neuron 14: 477-485.

[39] Compte A, Constaninidis C, Tegnér J, Raghavachari S, Chafee MV, Goldman-Rakic PS, Wang XJ (2003) Temporally irregular mnemonic persistent activity in prefrontal neurons of monkeys during a delayed response task. J Neurophysiol 90: 3441–3454.

[40] Kerr JND, de Kock CPJ, Greenberg DS, Bruno RM, Sakmann B, Helmchen F (2007) Spatial Organization of Neuronal Population Responses in Layer 2/3 of Rat Barrel Cortex. J Neuroscience 27(48): 13316-13328.

[41] Ohki K, Chung S, Ching YH, Kara P, Reid RC (2005) Functional imaging with cellular resolution reveals precise micro-architecture in visual cortex. Nature 433: 597-603.

[42] Bathellier B, Ushakova L, Rumpel S (2012) Discrete Neocortical Dynamics Predict Behavioral Categorization of Sounds. Neuron 76: 435-449.

[43] Rothschild, G, Nelken I, Mizrahi A (2010) Functional organization and population dynamics in the mouse primary auditory cortex. Nat Neurosci 13: 353–360.

[44] Arieli A, Sterkin A, Grinvald A, Aertsen A (1996) Dynamics of Ongoing Activity: Explanation of the Large Variability in Evoked Cortical Responses. Science 273: 1868-1871.

[45] Kenet T, Bibitchkov D, Tsodyks M, Grinvald A (2003) Spontaneously emerging cortical representations of visual attributes. Nature 425: 954-956.

[46] Muir DR, Da Costa NMA, Girardin CC, Naaman S, Omer DB, Ruesch E, Grinvald A, Douglas RJ (2011) Embedding of Cortical Representations by the Superficial Patch System. Cerebral Cortex, doi:10.1093/cercor/bhq290.

[47] Mountcastle V (1957) Modality and topographic properties of single neurons of cat's somatic sensory cortex. J Neurophysiol 20: 408-434.

[48] Hubel DH, Wiesel TN (1963) Shape and arrangement of columns in cat's striate cortex. J Physiol 165: 559-568

[49] Peters A, Yilmaz E (1993) Neurological organization in area 17 of cat visual cortex. Cereb Cortex 3: 49-68.

[50] Sato TR, Gray NW, Mainen ZF, Svoboda K (2007) The functional microarchitecture of the mouse barrel cortex. PloS Biol. 5, e189.

[51] Song S, Sjöström PJ, Reigl M, Nelson S, Chklovskii DB (2005) Highly Nonrandom Features of Synaptic Connectivity in Local Cortical Circuits. PLOS Biology 3 (39): 507-519.

[52] Yoshimura Y, Dantzker JL, Callaway EM (2005) Excitatory cortical neurons form fine-scale functional networks. Nature 433: 868-873.

[53] Kampa BM, Letzkus JJ, Stuart GJ (2006) Cortical feed-forward networks for binding different streams of sensory information. Nature Neuroscience 9 (12): 1472-1473.

[54] Perin R, Berger TK, Markram H (2011) A synaptic organizing principle for cortical neuronal groups. PNAS 108(13): 5419-5424.

[55] Rao SG, Williams GV, Goldman-Rakic PS (1999) Isodirectional Tuning of Adjacent Interneurons and Pyramidal Cells During Working Memory: Evidence for Microcolumnar Organization in PFC. J Neurophysiol 81: 1903-1916.

[56] Stettler D, Das A, Bennett J, Gilbert C (2002) Lateral connectivity and contextual interactions in macaque primary visual cortex. Neuron 14: 739–750.

[57] Binzegger T, Douglas RJ, Martin KAC (2009) Topology and dynamics of the canonical circuit of cat V1. Neural Networks, 1071-1078.

[58] Silverstein D, Lansner A (2011) Is Attentional Blink a Byproduct of Neocortical Attractors? Front Comput Neurosci 5 (2011): 1-14.

[59] Thomson AM, West DC, Wang Y, Bannister AP (2002) Synaptic connections and small circuits involving excitatory and inhibitory neurons in layers 2-5 of adult rat and cat neocortex: triple intracellular recordings and biocytin labelling in vitro. Cereb Cortex 12: 936-953.

[60] Pesaran B, Pezaris JS., Sahani M, Mitra PP, Andersen RA (2002) Temporal structure in neuronal activity during working memory in macaque parietal cortex. Nat Neurosci 5: 805-811.

[61] Gray CM, Singer W (1989) Stimulus-Specific Neuronal Oscillations in Orientation Columns of Cat Visual Cortex. PNAS 86: 1698-1702.

[62] Ward L.M (2003) Synchronous neural oscillations and cognitive processes. Trends Cogn. Sci. 7: 553-559.

[63] Tallon-Baudry C, Bertrand O, Peronnet F, Pernier J (1998) Induced gamma-band activity during the delay of a visual short-term memory task in humans. J Neurosci. 18: 4244-4254.

[64] Tallon-Baudry C, Bertrand O (1999) Oscillatory gamma activity in humans and its role in object representation. Trends in Cognitive Sciences 3: 151-162

[65] Fries P, Nikolic D, Singer W (2007) The gamma cycle. Trends Neurosci 30: 309–316.

[66] Fries P, Womelsdorf T, Oostenveld R, Desimone R (2008) The Effects of Visual Stimulation and Selective Visual Attention on Rhythmic Neuronal Synchronization in Macaque Area V4. J Neurosci 28: 4823-4835.

[67] Howard MW, Rizzuto DS, Caplan JB, Madsen JR, Lisman J., Aschenbrenner-Schreibe R, Schulze-Bonhage A, Kahana MJ (2003) Gamma Oscillations Correlate with Working Memory Load in Humans. Cereb Cortex 13: 1369-1374.

[68] Jacobs J, Kahana M (2009) Neural Representations of Individual Stimuli in Humans Revealed by Gamma-Band Electrocorticographic Activity. J Neurosci 29: 10203-10214.

[69] Brunel N, Hakim V (1999) Fast global oscillations in networks of integrate-and fire neurons with low firing rates. Neural Comput 11(7): 1621–71.

[70] Whittington MA, Traub RD, Kopell N, Ermentrout B, Buhl EH (2000) Inhibition-based rhythms: experimental and mathematical observations on network dynamics. Int J Psychophys 38: 315-36.

[71] Tsodyks MV, Sejnowski T (1995) Rapid state switching in balanced cortical network models. Network: Comput Neural Systems 6: 111–124.

[72] van Vreeswijk C, Sompolinsky H (1996) Chaos in neuronal networks with balanced excitatory and inhibitory activity. Science 274: 1724–1726.

[73] Vogels TP, Sprekeler H, Zenke F, Clopath C, Gerstner W (2011) Inhibitory Plasticity Balances Excitation and Inhibition in Sensory Pathways and Memory Networks. Science 334: 1569-1573.

[74] Joelving FC, Compte A, Constantinidis C (2007) Temporal properties of posterior parietal neuron discharges during working memory and passive viewing. J Neurophysiol 97: 2254–2266.

[75] Shafi M, Zhou Y, Quintana J, Chow C, Fuster J, et al. (2007) Variability in neuronal activity in primate cortex during working memory tasks. Neuroscience 146: 1082–1108.

[76] Tsodyks M, Pawelzik K, Markram H (1998) Neural networks with dynamical synapses. Neural Comp 10(4): 821-835.

[77] Axmacher N, Henseler MM, Jensen O, Weinreich I, Elger CE, Fell J (2010) Cross-frequency coupling supports multi-item working memory in the human hippocampus. PNAS 107 3228-3233.

[78] Canolty RT, Edwards E, Dalai SS, Soltani M, Nagarajan SS, Kirsch HE, Berger MS, Barbaro NM, Knight RT (2006) High Gamma Power Is Phase-Locked to Theta Oscillations in Human Neocortex. Science 313: 1626-1628.

[79] Jensen O, Colgin LL (2007) Cross-frequency coupling between neuronal oscillations. Trends Cogn Sci 11: 267-269.

[80] Palva JM, Palva S, Kaila K (2005) Phase synchrony among neural oscillations in the human cortex. J Neurosci. 25(15): 3962-3972.

[81] Kendrick KM, Zhan Y, Fisher H, Nicol AU, Zhang X, Feng J (2011) Learning alters the theta amplitude, theta-gamma coupling and neural synchronization in inferotemporal cortex. BMC, Neuroscience 12: 55.

[82] Raghavachari S, Kahana MJ, Rizzuto DS, Caplan JB, Kirschen MP, Bourgeois B (2001) Gating of human theta oscillations by a working memory task. J Neurosci 21: 3175–3183.

[83] Sederberg PB, Kahana MJ, Howard MW, Donner EJ, Madsen JR (2003) Theta and gamma oscillations during encoding predict subsequent recall. J Neurosci 23: 10809-10814.

[84] Fuentemilla L, Penny WD, Cashdollar N, Bunzeck N, Duzel E (2010) Theta-coupled periodic replay in working memory. Curr Biol 20: 1-7.

[85] Sirota A, Montgomery S, Fujisawa S, Isomura Y, Zugaro M, Buzsáki G (2008) Entrainment of neocortical neurons and gamma oscillations by the hippocampal theta rhythm. Neuron 60: 683–697.

[86] Huerta PT, Lisman JE (1993) Heightened synaptic plasticity of hippocampal CA1 neurons during a cholinergically induced rhythmic state. Nature 364: 723–725.

[87] Rutishauser U, Ross IB, Mamelak AN, Schuman EM (2010) Human memory strength is predicted by theta-frequency phase-locking of single neurons. Nature 464: 903–907.

[88] Bruederle et al. (2011) A comprehensive workflow for general-purpose neural modeling with highly configurable neuromorphic hardware systems. Biol Cybern 104: 263–296 DOI 10.1007/s00422-011-0435-9.

[89] Buffalo AE, Fries P, Landman R, Buschman TJ, Desimone R (2011) Laminar differences in gamma and alpha coherence in the ventral stream. PNAS 108 (27): 11262-11267.

[90] Pfurtscheller G, Stancak A, Neuper C (1996) Event-Related Synchronization (ERS) in the Alpha Band—An Electrophysiological Correlate of Cortical Idling: A Review. Int. J. Psychophysiol. 24: 39–46.

[91] Klimesch W, Sauseng P, Hanslmayr S (2007) EEG alpha oscillations: the inhibition-timing hypothesis. Brain Res Rev 53: 63-88.

[92] Brunel N, Wang XJ (2003) What determines the frequency of fast network oscillations with irregular neural discharges? I. Synaptic dynamics and excitation-inhibition balance. J Neurophysiol 90: 415-430.

[93] Wang XJ (1999) Synaptic basis of cortical persistent activity: the importance of NMDA receptors to working memory. J Neurosci 19: 9587–9603.

[94] Miller G (1956) The magical number seven, plus or minus two: some limits to our capacity to process information. Psychol Rev 63: 81-97.

[95] Cowan N (2001) Meta theory of storage capacity limits. Behavioral and Brain Sciences 24: 154-185.

[96] Lisman J, Idiart M (1995) Storage of 7 +/- 2 short-term memories in oscillatory subcycles. Science 267: 1512-1515.

[97] Wang Y, Markram H, Goodman PH, Berger TK, Ma J, Goldman-Rakic PS (2006) Heterogeneity in the pyramidal network of the medial prefrontal cortex. Nat Neurosci 9: 534-542.

[98] Meltzer JA, Zaveri HP, Goncharova II, Distasio MM, Papademetris X, Spencer SS, Spencer DD, and Constable RT (2008) Effects of working memory load on oscillatory power in human intracranial EEG. Cereb Cortex 18: 1843-1855.

[99] Mölle M, Marshall L, Fehm HL, Born J (2002) EEG theta synchronization conjoined with alpha desynchronization indicate intentional encoding. Eur J Neurosci 15: 923-928.

[100] Jensen O, Tesche CD (2002) Frontal theta activity in humans increases with memory load in a working memory task. Eur J Neurosci 15: 1395-1399.

[101] Shinomoto S, Shima K, Tanji J (2003) Differences in Spiking Patterns Among Cortical Neurons. Neural Comput 15(12): 2823–2842.

[102] Holt GR, Softky WR, Koch C, Douglas RJ (1996) Comparison of discharge variability in vitro and in vivo in cat visual cortex neurons. J Neurophysiol 75: 1806–1814.

[103] Shinomoto S, Miyazaki Y, Tamura H, Fujita I (2005) Regional and laminar differences in in vivo firing patterns of primate cortical neurons. J Neurophysiol 94: 567–575.

[104] Shinomoto S, Kim H, Shimokawa T, Matsuno N, Funahashi S, et al. (2009) Relating Neuronal Firing Patterns to Functional Differentiation of Cerebral Cortex. PLoS Comput Biol 5(7), e1000433.

[105] Tzeng OJL (1973) Positive recency effect in a delayed free recall. Journal of Verbal Learning and Verbal Behavior (12): 436–439.

[106] Beck DB, Kastner S (2009) Top-down and bottom-up mechanisms in biasing competition in human brain. Vision Res 49(10): 1154-1165.

[107] Broadbent DE, Broadbent MH (1987) From detection to identification: Response to multiple targets in rapid serial visual presentation. Perception & Psychophysics 42: 105–113.

[108] McArthur G, Budd T, Michie P (1999) The attentional blink and P300. Neuroreport 26: 3691–3695.

[109] Fell J, Klaver P, Elger CE, Fernández G (2002) Suppression of EEG Gamma Activity May Cause the Attentional Blink. Consciousness and Cognition 11: 114-122.

[110] Shapiro KL, Raymond JE, Arnell KM (1994) Attention to visual pattern information produces the attentional blink in rapid serial visual presentation. J Exp Psychol Hum Percept Perform 20: 357–371.

Chapter 10

Multi-Scale Information, Network, Causality, and Dynamics: Mathematical Computation and Bayesian Inference to Cognitive Neuroscience and Aging

Michelle Yongmei Wang

Additional information is available at the end of the chapter

http://dx.doi.org/10.5772/55262

1. Introduction

The human brain is estimated to contain 100 billion or so neurons and 10 thousand times as many connections. Neurons never function in isolation: each of them is connected to 10, 000 others and they interact extensively every millisecond. Brain cells are organized into neural circuits often in a dynamic way, processing specific types of information and providing the foundation of perception, cognition, and behavior. Brain anatomy and activity can be described at various levels of resolution and are organized on a hierarchy of scales, ranging from molecules to organisms and spanning 10 and 15 orders of magnitude in space and time, respectively. Different dynamic processes on local and global scales generate multiple levels of segregation and integration, and lead to spatially distinct patterns of coherence. At each scale, neural dynamics is determined by processes at the same scale, as well as smaller and larger scales, with no scale being privileged over others. These scales interact with each other and are mutually dependent; the coordinated action yields overall functional properties of cells and organisms.

An ultimate goal of neuroscience is to understand the brain's driving forces and organizational principles, and how the nervous systems function together to generate behavior. This raises a challenge issue for researchers in the neuroscience community: integrate the diverse knowledge derived from multiple levels of analyses into a coherent understanding of brain structure and function. The accelerating availability of neuroscience data is placing a huge need on mining and modeling methods. These data are generated at different description resolutions, for example, from neuron spike trains to electroencephalogram (EEG), magnetoencephalography (MEG), and functional magnetic resonance imaging (fMRI). A key theme in modern neuroscience is to move from localization of function to characterization of brain networks; mathematical approaches aiming at extracting directed causal connectivity from neural or neuroimaging signals are increasingly in demand. Despite differences in spatiotemporal scales of the brain signals, the data analysis and modeling share some fundamental computation strategies.

Among the diverse computational methods, probabilistic modeling and Bayesian inference play a significant role, and can contribute to neuroscience from different perspectives. Bayesian approaches can be used to analyze or decode brain signals such as spike trains and structural and functional neuroimaging data. Normative predictions can be made regarding how an ideal perceptual system integrate prior knowledge with sensory observations, and thus enable principled interpretations of data from behavioral and psychological experiments. Moreover, algorithms for Bayesian estimation could provide mechanistic interpretations of neural circuits and cognition in the brain. In addition, better understanding of the brain's computational mechanisms would have a synergistic impact on developing novel algorithms in Bayesian computation, resulting in new technologies and applications.

This chapter reviews and categorizes varieties of mathematical and statistical approaches for measuring and estimating information, networks, causality and dynamics in the multi-scale brain. Specifically, in Section 3, we introduce the fundamentals in information theory and the extended concepts and metrics for describing information processing in the brain, with validity and applications demonstrated on neural signals from multiple scales and aging research. Bayesian inference for neuroimaging data analysis, and cognition modeling of observations from psychological and behavioral experiments as well as the corresponding neural/neuronal underpinnings are provided in Section 4. Graphical models, Bayesian and dynamic Bayesian networks, and some new development, together with their applications in detecting causal connectivity and longitudinal morphological changes are presented in Section 5. We illustrate the attractor dynamics and the associated interpretations for aging brain in Section 6. Conclusions and future directions are given in Section 7.

2. Neuroscience data/signals and brain connectivity

2.1. Recording and imaging techniques at multiple scales

An important breakthrough regarding neuronal activity and neurotransmission is that electrophysiological recordings of single neurons were carried out in the intact brain of an awake or anesthetized animal, or in an explanted piece of tissue [1]. Such recordings have extremely high spatial (micrometer) and temporal (millisecond) resolution and allow direct observation of electrical currents and potentials generated by single nerve cells, which, however, at considerable cost since all cellular recording techniques are highly invasive, requiring surgical intervention and placement of recording electrodes within brain tissue. Neurons communicate via action potentials or spikes; neural recordings are usually transformed into series of discrete spiking events that can be characterized in terms of rate and timing. Less direct observations of electrical brain activity are electromagnetic potentials generated by combined electrical currents of large neuronal populations, i.e. electroencephalography (EEG) and magnetoencephalography (MEG). They are non-invasive as recordings are made through sensors placed on, or near, the surface of the head. EEG and MEG directly record signals of neuronal activity and thus have a high temporal resolution. But the spatial resolution is relatively poor as neither technique allows an unambiguous reconstruction of the electrical sources responsible for the recorded signal. EEG and MEG signals are often processed in sensor space as sources are difficult to localize in anatomical space.

With the development of magnetic resonance imaging (MRI) in 1980s [2], brain imaging took a huge step forward. The strong magnetic field and radiofrequency pulse used in MRI scanning are harmless, making this technique completely noninvasive. MRI is also extremely versatile: by changing the scanning parameters, we can acquire images based on a wide variety of different contrast mechanisms. For example, diffusion MRI is a MRI method allows the mapping of diffusion process of molecules, mainly water, in biological tissues, in vivo and non-invasively. Water molecule diffusion patterns can consequently reveal microscopic details about tissue architecture in the brain. Functional magnetic resonance imaging (fMRI) measures hemodynamic signals, only indirectly related to neural activity. These techniques allow the reconstruction of spatially localized signals at millimeter-scale resolution across the imaged brain volume. In fMRI, the primary measure of activity is the contrast between the magnetic susceptibility of oxygenated and deoxygenated hemoglobin within each voxel; so it is called the *blood oxygen level-dependent* (BOLD) signal. BOLD signal can only be viewed as an indirect measure of neural activity, In addition, the slow time constants of the BOLD response result in poor temporal resolution on the order of seconds. A critical objective of neuroimaging data analysis is the inference of neural processes responsible for the observed data, that is, the estimation of the hemodynamic response functions.

Neural signals recorded via the above techniques differ significantly in both spatial and temporal resolutions and in the directness with which neuronal activity is detected. Simultaneously using two more recording methods within the same experiment can reveal how different neural or metabolic signals are interrelated [3]. Each technique measures a different aspect of neural dynamics and organization, and interpreting neural data sets shall take these differences into account. All methods for observing brain structure and function have advantages but also disadvantages: some methods provide great structural detail but are invasive or cover only a small part of the brain, while others may be noninvasive but have poor spatial or temporal resolution. Nervous systems are organized at multiple scales, from synaptic connections between single cells, to the organization of cell populations within individual anatomical regions, and finally to the large-scale architecture of brain regions and their interconnections or network connectivity. Different techniques are sensitive to different levels of organization. The multi-scale aspect of the nervous system is an essential feature of its organization and network architecture [4].

2.2. Categorization of brain network connectivity

Given the diverse techniques for observing the brain, there are many different ways to describe and measure brain connectivity [5, 6]. Brain connectivity can be derived from histological sections revealing anatomical connections, from electrical recordings of single nerve cells, or from functional imaging of the entire brain. Even with a single recording technique, different ways of processing and analyzing neural data may result in different descriptions of the underlying network. Structural connectivity is a wiring diagram if physical links while functional connectivity describes dynamic interactions. A third class of brain networks is effective connectivity, which encompasses the network of directed interactions between neural elements. Effective connectivity goes beyond structural and functional connectivity by detecting patterns of causal influence among neural elements. These three main types of brain connectivity are defined more precisely as below.

Structural connectivity refers to a set of physical or structural (anatomical) connections that links neural elements. These anatomical connections range in scale from those of local circuits of single cells to large-scale networks of interregional pathways. Their physical pattern can be treated as relatively static at shorter time scales (seconds to minutes) but may be dynamic at longer time scales (hours to days). *Functional connectivity* describes patterns of deviations from statistical independence between distributed and often spatially remote neuronal units. The basis of functional connectivity is time series data from neural recordings such as cellular recording, EEG, MEG, and fMRI. Deviations from statistical independence typically indicates dynamic coupling and can be measured by estimating the correlation or covariance, spectral coherence, or other metrics. Functional connectivity is very time dependent, and can be statistically nonstationary. It is also modulated by external task demands and sensory stimulation, as well as internal state of the organism. But functional connectivity does not make any explicit reference to causal effects among neural elements. *Effective connectivity* captures the network causal effects between neural elements, and can be inferred through time series analysis, statistical modeling, or experimental perturbation. Same as functional connectivity, effective connectivity is also time dependent and can be rapidly modulated by external stimuli or tasks, and internal state. Some methods for effective connectivity inference are model-free without assuming anatomical pathways, while others require the specification of an explicit causal model including structural parameters. In general, the estimation of effective connectivity needs complex data processing and modeling techniques. Thus, in this chapter, regarding the networks, I mainly review strategies for estimation of effective connectivity or causal inference.

3. Information theory and processing

3.1. Fundamentals and definitions: Entropy, Kullback-Leibler divergence, and mutual information

A major objective of neuroscience is to understand how the brain processes information. Here we provide probabilistic notations and information-theoretic definitions that will be used in this section (definitions denoted with $\triangleq$). We define $x^n \triangleq x_1^n = (x_1, \ldots, x_n)$. More generally, for integers $i \leq j$, $x_i^j \triangleq (x_i, \ldots, x_j)$. For a random variable X, X corresponds to a measurable space that X takes values in, and $x \in \mathsf{X}$ are specific realizations. The probability mass function (PMF) of a discrete random variable X is defined as $P_X(x) \triangleq P(X = x)$, and the probability density function (PDF) of a continuous random variable is denoted as $p_X(x)$.

The *information* or *surprise* [7] of a discrete random variable is defined as:

$$\log \frac{1}{P_X(x)} = -\log P(X = x) \quad .$$

The choice of logarithmic base determines the unit. The most common unit of information is the *bit*, based on the binary logarithm. The information is zero for a fully predicted outcome x with $P(X = x) = 1$, and it increases as $P(X = x)$ decreases.

The *entropy* of a discrete random variable X is defined to be the average information from observing this variable:

$$H(X) = \sum_{x \in X} - P_X(x) \log P_X(x) \quad .$$

Entropy is a measure of randomness or uncertainty of the distribution: the more random the distribution, the more information is gathered by observing its value. Specifically, entropy is zero for a deterministic variable and is maximized for a uniform distribution. The conditional entropy is given as below:

$$H(Y \mid X) = \sum_{x \in X} \sum_{y \in Y} - P_{X,Y}(x, y) \log P_{Y \mid X}(y \mid x) \quad .$$

The chain rule for entropy is

$$H(X^n) = \sum_{i=1}^{n} H(X_i \mid X^{i-1}) \quad .$$

The *Kullback-Leibler* (KL) *divergence* (also called the relative entropy) between two probability distributions P and Q on X is defined as their average difference:

$$D(P \| Q) \triangleq E_P\left[\log \frac{P(X)}{Q(X)}\right] = \sum_{x \in X} P(x) \log \frac{P(x)}{Q(x)} \geq 0 \quad .$$

It is a measure of the difference of two distributions, but does not usually satisfy the symmetry condition, that is, $D(P \| Q) \neq D(Q \| P)$. So, it cannot be called “distance”.

The *Mutual information* of two discrete random variables X and Y is defined as:

$$I(X;Y) \triangleq D(P_{XY}(\bullet, \bullet) \| P_X(\bullet) P_Y(\bullet)) = E_{P_{XY}}\left[\log \frac{P_{Y \mid X}(Y \mid X)}{P_Y(Y)}\right]$$

$$= \sum_{x \in X} \sum_{y \in Y} P_{X,Y}(x, y) \frac{P_{Y \mid X}(Y \mid X)}{P_Y(Y)} = H(Y) - H(Y \mid X) \quad .$$

Intuitively, mutual information measures the information that X and Y share: it measures how much knowing one of the variables reduces uncertainty about the other. The mutual information is known to be symmetric: $I(X;Y) = I(Y;X)$. The chain rule for mutual information is

$$I(X^n; Y^n) = \sum_{i=1}^{n} I(Y_i; X^n \mid Y^{i-1}) \quad ,$$

with the conditional mutual information given as following:

$$I(X;Y \mid Z) = E_{P_{XYZ}}\left[\log \frac{P_{Y\mid X,Z}(Y \mid X, Z)}{P_{Y\mid Z}(Y \mid Z)}\right] .$$

3.2. Causal inference: Granger causality, transfer entropy, and directed information

Granger Causality: A widely-established technique for extracting causal relations or effective connectivity from data is *Granger causality* [8-11]. The principle of Granger causality is based on the concept of cross prediction. Accordingly, if incorporating the past values of times series X improves the future prediction of time series Y, the X is said to have a causal influence on Y [8]. Exploring Granger causality is closely related to analysis of vector autoregressive (VAR) models, by calculating the variances to correlation terms for autoregressive models. Using terminology introduced in [10], let $X=(X_i:i\geq 1)$ and $Y=(Y_i:i\geq 1)$ be the two time series for determining whether X causally influences Y. Y is first modeled as an univariate autoregressive series with error term V_i, and then modeled again using the X series as causal information. That is:

$$Y_i = \sum_{j=1}^{p} a_j Y_{i-j} + V_i \quad ,$$

$$Y_i = \sum_{j=1}^{p} b_j Y_{i-j} + c_j X_{i-j} + W_i \quad , \tag{1}$$

where W_i in Eq. (1) is the new error term. The number of time-lags or model order p can be a fixed prior or specified by minimizing a criterion (for example, Akaike information criterion [12] or Bayesian information criterion [13]) that balances the variance accounted for by the model, against the number of coefficients to be estimated. The Granger causality is defined as below, examining the ratio of the variances of the error terms:

$$G_{X\rightarrow Y} \triangleq \log \frac{\mathrm{var}(V)}{\mathrm{var}(W)} \quad .$$

If including X in the modeling decreases the variance of the error term, $G_{X\rightarrow Y}>0$. Typically by comparing $G_{X\rightarrow Y}$ and $G_{Y\rightarrow X}$, we determine the causal direction as the larger one. The directed transfer function transforms the autoregressive model into the spectral domain [14], and also uses multivariate models rather than univariate and bivariate models for each time series to consider the full covariance matrix for improved modeling. Granger causality, the directed transfer function, and their derivative methods are usually fast to calculate and easy to interpret. Despite the advantages, they may not be statistically suitable for inference questions associated with neural spike train data that are often modeled as point processes due to the sample-variance computation.

Transfer entropy is a measure of effective connectivity based on information theory [15, 16]. It does not require a model of interaction, is inherently non-linear, and thus provides a reasonable basis to precisely formulate causal hypotheses. Assume that the two time series $X=(X_i:i\geq 1)$ and $Y=(Y_i:i\geq 1)$ can be approximated by Markov processes:

http://dx.doi.org/10.5772/55262

$$P_{Y_{n+1}|Y^n,X^n}(y_{n+1} \mid y^n, x^n) = P_{Y_{n+1}|Y^n_{n-J+1},X^n_{n-K+1}}(y_{n+1} \mid y^n_{n-J+1}, x^n_{n-K+1}) ,$$

where J and K are respectively the orders (memory) of the Markov processes for X and Y. The transfer entropy is defined as conditional mutual information [15]:

$$T_{X \to Y}(i) = I(Y_{i+1}; X^i_{i-K+1} \mid Y^i_{i-J+1}) . \tag{2}$$

Transfer entropy is asymmetric and based on transition probabilities; it thus provides directional and dynamic information. The key feature of this information theoretic functional for identifying causality is that, theoretically, it does not assume any particular model for the interaction between the two time series. So, transfer entropy is sensitive to all order correlations, which makes it suitable for exploratory analyses over Granger causality or other model based approaches. This is especially advantages if some unknown non-linear interactions are embedded in the systems to be discovered. It is shown in [17] that for Gaussian variables, Granger causality and transfer entropy are equivalent, which bridges autoregressive and information-theoretic methods in causal inference. Another issue with transfer entropy is that its performance depends on the estimation of transitional probabilities; this requires the order selection for both the driven and driving systems.

Directed information, proposed by Marko [18] and re-formalized by others [19, 20], is more general for quantifying directional dependencies, and has recently attracted attention [10, 21]. It is modified from the mutual information to capture causal influences, denoted as $I(X \to Y)$ for two stochastic processes X and Y. For vectors X^n and Y^n, the mutual information can be shown to be:

$$\begin{aligned} I(X^n;Y^n) &= \sum_{i=1}^{n} I(X^n;Y_i \mid Y^{i-1}) \\ &= E\left[\sum_{i=1}^{n} \log \frac{P_{Y_i|Y^{i-1},X^n}(Y_i \mid Y^{i-1}, X^n)}{P_{Y_i|Y^{i-1}}(Y_i \mid Y^{i-1})}\right] \\ &= \sum_{i=1}^{n} D(P_{Y_i|Y^{i-1},X^n} \| P_{Y_i|Y^{i-1}}) . \end{aligned} \tag{3}$$

The mutual information is symmetric and only measures the correlation or statistical dependence between random processes, but cannot identify causal directionality. The directed information is defined as:

$$I(X^n \to Y^n) \triangleq \sum_{i=1}^{n} I(X^i; Y_i \mid Y^{i-1}) \tag{4}$$

$$=E\left[\sum_{i=1}^{n}\log\frac{P_{Y_i|Y^{i-1},X^i}(Y_i\mid Y^{i-1},X^i)}{P_{Y_i|Y^{i-1}}(Y_i\mid Y^{i-1})}\right] \quad (5)$$

$$=\sum_{i=1}^{n}D\left(P_{Y_i|Y^{i-1},X^i}\,\|\,P_{Y_i|Y^{i-1}}\right) \quad . \quad (6)$$

It can also be written as following with the chain rule for entropy:

$$I(X^n \to Y^n) = H(Y^n) - H(Y^n \| X^n) \ ,$$

where the $H(Y^n \| X^n)$ is the causally conditioned entropy given by [22]:

$$H\left(Y^n \| X^n\right) \triangleq \sum_{i=1}^{n} H(Y_i \mid Y^{i-1}, X^i) \ .$$

The difference between mutual information in Eq. (3) and directed information in Eq. (5) is that X^n is changed to X^i; so the causal influence of X on the current Y_i at each time i can be captured by directed information. Compared with Granger causality, directed information is a sum of divergences (Eq. (6)), and well-defined for any joint probability distributions including point processes. In addition, directed information is not tied to any particular statistical model; it operates on log likelihood ratios, and thus is more flexible and can be directly applied to varieties of modalities such as neural spike trains. By calculating the mutual information in bits, a degree of correlation (or statistical interdependence) is determined. Similarly, we can also quantify a degree of causation in bits through calculating the directed information. It is demonstrated by Amblard et al. [20]: for linear Gaussian processes, directed information and Granger causality are equivalent. Note that the transfer entropy defined in Eq. (2) is part of the sum terms in Eq. (4) for directed information. Amblard et al. also proved that for a stationary process, directed information rate can be decomposed into two parts: one is equivalent to a particular instance of the transfer entropy, and the other to the instantaneous information change rate. In fact, it has recently shown in [23] that transfer entropy is equal to the upper bound of directed information rate.

3.3. Applications and validity in neuroscience and aging research

Granger Causality: Li et al. [24] performed a longitudinal MRI study to examine the gray matter changes due to Alzheimer's disease (AD) progression. A standard voxel-based morphometry method was used to localize the abnormal brain regions, and the absolute atrophy rate in these regions was calculated with a robust regression method. The hippocampus and middle temporal gyrus (MTG) were identified as the primary foci of atrophy. A model based Granger causality approach was developed to examine the cause–effect relationship over time between these regions based on gray matter concentration. It is shown that primary pathological foci are in the hippocampus and entorhinal cortex in the earlier stages of AD, and appears to subsume the MTG subsequently. The causality results indicate that there are larger differences in MTG between AD and age-matched healthy control but little in hippocampus, which implies local pathology in MTG being the predominant progressive abnormality during intermediate stages of AD development. In [25], the authors would like to address ongoing issues regarding how the default-mode network (DMN) hubs, including posterior cingulate cortex (PCC), medial prefrontal cortex (MPFC) and inferior parietal cortex (IPC), interact to each other, and the altered pattern of hubs in AD. Causal influences were examined between any pair of nodes within the DMN using Granger causality analysis and graph-theoretic methods on resting-state fMRI of 12 young subjects, 16 old normal controls and 15 AD patients. Results support the hub configuration of the DMN from the perspective of causal relationship, and reveal abnormal pattern of the DMN hubs in AD. Findings from young subjects give additional evidence for the role of PCC/MPFC/IPC acting as hubs in the DMN. Compared to old control, MPFC and IPC lost their roles as hubs due to the obvious causal interaction disruption, and PCC was preserved as the only hub with significant causal relations with all other nodes. Deshpande et al. [11] proposed a combination of multivariate Ganger causality analysis through temporal down-sampling of fMRI time series, to investigate causal brain networks and their dynamics. The method was applied to study epoch-to-epoch changes in a hand-gripping, muscle fatigue experiment. Causal influences between the activated regions were analyzed by applying the directed transfer function analysis of multivariate Granger causality with the integrated epoch response as the input, to account for the effects of several relevant regions simultaneously. The authors separately modeled the early, middle, and late periods in the fatigue. The results demonstrate the temporal evolution of the network and reveal that motor fatigue leads to a disconnection in the associated neural network.

Transfer Entropy and Directed Information: Vicente et al. [16] investigated the applicability of transfer entropy as a measure to electrophysiological data from simulations and MEG recordings in a motor task. Specifically, they demonstrated that transfer entropy improved the effective connectivity identification for non-linear interactions, and for sensor level MEG signals where linear approaches are hampered by signal-cross-talk due to volume conduction. Utilizing transfer entropy at the source-level, Wibral et al. [26] analyzed MEG data from an auditory short-term memory experiments and found that changes in the network between different task types can be detected. Prominently involved areas for the changes include left temporal pole and cerebellum, which have previously been implied to be involved in auditory short-term or working memory. Amblard and Michel [20] extracted Granger causality graphs using directed information, and such techniques were shown to be necessary to analyze the structure of systems with feedback in general, and neural systems specifically. Quinn et al. [10] proposed a nonlinear robust extension of the linear Granger tools also based directed information. They used point process models of neural spike trains, performed parameter and model order selection with minimal description length, and applied the analysis to infer the interactions and dynamics of neural ensembles in the primary motor cortex (MI) of macaque monkeys.

Multi-Scale Information and Multi-Scale Entropy: There is increasing evidence that brain signals are expressed with variability of the neural network dynamics [27]. Effective characterization of this variability in the complex systems can bring new insight to empirical studies. A number of tools have recently been developed, integrating information theory, nonlinear dynamics, and complex systems, to support the empirical research and unravel the principles of brain dynamics [28]. In particular, approximate entropy and sample entropy were proposed to quantify the complexity of short and noisy time series, and with later correcting the bias effect in approximate entropy. Higher values of sample entropy are associated with the signals having more complexity and less regular patterns, while smaller values indicate less irregularity in their representation. Note that signaling in the brain is not instantaneous, and neural activity propagation takes time. Utilizing multiscale entropy (MSE) is a reasonable strategy to control for the embedding delay of the brain system. This can be achieved through down-sampling the original time series by factors 2, 4, 8, etc., which, would alleviate the effects of linear correlations between consecutive samples. A similar idea was previously introduced in [29], using a complexity measure based on the Shannon entropy at various scales. Some studies used the approximate and sample entropy statistics to quantify the brain signal variability for both the electrode measurements [30] and source dynamics [31]. In [32], in order to test the hypothesis that complexity of BOLD activity is reduced with aging and is correlated with cognitive performance in the elderly, the authors employed the MSE analysis, and investigated appropriate parameters for MSE calculation. Compared with younger subjects, the older group had the most significant reductions in MSE of BOLD signals in posterior cingulate gyrus and hippocampal cortex. MSE of BOLD signals from DMN areas were found to be positively correlated with major cognitive functions including attention, short-term memory and language, etc. The MSE approach was also applied to reveal the differences in the EEG signals, between normal subjects and patients with AD. The resting-state EEG was utilized in [33] with MSE curves (scales 1-16) averaged over channels and individuals for three groups: normal population, subjects with mild cognitive impairment (MCI), and AD patients. The three groups have some common features for the MSE curves, i.e. the sample entropy reached its maximum at scales 5-7 and then gradually decreased. Severe AD patients had a significantly lower level of sample entropy values than that of the normal group at scale 2-16. The maximal difference in the complexity was observed at scales 6-8. Between MCI and normal subjects, the main difference in the MSE curve was the shift of the peak in sample entropy toward coarse timescales for the MCI group.

4. Probabilistic modeling and Bayesian inference for neural computation, cognition, and behavior

4.1. Bayes' theorem and approximate inference

A generic problem in science is: given the observed data D and some knowledge of the underlying data generating mechanism, can you tell something about the variable θ? Based on Bayes' theorem, our interest is the quantity:

$$p(\theta \mid \mathrm{D}) = \frac{p(\mathrm{D} \mid \theta)p(\theta)}{p(\mathrm{D})} = \frac{p(\mathrm{D} \mid \theta)p(\theta)}{\int_\theta p(\mathrm{D} \mid \theta)p(\theta)d\theta}.$$

That is: from a *generative model* $p(\mathrm{D} \mid \theta)$ of dataset and a *prior* belief $p(\theta)$ about which variable values are appropriate, we can infer the *posterior* distribution $p(\theta \mid \mathrm{D})$ of the variable in light of the observed data. When a particular observation is made, $p(\mathrm{D} \mid \theta)$ is called the likelihood. The *maximum a posteriori* (MAP) estimate maximizes the posterior, $\theta_{*}=\mathrm{argmax}_{\theta} p(\theta \mid \mathrm{D})$. For a flat prior, i.e. for $p(\theta)$ being a constant, the MAP solution is equivalent to the *maximum likelihood*, with θ maximizing the likelihood $p(\mathrm{D} \mid \theta)$ of the model generating the observed data. The MAP can incorporate our prior knowledge about the variable, but it is still a point estimate. Bayesian estimate gives the full probability distribution or density of the posterior $p(\theta \mid \mathrm{D})$. For example, when the distribution is wide or even has multiple peaks, the corresponding outputs can be averaged to make a more conservative estimate instead of just using a single point estimate.

A key algorithm challenge for Bayesian inference is for many models of interest, analytical tractability of the above posterior is elusive due to the integral in the denominator. We therefore resort to approximation inference, where the approaches tend to fall into one of following two classes: 1) *Monte Carlo methods* [34] provide approximate answers with accuracy depending on the number of generated samples. Importance sampling is a simple Monte Carlo approximation while Markov chain Monte Carlo (MCMC) is more efficient and popular. MCMC generates each sample by making a random change to the preceding sample. So we can think of an MCMC algorithm as being in a particular current state specifying a value for every variable and generating a next state by making random changes to the current state. Special cases of MCMC include Gibbs sampling and the Metropolis-Hasting algorithm. 2) *Variational approximations* [35, 36] are a series of deterministic techniques that make approximate inference for the parameters in complex statistical models. Compared with MCMC, they are much faster, especially for large models, but limited in their approximation accuracy. The mean-field approximation is a simplest example, which exploits the law of large numbers to approximate large sums of random variable by their means. Variational parameters are introduced and iteratively updated so as to minimize the KL divergence between the approximate and true probability distributions. Updating the variational parameters becomes a proxy for inference. The mean-field approximation produces a lower bound on the likelihood. More sophisticated methods are possible, which give tighter lower (and upper) bounds.

4.2. Neuroimaging data analyses using Bayesian approaches

Here I focus on Bayesian inference in fMRI data analysis, mainly for activation detection and hemodynamic response function (HRF) estimation, although the key concepts of Bayesian methods have been applied to structural MRI images as well [37-39]. Graphical model based Bayesian and dynamic Bayesian networks and their applications will be discussed in Section 5.

Bayesian inference has taken fMRI analysis research into an area that classical frequentist statistics have difficulty to address because of some challenging issues associated with the data. For example, fMRI response to stimuli is not instantaneous, but lagged and damped by the hemodynamic response. Estimating HRFs has gained increasing interests, since it provides not only a deep insight into the underlying dynamics of human brain, but also a basis for making inference of brain activation regions. How do we account for the HRF properties such as the nonlinearities and variability over different brain regions? fMRI is a 4-dimensional signal though with spatial and temporal noise correlations [40, 41]. How to incorporate the modeling of the presence of these correlations into the data analysis, alongside considering the clustered pattern of activation? Moreover, group level statistical inference of fMRI time series is usually needed to answer imaging-based scientific questions. How to make valid, sensitive and robust estimation of activation effects in populations of subjects? In fMRI analysis, what we often do is taking acquired data plus a generative model and extracting pertinent information about the brain, i.e. making inference on the model and its parameters. Bayesian statistics requires a prior probabilistic belief about the model parameters to be specified. Such models are typically HRF models, spatial models, and hierarchical multi-subject models, to respectively address the challenges listed above.

HRF models can incorporate biophysical or regularization priors for flexible HRF modeling across brain voxels and over subjects. Several similar Bayesian approaches in the literature use parametric HRFs with parameters describing features such as time-to-peak and undershoot size [42, 43]. Priors placed on these HRF parameters can ensure biological plausibility and result in increased sensitivity. An early example of more advanced HRF modeling is in [44], which uses Bayes to infer on a fully Bayesian biologically informed generative model. The reason of introducing regularization priors is the models have too many parameters to infer stably without regularization. Bayesian regularization places priors on HRF parameters to encode the prior belief that HRF is smooth temporally without strong assumptions about the shape of the response function. Thus such priors are suitable for exploratory approaches or possibly abnormal HRFs. Regularization priors can also be achieved through semi-parametric Bayesian for HRF modeling [45-47]. In semi-parametric approaches, HRF does not have a fixed parametric format but can take any form with a parameter describing the HRF size at each time point.

Spatial models for regularization using spatial Markov random field (MRF) priors to tackle spatial correlation in fMRI were proposed in [38, 48, 49], followed by MCMC numerical integration for inference. To overcome the large computation cost for spatial model inference in MCMC, Variational Bayesian approaches were developed [50, 51] without time-consuming numerical integration. Variational Bayes approximate the true posterior distribution through estimation using a posterior factorized over subsets of the model parameters, which results in update equations with the desired approximate posterior distributions in a much more efficient way than techniques such as MCMC. MRF-based work has recently been extended to using more flexible spatial Gaussian Process priors, to allow for the modeling of spatial non-stationarities [52] and the combining of spatial and non-spatial prior information [53]. The hyperparameters of the spatial priors can be estimated via Bayesian inference together with the rest of the model, which is a key advantage of fully Bayesian methods. Some other spatial models include mixture models representing the active and non-active voxels [54-56] and a Bayesian wavelets approach [57]. The popular mixture modeling, however, can be hampered by the presence of structured noise artifacts (e.g. stimulus correlated motion, spontaneous networks of

http://dx.doi.org/10.5772/55262

activity) violating the distributional assumptions. More sophisticated modeling of structured noise could be needed to render the distributional assumptions valid. Recent development of nonparametric Bayes can also be used to handle the mixture modeling, though a massive number of model parameters need to be estimated. Infinite mixture models based on Dirichlet process priors [58] involve effectively an infinite number of distributions. An application of such methods in fMRI for activation regions is in [59] using a spatial mixture model.

Hierarchical models for group inference was first proposed in [60], which fit naturally into the Bayesian framework via a cascade of conditional probabilities to handle activation effects over multiple subjects. In classical fMRI analysis, group-level inferences are usually made using the results of separate first-level analyses to decrease computation cost. This is the so-called summary statistics approach. The widely-used frequentist group analysis in [61] employed parameter estimates from the general linear model regression as summary statistics, which however, was only optimal under certain conditions due to the required balanced designs. On the contrary, Woolrich et al. [55] utilized Bayes to incorporate the summary statistics without restrictions, with information regarding both the effect sizes from the lower levels and their variances passed up.

4.3. Bayesian brain: Cognition, perception, uncertainty, behavior and neural representations

The neuroscience principle that the nervous system of animals and humans is adapted to the statistical properties of the environment is reflected across all organizational levels, from the activity of single neurons to networks and behavior [62]. A critical aim of the nervous system is to estimate the world state from incomplete and noisy data. During such process, a challenge issue that brains must handle is uncertainty. For example, when we perceive the physical world, make a decision, and take an action, there is uncertainty associated with the sensory system, the motor apparatus, one's own knowledge, and the world itself. Probability has played a central role in perception and cognition modeling. Specifically, the Bayesian framework of statistical estimation provides a systematic way of dealing with these uncertainties for optimal estimation. Comparison between the optimal and actual behavior gives rise to better understanding about how the nervous system works. Bayesian models have been used to explain results in perception, cognition, behavior, and neural coding in diverse forms [63-67], with differences in distinct assumptions about the world variables and how they relate to each other. However, the same key idea shared by all these Bayesian models is that different sources of information can be integrated for estimation of the relevant variables. Thus the Bayesian approach unifies an enormous range of otherwise apparently disparate behavior within one coherent framework.

A key aim of cognitive science is to reverse-engineer the mind. Cognition modeling based on the probabilistic method begins by identifying ideal solutions to these inductive problems, and then uses algorithms to model the mental processes for approximating these solutions. Neural processes are viewed as mechanisms for implementing these algorithms. Probabilistic models of cognition pursue a top-down strategy, which begins with abstract principles allowing agents to solve problems posed by the world (i.e. the functions minds performing) and then aims to reduce these principles to psychological and neural processes. This analysis results in better flexibility in exploration of the representations and inductive biases underlying human cognition. On the contrary, connectionist models usually follow a bottom-up approach that starts with a neural mechanism characterization and explores what macro-level functional phenomena might emerge. With a formal characterization of an inductive problem, a probabilistic model specifies the hypotheses under investigation, the relation between these hypotheses and observable data, and the prior probability of each hypothesis. By assuming different prior distribution for the hypotheses, different inductive biases can be captured. Although the link between probabilistic inference and neural computation/function is drawing attention of modelers from different backgrounds, little is known concerning how these structured representations can be implemented in neural systems for high-level cognition.

Sufficient results in perception have shown that the nervous system represents its uncertainty about the true state of the world probabilistically and such representations are utilized in two related cognitive areas: information fusion and perceptual decision-making. To fuse information from different sources about the same object, inferences about the object should rely on these sources commensurate with their corresponding uncertainty, as demonstrated in multisensory integration [68, 69] with the sources of different sensory modalities, or between information coming from the senses and being stored in memory [70, 71]. With the Bayesian framework, the organism calculates probability distributions over parameters describing the state of the world, with computation based on sensory information and knowledge accrued from experience. Although the particular sensory information and prior knowledge are specific to the task, the computation follows the same probability rules. Psychological evidence at the behavior level that animals and humans represent uncertainty during perceptual processes caused research into the neural underpinnings of such probabilistic representations. That is: how neurons compute with sensory uncertainty information or even full probability distributions? One scheme is the probabilistic population coding [72] that involves making use of the likelihood function encoded in neural population activity (as described below). Beyond perception, the neural implementation of cognitive probabilistic models has basically not been explored yet [64, 73].

Neural/Neuronal Models of Probabilistic Computation (Probabilistic Population Coding): Perception modeling has the potential to constrain neural implementation of perceptual computation. In order to form a neural model from a behavioral model, one needs to first define the relevant level of neural variables. A common candidate is the level of spike counts in sensory and decision-making neurons. For example, an orientated stimulus s might elicit a set of spike counts $\mathbf{r}=(r_1, \ldots, r_n)$ in a population of orientation-tuned cells in primary visual cortex. There is trial-to-trial variability in the population activity, which can be described by a distribution $p(\mathbf{r}|s)$. The connection between **r** and s, is that the latter (the scalar stimulus in a behavioral model) is the value maximizing the neural likelihood function, $\mathrm{L}(s)=p(\mathbf{r}|s)$ [74]. The likelihood function $\mathrm{L}(s)$ has a width, σ, reflecting the observer's uncertainty about the stimulus. The variable **r**, is high-dimensional with sufficient degrees of freedom to encode σ on a trial-by-trial basis. With neural likelihood functions, Bayesian models of behavior can be mapped to neural operations. This scheme has been successfully applied to cue combination [72], decision-making [75], etc. Some alternative approaches for encoding likelihood functions or probability distributions using neurons have also been proposed in the literature [65, 66, 76, 77].

5. Graphical models, Bayesian and dynamic Bayesian networks

5.1. Mathematical description and solution

Graphical models, intersecting probability and graph theories, provide a natural tool for handling uncertainty and complexity that frequently occur in applied mathematics and engineering, and scientific domains involving computation. Many of the classical multivariate probabilistic techniques are special cases of the general graphical models, such as mixture models, factor analysis, hidden Markov models, Kalman filters and Ising models [35, 78, 79]. A graph consists of *nodes* connected by *links* (also called *arcs* or *edges*). The nodes in probabilistic graphical models represent random variables, and the links or arcs express probabilistic relationships between these variables. The lack-of-arcs represent conditional independence assumptions. This provides a compact representation of joint probability distributions over all of the random variables, which can be decomposed into a product of factors each depending on a subset of variables. One category of graphical models is *Markov Random Fields* (MRFs), also known as *undirected graphical models*, in which the links do not have arrows and thus do not provide directional significance. For example, two sets of nodes A and B are conditionally independent given a third set, C, if all paths between the nodes in A and B are separated by a node in C. The other major class is *Bayesian Networks* or *Belief Networks* (BNs), also known as *directed graphical models*, in which the links carry arrows indicating a particular directionality in the notion of independence. Despite the complexity, directed models do have several advantages compared to undirected models; and the most important is that they can express causal relationships between random variables, whereas undirected graphics are more suitable for soft constraints between random variables.

In Bayesian Networks, if there is an arrow from node X to node Y, X is said to be a *parent* of Y. Each node X_i is associated with a conditional probability distribution (CPD) $\mathrm{P}(X_i \mid Parents(X_i))$, quantifying the effect of the parents on the node. If the variables are discrete, it is represented as a table (CPT), listing the probability that the child node takes on each of its different values for each combination of its parents' values. The network in BNs can be viewed as a representation of the joint probability distribution (JPD), or as an encoding of a collection of conditional independence statements. Let the joint distribution be $\mathrm{P}(x_1, \ldots, x_n)$; and we have

$$\mathrm{P}(x_1, \ldots, x_n) = \prod_{i=1}^{n} \mathrm{P}(x_i \mid parents(X_i)) \ , \tag{7}$$

where $parents(X_i)$ denotes the values of $Parents(X_i)$ appearing in $x_1, \ldots, x_n$. The CPTs are essentially conditional probability tables based on Eq. (7). In general, given n binary nodes, the full joint would require O^{2^n} space to represent, but due to the presence of independence in the graphical modeling, the factored form would require O^{n2^k} space, where k is the maximum fan-in of a node. Fewer parameters make learning easier.

Note that Bayesian networks do not necessarily imply Bayesian statistics. In fact, it is common to use frequentists methods to estimate the parameters of the CPDs. They are so called because they use Bayes' rule for probabilistic inference. Nevertheless, Bayes net are a useful representation for hierarchical Bayesian models, which form the foundation of applied Bayesian statistics. Bayesian statistical methods in conjunction with Bayesian networks offer an efficient and principled approach for avoiding the data overfitting. Dynamic Bayesian Networks (DBNs) are directed graphical models of stochastic processes, and generalization of hidden Markov models (HMMs) and linear dynamical systems (LDSs). DBN represent the hidden (and observed) state in terms of state variables, which can have complex interdependencies. The simplest DBN is a HMM, with one discrete hidden node and one discrete or continuous observed node per slice. A LDS has the same topology as an HMM, but all the nodes are assumed to have linear-Gaussian distributions. Kalman filter is an online filtering of this model.

A graphical model specifies a complete JPD over all the variables; and all possible inference queries can be answered by marginalization, i.e. summing out over irrelevant variables. However, the JPD has size O^{2^n}, with n the number of nodes, and each node is assumed to have 2 states. So, summing over the JPD takes exponential time. More efficient methods are thus desirable, including variable elimination [80], dynamic programming [81], approximation algorithms [34, 35] (Monte Carlo methods, variational methods), etc. For the learning part, a BN has two components that need to be specified, i.e. the graph topology (structure) and the parameters (CPD of each node). It is possible to learn both of these from data, though learning structure is much harder than learning parameters. Also, learning when some of the nodes are hidden, or we have missing data, is much harder than when everything is observed. This gives rise to 4 cases and the respective algorithms: 1) known structure and full observability: Maximum Likelihood Estimation; 2) known structure and partial observability: Expectation Maximization (EM) algorithm; 3) unknown structure, full observability: search through model space; 4) unknown structure, partial observability: EM and search through model space.

5.2. Applications and validity in neuroimaging and aging research

Functional MRI: Bayesian networks (BNs) were used in [82] to learn the structure of effective connectivity involved in a fMRI experiment. The approach is exploratory, does not require a priori hypothesized model, and was validated using synthetic data and fMRI data collected in silent word reading and counting Stroop tasks. However, BNs provide a single snapshot of effective connectivity of the entire experiment and thus are not suitable for accurately inferring the temporal characteristics of connectivity. Dynamic Bayesian networks (DBNs) were then proposed [83] to learn the structure of effective brain connectivity in an exploratory way. A

http://dx.doi.org/10.5772/55262

Markov chain was employed to model fMRI time-series for discovery of temporal interactions among brain regions. DBNs yield more accurate and informative brain connectivity than earlier methods since temporal characteristics of time-series are explicitly accounted. The functional structures captured on two fMRI datasets are consistent with the previous literature findings and more accurate than those identified by BN. Li et al. [84] aimed to extrapolate BN results from one subject to an entire population while addressing inter-subject, within-group variability. The authors explored two group analysis approaches in fMRI using DBNs: constructing a group network based on a common structure assumption across individuals, and identifying significant structure features by examining DBNs individually-trained. The methods were validated on subjects performing a motor task at three progressive levels of difficulty, and statistically significant, biologically plausible connectivity was detected.

Structural MRI: Detecting interactions among brain regions from structural MRI presents a major challenge in computational neuroanatomy. Instead of traditional univariate analysis for brain morphometry, a network analysis based on a BN representation of variables was investigated in [85] to take into account interactions among brain structures in explaining a clinical outcome. Results on a cross-sectional study of mild cognitive impairment (MCI) demonstrated nonlinear and complex multivariate associations among morphological changes in the left hippocampus, the right thalamus, and the presence of MCI. This indicates that the BN has the potential to predict the presence of MCI from structural MRI. Chen et al. [86] proposed to use DBN to represent evolving inter-regional dependencies and identify longitudinal morphological changes in the human brain. The main advantage of DBN modeling is that it can represent complicated interactions among temporal processes. The approach wad validated by analyzing a simulated atrophy study: only a small number of samples were needed to detect the ground-truth temporal model. The method was also applied to a longitudinal study of normal aging and MCI — the Baltimore Longitudinal Study of Aging. It was shown that interactions among regional volume-change rates for the MCI group were different from those for the normal aging group.

Further Development of Sparse BNs and Time-Varying DBNs: There are some recent new development in the area of BNs and DBNs. Sparse BN for effective connectivity modeling was investigated in [87], with a novel formulation for the structure learning of BNs. A L1-norm penalty term imposes sparsity and another penalty ensures the learned networks to satisfy the required property of BNs (i.e. directed acyclic graph). Both theoretical analysis and experiments on moderate and large benchmark networks demonstrate that the approach has enhanced learning accuracy and scalability compared with existing algorithms. The authors also applied the proposed method to brain images of 42 Alzheimer's disease (AD) and 67 normal controls (NC); the revealed effective connectivity of AD was shown to be different from that of NC, for example, in the global-scale effective connectivity, intra-lobe, inter-lobe, and inter-hemispheric effective connectivity distributions, and the effective connectivity corresponding to specific brain regions. Graphical model results are often based on static networks, assuming networks with invariant topology. For certain situations, it is desirable to understand and quantitatively model the dynamic topological and functional properties of biological or brain networks. This yields time or condition specific time-varying or non-stationary networks. In order to capture the dynamic causal influences between covariates, time-varying dynamic Bayesian networks (TV-DBNs) was proposed [88]. It models the varying directed dependency structures underlying non-stationary biological/neural time series. A kernel reweighted L1-regularized auto-regressive procedure was employed, with desirable properties including computational efficiency and asymptotic consistency. Application of the TV-DBNs to simulated data and brain EEG signals to visual stimuli show that the technique can identify temporally rewiring networks due to system dynamic transformation.

6. Dynamical brain system

6.1. Attractors and brain dynamics

Computational neuroscience illustrates the network dynamics of neurons and synapses with models to reproduce emergent properties or predict observed neurophysiology (e.g. single- and multiple-cell recordings, EEG, MEG, fMRI) and associated behavior [27]. Attractor theory [89] is a powerful theoretical framework that can capture the neural computations inherence in cognitive functions such as attention, memory, and decision making. It is based on mathematical models formulated at the level of neuronal spiking and synaptic activity. An attractor of a dynamical system is a subset of the state space to which orbits originating from typical initial conditions evolve over time. It is common for dynamical system to have more than one attractor. For each such attractor, its *basin of attraction* is the set of initial conditions that give rise to long-time behavior approaching that attractor. Reduced depths in the basins of attraction of prefrontal cortical networks and the noise effects could result in some cognitive symptoms like poor short-term memory and attention. The hypothesis is that reduced depth in the basins of attraction would make short-term memory unstable. Hence the continuing firing of neurons implementing short-term memory sometimes would cease, and the system under noise influence would fall back out of the short-term memory state into spontaneous firing. Top-down attention requires a short-term memory to hold the object of attention in mind. This is the source of the top-down attentional bias that influences competition in other networks receiving incoming signals. Therefore, disruption of short-term memory is also predicted to impair the attention stability.

6.2. Attractors dynamics in aging

The stochastic dynamical theory to brain function given above has implications in aging research. In the following, we describe effects of these factors and the associated hypotheses to aging [90]. The stochastic dynamic approach to aging can provide a way to test combinations of pharmacological treatments, which may together help to minimize the cognitive symptoms of aging.

NMDA Receptor Hypofunction: NMDA receptor functionality tends to decrease with aging [91]. This would act to reduce the depth of the basins of attraction, by reducing firing rate of the neurons in the active attractor, and by decreasing the strength of the potentiated synaptic connections that support each attractor. The reduced depth in the basins of attraction could have several effects to cognitive changes in aging. First, the stability of short-term memory networks would be impaired, which may cause difficulty in hold items in short-term memory for long. Second, top-down attention would be impaired. Third, the recall of information from episodic memory systems in the temporal lobe would be impaired [92]. Lastly, any reduction of the firing rate of the pyramidal cells caused by NMDA receptor hypofunction would itself be likely to impair new learning involving long-term potentiation (LTP).

Dopamine: D1 receptor blockade in the prefrontal cortex can impair short-term memory [93]. Partial reason for this may be that D1 receptor blockade can decrease NMDA receptor activated ion channel conductances. Hence part of the role of dopamine in prefrontal cortex in short-term memory can be accounted for by a decreased depth in the basins of attraction of prefrontal attractor networks [94]. The decreased depth would be caused by both the decreased firing rate of the neurons, and the reduced efficacy of the modified synapse since their ion channels would be less conductive. Dopaminergic function in the prefrontal cortex may decline with aging [95], which could contribute to the reduced short-term memory and attention in aging.

Impaired Synaptic Modification: Long-lasting associative synaptic modification may also contribute to the cognitive changes in aging, as LTP is more difficult to achieve in older animals and decays more quickly [91, 96]. This would tend to make the synaptic strengths support an attractor weaker and weaken further over time, and thus directly reduces the depth of the attractor basins. This would impact episodic memory, the memory for particular past episodes. The reduction of synaptic strength over time could also affect short-term memory, which requires the synapses supporting a short-term memory attractor be modified in the first place using LTP, before the attractor is used [97].

Cholinergic Function: Acetylcholine in the neocortex has its origin largely in the cholinergic neurons in the basal magnocellular forebrain nuclei of Meynert. The correlation of clinical dementia ratings with the reductions in a number of cortical cholinergic markers such as choline acetyltransferase, muscarinic and nicotinic acetylcholine receptor binding, as well as levels of acetylcholine, implied an association of cholinergic hypothesis of memory dysfunction in senescence and AD [98]. Cholinergic system could also alter the cerebral cortex function in ways that can be illuminated by stochastic neurodynamics [99]. Enhancing cholinergic function will likely help to reduce the instability of attractor networks involved in short-term memory and attention that may occur in aging.

7. Conclusions

Brain structure and activity can be described at various levels of resolution. Recent developments in biotechnology have provided us the ability to measure and record population neuronal activity with more precision and accuracy than ever before, allowing researchers to study and perform detailed analyses which may have been impossible just a few years ago. Brain imaging techniques, such as EEG, MEG, and structural/functional MRI, open macroscopic windows on processes in the working brain. These methods yield high dimensional data sets that are organized in space and time [100]. This creates a huge analysis need to extract interpretable signals and information from the big data, harvesting the full richness of the multi-modality measurements of the multi-scale brain. One of the future directions on the computation side is to develop high-dimensional analysis methods for mining and modeling of the neuroscience data, and thus to assess and interpret properties in the joint data set combining imaging and behavior/stimulus measurements. The objective is to further our understanding about how neural structures of humans and other animals develop, are aged, and create systems able to accomplish basic and complex behavioral tasks.

Acknowledgements

Preparation of this chapter is supported in part by a grant from the National Institute of Aging, K25AG033725.

Author details

Michelle Yongmei Wang*

Address all correspondence to: ymw@illinois.edu

Departments of Statistics, Psychology, and Bioengineering, Beckman Institute, University of Illinois at Urbana-Champaign, U.S.A.

References

[1] Purves, D., Augustine, G. J., Fitzpatrick, D., Hall, W. C., LaMantia, A.-S., & White, L. E. *Neuroscience*, Sinauer Associates, Inc., (2008).

[2] Ramachandran, V. S. *Encyclopedia of the Human Brain*, (2002), 3.

[3] Logothetis, N. K., Pauls, J., Augath, M., Trinath, T., & Oeltermann, A. Neurophysiological investigation of the basis of the fMRI signal, *Nature*, (2001), 412: 150-157.

[4] Sporns, O. *Networks of the Brain*, Massachusetts Institute of Technology, (2011).

[5] Friston, K. J. Functional and effective connectivity: a review, *Brain Connectivity*, (2011), 1: 13-36.

[6] Sporns, O. *Discovering the Human Connectome*, Massachusetts Institute of Technology, (2012).

[7] Shannon, C. E. A mathematical theory of communication, *Bell System Technical Journal*, (1948), 27: 379-423.

[8] Granger, C. Investigating causal relations by econoetric models and cross-spectral methods, *Econometrica,* (1969), 37: 424-438.

[9] Seth, A. K. A MATLAB toolbox for Granger causal connectivity analysis, *J Neurosci Methods,* (2010), 186: 262-273.

[10] Quinn, C. J., Coleman, T. P., Kiyavash, N., & Hatsopoulos, N. G. Estimating the directed information to infer causal relationships in ensemble neural spike train recordings, *J Comput Neurosci,* (2011), 30: 17-44.

[11] Deshpande, G., LaConte, S., James, G. A., Peltier, S., & Hu, X. Multivariate Granger causality analysis of fMRI data, *Hum Brain Mapp, (2009),* 30: 1361-1373.

[12] Akaike, H. A new look at the statistical model identification, *IEEE Transactions on Automatic Control,* (1974), 19: 716-723.

[13] Schwartz, G. Estimating the dimension of a model, *Annals of Statistics,* (1978), 5: 461-464.

[14] Kaminski, M., Ding, M., Truccolo, W. A., & Bressker, S. L. Evaluating causal relations in neural systems: Granger causality, directed transfer function and statistical assessment of significance, *Biological Cybernetics,* (2001), 85: 145-157.

[15] Schreiber, T. Measuring information transfer, *Phys Rev Lett,* (2000), 85: 461-464.

[16] Vicente, R., Wibral, M., Lindner, M., & Pipa, G. Transfer entropy--a model-free measure of effective connectivity for the neurosciences, *J Comput Neurosci,* (2011), 30: 45-67.

[17] Barnett, L., Barrett, A. B., & Seth, A. K. Granger causality and transfer entropy are equivalent for Gaussian variables, *Phys Rev Lett,* (2009), 103: 238701.

[18] Marko, H. The bidirectional communication theory- a generalization of information theory, *IEEE Transactions on Communications,* (1973), 21: 1345-1351.

[19] Massey, G. Causality, feedback and directed information, in *Proceedings of International Symposium on Information Theory and Its Applications,* (1990), pp. 27-30.

[20] Amblard, P. O., & Michel, O. J. On directed information theory and Granger causality graphs, *J Comput Neurosci,* (2011), 30: 7-16.

[21] Seghouane, A. K., & Amari, S. Identification of directed influence: Granger causality, Kullback-Leibler divergence, and complexity, *Neural Comput,* (2012), 24: 1722-1739.

[22] Kramer, G. *Directed Information for Channels with Feedback,* Ph.D. Thesis, University of Manitoba, Canada, (1998).

[23] Liu, Y., & Aviyente, S. The relationship between transfer entropy and directed information, in *IEEE Statistical Signal Processing Workshop,* (2012), pp. 73-76.

[24] Li, X., Coyle, D., Maguire, L., Watson, D. R., & Mcginnity, T. M. Gray matter concentration and effective connectivity changes in Alzheimber's disease: a longitudinal structural MRI study, *Diagnostic Neuroradiology,* (2011), 53: 773-748.

[25] Miao, X., Wu, X., Li, R., Chen, K., & Yao, L. Altered connectivity pattern of hubs in default-mode network with Alzheimer's disease: an Granger causality modeling approach, *PLoS One,* (2011), 6: e25546.

[26] Wibral, M., Rahm, B., Rieder, M., Lindner, M., Vicente, R., & Kaiser, J. Transfer entropy in magnetoencephalographic data: quantifying information flow in cortical and cerebellar networks, *Prog Biophys Mol Biol,* (2011), 105: 80-97.

[27] Rabinovich, M. I., Friston, K. J., & Varona, P. *Principles of Brain Dynamics,* Massachusetts Institute of Technology, (2012).

[28] Vakorin, V. A., Ross, B., Krakovska, O., Bardouille, T., Cheyne, D., & Mcintosh, A. R. Complexity analysis of source activity underlying the neuromagnetic somatosensory steady-state response, *Neuroimage,* (2010), 51: 83-90.

[29] Zhang, Y.-C. Complexity and 1/f noise. A phase space approach, *Journal of Physique I France,* (1991), 1: 971-977.

[30] Abasolo, D., Hornero, R., Espino, P., Alvarez, D., & Poza, J. Entropy analysis of the EEG background activity in Alzheimer's disease patients, *Physiological Mesurement,* (2006), 27: 241-253.

[31] Misic, B., Mills, T., Taylor, M. J., & Mcintosh, A. R. Brain noise is task-dependent and region-specific, *Journal of Neurophysiology,* (2010), 104: 2667-2676.

[32] Yang, A. C., Huang, C.-C., Yeh, H.-L., Liu, M.-E., Hong, C.-J., & Tu, P.-C. Complexity of spontaneous BOLD activity in default mode network is correlated with cognitive function in normal male elderly: a multiscale entropy analysis, *Neurobiology of Aging,* (2013), 34: 428-438.

[33] Park, J. H., Kim, S., Kim, C. H., Cichocki, A., & Kim, K. Multiscale entropy analysis of EEG from patients under different pathological conditions, *Fractals,* (2007), 15: 399-404.

[34] Robert, C., & Casella, G. *Monte Carlo Statistical Methods,* Berlin: Springer-Verlag, (2004).

[35] Jordan, M., Ghahramani, Z., Jaakkola, T., & Saul, L. An introduction to variational methods for graphical models, *Machine Learning,* (1999), 37: 183-233.

[36] Ormerod, J. T., & Wand, M. P. Explaining variational approximations, *The American Statistician,* (2010), 64: 140-153.

[37] Wang, Y. *Statistical Shape Analysis for Image Segmentation and Physical Model-Based Non-Rigid Registration,* Ph.D. Thesis, Department of Electrical Engineering, Yale University, (1999).

[38] Woolrich, M. W., Jbabdi, S., Patenaude, B., Chappell, M., Makni, S., & Behrens, T. Bayesian analysis of neuroimaging data in FSL, *Neuroimage,* (2009), 45: S173-S186.

[39] Wang, Y, & Staib, L. H. Boundary finding with prior shape and smoothness models, *IEEE Trans. on Pattern Analysis and Machine Intelligence,* (2000), 22: 738-743.

[40] Wang, Y. M., & Xia, J. Unified framework for robust estimation of brain networks from fMRI using temporal and spatial correlation analyses, *IEEE Transactions on Medical Imaging,* (2009), 28: 1296-1307.

[41] Wang, Y. M. Modeling and nonlinear analysis in fMRI via statistical learning, in *Advanced Image Processing in Magnetic Resonance Imaging*, Landini, L. Positano, V., & Santarelli, M. F., Eds., Marcel Dekker International Publisher, (2005), pp. 565-586.

[42] Genovese, C. A Bayesian time-course model for functional magnetic resonance imaging data (with discussion), *Journal of the American Statistical Association,* (2000), 95: 691-703.

[43] Gossl, C., Fahrmeir, I., & Auer, D. P. Bayesian modeling of the hemodynamic response function in bold fmri, *Neuroimage,* (2001), 14: 140-148.

[44] Friston, K. J. Bayesian estimation of dynamical systems: an application to fmri, *Neuroimage,* (2002), 16: 513-530.

[45] Ciuciu, P., Poline, J. B., Marrelec, G., Idier, J., Pallier, C., & Benali, H. Unsupervised robust nonparametric estimation of the hemodynamic response function for any fmri experiment, *IEEE Transactions on Medical Imaging,* (2003), 22: 1235-1251.

[46] Goutte, C., Nielsen, F. A, & Hansen, L. K. Modeling the haemodynamic response in fmri using smooth fir filters, *IEEE Transactions on Medical Imaging,* (2000), 19: 1188-1201.

[47] Marrelec, G., Benali, H., Ciuciu, P., Pelegrini-Issac, M., & Poline, J. B. Robust Bayesian estimation of the hemodynamic response function in event-related bold fmri using basic physiological information, *Human Brain Mapping,* (2003), 15: 1-25.

[48] Gossl, C., Auer, D. P., & Fahrmeir, L. Bayeisan spatiotemporal inference in functional magnetic resonance imaging, *Biometrics,* (2001), 57: 554-562.

[49] Xia, J., Liang, F., & Wang, Y. M. FMRI analysis through Bayesian variable selection with a spatial prior, in *IEEE International Symposium on Biomedical Imaging,* (2009), pp. 714-717.

[50] Penny, W. D., Trujillo-Barreto, N. J, & Friston, K. J. Bayesian fmri time series analysis with spatial priors, *Neuroimage,* (2005), 24: 350-362.

[51] Woolrich, M., Behrens, T., & Smith, S. Constrained linear basis sets for HRF modeling using variational Bayes, *Neuroimage,* (2004), 21: 1748-1761.

[52] Harrison, L. M., Penny, W. D., Ashburner, J., Trujillo-Barreto, N., & Friston, K. J. Diffusion-based spatial priors for imaging, *Neuroimage,* (2007), 38: 677-695.

[53] Groves, A. R., Chappell, M. A., & Woolrich, M. W. Combined spatial and non-spatial prior for inference on MRI time-series, *Neuroimage,* (2009), 45: 795-809.

[54] Hartvig, N. V., & Jensen, J. L. Spatial mixture modeling of fMRI data, *Hum Brain Mapp,* (2000), 11: 233-248.

[55] Woolrich, M., Behrens, T, Beckmann, C, & Smith, S. Mixture models with adaptive spatial regularization for segmentation with an application to fmri data, *IEEE Transactions on Medical Imaging,* (2005), 24: 1-11.

[56] Xia, J., Liang, F., & Wang, Y. M. On clustering fMRI using Potts and mixture regression models, in *IEEE Engineering in Medicine and Biology Society Conference,* (2009), pp. 4795-4798.

[57] Flandin, G., & Penny, W. D. Bayesian fMRI data analysis with sparse spatial basis function priors, *Neuroimage,* (2007), 34: 1108-1125.

[58] Fergusson, T. A Bayesian analysis of some nonparametric problems, *Annals of Statistics,* (1973), 1: 209-230.

[59] Kim, S., & Smyth, P. Hierarchical Dirichlet Processes with random effects, in *Neural Information Processing Systems,* (2006), pp. 697-704.

[60] Friston, K. J., Penny, W., Phillips, C., Kiebel, S., Hinton, G., & Ashburner, J. Classical and Bayesian inference in neuroimaging: theory, *Neuroimage,* (2002), 16: 465-483.

[61] Holmes, A., & Friston, K. Generalisability, random effects & population inference, in *Fourth International Conference on Functional Mapping of the Human Brain: Neuroimage,* (1998), pp. S754.

[62] Geisler, W. S., & Diehl, R. L. Bayesian natural selection and the evolution of perceptual systems, *Philos Trans R Soc Lond B Biol Sci,* (2002), 357: 419-448.

[63] Ma, W. J. Organizing probabilistic models of perception, *Trends Cogn Sci,* (2012), 16: 511-518.

[64] Griffiths, T. L., Chater, N., Kemp, C., Perfors, A., & Tenenbaum, J. B. Probabilistic models of cognition: exploring representations and inductive biases, *Trends Cogn Sci,* (2010), 14: 357-364.

[65] Fiser, J., Berkes, P., Orban, G., & Lengyel, M. Statistically optimal perception and learning: from behavior to neural representations, *Trends Cogn Sci,* (2010), 14: 119-130.

[66] Vilares, I., & Kording, K. Bayesian models: the structure of the world, uncertainty, behavior, and the brain, *Ann N Y Acad Sci,* (2011), 1224: 22-39.

[67] Knill, D. C., & Pouget, A. The Bayesian brain: the role of uncertainty in neural coding and computation, *Trends Neurosci,* (2004), 27: 712-719.

[68] Atkins, J. E., Fiser, J., & Jacobs, R. A. Experience-dependent visual cue integration based on consistencies between visual and haptic percepts, *Vision Res,* (2001), 41: 449-461.

[69] Ernst, M. O., & Banks, M. S. Humans integrate visual and haptic information in a statistically optimal fashion, *Nature,* (2002), 415: 429-433.

[70] Weiss, Y., Simoncelli, E. P., & Adelson, E. H. Motion illusions as optimal percepts, *Nat Neurosci,* (2002), 5: 598-604.

[71] Kording, K. P., & Wolpert, D. M. Bayesian integration in sensorimotor learning, *Nature,* (2004), 427: 244-247.

[72] Ma, W. J., Beck, J. M., Latham, P. E., & Pouget, A. Bayesian inference with probabilistic population codes, *Nat Neurosci,* (2006), 9: 1432-1438.

[73] Shi, L., Griffiths, T. L., Feldman, N. H., & Sanborn, A. N. Exemplar models as a mechanism for performing Bayesian inference, *Psychon Bull Rev,* (2010), 17: 443-464.

[74] Sanger, T. D. Probability density estimation for the interpretation of neural population codes, *J Neurophysiol,* (1996), 76: 2790-2793.

[75] Huys, Q. J. M., Zemel, R. S., Natarajan, R., & Dayan, P. Fast population coding, *Neural Computation,* (2007), 19: 404-441.

[76] Deneve, S. Bayesian spiking neurons I: inference, *Neural Comput,* Jan (2008). , 20, 91-117.

[77] Jazayeri, M., & Movshon, J. A. Optimal representation of sensory information by neural populations, *Nat Neurosci,* (2006), 9: 690-696.

[78] Murphy, K. P. *Dynamic Bayesian Networks: Representation, Inference and Learning,* Ph.D. Thesis, Department of Computer Science, University of California, Berkeley, (2002).

[79] Bishop, C. M. *Pattern Recognition and Machine Learning,* Springer Science + Business Media, LLC, (2006).

[80] Kschischang, F. R., Frey, B. J., & Loeliger, H.-A. Factor graphs and the sum-product algorithm, *IEEE Transactions on Information Theory,* (2001), 47: 498-519.

[81] Peot, M. A., & Shachter, R. D. Fusion and propagation with multiple observations in belief networks, *Artificial Intelligence,* (1991), 48: 299-318.

[82] Zheng, X., & Rajapakse, J. C. Learning functional structure from fMR images, *Neuroimage,* (2006), 31: 1601-1613.

[83] Rajapakse, J. C., & Zhou, J. Learning effective brain connectivity with dynamic Bayesian networks, *Neuroimage,* (2007), 37: 749-760.

[84] Li, J., Wang, Z. J., & Mckeown, M. J. Multi-subject, A. dynamic Bayesian networks (DBNs) framework for brain effective connectivity, in *IEEE International Conference on Acoustics, Speech and Signal Processing*, (2007). pp. I-429 – I-432.

[85] Chen, R., & Herskovits, E. H. Network analysis of mild cognitive impairment, *Neuroimage,* (2006), 29: 1252-1259.

[86] Chen, R., Resnick, S. M., Davatzikos, C., & Herskovits, E. H. Dynamic Bayesian network modeling for longitudinal brain morphometry, *Neuroimage,* Feb 1 (2012). , 59, 2330-2338.

[87] Huang, S., Li, J., Ye, J., Fleisher, A., Chen, K., & Wu, T. Brain effective connectivity modeling for Alzheimer's disease study by sparse Bayesian network, in *The Seventeenth ACM SIGKDD International Conference On Knowledge Discovery and Data Mining* (2011), pp. 931-939.

[88] Song, L., Kolar, M., & Xing, E. P. Time-varying dynamic Bayesian networks, in *Proceeding of the 23rd Neural Information Processing Systems,* (2009), pp. 1732-1740.

[89] Brunel, N., & Wang, X. J. Effects of neuromodulation in a cortical network model of object working memory dominated by recurrent inhibition, *J Comput Neurosci,* (2001), 11: 63-85.

[90] Rolls, E. T., Deco, G., & Loh, M. *A Stochastic Neurodynamics Approach to the Changes in Cognition and Memory in Aging,* (2010).

[91] Kelly, K. M., Nadon, N. L., Morrison, J. H., Thibault, O., Barnes, C. A., & Blalock, E. M. The neurobiology of aging, *Epilepsy Res,* Suppl 1, 2006), 68: S5-20.

[92] Dere, E., Easton, A., Nadel, I., & Huston, J. P. *Handbook of Episodic Memory*, Elsevier, Amsterdam, (2008).

[93] Goldman-Rakic, P. S. The physiological approach: functional architecture of working memory and disordered cognition in schizophrenia, *Biol Psychiatry,* (1999), 46: 650-661.

[94] Loh, M., Rolls, E. T., & Deco, G. Statistical fluctuations in attractor networks related to schizophrenia, *Pharmacopsychiatry,* (2007), 40: S78-S84.

[95] Sikstrom, S. Computational perspectives on neuromodulation of aging, *Acta Neurochir Suppl,* (2007), 97: 513-518.

[96] Burke, S. N., & Barnes, C. A. Neural plasticity in the ageing brain, *Nat Rev Neurosci,* (2006), 7: 30-40.

[97] Kesner, R. P., & Rolls, E. T. Role of long-term synaptic modification in short-term memory, *Hippocampus,* (2001), 11: 240-250.

[98] Schliebs, R., & Arendt, T. The significance of the cholinergic system in the brain during aging and in Alzheimer's disease, *J Neural Transm,* (2006), 113: 1625-1644.

[99] Rolls, E. T., & Deco, G. *The Noisy Brain: Stochastic Dynamics as a Principle of Brain Function*, Oxford University Press, (2012).

[100] Wang, M. Y., Zhou, C., & Xia, J. Statistical analysis for recovery of structure and function from brain images, in *Biomedical Engineering, Trends, Researches and Technologies*, Komorowska, M. A. & Olsztynska-Janus, S., Eds., (2011), pp. 169-196.

Chapter 11

The Crossmodal Influence of Odor Hedonics on Facial Attractiveness: Behavioural and fMRI Measures

Francis McGlone, Robert A. Österbauer,
Luisa M. Demattè and Charles Spence

Additional information is available at the end of the chapter

http://dx.doi.org/10.5772/56504

1. Introduction

Facial attractiveness is a highly relevant social cue, readily assessed by human observers. Facial attractiveness significantly impact on success in both work and social environments [1, 2]. Taking a Darwinian perspective, Perrett at al. [3] have argued that the physical structure of beautiful faces – as judged by others – provide salient signals of mate value that motivate behavior in others. Several general features have been shown to contribute to the perceived attractiveness of a face, including both facial symmetry and the extent to which an individual face conforms to an average prototype [4, 5, 6]. Additionally, faces displaying various emotional expressions (e.g., joy, anger, etc.) have been used to investigate the brain regions involved in the coding of affect [7, 8, 9, 10, 11], such as the orbitofrontal cortex (OFC), the insular cortex, and the amygdala.

At both an explicit and implicit level, humans through the ages have devised means by which to enhance facial attractiveness (a multibillion dollar cosmetic industry attests to this fact). An equally lucrative fragrance industry exploits the hedonic primacy of odors in the human brain, yet it remains unclear whether the presence of odors can modulate the perceived attractiveness of faces.

A pioneering positron emission tomography (PET) study by Nakamura and colleagues [12] demonstrated that activity in left frontal brain regions correlates with perceived facial attractiveness in humans. Furthermore, functional magnetic resonance imaging (fMRI) has been used to show that the viewing of attractive female faces by male participants activates reward circuitry in the brain, in particular, the nucleus accumbens and the OFC [13, 14].

A recent study investigated the neural circuitry involved in the perception of facial attractiveness more directly by presenting participants with faces of varying attractiveness, while they performed a gender discrimination task [15]. Correlation analysis with ratings of attractiveness for the presented faces revealed a region in the medial orbitofrontal cortex (OFC) that responded specifically to facial attractiveness.

Physical attractiveness is not, however, solely dependent upon the visual aspects of appearance, but is often modulated by other sensory cues. For example, a person's voice has been shown to influence a speaker's perceived attractiveness [16, 17]. Similarly, a person's body odor also influences their perceived attractiveness [18]. The notion that odors can exert an influence over the perception of facial characteristics is also supported by the observation that the perceived masculinity/femininity of faces may be modulated by the presence of human sex hormone-like chemicals [19]. Additionally, the presence of a malodor can negatively influence the perceived attractiveness of male faces as rated by female observers in a psychophysical judgment task [20].

Only a few neuroimaging experiments have simultaneously presented odors and faces to participants, but none have directly assessed the impact of odor valence on facial attractiveness. For example, an fMRI study conducted by Gottfried and colleagues [21] paired faces with either a pleasant, unpleasant, or neutral odor, in an associative learning paradigm. Their results suggest that the brain regions involved in the processing of positive and negative affect, such as OFC, nucleus accumbens, and amygdala, are engaged during the appetitive and aversive learning process. Additionally, those brain areas previously found to participate in low-level odor processing, such as the piriform cortex and the caudal OFC, were also found to play an active role in the transfer of affective value between the olfactory and visual modalities. However, since no measure of the attractiveness of the faces was obtained, it remains unclear whether odor valence actually influenced the participants' perception of the faces.

Finally, it could be argued that odors do not necessarily modulate facial attractiveness *per se*, but rather other affective components of interpersonal perception such as, for example, perceived sympathy [22]. Alternatively, however, the presentation of the odor could also induce a general change in a person's mood (or emotional state) that might also be expected to alter facial attractiveness. Indeed, the psychological and physiological literature published to date supports the view that visual stimuli can influence olfactory perception while olfactory cues rarely influence visual perception [23, 24, 25, 26]. It thus appears reasonable to assume that the simultaneous presentation of an odor will not change the visual characteristics of a face as such, but rather will primarily just changes people's affective reaction to it.

The main aim of the present study was therefore to investigate, both behaviorally and using fMRI, whether olfactory cues can modulate visual judgments of facial attractiveness. In particular, we investigated whether olfactory cues of differing hedonic value (i.e., pleasant vs. unpleasant) enhance and/or reduce the perceived attractiveness of male faces to female participants. Additionally, we selected an artificial body odor and a common male fragrance as the olfactory stimuli for their ecological relevance when paired with human faces. We hypothesized that the OFC, in particular, would show differential responses depending on the perceived attractiveness of the stimuli presented, since this brain region

http://dx.doi.org/10.5772/56504

is activated by pleasant / unpleasant smells [27, 28, 29, 21, 30], and is also known to encode facial attractiveness [31, 15].

2. Material and methods

2.1. Participants

Twenty-one healthy right-handed female volunteers participated in this study (mean age 23 years, age range 19-29 years). All of the participants were non-smoking, had no history of nasal dysfunction or allergies to odors and each gave written informed consent after having received the written instructions concerning the study. Three participants had to be removed from the data analysis because of excessive head motion during the brain scanning session, and the data from two participants were discarded because they were unable to detect the presence versus absence of the odors at above chance levels (44% and 53% correct, respectively). Consequently, the data analysis at the group level included a total of 16 datasets. The study was approved by the Central Oxford Research Ethics Committee (C99.179).

2.2. Stimuli and task

Two odorants were used in this study, an artificial body odor (Thiol compound) and a popular male fragrance. The odors were diluted in 30ml of dipropylene glycol at concentrations of 0.0033% for the body odor and 0.5% for the male fragrance. The olfactory stimuli were delivered with a custom-built, computer-controlled olfactometer at a flow rate of 4 liters/ second, through Teflon tubes placed directly under the participant's nose. The participants were asked to breathe normally through their nose and to refrain from making any unduly strong sniffing movements. Clean medical air was delivered continuously through the olfactometer except during the delivery of the olfactory stimuli.

Twenty male faces taken from the standardized database developed by Perrett and his colleagues [3] were used as the visual stimuli. These faces have previously been rated for attractiveness on a 5-point rating scale. We used a subset of these faces, consisting of the 10 faces with the highest attractiveness ratings and the 10 faces with the lowest attractiveness ratings. Full screen color images of the faces were generated using a video projector located outside the scanner room and projected onto a translucent screen placed directly outside the bore of the magnet. A mirror fixed on the head coil allowed the participants to view the screen while lying in the scanner.

Each of the 20 faces was presented three times, once together with each of the two odors and once in the absence of any odor, resulting in the three conditions 'face-pleasant odor', 'face-unpleasant odor' and 'face-no odor'. Additionally, each odor was presented 10 times in the absence of any visual stimulus, resulting in a total of 80 trials being presented to each participant. The order of trials was randomized for each participant, with the sole constraint that the same face was never presented consecutively.

At the beginning of each trial, the participants were visually cued by the presentation of a fixation cross to breathe in and detect the presence or absence of an odor which was delivered for 2500ms following the onset of the visual cue (Figure 1). The faces were presented for 1000ms starting 1500ms after the onset of the odor stimuli. This lag between visual and olfactory stimuli was chosen on the basis of the results of a pilot study which had established that participants perceived the onset of both stimuli as concurrent when presented at this temporal delay.

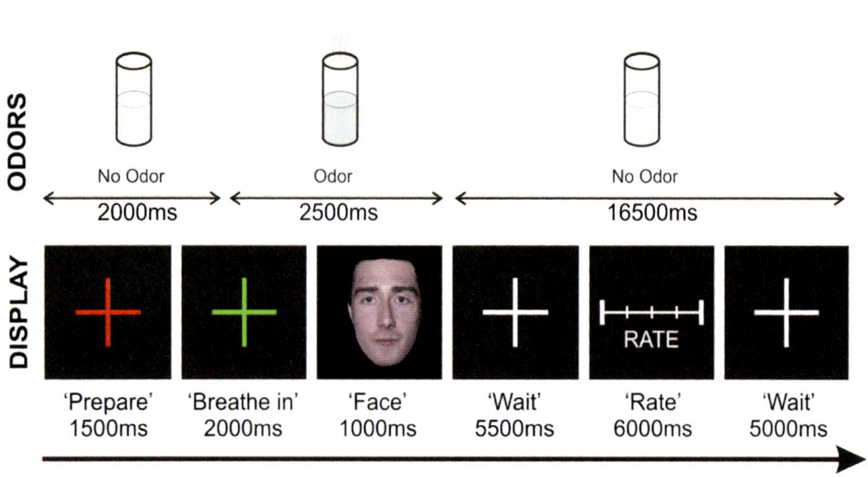

Figure 1. Participants were cued visually with a fixation cross that changed color from red to green to breathe-in and detect the presence or absence of an odor. In the trials where a face was presented, it was shown for 1000ms, beginning 2000ms after the cue to breathe in. After a rest period of 5500ms, the participants had to rate the attractiveness of the face on a 5-point rating scale. When odors were presented in the same trial, odor stimulation started 500ms after the onset of the cue to breathe-in and lasted for 2500ms, terminating together with the face. When odors were presented without a face, the cue to breathe in was displayed for 3000ms and the participants had simply to rate the pleasantness of the odor.

Following the presentation of the face, the participants rated its attractiveness on a rating scale ranging from 1='very unattractive' to 5='very attractive' with 3 as the neutral point. For the odor only trials, the participants had to rate the pleasantness of the odor on a similar scale ranging from 1='very unpleasant' to 5='very pleasant'. Behavioral measures relating to odor detection as well as the ratings were collected using a custom build button-box. The E-Prime software [32] was used to control stimulus presentation and to collect responses from the participants.

2.3. Data acquisition and analysis

Both functional and structural MRI images were acquired using a 3T Sonata Siemens scanner fitted with an 8-channel head coil (Siemens Medical Solutions, Erlangen, Germany) based at the University of Oxford Centre for Clinical Magnetic Resonance Research (OCMR). For the

http://dx.doi.org/10.5772/56504

functional data series, a total of 1120 T2* weighted echo-planar imaging (EPI) volumes were taken over a time period of 28 min.

Each volume consisted of 27 continuous oblique (tilted approximately 20º upward from the anterior to posterior commissure line, so as to be aligned with the temporal lobes) slices of 3mm thickness with an in-plane resolution of 3×3mm. These imaging parameters allowed us to image the ventral two thirds of the brain until approximately Z-coordinate of +50 of the Montreal Neurological Institute (MNI) 152 standard brain space, to include all primary and secondary olfactory areas in the temporal lobes and OFC, as well as the visual cortex. Other imaging parameters were: TR=1.5s, 64x64 matrix, FOV 192×192 mm, TE=30ms and, flip angle = 90º.

After acquisition of the functional volumes, a B_0 field map was acquired using a combined symmetric and asymmetric spin echo sequence. For registration into standard anatomical space, a single whole brain EPI volume (50 slices, TR=5s, other imaging parameters as above) as well as a high-resolution, whole-brain T1 weighted morphological scan (inversion-recovery fast gradient echo, 1 mm slice thickness, 1mm×1mm in-plane resolution) was acquired after the experimental paradigm had been completed.

Statistical image analysis of the functional dataset was carried out using the FMRIB Expert Analysis Tool (FEAT; www.fmrib.ox.ac.uk/fsl). The following pre-processing was applied: motion correction using MCFLIRT [33]; spatial smoothing using a Gaussian kernel of FWHM 5mm; mean-based intensity normalization of all volumes by the same factor; non-linear high-pass temporal filtering (Gaussian-weighted LSF straight line fitting, sigma=25s). A general linear model using the conditions Face-No odor/Face-Body odor/Face-Fragrance/Body odor/Fragrance as explanatory variables was fitted to the time course at each voxel. Statistical analysis for each experimental run was carried out using FMRIB's Improved Linear Model (FILM) with local autocorrelation correction [34].

For group analysis, the individual results were registered both to high-resolution anatomical MR images and to the Montreal Neurological Institute (MNI) 152 standard image. Registration to high resolution and standard images was carried out using FMRIB's Linear Image Registration Tool (FLIRT) [33]. Mixed-effects (often referred to as 'random-effects') group analysis was carried out using FMRIB's Local Analysis of Mixed Effects (FLAME) software [35] with a cluster threshold of Z>2.0 and a cluster significance threshold of p=.05 (corrected for multiple comparisons) [36, 37, 38].

3. Results

3.1. Behavioral

Comparison of the pleasantness ratings when the two odors were presented in isolation confirmed that the body odor was indeed perceived as significantly [$t(15) = 8.04$; $p < .001$] less pleasant ($M = 1.78$; $SEM = 0.14$) than the fragrance ($M = 3.68$; $SEM = 0.22$), as expected. The rating data for facial attractiveness were analyzed using a repeated-measures analysis of variance (ANOVA) with the factors of facial attractiveness (low vs. high) and odor condition (pleasant, unpleasant, or odorless). As expected, the results revealed a significant main effect of facial attractiveness, [$F(1,15) = 138.23$, $p < .001$], with participants judging the pre-selected attractive faces as being more attractive ($M = 3.56$; $SEM = 0.11$) than those faces pre-selected to be less attractive ($M = 2.15$; $SEM = 0.1$). Crucially, the main effect of odors on ratings of facial attractiveness was also significant [$F(2,14)= 9.17$, $p < .01$], demonstrating that the odors affected the perceived attractiveness of the male faces to the female participants. Post-hoc comparisons (Bonferroni corrected) of the 3 odor conditions revealed that participants rated the same faces as being significantly less attractive when presented together with the unpleasant body odor ($M = 2.60$; $SEM = 0.09$) than when presented together with the pleasant odor ($M = 2.99$; $SEM = 0.11$; $p < .01$), or in the absence of any odor ($M = 2.97$; $SEM = 0.1$; $p < .01$; see Figure 2). The analysis of this behavioral data revealed no significant difference in mean facial attractiveness ratings between the pleasant versus odorless conditions, nor any interaction between facial attractiveness and odor pleasantness [$F(2,14) < 1$; *n.s.*].

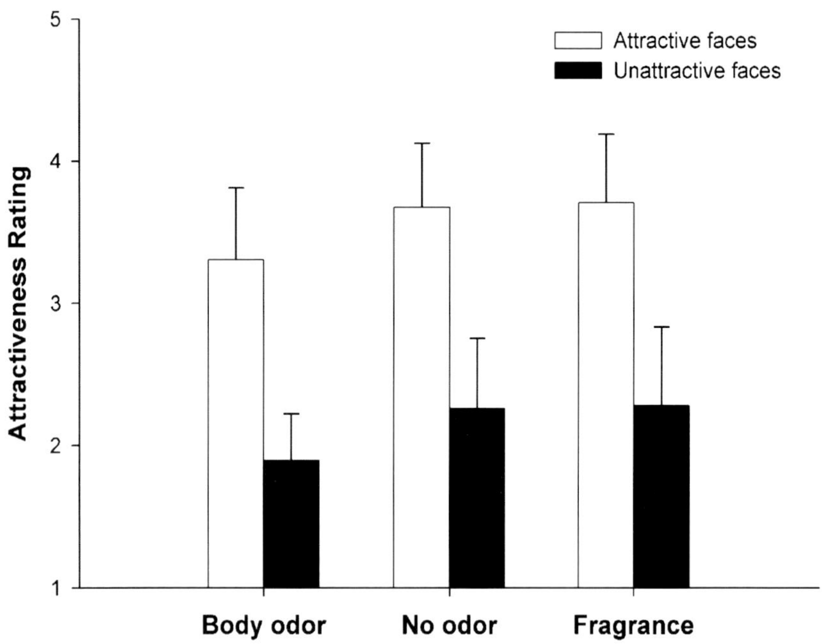

Figure 2. The average attractiveness ratings (n=16 participants) for the same 10 faces a-priori assumed to be of high attractiveness compared to the 10 low attractiveness faces are shown when either presented with an unpleasant body odor, a pleasant fragrance, or in the absence of any specific odor. The difference in ratings between the attractive and unattractive faces was significant (paired t-test, p <.05) in each odor group. Additionally, faces presented together with the body odor were rated as significantly less attractive than those presented with the fragrance or those presented in the absence of any odor (paired t-test, p <.05) for both high and low attractive faces.

3.2. Neuroimaging data

3.2.1. Odor valence

We first investigated those brain regions involved in encoding odor valence (pleasant vs. unpleasant) in the absence of any visual stimuli (i.e., faces). For this purpose, we computed two contrasts between the unimodal odor presentations, which were [Fragrance > Body odor] and [Body odor > Fragrance]. Results from the first contrasts showed several regions within the OFC to be more strongly activated by the pleasant fragrance as compared to the unpleasant odor (see Figure 3). These were located bilaterally in the medial OFC along the olfactory sulcus (*x/y/z* = 12/44/-18; *z-score* = 2.62 and *x/y/z* = -14/44/-14; *z-score* = 2.55), and in the lateral OFC in the right hemisphere only (*x/y/z* = 22/50/-8; *z-score* = 2.63). Additionally, a small cluster was detected in the right inferior frontal gyrus pars triangularis (*x/y/z* = 32/34/2; *z-score* = 2.36).

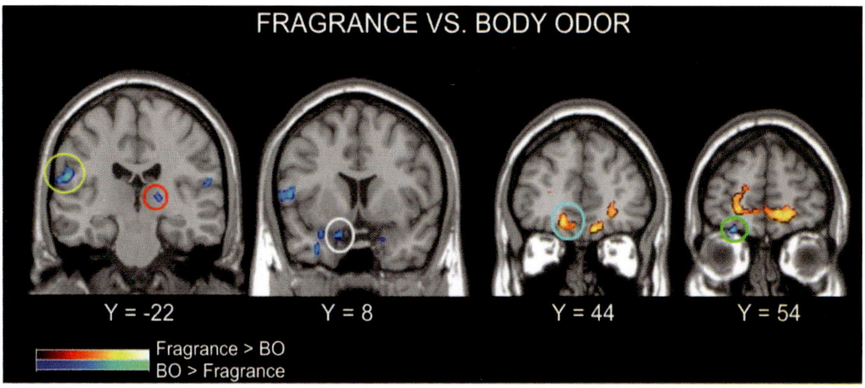

Figure 3. Group results (n=16 participants) for brain regions showing differences in brain activation relating to the pleasantness of the odors are shown on coronal slices at different y-coordinates in the canonical MNI 152 space. The contrast [Fragrance > BO] is rendered in orange/yellow and the contrast [BO > Fragrance] is rendered in blue. The unpleasant BO elicited stronger responses in the supramarginal gyrus (yellow), thalamus (red), piriform cortex (white), and lateral OFC (green). In contrast, the pleasant fragrance caused stronger activation primarily in medial OFC (turquoise). The right side of each slice corresponds to the right side of the brain.

Conversely, within the OFC, the unpleasant odor activated more strongly only in the left lateral orbital gyrus (*x/y/z* = -24/54/-18; *z-score* = 2.51). However, activation was stronger in the primary sensory olfactory areas in the piriform cortex/amygdaloid area bilaterally (*x/y/z* = 20/10/-26; *z-score* = 2.13 and *x/y/z* = -16/6/22; *z-score* = 2.28) and in the frontal operculum (*x/y/z* = 58/0/10; *z-score* = 2.13 and *x/y/z* = -54/8/8; *z-score* = 2.33). Activation differences were also detected bilaterally in the supramarginal gyrus (*x/y/z* = 58/-20/16; *z-score* = 2.27 and *x/y/z* = -56/-22/22; *z-score* = 2.52) and in the right thalamus (*x/y/z* = 18/-22/6; *z-score* = 2.30).

3.2.2. Facial attractiveness

In order to highlight those brain areas involved in encoding the attractiveness of the face stimuli independently of odors, we compared the responses to faces with high vs. low attractiveness. For these contrasts, no distinction was made between the various odor conditions (Fragrance, Body odor and clean air), which were grouped together. The results revealed that irrespective of the odor condition, the presentation of the more attractive faces led to increased BOLD signal amplitude in the medial OFC in both hemispheres (*x/y/z* = 4/36/-8; *z-score* = 2.60 and *x/y/z* = -2/36/-4; *z-score* = 2.96, see Figure 4). Two other brain regions also showed stronger activation in response to the more attractive faces, namely the left nucleus accumbens (*x/y/z* = -6/8/-18; *z-score* = 2.93) and the hypothalamus (*x/y/z* = 0/-6/-18; *z-score* = 2.69). Conversely, the presentation of the unattractive faces resulted in stronger activation bilaterally in the amygdala (*x/y/z* = 22/0/-12; *z-score* = 2.19 and *x/y/z* = -22/-4/-14; *z-score* = 2.45) as well as in the right pallidum (*x/y/z* = 26/-10/-6; *z-score* = 2.99). Interestingly, the unattractive faces also elicited stronger activation in visual areas in the left inferior occipital gyrus (*x/y/z* = -16/-96/-8; *z-score* = 2.61).

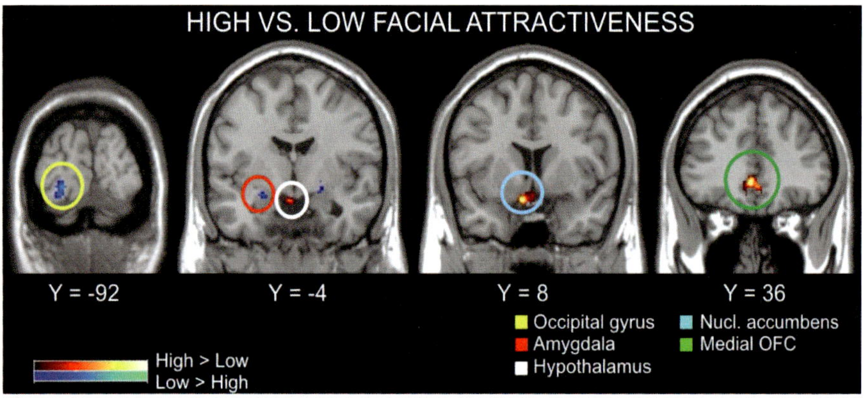

Figure 4. Group results (n=16 participants) for brain regions showing differences in brain activation relating to the attractiveness of the faces (high vs. low) are shown on coronal slices at different y-coordinates in the canonical MNI 152 space. The contrast [High > Low] is rendered in orange/yellow and the contrast [Low > High] is rendered in blue. Attractive faces preferentially engaged the medial OFC, whereas the less attractive faces led to stronger activation in the amygdala. The right side of each slice corresponds to the right side of the brain.

3.2.3. Odor-face interactions

The primary interest of the present study was to address the question of whether or not odor hedonics would influence the perceived or implicit attractiveness of male faces to female participants. The behavioral results confirmed that the same set of faces was rated as being significantly more attractive when accompanied by the pleasant odor as compared to the unpleasant odor. We were specifically interested in the brain regions associated with this effect and therefore contrasted those trials in which the faces were presented with the pleasant male fragrance to those where the same faces were presented with the unpleasant body odor. Similar to the unisensory effects of pleasant vs. unpleasant odors and attractive vs. unattractive faces, the face stimuli caused significantly stronger activation in the medial (*x/y/z* = -6/44/-24; *z-*

http://dx.doi.org/10.5772/56504

score = 2.64) and lateral (*x/y/z* = -38/54/-16; *z-score* = 2.93) OFC as well as in the ventral striatum (*x/y/z* = -2/12/-16; *z-score* = 2.63), when they were presented together with the pleasant odor (see Figure 5). A further analysis of the percentage BOLD signal change in the peak activated voxels in the left OFC (see Figure 6) revealed positive signal changes only when faces were presented with the fragrance or in the absence of odors. The responses in these regions to all other stimuli were either close to zero or slightly negative.

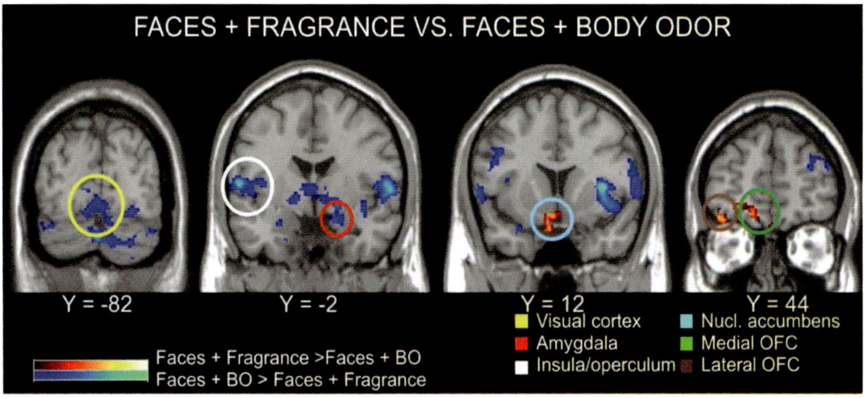

Figure 5. Group results (n=16 participants) for brain regions showing differences in brain activation when the same set of faces was presented together with the pleasant fragrance compared to the unpleasant body odor. The contrast [Faces + Fragrance > Faces + BO] is rendered in orange/yellow and the contrast [Faces + BO > Faces + Fragrance] is rendered in blue. The presence of the fragrance preferentially engaged the OFC and ventral striatum. Conversely, the unpleasant odor caused stronger activation in the amygdala, insular cortex, and visual cortex. The right side of each slice corresponds to the right side of the brain.

Conversely, a different network of brain regions responded more strongly when the faces were presented together with the unpleasant body odor. The presence of the unpleasant odor caused significantly stronger activation in the amygdala (*x/y/z* = 20/-8/-16; *z-score* = 3.03 and *x/y/z* = -18/-6/-16; *z-score* = 2.65) and anterior insular cortex (*x/y/z* = 36/12/6; *z-score* = 3.95 and *x/y/z* = -32/24/0; *z-score* = 3.01). Furthermore, we observed significantly stronger responses in the thalamus (*x/y/z* = 12/-16/4; *z-score* = 3.95 and *x/y/z* = -6/-20/4; *z-score* = 3.39) and an extensive cluster located at the junction of the rolandic operculum with the superior temporal sulcus (*x/y/z* = 60/-22/18; *z-score* = 4.06 and *x/y/z* = -62/-20/-14; *z-score* = 3.79). The only differences in frontal brain regions was found in the right medial frontal gyrus (*x/y/z* = 30/28/30; *z-score* = 2.69). Interestingly, both visual cortical areas (*x/y/z* = -2/-86/-10; *z-score* = 3.02) as well as the cerebellum (x/y/z = 12/-56/-14; z-score = 3.50 and x/y/z = -20/-60/-20; z-score = 3.97) also displayed stronger activation when the faces were accompanied by the unpleasant odor. A further analysis of the percentage BOLD signal change in the peak activated voxels in the amygdala (see Figure 7) revealed positive signal changes for all conditions.

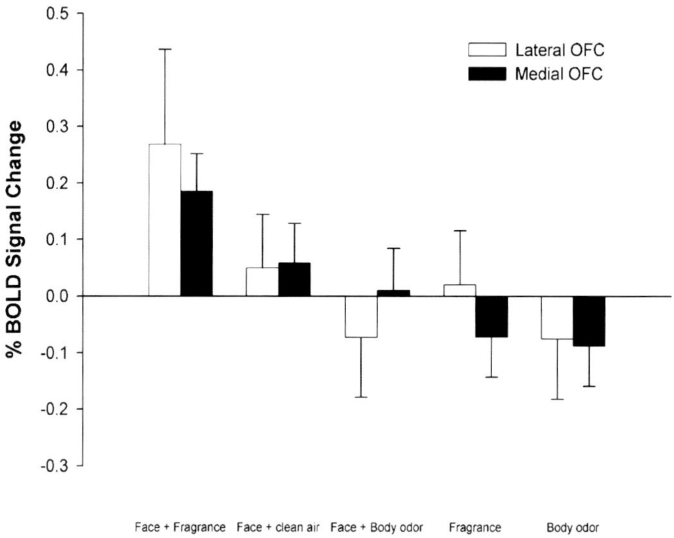

Figure 6. The average (n=16 participants) percentage BOLD signal change in the peak voxels in both medial and lateral OFC are shown for each of the five experimental conditions. Error bars depict the standard error.

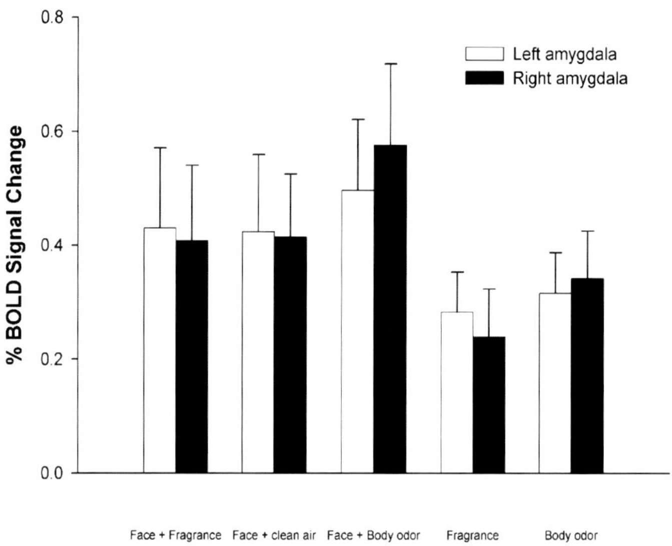

Figure 7. The average (n=16 participants) percentage BOLD signal change from baseline in the peak voxels in both the left and right amygdala are shown for each of the five experimental conditions. Error bars depict the standard error.

4. Discussion

The principal aim of the present study was to determine whether specific pleasant vs. unpleasant odors can exert a significant influence on the perception of facial attractiveness. Behavioral results confirmed that the two odors used in this study (a male fragrance and a synthetic body odor) were indeed perceived as different with respect to their pleasantness. Significantly, when briefly presented with the same set of male faces, the female participants in this study judged the faces accompanied by the pleasant fragrance as more attractive than when the faces were presented with an unpleasant synthetic body odor. This effect was related to a modulatory effect exerted by the unpleasant odor, as no significant difference in facial attractiveness *ratings* was found between the pleasant odor and a 'no odor' control condition.

In agreement with the behavioral data, the pleasant fragrance activated the medial OFC, a region that encodes the reward value of stimuli across a variety of sensory modalities including olfaction [27, 30, 39, 40]. Conversely, the unpleasant odor activated a different network or brain regions, including the amygdala which has previously been implicated in the processing of aversive stimuli [30, 41, 42].

There is currently some controversy over the role of the amygdala in the processing of odor hedonics, since the established view that this region specifically encodes aversive odors [43, 42] has been challenged by several more recent studies. For example, Anderson and colleagues [27] used the pleasant odor citral (which has a lemon smell) and the unpleasant odor valeric acid (a rancid smell) in high and low concentrations so that they could vary the valence and intensity of these stimuli. They found that amygdala activation was associated with odor intensity, but was independent of valence. Conversely, activity in the OFC was associated with odor valence, independent of intensity. In a similar study using a greater number of odors (3 pleasant and 3 unpleasant), Rolls and colleagues [40] found that ratings of odor intensity were correlated with the magnitude of the BOLD signal in medial olfactory cortical areas (including the piriform and anterior entorhinal cortex), but not in the OFC. In contrast, pleasant odors were found to activate a medial region of the OFC, whereas unpleasant odors activated the left lateral OFC, irrespective of odor intensity. Activation of this area have also been reported after monetary losses, unattractiveness in face stimuli, and the presentation of aversive odors [39, 44, 45, 46]. Since the odors used in the present study were matched with respect to their intensities, this supports the notion that stimulus aversiveness is encoded in the human amygdala. This view is also supported by the results of a recent study demonstrating that the amygdala does not encode odor valence or intensity *per se*, but rather appears to contain a general representation of the emotional value of a stimulus [47].

When the activation seen in response to more attractive faces was compared to that seen in response to relatively less attractive faces, it was found that the former engaged a reward circuit consisting of the medial OFC and nucleus accumbens, consistent with previous studies [31, 14, 15]. By contrast, relatively less attractive faces gave rise to stronger activation in the amygdala, a region implicated in the processing of the emotional expression of faces [48, 49] particularly when the expression is negative (fear, anger). The results presented here suggest that less attractive faces produce a similar neural response to that elicited by faces displaying negative emotions.

The main finding to emerge from this study was that the presence of odors with different hedonic characteristics altered the perception of male facial attractiveness in female participants. Under such conditions of bimodal stimulation, we found that when the faces were presented together with a pleasant fragrance, increased BOLD activation was predominantly observed in the OFC and ventral striatum (i.e. in the same regions that are engaged when viewing attractive faces). It appears that the positive valence of the odor interacted with the representation (itself not unpleasant), with the neuroimaging data providing a more in these regions, leading to an overall positive emotional response to the multisensory combination of stimuli (i.e., face plus odor). This observation is consistent with previous studies that have implicated these regions in the processing of facial attractiveness [31, 14, 15] and positively valenced odors [27, 40, 47]. Despite the observation that attractiveness *ratings* were no different when faces were presented together with the pleasant odor compared to faces presented in the absence of odors, significantly positive BOLD responses within the OFC were only observed in the former condition. This may suggest that even though the pleasant odor did not increase the consciously perceived and reported visual attractiveness of the faces *per se*, the medial OFC did and here we conjecture that this effect engaged more implicit affective processes that participants were unable to access consciously, but would nonetheless impact on mechanisms underpinning liking.

In contrast, when the male faces were presented with the unpleasant body odor, ratings of facial attractiveness were significantly reduced, compared to the pleasant odor and the odorless condition. The presence of the unpleasant odor caused significantly stronger activation in the insular cortex and the amygdala, both of which have previously been implicated in the representation of negative affect [50, 51, 52] and facial unattractiveness [15]. It thus appears that the aversiveness of the body odor negatively influences the emotional response to a face, leading to a decrease in its perceived attractiveness, an effect that was observed for faces of both high and low attractiveness. Several factors might explain the observation that the body odor influenced the ratings and brain activation more strongly than the fragrance. First, the hedonic difference of the body odor from hedonically neutral was greater than that of the fragrance (rating of 1.78 for body odor versus. 3.68 for fragrance with 3 being 'neutral'), so that a stronger effect might be expected on that basis alone.

In conclusion, even though the behavioral response (as measured by overt rating of facial attractiveness) in the presence of the pleasant odor, or no odor, condition did not influence facial attractiveness, results from the neuroimaging component of the study did show activations in the reward processing areas of OFC and ventral striatum. Reward region activity as evaluated using fMRI did not therefore follow the results of the behavioural task. The latter, we suggest, lacked the sensitivity required to dissociate between the fragrance and clean air (itself not unpleasant) of facial attractiveness with the neuroimaging data providing a more sensitive measure of affective state. For the unpleasant body odor, our findings support the notion that in the context of facial beauty, unpleasant odors have higher overt emotional salience than pleasant odors.

http://dx.doi.org/10.5772/56504

Acknowledgements

We would like to thank Unilever Research for supporting this research.

Author details

Francis McGlone[1], Robert A. Österbauer[2], Luisa M. Demattè[3] and Charles Spence[3]

1 School of Natural Sciences and Psychology, Liverpool John Moores University, UK

2 Oxford Centre for Functional Magnetic Resonance Imaging of the Brain, John Radcliffe Hospital, University of Oxford, Oxford, UK

3 Crossmodal Research Laboratory, Department of Experimental Psychology, University of Oxford, Oxford, UK

References

[1] Frieze IH, Olson JE and, Good DC, Perceived and actual discrimination in the salaries of male and female managers. *J. Appl. Soc. Psychol* 20: 46–67, 1990

[2] Marlowe CM, Schneider SL, and Nelson CE. Gender and attractiveness biases in hiring decisions are more experienced managers less biased? *J. Appl. Psychol* 81: 11–21, 1996

[3] Perrett DI, Lee KJ, Penton-Voak I, Rowland D, Yoshikawa S, Burt DM, Henzi SP, Castles DL, and Akamatsu S. Effects of sexual dimorphism on facial attractiveness. *Nature* 394: 884-887, 1998.

[4] Grammer K, and Thornhill R. Human (Homo sapiens) facial attractiveness and sexual selection: the role of symmetry and averageness. *J Comp Psychol* 108: 233-242, 1994.

[5] Hoss RA, Ramsey JL, Griffin AM, and Langlois JH. The role of facial attractiveness and facial masculinity/femininity in sex classification of faces. *Perception* 34: 1459-1474, 2005.

[6] Perrett D, May K, and Yoshikawa S. Facial shape and judgments of female attractiveness. *Nature 368*: 239–242, 1994.

[7] Adolphs R, Tranel D, Damasio H, and Damasio A. Impaired recognition of emotion in facial expressions following bilateral damage to the human amygdala. *Nature* 372: 669-672, 1994.

[8] Blair RJ, Morris JS, Frith CD, Perrett DI, and Dolan RJ. Dissociable neural responses to facial expressions of sadness and anger. *Brain* 122: 883-893, 1999.

[9] Haxby JV, Hoffman EA, and Gobbini MI. Human neural systems for face recognition and social communication. *Biol Psychiatry* 51: 59-67, 2002.

[10] Morris JS, Frith CD, Perrett DI, Rowland D, Young AW, Calder AJ, and Dolan RJ. A differential neural response in the human amygdala to fearful and happy facial expressions. *Nature* 383: 812-815, 1996.

[11] Posamentier MT, and Abdi H. Processing faces and facial expressions. *Neuropsychol Rev* 13: 113-143, 2003.

[12] Nakamura K, Kawashima R, Nagumo S, Ito K, Sugiura M, Kato T, Nakamura A, Hatano K, Kubota K, Fukuda H, and Kojima S. Neuroanatomical correlates of the assessment of facial attractiveness. *Neuroreport* 9: 753-757, 1998

[13] Aharon I, Etcoff N, Ariely D, Chabris CF, O'Connor E, and Breiter HC. Beautiful faces have variable reward value: fMRI and behavioral evidence. *Neuron* 32: 537-551, 2001.

[14] Kampe KK, Frith CD, Dolan RJ, and Frith U. Reward value of attractiveness and gaze. *Nature* 413: 589, 2001.

[15] O'Doherty J, Winston J, Critchley H, Perrett D, Burt DM, and Dolan RJ. Beauty in a smile: the role of medial orbitofrontal cortex in facial attractiveness. *Neuropsychologia* 41: 147-155, 2003.

[16] Casey SJ, Woods AT, and Newell FN. Is beauty in the eyes and ear of the beholder? In: *7th Annual Meeting of the International Multisensory Research Forum*. Dublin, Ireland: 200

[17] Zuckerman M, Miyake K, and Hodgins HS. Cross-channel effects of vocal and physical attractiveness and their implications for interpersonal perception. *J Pers Soc Psychol* 60: 545-554, 1991.

[18] Rikowski A, and Grammer K. Human body odour, symmetry and attractiveness. *Proc Biol Sci* 266: 869-874, 1999.

[19] Kovács G, Gulyas B, Savic I, Perrett DI, Cornwell RE, Little AC, Jones BC, Burt DM, Gal V, and Vidnyanszky Z. Smelling human sex hormone-like compounds affects face gender judgment of men. *Neuroreport* 15: 1275-1277, 2004.

[20] Dematte ML, Osterbauer R, and Spence C. Olfactory cues modulate facial attractiveness. *Chem Senses* 32: 603-610, 2007.

[21] Gottfried JA, O'Doherty J, and Dolan RJ. Appetitive and aversive olfactory learning in humans studied using event-related functional magnetic resonance imaging. *J Neurosci* 22: 10829-10837, 2002.

[22] König R. Kulturanthropologische Betrachtungen zum Problem der Parfmierung [A cultural anthropological consideration of the problem of perfume]. *J Cosmet Sci* 23: 823-829, 1972.

[23] Gottfried JA, and Dolan RJ. The nose smells what the eye sees: crossmodal visual facilitation of human olfactory perception. *Neuron* 39: 375-386, 2003

[24] Morrot G, Brochet F, and Dubourdieu D. The color of odors. *Brain Lang* 79: 309-320, 2001.

[25] Österbauer RA, Matthews PM, Jenkinson M, Beckmann CF, Hansen PC, and Calvert GA. Color of scents: chromatic stimuli modulate odor responses in the human brain. *J Neurophysiol* 93: 3434-3441, 2005.

[26] Zellner DA, Bartoli AM, and Eckard R. Influence of color on odor identification and liking ratings. *Am J Psychol* 104: 547-561, 1991.

[27] Anderson AK, Christoff K, Stappen I, Panitz D, Ghahremani DG, Glover G, Gabrieli JD, and Sobel N. Dissociated neural representations of intensity and valence in human olfaction. *Nat Neurosci* 6: 196-202, 2003.

[28] de Araujo IE, Rolls ET, Kringelbach ML, McGlone F, and Phillips N. Taste-olfactory convergence, and the representation of the pleasantness of flavour, in the human brain. *Eur J Neurosci* 18: 2059-2068, 2003.

[29] de Araujo IE, Rolls ET, Velazco MI, Margot C, and Cayeux I. Cognitive modulation of olfactory processing. *Neuron* 46: 671-679, 2005.

[30] Gottfried JA, O'Doherty J, and Dolan RJ. Encoding predictive reward value in human amygdala and orbitofrontal cortex. *Science* 301: 1104-1107, 2003.

[31] Ishai A. Sex, beauty and the orbitofrontal cortex. *Int J Psychophysiol* 63: 181-185, 2006

[32] Schneider W, Eschman A, and Zuccolotto A. *E-Prime reference guide. Pittsburgh, PA: Psychology Software Tools Inc.* 2002.

[33] Jenkinson M, Bannister P, Brady M, and Smith S. Improved optimization for the robust and accurate linear registration and motion correction of brain images. *Neuroimage* 17: 825-841, 2002.

[34] Woolrich MW, Ripley BD, Brady M, and Smith SM. Temporal autocorrelation in univariate linear modeling of FMRI data. *Neuroimage* 14: 1370-1386, 2001.

[35] Beckmann CF, Jenkinson M, and Smith SM. General multilevel linear modeling for group analysis in FMRI. *Neuroimage* 20: 1052-1063, 2003.

[36] Forman SD, Cohen JD, Fitzgerald M, Eddy WF, Mintun MA, and Noll DC. Improved assessment of significant activation in functional magnetic resonance imaging (fMRI): use of a cluster-size threshold. *Magn Reson Med* 33: 636-647, 1995.

[37] Friston KJ, Worsley KJ, Frakowiak RSJ, Mazziotta JC, and Evans AC. Assessing the significance of focal activations using their spatial extent. *Hum Brain Mapp* 1: 214-220, 1994.

[38] Worsley KJ, Evans AC, Marrett S, and Neelin P. A three-dimensional statistical analysis for CBF activation studies in human brain. *J Cereb Blood Flow Metab* 12: 900-918, 1992.

[39] O'Doherty J, Rolls ET, Francis S, Bowtell R, and McGlone F. Representation of pleasant and aversive taste in the human brain. *J Neurophysiol* 85: 1315-1321, 2001.

[40] Rolls ET, Kringelbach ML, and de Araujo IE. Different representations of pleasant and unpleasant odours in the human brain. *Eur J Neurosci* 18: 695-703, 2003.

[41] Zald DH, Lee JT, Fluegel KW, and Pardo JV. Aversive gustatory stimulation activates limbic circuits in humans. *Brain* 121: 1143-1154, 1998.

[42] Zald DH, and Pardo JV. Emotion, olfaction, and the human amygdala: amygdala activation during aversive olfactory stimulation. *Proc Natl Acad Sci USA* 94: 4119-4124, 1997.

[43] Royet JP, Hudry J, Zald DH, Godinot D, Gregoire MC, Lavenne F, Costes N, and Holley A. Functional neuroanatomy of different olfactory judgments. *Neuroimage* 13: 506-519, 2001.

[44] Ursu, S. and Carter, C. S. Outcome representations, counterfactual comparisons and the human orbitofrontal cortex: implications for neuroimaging studies of decision-making. *Cogn Brain Res*, 23(1), 51-60, 2005

[45] Liu X, Powell DK, Wang H, Gold BT, Corbly CR, and Joseph JE. Functional dissociation in frontal and striatal areas for processing of positive and negative reward information. *J Neurosci* 27:4587– 4597, 2007

[46] Elloit R, Agnew Z, and Deakin B. Hedonic and Informational Functions of the Human Orbitofrontal Cortex. *Cerebral Cortex* 20(1): 198-204, 2010

[47] Winston JS, Gottfried JA, Kilner JM, and Dolan RJ. Integrated neural representations of odor intensity and affective valence in human amygdala. *J Neurosci* 25: 8903-8907, 2005.

[48] Dolan RJ, Morris JS, and de Gelder B. Crossmodal binding of fear in voice and face. *Proc Natl Acad Sci USA* 98: 10006-10010, 2001.

[49] Kesler-West ML, Andersen AH, Smith CD, Avison MJ, Davis CE, Kryscio RJ, and Blonder LX. Neural substrates of facial emotion processing using fMRI. *Brain Res Cogn Brain Res* 11: 213-226, 2001.

[50] Nitschke JB, Sarinopoulos I, Mackiewicz KL, Schaefer HS, and Davidson RJ. Functional neuroanatomy of aversion and its anticipation. *Neuroimage* 29: 106-116, 2006.

[51] Sato W, Yoshikawa S, Kochiyama T, and Matsumura M. The amygdala processes the emotional significance of facial expressions: an fMRI investigation using the interaction between expression and face direction. *Neuroimage* 22: 1006-1013, 2004.

[52] Wicker B, Keysers C, Plailly J, Royet JP, Gallese V, and Rizzolatti G. Both of us disgusted in my insula: the common neural basis of seeing and feeling disgust. *Neuron* 40: 655-664, 2003.

Chapter 12

Seeing with Two Eyes: Integration of Binocular Retinal Projections in the Brain

Tenelle A. Wilks, Alan R. Harvey and Jennifer Rodger

Additional information is available at the end of the chapter

http://dx.doi.org/10.5772/56491

1. Introduction

In the visual system, accurate representation of images throughout each stage of processing requires the maintenance of topography in different but interconnected brain regions [1]. Topographic organisation also allows information from both eyes to be precisely integrated, underpinning depth perception and interpretation of the visual world. In the absence of this organisation within and between eye-specific projections, visual information becomes scrambled within the brain and function is compromised [2,3]. Despite advances in recent years that have given insight into the mechanisms responsible for topographic mapping of visual projections within the brain, comparatively less is known about the mechanisms that underpin the integration of binocular pathways. The aim of this review is to summarise what is known about the developmental processes that establish topography in binocular projections in key animal models. We review experiments in mice that examine the development of binocular projections to the superior colliculus and address the role of molecular guidance cues. We will also describe experiments in Siamese cats that shed light on the organisation of binocular projections to the lateral geniculate nucleus and visual cortex. Finally, we will discuss this research in the context of early diagnosis and rehabilitation strategies of loss of binocular vision in humans.

We will first describe the development and organisation of contralateral (crossed) and ipsilateral (uncrossed) visual projections to the major visual brain centres: the superior colliculus (SC), dorsal lateral geniculate nucleus (dLGN) and primary visual cortex (V1), with focus on their integration in relation to visual space. We will then consider how topography is established in the ipsilateral retinocollicular projection; specifically we will review recent evidence for the role of axon guidance molecules in organising the ipsilateral projection [2,3] in the context of early experiments which explored the role of the contralateral retinal projection in integrating binocular projections [4,5].

2. Visual system circuitry in the brain

Light casts an image onto the retina, is transduced into electrical signals by photoreceptors, and after intra-retinal processing the information is sent to the brain by the only efferent cells of the retina, the retinal ganglion cells (RGCs). Two of the major RGC outputs in the mouse are to the contralateral superior colliculus (SC) in the midbrain (the mammalian homologue of the optic tectum) and to the contralateral dorsal lateral geniculate nucleus (dLGN) of the thalamus. Neurons in the dLGN that receive retinal input then project to the ipsilateral primary visual cortex (V1). In addition, a subset of retinal ganglion cells project to the ipsilateral LGN and SC, approximately 3% of all RGCs in pigmented mice [6] and rats [7]. This circuitry is summarised in Figure 1. Our focus is the integration of ipsilateral and contralateral projections within the SC, LGN and visual cortex to provide the basis for binocular vision. This is key for processes such as depth perception and acuity in the frontal visual field. Other visual projections, although important in vision (reviewed extensively in Sefton et al., 2004), are not considered further here.

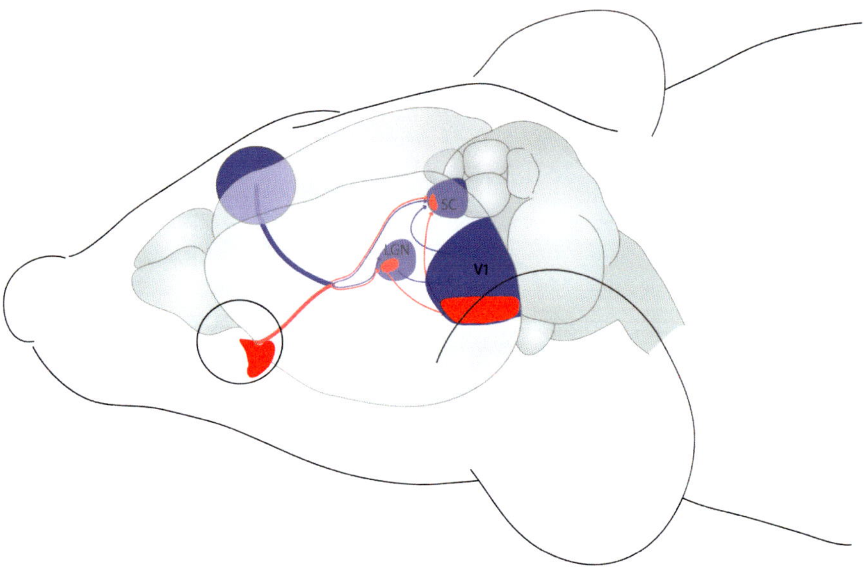

Figure 1. A schematic diagram of the main visual system circuitry in the mouse. dLGN= dorsal lateral geniculate nucleus, SC= superior colliculus, V1=primary visual cortex.

3. Retinal origin of ipsilateral projections

In most species, the number and distribution of ipsilateral RGCs within the retina correlates with binocular overlap and the orientation of the orbits [8]. Mice have laterally placed eyes and limited binocular vision; in pigmented mice, ipsilaterally projecting RGCs represent about 3% of the total RGCs population and are located in a temporo-ventral cresent, interspersed among a majority of contralaterally projecting cells [6]. Albino mice have an even smaller proportion with between 0.5-2% of the total RGC population projecting ipsilaterally [9]. This arrangement provides binocular vision in a 40-60° strip within the superficial visual field [10, 11]. In normal cats, the proportion of ipsilaterally projecting RGCs is 17% [12], but is reduced to about 13% (variable) in Siamese cats [13]. By contrast, in primates (including humans) with frontally oriented eyes, about 50% of RGCs project ipsilaterally, and this figure is also thought to be reduced in albinos [14]. Unlike in mice, in cats and primates, there is a strict vertically oriented zone of transition at the area centralis/fovea between the purely contralateral projection found in nasal retina to the predominantly ipsilateral projection in temporal retina [13], although in Siamese cats, this zone of transition is shifted towards temporal retina [13]. In both species, the resulting binocular field is extensive and oriented towards the frontal field (120° in cats, 140° in primates; [8].

4. The horopter and Panum's fusional area

Stereopsis is the ability to perceive depth based on the differences between the information arriving on the two retinae [15], A key concept in stereopsis is that of the horizontal horopter [16], the collection of points in visual space at which objects are detected by corresponding (anatomically identical) points in the two retinae [17]. In species with frontally placed eyes and large binocular overlap the horopter takes the shape of a curved line running through the fixation point and fusion of images occurs only in a small volume of visual space around the horopter, known as "Panum's fusional area" [18]. Points in this area fall on slightly different retinal locations and thus lead to "retinal disparity", the basis of quantitative stereoscopic depth discrimination [17]. Species with frontally oriented eyes often have the ability to improve depth perception by fixating, or moving the eyes, so that the two foveae or areae centralis (the retinal regions of highest visual acuity in primates and cats respectively) are aimed at the object of interest [17]. In humans, fixation allows the perception of depth differences of up to 0.0014 degrees [17].

Binocular vision or stereopsis occurs when neural circuits use the disparity (parallax) information to compute depth [15]. In order for these computations to occur, the projections (ipsilateral and contralateral projections) from each eye that carry information from Panum's area must be brought together in the same brain regions and on to binocularly driven, disparity sensitive neurons, a phenomenon that occurs in steps as information is passed along the visual pathway via the dLGN [19].

5. Integrating binocular projections

There is an organisational challenge in the integration of ipsilateral and contralateral projections within visual brain centres. The eyes are reflectively symmetrical across the midline and RGCs map based on their position to the nose, therefore visual space is mapped in opposite orientations in each hemisphere (Fig 2A). For example, in the SC, nasal retina maps to caudal SC and temporal retina maps to rostral SC using gradients of ephrin guidance cues (amongst other molecules, discussed below; [20]. Therefore, in order to integrate the ipsilateral projection with the contralateral one and maintain a continuous and coherent representation of visual space, the ipsilateral projection must "flip" relative to the contralateral one (fig 2B; [5,6,21]. Note that this holds true not only for mice with laterally positioned eyes, but also for cats and humans with frontally positioned eyes [22].

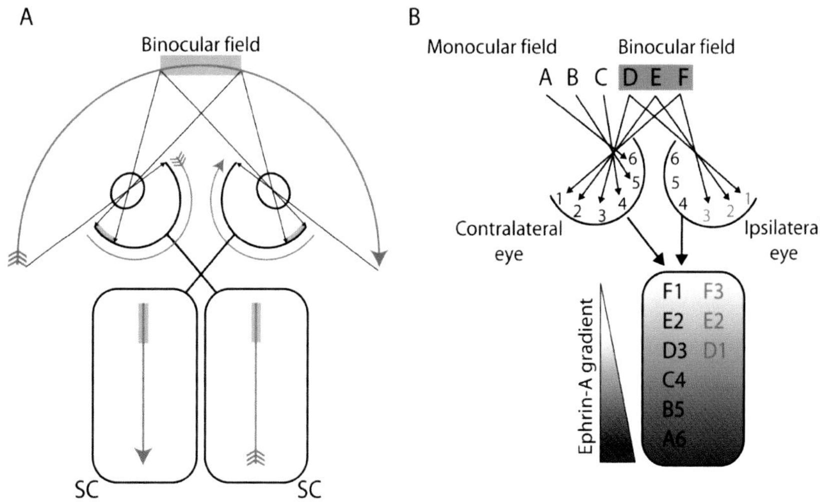

Figure 2. Monocular and binocular representation of the visual field in the superior colliculus (SC) in mice, modified from [2]. A: diagrammatic representation of visual field mapping across both SCs. B Diagrammatic representation of the integration of the ipsilateral and contralateral retinal projections within a single SC, and the resulting representation of visual field information. Letters represent visual field information and numbers represent RGCs within the retina and their terminations within the SC. In mice, the ipsilateral and contralateral retinal axons (numbers) project in reverse orientation relative to each other within the SC, providing a continuous representation of the binocular visual field (letters).

The reversal of the orientation of the ipsilateral relative to the contralateral map is also observed in the dLGN as illustrated by the Siamese cat experiments (see below). This organisation raises several possibilities of the mechanisms underpinning the organisation of the ipsilateral projection. One possibility is that unique guidance cues that are specific to the uncrossed projection might be expressed on RGC axons or within the SC. Alternatively, the same molecular cues might differentially guide ipsilateral and contralateral RGCs. A third possibil-

http://dx.doi.org/10.5772/56491

ity is that the ipsilateral projection maps onto the contralateral projection by activity-dependent mechanisms based on the similarity of visual information from both eyes. We will describe the development of both structures (SC and dLGN) and for each, review experiments that address the possible mechanisms of integration of ipsilateral and contralateral projections.

6. Development of the contralateral and ipsilateral retinal projections in mice

Retinal ganglion cells are generated between embryonic (E) days 11-19 in pigmented mice [23]. Contralaterally and ipsilaterally projecting RGCs are generated at the same time, though not on the same timetable; cells which cross at the optic chiasm are generated throughout this period, whereas cells that do not cross are generated within ventro-temporal retina mostly between E11-E16 [23]. Murine RGC axons reach the optic chiasm by E14 [24] where they make the decision to cross (contralateral RGCs) or not (ipsilateral RGCs; [25]).

6.1. Development of the superior colliculus in mice

The superior colliculus of the midbrain has an important role in integrating cortical and retinal inputs, and functionally is involved in recognition, localization and responsiveness to novel stimuli (Sefton et al., 2004). The majority of visually driven input to the superficial layers of the SC is from the retina and the primary visual cortex and, as for the dLGN, mapping of the ipsilateral and contralateral visual projections provides a continuous representation of the visual field even though the inputs are anatomically segregated. There are also auditory and somatosensory inputs to intermediate and deep SC layers as well as input from secondary visual cortices, parabigeminal nucleus, and a large number of nuclei in the brainstem [26,27]. Major outputs are to the thalamus, the pons, as well as brainstem nuclei and spinal cord segments involved in the control of head and neck movements [10,26,27,28,29].

There are seven layers in the superior colliculus in mammals. The most superficial three layers primarily receive retinal input: the *stratum zonale, stratum griseum superficiale* and the *stratum opticum* [26,30,31]. The superficial layers receive also inputs from the visual cortex and the intermediate and deep layers receive input from other cortical areas [32].

The neurons of the SC in the mouse are produced between E11-E13, with the most superficial layers being produced last [33]. Layers resembling those seen in the mature mouse are present by postnatal (P) day 6 [33,34]. Contralateral RGC axonal outgrowth is present in the SC by E15 and continues after birth [24,33,34,35]. Ipsilateral fibres appear later, around E19 until P3 [24]. Incoming contralateral [36] and ipsilateral [37] axons all extend past their appropriate termination zones and as a result, input is initially scattered and widespread [38], with only rough retinotopic topography and without segregation of ipsilateral and contralateral fibres. Refinement of the projections (topography and eye-specific) occurs by the formation along the rostrocaudal axis of interstitial branches that are targeted to the location of the topographically appropriate termination zone [39]. There is evidence for the interaction between TrkB/BDNF and ephrin-A ligands to promote topographic specific branching [40]. These branches form dense arborisations within the superficial grey layer of the SC and any ectopic branches and overshooting axons are removed [41,42,43,44]. Pruning begins to occur by P4 and is complete by P8-P11 for both contralateral and ipsilateral projections [24,37]. As a result, the retinocollicular map is established and refined in the first two postnatal weeks [45] such that temporal retinal axons project to rostral SC and nasal retinal axons project to caudal SC. The ipsilateral axons terminate in small patches that are within the rostro-medial superficial grey but located slightly deeper than the contralaterally projecting axons [10].

6.2. Development of the LGN and visual cortex

In the mouse, contralateral RGC axons arrive in the dLGN by E16 and ipsilateral axons by E18 [24]. Mature retinotopy in the dLGN is mapped such that temporal axons project to dorsomedial dLGN and nasal axons project to ventrolateral dLGN. There is overlap of contralateral and ipsilateral fibres during the first postnatal week; segregation occurs before the eyes open and is complete by the end of the second postnatal week (P12-14) [41,46] with the ipsilateral terminals being restricted to an isolated roughly trapezoid shape patch within the contralateral terminals [47,48]. Carnivorous mammals such as cats, ferrets and shrews, as well as primates, have more complex layering and segregation within the dLGN based on the characteristics of the RGC inputs [49], reflecting their more sophisticated thalamo-cortical visual processing circuitries.

From the LGN, information from both eyes is carried to neurons in layer 4 of primary visual cortex. In cats and primates [50,51], ipsilateral and contralateral inputs are segregated into ocular dominance columns in layer 4 throughout V1. By contrast in rodents, only lateral visual cortex receives binocular inputs with the medial part being purely monocular [52,53,54]. Nonetheless, in all mammals, ipsilateral and contralateral inputs converge on neurons in layer 2/3, where processing of binocular disparity and thus stereopsis occurs.

7. Visual maps — Molecular mechanisms of topography

The circuitry of the visual system is established via complex guidance mechanisms that involve responses to molecular cues, and interactions between projections by activity-dependent mechanisms [1,55,56]. During development, newly-generated neurons send out developing axons that are guided in their outgrowth via cues which may be diffusible or cell-surface bound, and which may attract or repulse actively growing processes [56]. These various molecular cues assist in targeting, axon fasciculation, and the pruning of inappropriate axonal arbours. Targeting is both structural (in assisting the axon to locate the correct structure within the brain) and detailed (so that the connections are to the correct postsynaptic cell in the appropriate cell layer). In addition, activity dependent pruning further refines the developing projections such that accuracy is maximised [57,58,59]. This review will focus on Eph/ephrin interactions and Teneurins since these proteins have been shown to be important in establishing topography within the ipsilateral as well as the contralateral projection [2,3]. Other guidance cues for example semaphorins, engrailed and L1 are crucial for the contralateral projection [60,61,62] In addition other molecules that have been implicated in eye specific segregation and terminal arborisation, but not in fundamental topographic organisation of the ipsilateral projection, such as BDNF, nitric oxide and the NMDA receptor [63,64,65] will not be discussed further.

7.1. Ephrins and Teneurins guide topography within the ipsilateral projection

The property which makes ephrins and Teneurins unique and ideally suited to topographic mapping between brain regions is their graded expression patterns. This mechanism of action is consistent with the 'chemoaffinity hypothesis', first proposed by Sperry [66] some time before the molecules were identified. This theory predicted that topographic mapping would require unique cytochemical cues expressed by each RGC and its target neuron in the SC. Within the visual system, the Eph/ephrin and teneurin proteins fulfilled this prediction by their graded expression across the origin and target structures in interconnected regions (retina – SC ; retina – dLGN – visual cortex) [55], conferring a unique coordinate in each structure by amount of protein [3,67,68,69].

7.1.1. Ephs and Ephrins

Ephrins are cell-surface bound ligands that bind to Eph receptors, which are receptor tyrosine kinases. The Eph/ephrin interaction is involved in cell-contact mediated signalling that aids cell and tissue organisation [70,71] There are two classes of ephrin ligands, ephrin-A and ephrin-B, classified according to mechanisms of membrane attachment. The members of the ephrin-A class are linked to the membrane by a glycerophospholipid and the ephrin-B class ligands are transmembrane molecules [72]. There are multiple ephrins and Eph receptors in the two classes; with some exceptions [73], ephrin-As will only bind to EphA receptors though binding within each class is non-specific and ligands are able to bind to multiple receptors [70].

Ephs and ephrins are expressed during nervous system development by the target tissue and growth cones of the developing axon. Following Eph-ephrin binding, the growth cone can be attracted (primarily through EphB-ephrin-B signalling) or repulsed (EphA-ephrin-A signalling) directing axons into appropriate regions within brain structures and setting up tissue boundaries and internal organisation [74,75]. The mechanism of growth cone stabilisation or collapse is by modulation of the cytoskeleton [76,77] and can occur bidirectionally via the ephrin and/or the Eph receptor [78,79]. In addition, both receptors and ligands are found to be expressed in the tissue of origin and in the target cells, further regulating the signal transduction process and sensitivity to target guidance cues [80,81,82].

7.1.2. Eph/ephrins in mapping visual projections

During development retinal ganglion cells make a crucial choice at the chiasm. The partial decussation of retinal axons at the optic chiasm is thought to be due to the action of ephrin-B ligands, specifically ephrin-B2 [83] which is expressed on specialised radial glial cells that are situated each side of the midline at the base of the third ventricle [84]. This localised ephrin-

B1 at the chiasm causes repulsion of ipsilaterally projecting RGC axons which express EphB1 [85,86,87] and as a result they do not cross but remain on the same side of the brain. However, EphB triple knockout mice retain some ipsilaterally projecting axons, suggesting that other molecules, such as Nogo [88,89] may also play a role.

Within the LGN, ephrin ligands and Eph receptors are expressed as gradients correlating topographic organisation of the contralateral projection [41]. During postnatal development, there is a correlation between a peak of ephrin expression and the segregation of eye-specific input to the dLGN when expression becomes restricted to the contralateral eye input areas of the dLGN, but no evidence that Eph/ephrin interactions regulate mapping of the ipsilateral retinogeniculate projection [41]. Similarly in visual cortex, there is evidence for a role of Eph/ephrin interactions in establishing contralateral but not ipsilateral topography [41,58].

By contrast, there is strong evidence for a role of Eph/ephrin interactions in establishing ipsilateral topography in the SC. Graded expression of ephrin ligands was first demonstrated in the tectum of the chick [67,68] and knockout mice subsequently confirmed the key role of these proteins in mapping the contralateral visual projection [45,90]. More recently, a role for ephrins in mapping the ipsilateral projection in the superior colliculus was demonstrated by anatomical tracing and electrophysiological experiments which compared the distribution of ipsilateral and contralateral projections [2]. The ipsilateral projection was expanded to fill the full extent of the SC and the organisation of the projection was highly abnormal and misaligned with the contralateral one. Furthermore, the study showed a behavioural deficit that could be rescued by blocking the input to one eye, confirming that although small in size, the ipsilateral projection has significant functional impact [2].

7.1.3. Teneurins

In most species studied to date, the Teneurin family contains four members (Ten-m1-4; [91], which are large transmembrane proteins that are found as homo or heterodimers [92,93]. They are believed to interact with Ten-m molecules on other cells via homophilic or heterophilic interactions [92,94].

Like Ephs and ephrins, Teneurins are expressed as gradients within many regions of the developing brain [95] and relevant to this chapter, have matching gradients across the interconnected visual brain regions (retina, dLGN, SC and visual cortex; [3,96]. However, in contrast to the Ephs and ephrins, very little is known about how the Teneurins exert their guidance activity. In response to binding, Teneurins have several potential signalling methods involving the extracellular and intracellular domains. The C-terminus (extracellular domain) of Teneurins can be cleaved by furin to produce a peptide with homology to the corticotrophin releasing factor (CRF; [97,98]) that has been shown to influence neurite extension and anxiety-related behaviours [99,100]. In addition, the intracellular domain has multiple tyrosine phosphorylation sites, calcium binding motifs and two SH3 binding sites, providing opportunities to interact with many signalling pathways as well as the cytoskeleton [101]. Furthermore, the intracellular domain has been shown to translocate to the nucleus and regulate transcription [101,102].

7.1.4. Ten_m3 in mapping visual projections

One of the Teneurin family members, Ten_m3, has been shown to play a key role in the organisation of eye specific inputs in the dLGN and visual cortex [3,103] and similar to the ephrins, is expressed in matching gradients across the retina and visual brain regions [3]. However, unlike Eph/ephrin interactions, Ten_m3 appears to have no impact on the contralateral projection. Expression peaks during early postnatal development and is highest in regions of the visual pathway associated with the ipsilateral projection. The role of Ten_m3 in mapping the ipsilateral projection was demonstrated in Ten_m3 knockout mice, in which normal numbers of ipsilaterally projecting RGCs are present, but their terminals extend abnormally broadly within the dLGN, covering the full dorso-medial to ventrolateral extent of the nucleus and invading regions that are normally monocular (contralateral) [3]. Normal segregation of the eye-specific inputs in these mice combined with normal contralateral topography further confirmed a specific effect of Ten_m3 on topographic mapping of ipsilateral projections. Aberrant projections were also observed in visual cortex, where ipsilateral input was not restricted to the laterally located binocular zone, but rather formed patches within the monocular region that are reminiscent of ocular dominance domains [103]. Furthermore, recording from cortical cells confirmed that binocular stimulation leads to functional suppression of mismatched binocular inputs [103]. Similar to results with ephrin-A knockout mice, Ten_m3 have abnormal visual function that can be rescued by blocking the input from one eye by injecting tetrodotoxin [3]. Ten_m3 is also implicated in mapping the ipsilateral projection within the SC [37] with knockout mice displaying mapping errors in both horizontal and azimuthal axes of the representation of the visual field. This study also examined for the first time the developmental time-course of ipsilateral retinocollicular projections relative to contralateral ones.

7.2. Research methodologies/tools

For the Ephs and ephrins, an important tool used to study this graded expression pattern was the stripe assay, which studied the growth behaviours of RGCs from different retinal locations on substrates made up of collicular membranes [104,105]. Temporal axons were more inhibited than nasal axons, and though they would grow on both anterior and posterior collicular membranes, they showed a preference for anterior membranes, their natural target [106]. Nasal axons did not show a consistent preference (although see [107]). Perhaps surprisingly, Ten-ms have not been studied in the stripe assay, possibly because the technique has not been used in recent years: although membrane stripe assays provided a foundation for understanding how the retinotopic map develops, there are limitations with these studies. The artificial *in vitro* conditions, sometimes using lysed or non-neuronal cells, did not reproduce the complex environment of the developing brain and may have adversely affected retinal explant outgrowth. These initial studies also failed to identify the importance of the concentration gradient itself [69,108,109] or the complexity of the multiple interactions between ephrins and other proteins that have since been elucidated [43,110,111]. However, such studies provided the useful background for studying topographical development *in vivo*. A particular limitation has been in the study of ipsilaterally projecting RGCs which represent such a small proportion of the total RGCs that their behaviour, even if different from that of contralaterally projecting cells, would not have been noted.

For both molecules, transgenic mice have been key tools in elucidating their role in guiding visual projections, in particular single, double and triple ephrin-A knockout mice [45,112,113], as well as Ten_m3 knockout mice [3,37], which provide much of the data reviewed below. Other Eph transgenic mice have been useful in elucidating the principles of topographic mapping by Ephs, in particular an elegant study by Brown and colleagues which demonstrates the importance of graded expression in point to point mapping [69].

8. Mechanisms of ipsilateral mapping in the superior colliculus: enucleation model

As reviewed above, the development of the ipsilateral retinocollicular projection is at least in part regulated by molecular guidance cues. However, studies that removed one eye at birth have indicated that the contralateral projection has an influence on the development of the ipsilateral projection. In monocular enucleation, one eye is removed at, or in some cases, before birth [114,115]. The age of enucleation has a significant effect on the surviving ipsilateral pathway. Rats enucleated at birth have an expanded uncrossed retinofugal pathway whereas those enucleated prenatally (E16.5) develop a smaller pathway than normal [114]; there is a greater number of retinal ganglion cells which project ipsilaterally and this seems to be due to an increase in survival of those retinal ganglion cells which would die under normal conditions [7]. A similar effect is seen in pigmented mice enucleated *in utero* [5,116] as well as in other species when prenatal and neonatal enucleation time-points are compared [117]. It seems that the two events which affect this outcome are whether the fibres have reached the chiasm and terminal location at enucleation [114].

The main change in the surviving ipsilateral RGC pathway is in the failure of retraction of growth into more caudally located regions of the superior colliculus that are normally occupied by terminations from the contralateral eye. In rats enucleated on at birth and then examined as adults, functional terminations were recorded in locations more caudal relative to their retinal position than seen in the ipsilateral projections of normal rats [5]. Crucially, the topography of this projection is as per the normal (non-enucleated) ipsilateral pattern. A similar result was obtained in the dLGN following enucleation in rats [118]. However, when rats were enucleated before birth, there was a reversal in the polarity of rostral-caudal mapping in the SC [5]. This suggests the importance of prior innervation of contralateral axons to the SC in the final distribution of ipsilateral terminations as contralateral RGC axons enter the SC prior to birth, whereas the ipsilateral axons arrive later [24].

The finding of normal ipsilateral topography in the SC following monocular enucleation at birth is particularly interesting when considered in the context of how RGC axons respond to the ephrin gradient. Typically, temporal RGC axons terminate in the contralateral rostral superior colliculus. However, those that project ipsilaterally terminate in more caudal positions, suggesting they either ignore or respond differently to the repulsive ephrin gradient that restricts contralateral temporal axons to rostral SC (Figure 2). Moreover, the results highlight that ipsilateral RGC axons can terminate in topographically appropriate locations even in the absence of the contralateral retinocollicular topographic map.

9. Mechanisms of ipsilateral mapping in dLGN and V1: Siamese cats

A key model that has provided insight into the organisation of the ipsilateral projection in the LGN and visual cortex is the Siamese cat. As described by several groups, the visual system of the Siamese cat has a reduced ipsilateral retinal projection, resulting in significant reorganisation within the dLGN and visual cortex [119,120,121]. The abnormality has been definitively linked to a homozygous mutation at the albino locus[122] which affects chiasm crossing by RGC axons [123]. Interestingly, at least in the cat, the extent of ipsilateral and contralateral projections is different for different RGC subtypes [124,125]. It remains unclear to this day how changes in pigmentation affect this specific aspect of axonal guidance [126].

In Siamese cats, retinogeniculate fibers representing about the first 20 degrees of ipsilateral visual field in each eye cross aberrantly in the optic chiasm, providing a larger retinal input to the contralateral dLGN [119]. There is not sufficient space for these aberrant fibres to terminate in the A lamina of the dLGN where contralateral fibres would normally arrive. Therefore they overflow into the A1 lamina of the dLGN that normally receives ipsilateral input [119,127]. Furthermore, anatomical and physiological studies of the LGN confirm that this additional projection aligns itself with the topography of the ipsilateral but not contralateral projections, resulting in a "mirror image" of the normal representation [119].

The organisation of ipsilateral projections within the dLGN is thus severely disordered and predictably results in downstream rearrangement of visual pathways in the geniculocortical [121,128], corticogeniculate [129,130] and callosal projections [131,132], as well as cortical associational pathways [130]. Interestingly, when an albino-like representation of the ipsilateral hemifield is induced in the visual cortex of normally pigmented cats, these downstream defects are also observed, suggesting that they are secondary to the initial misrouting of ganglion cells at the optic chiasm [133] rather than a direct consequence of the albino mutation [134].

Most attention has been focused on the geniculocortical pathway, where previous work has reported two distinct modes of processing the aberrant retinal input to the LGN [135]. Work carried out at Harvard defined the "Boston" variety of Siamese cat [121], in which the input that arises from the abnormal section of the dLGN is modified to integrate into cortical map and provide a continuous topographic representation of the visual field. By contrast, work in a Chicago laboratory defined the "Midwestern" Siamese cat [128], in which the abnormal input from the dLGN is silenced. Importantly, these two models provided an opportunity to examine the behavioural consequences of abnormal binocular inputs to LGN and visual cortex. In agreement with the low numbers of binocularly driven cells in visual cortex [136], stereoscopic depth perception and binocular summation in contrast sensitivity have been found to be impaired in Siamese cats [137,138]. However, there was no correlation between squint and the extent of ipsilateral visual field represented in the visual cortex for either variety of Siamese cat [127].

10. Implications for human pathologies

The importance of binocular integration in the visual centres is evidenced by the loss of visual acuity that can occur in amblyopic individuals. Amblyopia is a broad pathological condition where there is dysfunction in the processing of visual information [139]. It can be caused by misalignment of the retinal output to the brain, in disorders such as strabismus (ocular misalignment, such as in 'lazy eye' syndromes), anisometropia (differences in refractive error), and monocular deprivation [139]. The downstream effects of such pathologies involve a degradation of visual acuity and other visual functions associated with binocular processing due to misalignment of retinal inputs.

A more complete loss of visual function occurs with monocular enucleation in which one eye is removed, and provides a unique opportunity to study the importance of binocularity in humans. In such cases, both motion processing and oculomotor behaviour are reduced in enucleated individuals [140]. This processing occurs in the associative visual cortex areas and in the midbrain and suggests the importance of binocular summation in these tasks. However, in some tests related to spatial acuity, enucleated individuals performed better than normally sighted people, although this was strongly related to the age at which enucleation occurred. This may be due to the adaptable nature of the cortex, with incoming connections from the intact eye taking up a relatively larger area of the cortex.

Although rodents are often used as models for the study of the visual system, the crossover at the optic chiasm (3%) is considerably less than that of humans (50%). However, the treatment paradigms which have been studied in rodents may still be applicable to humans due to the similarities in the plastic nature of the visual cortex. The visual cortex is especially sensitive to external influences such as amblyopic pathologies during the critical period. This can last up to 7 years in humans, but only 5 weeks in mice (~32 days [141]; rats [142]). During this time, if there are any abnormalities, they can be successfully treated by intervention because the neuronal connections are still developing. The task becomes considerably harder once the critical period has closed, but work in rodents can help to study treatments which may work in older individuals in recovering visual acuity.

Loss of visual acuity can be induced in a rodent model of through the use of monocular deprivation, in which one eyelid is sutured during the critical period of postnatal development and the remaining eye then becomes dominant in the visual cortex, a phenomenon first described in cats [143]. Typically, such a condition can be reversed if the deprivation effects are terminated during the critical period [144,145,146,147] and, though it is possible, there is less chance of recovery if not treated until adulthood [148]. In addition to pharmacological interventions, which at present lack clinical feasibility [149], a promising experimental treatment recently described in the rodent model involves environmental enrichment, which

http://dx.doi.org/10.5772/56491

has been shown to rescue the visual acuity of amblyopic rats in adulthood if there is damage to one eye [150].

11. Conclusion

Binocular vision requires integration of the inputs from both eyes onto neurons in the major visual brain centres. There is a challenge to understanding how these distinct inputs map the binocular field because the ipsilateral projection maps in the opposite direction relative the contralateral one. Most of the known cues which guide the development of visual mapping in the brain relate to the contralateral eye only, with little known about ipsilateral mapping. Animal models, especially in cat and rodents, have been used to study both normal and abnormal integration of the two eyes and to elucidate the mechanisms underpinning this process. There is also the capacity for further work in animal models, especially with regard to possible interventions for disorders of binocular integration such as amblyopia.

Acknowledgements

We are grateful to Marissa Penrose for figure production. JR is a National Health and Medical Research Council Australia Senior Research Fellow.

Author details

Tenelle A. Wilks, Alan R. Harvey and Jennifer Rodger

Schools of Animal Biology and Anatomy, Physiology and Human Biology, The University of Western Australia, Crawley WA, Australia

References

[1] McLaughlin T, O'Leary DD. Molecular gradients and development of retinotopic maps. Annu Rev Neurosci 2005; 28 327-355.

[2] Haustead D, Lukehurst S, Clutton GB, Dunlop S, Arrese CA, Sherrard RM, Rodger J. Functional topography and integration of the contralateral and ipsilateral retinocollicular projections in ephrin-A-/- mice. J Neurosci 2008; 28 (29): 7376-7386.

[3] Leamey CA, Merlin S, Lattouf P, Sawatari A, Zhou X, Demel N, Glendining KA, Oohasi T, Sur M, Fassler R. Ten_m3 regulates eye-specific patterning in the mammalian

visual pathway and is required for binocular vision. PLoS Biology 2007; 5 (9): 2077-2092.

[4] Bishop PO, Pettigrew JD. Neural mechanisms of binocular vision. Vision Res 1986; 26 (9): 1587-1600.

[5] Jeffery G, Thompson ID. The effects of prenatal and neonatal monocular enucleation on visual topography in the uncrossed retinal pathway to the rat superior colliculus. Exp Brain Res 1986; 63 (2): 351-363.

[6] Drager UC, Olsen JF. Origins of crossed and uncrossed retinal projections in pigmented and albino mice. J Comp Neurol 1980; 191 (3): 383-412.

[7] Jeffery G. Retinal ganglion cell death and terminal field retraction in the developing rodent visual system. Brain Res 1984; 315 (1): 81-96.

[8] Heesy C. On the relationship between orbit orientation and binocular visual field overlap in mammals. Anat Record 2004; 281A 1104-1110.

[9] Balkema GW, Pinto LH, Drager UC, Vanable JW. Characterisation of abnormalities in the visual system of the mutant mouse pearl. J Neurosci 1981; 1 (11): 1320-1329.

[10] Sefton AJ, Dreher B, Harvey AR (2004) Visual System. In: Paxinos G, editor. The Rat Nervous System. 3rd ed. San Diego: Elsevier Academic Press. pp. 1083-1165.

[11] Hughes A (1977) The topography of vision in mammals. In: Crescitelli C, editor. Handbook of Sensory Physiology. Heidelberg: Springer Verlag. pp. 615-756.

[12] Illing RB, Wassle H. The retinal projection to the thalamus in the cat: a quantitative investigation and a comparison with the retinotectal pathway. J Comp Neurol 1981; 202 (2): 265-285.

[13] Stone J, Campion JE, Leicester J. The nasotemporal division of retina in the Siamese cat. J Comp Neurol 1978; 180 (4): 783-798.

[14] Morland AB, Hoffmann MB, Neveu M, Holder GE. Abnormal visual projection in a human albino studied with functional magnetic resonance imaging and visual evoked potentials. J Neurol Neurosurg Psychiatry 2002; 72 (4): 523-526.

[15] Cumming BG, DeAngelis GC. The physiology of stereopsis. Annu Rev Neurosci 2001; 24 203-238.

[16] Wheatstone C. Contributions to the physiology of vision.-Part the First. On some remarkable, and hitherto unobserved, phænomena of binocular vision. Philosophical Transactions of the Royal Society of London 1838; 128 371–394.

[17] Ponce CR, Born RT. Stereopsis. Curr Biol 2008; 18 (18): R845-850.

[18] Panum P Physiologische Untersuchungen über das Sehen mit zwei Augen. 1858. Kiel: Schwersscher Buchhandlung.

[19] Gonzalez F, Perez R. Neural mechanisms underlying stereoscopic vision. Prog Neurobiol 1998; 55 (3): 191-224.

[20] McLaughlin T, Hindges T, O'Leary DDM. Regulation of axial patterning of the retina and its topographic mapping in the brain. Curr Op Neurobiol 2003; 13 57-69.

[21] Leamey CA, Wart AV, Sur M. Intrinsic patterning and experience-dependent mechanisms that generate eye-specific projections and binocular circuits in the visual pathway. Current Opinion in Neurobiology 2009; 19 (2): 181-187.

[22] Lambot MA, Depasse F, Noel JC, Vanderhaeghen P. Mapping labels in the human developing visual system and the evolution of binocular vision. J Neurosci 2005; 25 (31): 7232-7237.

[23] Drager U. Birth dates of retinal ganglion cells giving rise to the crossed and uncrossed optic projections in the mouse. Proc R Soc Lond B Biol Sci 1985; 224 57-77.

[24] Godement P, Salaun J, Imbert M. Prenatal and postnatal development of retinogeniculate and retinocollicular projections in the mouse. J Comp Neurol 1984; 230 (4): 552-575.

[25] Jeffery G. Architecture of the optic chiasm and the mechanisms that sculpt its development. Physiological Reviews 2001; 81 (4): 1393-1414.

[26] Drager UC, Hubel DH. Responses to visual stimulation and relationship between visual, auditory, and somatosensory inputs in mouse superior colliculus. Journal of Neurophysiology 1975; 28 (3): 690.

[27] Drager UC, Hubel DH. Topography of visual and somatosensory projections to mouse superior colliculus. J Neurophysiol 1976; 39 (1): 91-101.

[28] Westby GWM, Keay KA, Redgrave P, Dean P, Bannister M. Output pathways from the rat superior colliculus mediating approach and avoidance have different sensory properties. Experimental Brain Research 1990; 81 (3): 626-638.

[29] Mooney RD, Nikoletseas MM, Hess PR, Allen Z, Lewin AC, Rhoades RW. The projection from the superficial to the deep layers of the superior colliculus: An intracellular horseradish peroxidase injection study in the hamster. The Journal of Neuroscience 1998; 8 (4): 1384-1399.

[30] Chalupa LM, Williams RW, editors (2008) Eye, retina and visual system of the mouse. Cambridge, Massachusetts: MIT Press.

[31] Stein BE. Development of the superior colliculus. Annual Review of Neuroscience 1984; 7 95-125.

[32] Lund RD. The occipitotectal pathway of the rat. J Anat 1966; 100 (Pt 1): 51-62.

[33] Edwards MA, Caviness Jr. VS, Schneider GE. Development of cell and fiber lamination in the mouse superior colliculus. Journal of Comparative Neurology 1986; 248 (248): 395-409.

[34] Edwards MA, Schneider GE, Caviness Jr. VS. Development of the crossed retinocollicular projection in the mouse. Journal of Comparative Neurology 1986; 248 (3): 410-421.

[35] Dallimore EJ, Park KK, Pollett MA, Taylor JS, Harvey AR. The life, death and regenerative ability of immature and mature rat retinal ganglion cells are influenced by their birthdate. Exp Neurol 2010; 225 (2): 353-365.

[36] Simon DK, O'Leary DD. Development of topographic order in the mammalian retinocollicular projection. J Neurosci 1992; 12 (4): 1212-1232.

[37] Dharmaratne N, Glendining KA, Young TR, Tran H, Sawatari A, Leamey CA. Ten-m3 Is Required for the Development of Topography in the Ipsilateral Retinocollicular Pathway. PLoS ONE 2012; 7 (9): e43083.

[38] Lund RD, Bunt AH. Prenatal development of central optic pathways in albino rats. J Comp Neurol 1976; 165 (2): 247-264.

[39] Yates PA, Roskies AL, McLaughlin T, O'Leary DDM. Topographic-specific axon branching controlled by ephrin-As is the critical event in retinotectal map development. Journal of Neuroscience 2001; 21 (21): 8548–8563.

[40] Marler KJ, Becker-Barroso E, Martinez A, Llovera M, Wentzel C, Poopalasundaram S, Hindges R, Soriano E, Comella J, Drescher U. A TrkB/EphrinA interaction controls retinal axon branching and synaptogenesis. J Neurosci 2008; 28 (48): 12700-12712.

[41] Pfeiffenberger C, Cutforth T, Woods G, Yamada J, Renteria RC, Copenhagen DR, Flanagan JG, Feldheim DA. Ephrin-As and neural activity are required for eye-specific patterning during retinogeniculate mapping. Nature Neuroscience 2005; 8 (8): 1022-1027.

[42] Huberman AD. Mechanisms of eye-specific visual circuit development. Current Opinion in Neurobiology 2007; 17 (1): 73-80.

[43] Nicol X, Muzerelle A, Rio J, Metin C, Gaspar P. Requirement of Adenylate Cyclase 1 for the ephrin-A5-dependent retraction of exuberant retinal axons. J Neurosci 2006; 26 (3): 862-872.

[44] Nicol X, Voyatzis S, Muzerelle A, Narboux-Neme N, Sudhof T, Miles R, Gaspar P. cAMP oscillations and retinal activity are permissive for ephrin signalling during the establishment of the retinotopic map. Nat Neurosci 2007; 10 (3): 340-347.

[45] Frisen J, Yates PA, McLaughlin T, Friedman GC, O'Leary DD, Barbacid M. Ephrin-A5 (AL-1/RAGS) is essential for proper retinal axon guidance and topographic mapping in the mammalian visual system. Neuron 1998; 20 (2): 235-243.

[46] Jaubert-Miazza L, Green E, Lo F-S, Bui K, Mills J, Guido W. Structural and functional composition of the developing retinogeniculate pathway in the mouse. Visual Neuroscience 2005; 22 (5): 661-676.

[47] Lund RD, Lund J, S., Wise RP. The organization of the retinal projection to the dorsal lateral geniculate nucleus in pigmented and albino rats. Journal of Comparative Neurology 1974; 158 (4): 383-404.

[48] Godement P, Saillour P, Imbert M. The ipsilateral optic pathway to the dorsal lateral geniculate nucleus and superior colliculus in mice with prenatal or postnatal loss of one eye. Journal of Comparative Neurology 1980; 190 (4): 611-626.

[49] Sillito AM, Jones HE. Corticothalamic interactions in the transfer of visual information. Philosophical Transactions: Biological Sciences 2002; 357 (1428): 1739-1752.

[50] Hubel DH, Wiesel TN. Receptive fields, binocular interaction and functional architecture in the cat's visual cortex. J Physiol 1962; 160 (1): 106-154.

[51] Gattass R, Nascimento-Silva S, Soares JG, Lima B, Jansen AK, Diogo AC, Farias MF, Botelho MM, Mariani OS, Azzi J, Fiorani M. Cortical visual areas in monkeys: location, topography, connections, columns, plasticity and cortical dynamics. Philos Trans R Soc Lond B Biol Sci 2005; 360 (1456): 709-731.

[52] Adams AD, Forrester JM. The projection of the rat's visual field on the cerebral cortex. Q J Exp Physiol Cogn Med Sci 1968; 53 (3): 327-336.

[53] Montero VM. Evoked responses in the rat's visual cortex to contralateral, ipsilateral and restricted photic stimulation. Brain Res 1973; 53 (1): 192-196.

[54] Thurlow GA, Cooper RM. Metabolic activity in striate and extrastriate cortex in the hooded rat: contralateral and ipsilateral eye input. J Comp Neurol 1988; 274 (4): 595-607.

[55] Goodhill G, Richards L. Retinotectal maps: molecules, models and misplaced data. Trends in Neuroscience 1999; 22 (12): 529-534.

[56] Feldheim DA, O'Leary DD. Visual map development: bidirectional signaling, bifunctional guidance molecules, and competition. Cold Spring Harb Perspect Biol 2010; 2 (11): a001768.

[57] McLaughlin T, Hindges R, O'Leary DDM. Regulation of axial patterning of the retina and its topographic mapping in the brain. Current Opinion in Neurobiology 2003; 13 (1): 57-69.

[58] Cang J, Kaneko M, Yamada J, Woods G, Stryker MP, Feldheim DA. Ephrin-As guide the formation of functional maps in the visual cortex. Neuron 2005; 48 (4): 577-589.

[59] Mrsic-Flogel TD, Hofer SB, Creutzfeldt C, Cloez-Tayarani I, Changeux J-P, Bonhoeffer T, Hubener M. Altered map of visual space in the superior colliculus of mice lacking early retinal waves. The Journal of Neuroscience 2005; 25 (29): 6921- 6928.

[60] Claudepierre T, Koncina E, Pfrieger FW, Bagnard D, Aunis D, Reber M. Implication of neuropilin 2/semaphorin 3F in retinocollicular map formation. Dev Dyn 2008; 237 (11): 3394-3403.

[61] Wizenmann A, Brunet I, Lam JS, Sonnier L, Beurdeley M, Zarbalis K, Weisenhorn-Vogt D, Weinl C, Dwivedy A, Joliot A, Wurst W, Holt C, Prochiantz A. Extracellular Engrailed participates in the topographic guidance of retinal axons in vivo. Neuron 2009; 64 (3): 355-366.

[62] Demyanenko GP, Maness PF. The L1 cell adhesion molecule is essential for topographic mapping of retinal axons. J Neurosci 2003; 23 (2): 530-538.

[63] Rodger J, Frost DO. Effects of trkB knockout on topography and ocular segregation of uncrossed retinal projections. Exp Brain Res 2009; 195 (1): 35-44.

[64] Ernst AF, Wu HH, El-Fakahany EE, McLoon SC. NMDA receptor-mediated refinement of a transient retinotectal projection during development requires nitric oxide. J Neurosci 1999; 19 (1): 229-235.

[65] Mize RR, Wu HH, Cork RJ, Scheiner CA. The role of nitric oxide in development of the patch-cluster system and retinocollicular pathways in the rodent superior colliculus. Prog Brain Res 1998; 118 133-152.

[66] Sperry R. Chemoaffinity in the orderly growth of nerve fiber patterns and connections. Proc Natl Acad Sci USA 1963; 50 703-710.

[67] Cheng H-J, Flanagan J. Identification and cloning of ELF-1, a developmentally expressed ligand for the Mek4 and Sek receptor tyrosine kinases. Cell 1994; 79 (1): 157-168.

[68] Cheng H-J, Nakamoto M, Bergemann A, Flanagan J. Complementary gradients in expression and binding of ELF-1 and Mek4 in development of the topographic retinotectal projection map. Cell 1995; 82 (3): 371-381.

[69] Brown A, Yates PA, Burrola P, Ortuño D, Vaidya A, Jessell TM, Pfaff SL, OLeary DDM, Lemke G. Topographic mapping from the retina to the midbrain Is controlled by relative but not absolute levels of EphA receptor signaling. Cell 2000; 102 (1): 77-88.

[70] Wilkinson DG. Multiple roles of Eph receptors and ephrins in neural development. Nat Rev Neurosci 2001; 2 (3): 155-164.

[71] Triplett JW, Feldheim DA. Eph and ephrin signaling in the formation of topographic maps. Seminars in Cell & Developmental Biology 2012; 23 (1): 7-15.

[72] Pasquale EB. The Eph family of receptors. Current Opinion in Cell Biology 1997; 9 (5): 608-615.

[73] Himanen JP, Chumley MJ, Lackmann M, Li C, Barton WA, Jeffrey PD, Vearing C, Geleick D, Feldheim DA, Boyd AW, Henkemeyer M, Nikolov DB. Repelling class

discrimination: ephrin-A5 binds to and activates EphB2 receptor signaling. Nat Neurosci 2004; 7 (5): 501-509.

[74] Rodger J, Salvatore L, Migani P. Should I stay or should I go? Ephs and ephrins in neuronal migration. Neurosignals 2012; 20 (3): 190-201.

[75] North HA, Clifford MA, Donoghue MJ. 'Til Eph Do Us Part': Intercellular signaling via eph receptors and ephrin ligands guides cerebral cortical development from birth through maturation. Cerebral Cortex 2012.

[76] Davenport R, Thies E, Cohen M. Neuronal growth cone collapse triggers lateral extensions along trailing axons. Nature Neuroscience 1999; 2 254-259.

[77] Sahin M, Greer PL, Lin MZ, Poucher H, Eberhart J, Schmidt S, Wright TM, Shamah SM, O'Connell S, Cowan CW, Hu L, Goldberg JL, Debant A, Corfas G, Krull CE, Greenberg ME. Eph-dependent tyrosine phosphorylation of ephexin1 modulates growth cone collapse. Neuron 2005; 46 (2): 191-204.

[78] Davy A, Gale NW, Murray EW, Klinghoffer RA, Soriano P, Feuerstein C, Robbins SM. Compartmentalised signaling by GPI-anchored eprhin-A5 requires the Fyn tyrosine kinase to regulate cellular adhesion. Genes and Development 1999; 13 (23): 3125-3135.

[79] Davy A, Soriano P. Ephrin signaling in vivo: look both ways. Dev Dyn 2005; 232 (1): 1-10.

[80] Hornberger MR, Dutting D, Ciossek T, Yamada T, Handwerker C, Lang S, Weth F, Huf J, Weßel R, Logan C, Tanaka H, Drescher U. Modulation of EphA receptor function by coexpressed ephrinA ligands on retinal ganglion cell axons. Neuron 1999; 22 (4): 731-742.

[81] Marquardt T, Shirasaki R, Ghosh S, Andrews SE, Carter N, Hunter T, Pfaff SL. Coexpressed EphA receptors and ephrin-A ligands mediate opposing actions on growth cone navigation from distinct membrane domains. Cell 2005; 121 (1): 127-139.

[82] Carvalho RF, Beutler M, Marler KJM, Knoll B, Becker-Barroso E, Heintzmann R, Ng T, Drescher U. Silencing of EphA3 through a cis interaction with ephrin A5. Nature Neuroscience 2005; 9 (3): 322-330.

[83] Williams SE, Mason CA, Herrera E. The optic chiasm as a midline choice point. Current Opinion in Neurobiology 2004; 14 (1): 51-60.

[84] Marcus RC, Blazeski R, Godement P, Mason CA. Retinal axon divergence in the optic chiasm: uncrossed axons diverge from crossed axons within a midline glial specialization. J Neurosci 1995; 15 (5 Pt 2): 3716-3729.

[85] Nakagawa S, Brennan C, Johnson KG, Shewan D, Harris WA, Holt CE. Ephrin-B regulates the ipsilateral routing of retinal axons at the optic chiasm. Neuron 2000; 25 (3): 599-610.

[86] Williams SE, Mann F, Erskine L, Sakurai T, Wei S, Rossi DJ, Gale NW, Holt CE, Mason CA, Henkemeyer M. Ephrin-B2 and EphB1 mediate retinal axon divergence at the optic chiasm. Neuron 2003; 39 (6): 919-935.

[87] Petros TJ, Bryson JB, Mason C. Ephrin-B2 elicits differential growth cone collapse and axon retraction in retinal ganglion cells from distinct retinal regions. Dev Neurobiol 2010; 70 (11): 781-794.

[88] Wang J, Chan CK, Taylor JS, Chan SO. The growth-inhibitory protein Nogo is involved in midline routing of axons in the mouse optic chiasm. J Neurosci Res 2008; 86 (12): 2581-2590.

[89] Fabre PJ, Shimogori T, Charron F. Segregation of ipsilateral retinal ganglion cell axons at the optic chiasm requires the Shh receptor Boc. J Neurosci 2010; 30 (1): 266-275.

[90] Feldheim DA, Kim Y-I, Bergemann AD, Frisen J, Barbacid M, Flanagan JG. Genetic analysis of ephrin-A2 and ephrin-A5 shows their requirement in multiple aspects of retinocollicular mapping. Neuron 2000; 25 (3): 563-574.

[91] Tucker RP, Chiquet-Ehrismann R. Teneurins: a conserved family of transmembrane proteins involved in intercellular signaling during development. Dev Biol 2006; 290 (2): 237-245.

[92] Oohashi T, Zhou XH, Feng K, Richter B, Morgelin M, Perez MT, Su WD, Chiquet-Ehrismann R, Rauch U, Fassler R. Mouse ten-m/Odz is a new family of dimeric type II transmembrane proteins expressed in many tissues. J Cell Biol 1999; 145 (3): 563-577.

[93] Feng K, Zhou XH, Oohashi T, Morgelin M, Lustig A, Hirakawa S, Ninomiya Y, Engel J, Rauch U, Fassler R. All four members of the Ten-m/Odz family of transmembrane proteins form dimers. J Biol Chem 2002; 277 (29): 26128-26135.

[94] Rubin BP, Tucker RP, Brown-Luedi M, Martin D, Chiquet-Ehrismann R. Teneurin 2 is expressed by the neurons of the thalamofugal visual system in situ and promotes homophilic cell-cell adhesion in vitro. Development 2002; 129 (20): 4697-4705.

[95] Kenzelmann D, Chiquet-Ehrismann R, Leachman NT, Tucker RP. Teneurin-1 is expressed in interconnected regions of the developing brain and is processed in vivo. BMC Dev Biol 2008; 8 30.

[96] Leamey CA, Glendining KA, Kreiman G, Kang ND, Wang KH, Fassler R, Sawatari A, Tonegawa S, Sur M. Differential gene expression between sensory neocortical areas: potential roles for Ten_m3 and Bcl6 in patterning visual and somatosensory pathways. Cereb Cortex 2008; 18 (1): 53-66.

[97] Wang L, Rotzinger S, Al Chawaf A, Elias CF, Barsyte-Lovejoy D, Qian X, Wang NC, De Cristofaro A, Belsham D, Bittencourt JC, Vaccarino F, Lovejoy DA. Teneurin proteins possess a carboxy terminal sequence with neuromodulatory activity. Brain Res Mol Brain Res 2005; 133 (2): 253-265.

[98] Lovejoy DA, Rotzinger S, Barsyte-Lovejoy D. Evolution of complementary peptide systems: teneurin C-terminal-associated peptides and corticotropin-releasing factor superfamilies. Ann N Y Acad Sci 2009; 1163 215-220.

[99] Al Chawaf A, Xu K, Tan L, Vaccarino FJ, Lovejoy DA, Rotzinger S. Corticotropin-releasing factor (CRF)-induced behaviors are modulated by intravenous administration of teneurin C-terminal associated peptide-1 (TCAP-1). Peptides 2007; 28 (7): 1406-1415.

[100] Tan LA, Xu K, Vaccarino FJ, Lovejoy DA, Rotzinger S. Teneurin C-terminal associated peptide (TCAP)-1 attenuates corticotropin-releasing factor (CRF)-induced c-Fos expression in the limbic system and modulates anxiety behavior in male Wistar rats. Behav Brain Res 2009; 201 (1): 198-206.

[101] Nunes SM, Ferralli J, Choi K, Brown-Luedi M, Minet AD, Chiquet-Ehrismann R. The intracellular domain of teneurin-1 interacts with MBD1 and CAP/ponsin resulting in subcellular codistribution and translocation to the nuclear matrix. Exp Cell Res 2005; 305 (1): 122-132.

[102] Bagutti C, Forro G, Ferralli J, Rubin B, Chiquet-Ehrismann R. The intracellular domain of teneurin-2 has a nuclear function and represses zic-1-mediated transcription. J Cell Sci 2003; 116 (Pt 14): 2957-2966.

[103] Merlin S, Horng S, Marotte LR, Sur M, Sawatari A, Leamey CA. Deletion of Ten-m3 Induces the Formation of Eye Dominance Domains in Mouse Visual Cortex. Cereb Cortex 2012; Doi: 10.1093/cercor/bhs030.

[104] Baier H, Bonhoeffer F. Axon guidance by gradients of a target-derived component. Science 1992; 255 (5043): 472-475.

[105] Walter J, Kern-Veits B, Huf J, Stolze B, Bonhoeffer F. Recognition of position-specific properties of tectai cell membranes by retinal axons in vitro. Development 1987; 101 (4): 685-696.

[106] Walter J, Henke-Fahle S, Bonhoeffer F. Avoidance of posterior tectal membranes by temporal retinal axons. Development 1987; 101 (4): 909-913.

[107] von Boxberg Y, Deiss S, Schwarz U. Guidance and topographic stabilization of nasal chick retinal axons on target-derived components in vitro. Neuron 1993; 10 (3): 345-357.

[108] Hansen MJ, Dallal GE, Flanagan JG. Retinal axon response to ephrin-as shows a graded, concentration-dependent transition from growth promotion to inhibition. Neuron 2004; 42 (5): 717-730.

[109] Rosentreter SM, Davenport RW, Loschinger J, Huf J, Jung J, Bonhoeffer F. Response of retinal ganglion cell axons to striped linear gradients of repellent guidance molecules. J Neurobiol 1998; 37 (4): 541-562.

[110] Poopalasundaram S, Marler KJ, Drescher U. EphrinA6 on chick retinal axons is a key component for p75(NTR)-dependent axon repulsion and TrkB-dependent axon branching. Mol Cell Neurosci 2011; 47 (2): 131-136.

[111] Fitzgerald M, Buckley A, Lukehurst SS, Dunlop SA, Beazley LD, Rodger J. Neurite responses to ephrin-A5 modulated by BDNF: evidence for TrkB-EphA interactions. Biochem Biophys Res Commun 2008; 374 (4): 625-630.

[112] Feldheim D, Vanderhaeghen P, Hansen M, Frisen J, Lu Q, Barbacid M, Flanagan J. Topographic guidance labels in a sensory projection to the forebrain. Neuron 1998; 21 (6): 1303-1313.

[113] Cang J, Niell C, Liu X, Pfeiffenberger C, Feldheim D, Stryker M. Selective disruption of one cartesian axis of cortical maps and receptive fields by deficiency in ephrin-As and structured activity. Neuron 2008; 57 (4): 511-523.

[114] Chan SO, Guillery RW. Developmental changes produced in the retinofugal pathways of rats and ferrets by early monocular enucleations: the effects of age and the differences between normal and albino animals. J Neurosci 1993; 13 (12): 5277-5293.

[115] Land PW, Lund RD. Development of the rat's uncrossed retinotectal pathway and its relation to plasticity studies. Science 1979; 205 (4407): 698-700.

[116] Chan SO, Chung KY, Taylor JSH. The effects of early prenatal monocular enucleation on the routing of uncrossed retinofugal axons and the cellular environment at the chiasm of mouse embryos. European Journal of Neuroscience 1999; 11 (9): 3225-3235.

[117] Coleman L-A, Beazley LD. Retinal ganglion cell number is unchanged in the remaining eye following early unilateral eye removal in the wallaby Setonix brachyurus, quokka. Developmental Brain Research 1989; 48 (2): 293-307.

[118] Reese B. The topography of expanded uncrossed retinal projections following neonatal enucleation of one eye: differing effects in dorsal lateral geniculate nucleus and superior colliculus. J Comp Neurol 1986; 250 (1): 8-32.

[119] Guillery RW, Kaas JH. A study of normal and congenitally abnormal retinogeniculate projections in cats. J Comp Neurol 1971; 143 (1): 73-100.

[120] Kalil RE, Jhaveri SR, Richards W. Anomalous retinal pathways in the Siamese cat: an inadequate substrate for normal bioncular vision. Science 1971; 174 (4006): 302-305.

[121] Hubel DH, Wiesel TN. Aberrant visual projections in the Siamese cat. J Physiol 1971; 218 (1): 33-62.

[122] Creel DJ. Visual system anomaly associated with albinism in the cat. Nature 1971; 231 (5303): 465-466.

[123] Rice DS, Goldowitz D, Williams RW, Hamre K, Johnson PT, Tan SS, Reese BE. Extrinsic modulation of retinal ganglion cell projections: analysis of the albino mutation in pigmentation mosaic mice. Dev Biol 1999; 216 (1): 41-56.

[124] Kirk DL, Levick WR, Cleland BG. The crossed or uncrossed destination of axons of sluggish-concentric and non-concentric cat retinal ganglion cells, with an overall synthesis of the visual field representation. Vision Res 1976; 16 (3): 233-236.

[125] Kirk DL, Levick WR, Cleland BG, Wassle H. Crossed and uncrossed representation of the visual field by brisk-sustained and brisk-transient cat retinal ganglion cells. Vision Res 1976; 16 (3): 225-231.

[126] Guillery RW. Why do albinos and other hypopigmented mutants lack normal binocular vision, and what else is abnormal in their central visual pathways? Eye (Lond) 1996; 10 (Pt 2) 217-221.

[127] Shatz C. A comparison of visual pathways in Boston and Midwestern Siamese cats. J Comp Neurol 1977; 171 (2): 205-228.

[128] Kaas J, Guillery R. The transfer of abnormal visual field representations from lateral geniculate nucleus to the visual cortex in siamese cats. Brain Research 1973; 59 61-95.

[129] Montero VM, Guillery RW. Abnormalities of the cortico-geniculate pathway in Siamese cats. J Comp Neurol 1978; 179 (1): 1-12.

[130] Shatz CJ, LeVay S. Siamese cat: altered connections of visual cortex. Science 1979; 204 (4390): 328-330.

[131] Shatz C. Abnormal interhemispheric connections in the visual system of Boston Siamese cats: a physiological study. J Comp Neurol 1977; 171 (2): 229-245.

[132] Shatz CJ. Anatomy of interhemispheric connections in the visual system of Boston Siamese and ordinary cats. J Comp Neurol 1977; 173 (3): 497-518.

[133] Kliot M, Shatz CJ. Abnormal development of the retinogeniculate projection in Siamese cats. J Neurosci 1985; 5 (10): 2641-2653.

[134] Schall JD, Ault SJ, Vitek DJ, Leventhal AG. Experimental induction of an abnormal ipsilateral visual field representation in the geniculocortical pathway of normally pigmented cats. J Neurosci 1988; 8 (6): 2039-2048.

[135] Cooper ML, Blasdel GG. Regional variation in the representation of the visual field in the visual cortex of the Siamese cat. J Comp Neurol 1980; 193 (1): 237-253.

[136] Di Stefano M, Bedard S, Marzi CA, Lepore F. Lack of binocular activation of cells in area 19 of the Siamese cat. Brain Res 1984; 303 (2): 391-395.

[137] Girelli M, Campara D, Tassinari G, Marzi CA. Abnormal spatial but normal temporal resolution in the Siamese cat: a behavioral correlate of a genetic disorder of the parallel visual pathways. Can J Physiol Pharmacol 1995; 73 (9): 1348-1351.

[138] Marzi CA. Vision in siamese cats. TRENDS in Neurosciences 1980; 3 (7): 165-169.

[139] Holmes JM, Clarke MP. Amblyopia. Lancet 2006; 367 (9519): 1343-1351.

[140] Steeves JKE, Gonzales EG, Steinbach MJ. Vision with one eye: a review of visual function following unilateral enucleation. Spatial Vision 2008; 21 (6): 509-529.

[141] Gordon JA, Stryker MP. Experience-dependent plasticity of binocular responses in the primary visual cortex of the mouse. J Neurosci 1996; 16 (10): 3274-3286.

[142] Fagiolini M, Pizzorusso T, Berson D, Domenicia L, Maffei L. Functional postnatal development of the rat primary visual cortex and the role of visual experience: dark rearing and monocular deprivation. Vision Research 1994; 34 (6): 709-720.

[143] Wiesel TN, Hubel DH. Single-cell responses in striate cortex of kittens deprived of vision in one eye. Journal of Neurophysiology 1963; 26 1003-1017.

[144] Blakemore C. The development of stereoscopic mechanisms in the visual cortex of the cat. Proc R Soc Lond B Biol Sci 1979; 204 (1157): 477-484.

[145] Kind PC, Mitchell DE, Ahmed B, Blakemore C, Bonhoeffer T, Sengpiel F. Correlated binocular activity guides recovery from monocular deprivation. Nature 2002; 416 (6879): 430-433.

[146] Blakemore C, Garey LJ, Vital-Durand F. The physiological effects of monocular deprivation and their reversal in the monkey's visual cortex. J Physiol 1978; 283 223-262.

[147] Blakemore C, Van Sluyters RC. Reversal of the physiological effects of monocular deprivation in kittens: further evidence for a sensitive period. J Physiol 1974; 237 (1): 195-216.

[148] Smith DC, Spear PD, Kratz KE. Role of visual experience in postcritical-period reversal of effects of monocular deprivation in cat striate cortex. Journal of Comparative Anatomy 1978; 178 (2): 313-328.

[149] Pizzorusso T, Medini P, Landi S, Baldini S, Berardi N, Maffei L. Structural and functional recovery from early monocular deprivation in adult rats. Proc Natl Acad Sci U S A 2006; 103 (22): 8517-8522.

[150] Tognini P, Manno I, Bonaccorsi J, Cenni MC, Sale A, Maffei L. Environmental enrichment promotes plasticity and visual acuity recovery in adult monocular amblyopic rats. PLoS One 2012; 7 (4).

Chapter 13

The Role of Cortical Feedback Circuitry on Functional Maps of V2 in Primates: Effects on Orientation Tuning and Direction Selectivity

Ana Karla Jansen-Amorim, Cecilia Ceriatte,
Bruss Lima, Juliana Soares, Mario Fiorani and
Ricardo Gattass

Additional information is available at the end of the chapter

http://dx.doi.org/10.5772/56497

1. Introduction

Extensive work in anatomy, neurophysiology and brain imaging has approached the challenge of understanding visual processing in human and non-human primate brains. This approach has been very successful in generating a roadmap of the primate brain: identifying a large number of different cortical areas associated with different functions and cognitive skills. Recent developments in multi-unit recordings combined with inactivation paradigms have provided powerful methods for the study of cortical circuits and novel insights into cortical dynamics.

In monkeys, visual cortical information has been considered to be the result of ascending projections and local processing through a series of hierarchical cortical visual areas [1]. At each station, horizontal connections reinforce the interplay between groups of neurons with similar properties [2]. Both feed-forward and intrinsic circuits contribute to the extraction of complex attributes of the visual scene at each successive processing stage. The feed-forward connections are excitatory and make non-specific synaptic contacts with different compartments of post-synaptic cells [3]. These connections are visuotopically organized, converging in clusters, and they are paramount for the receptive field properties of post-synaptic neurons [4,5]. Indirect feed-forward projections to area MT (via V2 and V3) contribute to the response to fast moving stimuli and for binocular disparity tuning [6,7]. The role of caudally directed (feedback) projections is less clear. The exuberance of the feedback connections between different cortical areas, the speed of electric signal propagation along these connections, and the latency of visual response all suggest that feedback connections could affect the functional performance of neurons beyond a "modulatory" role [8-11]. Some studies have demonstrated the influence of feedback circuits on the receptive field properties of target neurons [8,12-14,17], whereas others have not found any influence [18,19].

In primates, the second visual area (V2) is the largest extrastriate area. The visuotopic organization of V2 in *Cebus apella* was described using extracellular recordings. V2 area is located in the opercular region of the occipital pole. V2 forms a continuous belt of variable width around the primary visual area (V1) except at the most anterior portion of the calcarine sulcus. It contains a complete visuotopic representation of the contralateral visual hemifield [20]. V1 and V2 are part of both dorsal and ventral pathways of visual information processing.

The prestriate visual area MT is an area of the dorsal stream of visual information processing. It is strongly involved in motion and depth perception and it contains an abundance of motion-coding cells. The medial temporal area is a small area that exists in the temporal lobe of all primates, including human [21]. In *Cebus*, MT is an oval area located mainly in the posterior bank of the superior temporal sulcus (STS). MT contains a continuous representation of the coarse and contralateral segment binocular visual field. As in V1 and V2, the superior field is located ventrally and the lower field is located dorsally. the representation of the fovea is located at the lateral posterior bank of the superior temporal sulcus while the periphery is located medially. The average area of MT is 70 mm^2 [22].

The prestriate visual area V4 is an area of the ventral stream of visual information processing. It is strongly involved in shape and color perception and it contains an abundance of color-coding cells [23,24]. It is defined as a strip of cortex from 10 to 12 mm in width anterior to V3 that extends dorsally from the anterior margin of the lunate sulcus. V4 contains a topographically organized representation central of 35° 40° of the visual field. The representation of the central portion of the visual field is greatly expanded compared to the periphery. The receptive field size increases with increasing eccentricity, while the cortical magnification factor decreases [25,26].

The pulvinar nucleus is a diencephalic structure located in the posterior region of the thalamus whose evolutionary development occurred in parallel with the expansion and differentiation of the temporo-parieto-occipital cortex. Its involvement with visual function has been demonstrated by the presence of a retinotopic organization, and by its connections with the different cortical visual areas.

It has been suggested that some receptive field properties of cortical neurons, such as orientation selectivity and direction selectivity, may be attributed to the inhibitory influence of intrinsic circuits on incoming information [30,31]. The inactivation of intrinsic inhibitory processes impairs both orientation and direction selectivity [32,33]. In primary (V1) and secondary (V2) visual areas of monkeys and cats, the orientation and direction selectivity depend on the inhibitory influence of basket cells projecting to orientation- and direction-selective functional modules [30,31,34-36]. However, evidence indicates that excitatory intrinsic inputs also contribute to V1 orientation selectivity and direction selectivity [30,36]. We have investigated whether feedback projections from area MT, V4 or pulvinar directly interfere with the orientation and direction selectivity of V2 neurons. We studied the receptive field properties of V2 neurons before and after the inactivation of a large topographically corresponding portion of area MT, V4 or pulvinar in the capuchin monkey (*Cebus apella*). Several aspects of the visual system of this New World monkey, including photoreceptor distribution [37], ganglion cell topography [38], thalamic organization [39-41], morphology and physiology of the M and P ganglion cells [42-44], intrinsic circuitry of V1 [45-47] and the topographical characteristics of areas V1, V2, MT, and V4 [20,22,26,48,49] have been studied for almost two decades, making this monkey a suitable experimental model.

In this chapter we will describe the role of feedback circuits to V2 from two cortical visual areas and one subcortical nucleus and compare these inactivation results with the direct inactivation of V2. We will also address the cortical dynamics using an illusory motion paradigm.

We have also investigated feedback influence on early visual cortices related to perception of illusory motion stimulus. Mapping of cortical visual areas suggests that cortical feedback from higher visual areas induces a selective increase of activity in the early visual stage along the corticalrepresentation of illusory stimuli [27-29].

2. Inactivation paradigm

The stimulus consisted of a thin white bar (18 x 0.5 degrees) that appeared in four random orientations (0°, 45°, 90°, or 135°), crossed the screen in a direction perpendicular to its orientation at a velocity of 10 degrees/sec, and passed through the receptive fields of all the recorded neurons. We continuously tested the direction of motion selectivity before and after GABA injection. We did not segregate orientation selectivity from axis-of-movement selectivity.

To locate the topographically corresponding portions of areas MT, V4, pulvinar and V2, we penetrated the cortex with 1MΩ-impedance tungsten microelectrodes, using stereotaxic coordinates and sulcal landmarks [20,22,26,39,50].

Areas MT, V4 and the pulvinar were individually inactivated by pressure injections of GABA 0.25 M until virtually all recorded activity at the injection site in these areas were silenced. Data collection resumed immediately before and after the injection, and several blocks of recording protocols were acquired until recovery of MT, V4 and pulvinar cellular activity. The recording sessions typically continued for 24–30 h.

After the corresponding topographical site was localized in area V2, a single microelectrode was replaced by a two-electrode recording system, with the electrodes placed 800 mm apart, to record V2 neuron activity. Single-unit activity from area V2 was recorded using tungsten microelectrodes. The activity was amplified and filtered, and single spikes were sampled by a waveform discriminator system (SPS-8701, Signal Processing System, Malvern, VIC, AU). Extracellular single-unit spike events were stored using the CORTEX software (Laboratory of Neuropsychology, NIMH/NIH, Bethesda, MD, USA) for offline analysis (MATLAB toolbox, Mathworks Inc., Natick, USA). The receptive fields were initially localized and mapped using a hand-plot mapping procedure. To determine the statistical significance of the effects on V2 neuron direction selectivity before and after GABA injection into area MT, V4 or pulvinar, the cell activity under each condition was analyzed using a two-way ANOVA. We also performed a statistical evaluation of the recovery after GABA injection by evaluating the cell activity in the control condition, before GABA injection and after the GABA-induced effects had vanished, using a two-way ANOVA. Selectivity of the neurons was examined with a standard test of circular tuning in order to determine the magnitude of the GABA-induced changes in both direction and orientation selectivity across the population.

The receptive field automatic mapping procedure was based on computing the latency-corrected neuronal activity in response to elongated bars moving in one of eight directions of motion. Initially, Peristimulus Time Histograms (PSTHs) were computed based on 10 stimulus presentations, using a bin width of 10 ms. Single-trial spike trains used to produce the PSTHs were aligned to stimulus onset. The PSTHs were then smoothed, using a normal convolution filter of 200 ms time-window, resulting in the Time Spike Density Function (TSDF). The TSDF characterizes the dynamics of neuronal firing pattern well, as it is a continuous and derivable function [51].

3. Evaluation of the early and late effects of GABA inactivation

GABA inactivation of area MT produced an early and short (10-30 min) decrease in both spontaneous activity and responsiveness followed by a transitory change in the V2 neuronal direction selectivity. The difference in the time course of these effects resulted in an intermediate improvement (20-40 min) of the signal-to-noise ratio of the stimulus driven activity. After a variable time period, this improvement disappeared. GABA inactivation in area MT produced either an inhibitory effect, a significant change of direction tuning or a complete loss of directional selectivity in most (72%) of the V2 neurons. During the 15 min following GABA inactivation, a clear inhibitory trend in the response pattern was observed. Additionally, 56% of the V2 neurons exhibited a significant change in directional selectivity. For 6% of the V2 neurons, a general suppression of activity was observed after GABA injection into area MT - even though no change in direction selectivity was observed. In 3 cells, GABA inactivation had no discernable effect on the direction or orientation selectivity.

GABA inactivation of V4 induced a statistically significant effect in the majority (72%) of V2 neurons studied. Statistical analysis of the first five minutes of the response of the V2 neurons after GABA inactivation of V4 showed a change in direction selectivity in 46% of these neurons; of these, 23% showed a change from pandirectionality to directional selectivity. The remaining 23% showed a change from directional selectivity to pandirectionality. In seven neurons, there was no change of direction selectivity, although there was a statistically significant effect on the strength of the response. There was no significant effect in the remaining three cells.

In the pulvinar nucleus, GABA injections resulted in a significant decrease of cellular activity, and 5 minutes after the injection the activity was, in average, 40% that of the initial level. We studied 33 cells in V2 before and after GABA injections in the pulvinar. All cells had their receptive fields within 10 degrees of the representation of the central visual field. Most cells studied in V2 (67%) during pulvinar inactivation showed changes in the response to visual stimuli and/or in the spontaneous activity. We observed a change in the direction and/or orientation selectivity in 91% of the cells during pulvinar inactivation. Most of these cells (55%) showed changes in both directional index (DI) and orientation index (OI), while 15% showed changes only in DI and 21% only in OI.

Figure 1 shows an example of a V2 cell after inactivation of visual area V4. The cell was pan-directional with good response to virtually all directions. One minute after inactivation the spontaneous activity and the driven activity were drastically reduced.

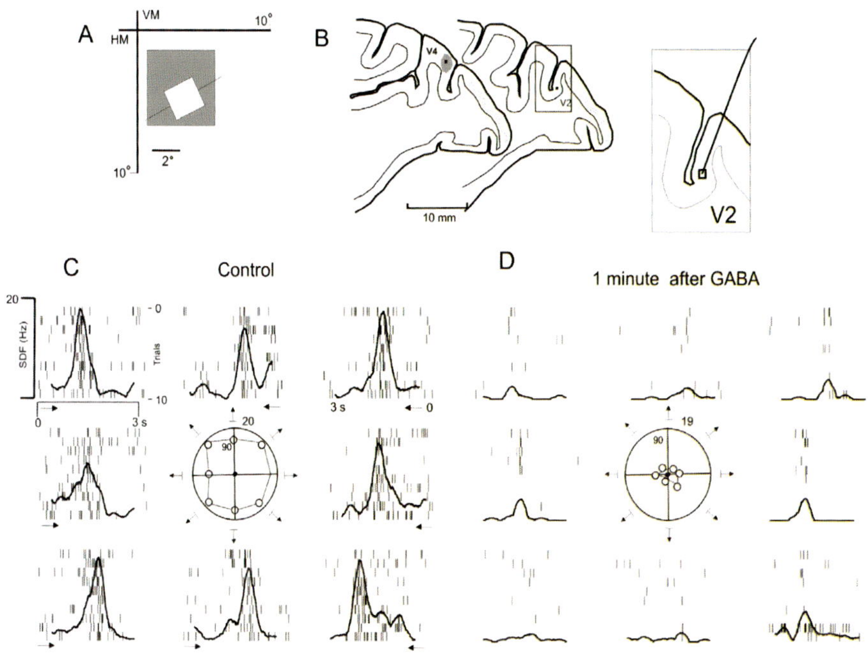

Figure 1. The effect of GABA inactivation of a portion of V4 in the visual response of a V2 neuron. A: The visual field location of the receptive fields of the neurons of V4 and V2 that were studied in this experiment. The large and small rectangles correspond to the V4 and V2 receptive fields, respectively. The approximate positions of the recordings sites are indicated by small rectangles; B: Parasagittal sections of the Cebus brain, showing the locations of V4 and V2. The approximate positions of the recordings sites are indicated by small rectangles; C: A pandirectional selective V2 neuron ($p < 0.05$) recorded at the V2 site. The polargrams depicted at left illustrate the V2 neuron mean firing rate elicited by bars moving in eight directions orthogonal to its preferred orientation before (control condition, polargram at the top) and one minute after GABA (D) ($p < 0.05$). The polargrams represent the response magnitude relative to each direction of motion. These SDFs represent the cellular activity in the space domain. The vertical ticks represent spikes, and each line of spikes corresponds to the total span of visual stimulation during each trial.

GABA inactivation of area MT, V4 and pulvinar produced early (up to 20 min) and late (from 20 to 160 min after GABA injection) effects on V2 neurons. These effects consisted of an early general decrease in neuronal excitability, which corresponded to a depression in the spontaneous and driven activities, and late effects, which generally reflected changes in the orientation and/or direction selectivity of the V2 neurons. In general, a loss of direction or orientation selectivity was observed during the 25 min after GABA inactivation. As an intermediate effect, an improvement in the amount of driven activity inside the classical receptive field relative to that outside the classical receptive field was observed 15 to 25 min after GABA inactivation. This effect was transient and was followed by a longer-lasting decrease in neuronal excitability.

The greater the amount of GABA injected the longer the inactivation duration period and the time needed for the neurons to recover [52]. This last result is in agreement with our observations for MT, V4 and pulvinar. Neurons required 40 min to recover to baseline after a 0.9-μL injection of GABA 0.1M [19]. This recovery period coincided with the time required by V2 neurons to regain baseline activity after a 0.8-1.0 μL GABA (0.25 mol/L) injection into area MT and V4. Considering the extent of area MT and V4 [22,26], we extended preceding predictions [52] regarding the relationship of the injected volume and occupied extracellular volume. We predicted that injection volumes between 0.8 and 10 μL would inactivate between 2.3 and 33.3% of area MT and 0.7–3.22% of area V4.

4. Population circular tuning when areas MT, V4, pulvinar or intrinsic V2 were inactivated

When area MT was inactivated, both increase (62%) and decrease (38%) of direction circular tuning was observed in the V2 neurons. In addition, some cells significantly changed their orientation selectivity. However, a significant change in the mean orientation circular tuning of the V2 neurons was not observed after GABA inactivation in area MT. When a change greater than 0.2 was used as criterion, only 38% of the neurons altered their direction or orientation circular tuning.

When area V4 was inactivated both increase (72.2%) and decrease (27.7%) of direction circular tuning were observed in the V2 neurons. In addition, we found that 72.2% of these cells decreased while 27.7% increased their orientation selectivity, thus presenting an opposite effect for direction and orientation circular tuning. When changes greater than 0.2 were used as criterion, only 25% of the neurons changed their direction or orientation circular tuning. There was no statistical segregation of GABA effect for directional or orientation index in this sample (χ^2 test p=0.1). Although the number of cells that increased OI is similar to the number that decreased DI, there was no bias toward increase or decrease in the sample (χ^2 test p=0.1).

GABA and lidocaine-induced inactivation of the area V2 changed direction and orientation tuning in 37.4% of V2 cells. When changes greater than 0.2 were used as criterion, 29.2% of the neurons changed their direction or orientation circular tuning. There was no trend in the sample of cells toward increase or decrease in selectivity. Sixteen percent of V2 neurons increased while 20.8% decreased their direction selectivity after injections of GABA or lidocaine. In addition, some cells decreased (2/24) while others increased (3/24) their orientation selectivity. The effect of intrinsic inactivation of V2, unlike the effect produced by inactivation of MT and V4 areas, decreased the indices of orientation or direction circular tuning.

GABA inactivation of the pulvinar induced both excitatory and inhibitory change in the V2 neuronal activity and produced a decrease in orientation selectivity. The effects of inactivation of the visual area MT are quantitatively different from those of inactivation of area V4. While inactivation of MT, on average, decreases DI, the inactivation of V4 increases DI [51,53]. In addition, inactivation of MT, on average, increases OI, while inactivation of V4 or the pulvinar decreases OI [51,53,54]. Thus, the feedback connections of MT are different from those of V4, but both promote inhibitory modulations in V2, while the projection of pulvinar produces both excitatory and inhibitory modulations on the target cells in V2.

4.1. V2 neurons that became selective with GABA

There have been some neurons that became direction and orientation selective with GABA injection in areas MT, V4 or pulvinar. There was a pan-directional V2 neuron that had high spontaneous activity before GABA injection in MT. It became directionally selective 1 min after a 10-μL injection of 0.25 M GABA into area MT. Under GABA-induced inactivation, the unit acquired a bi-directional response pattern ($p<0.01$), and an inhibitory flank could be observed when a bar moving at 180° was presented.

4.2. V2 neurons that lost direction or orientation selectivity with GABA

The loss of selectivity was the most frequently detected receptive field alteration in the V2 neurons after GABA inactivation in areas MT, V4 or pulvinar. Two V2 neurons lost their direction selectivity after GABA-induced inactivation in area MT ($p<0.01$). These cells exhibited directional selectivity during the control condition and became pan-directional 1 min after GABA injection ($p=0.9$ and $p=0.7$ respectively). After 14-15 min, the cells recovered their directional selectivity ($p<0.01$).

4.3. Hypothetical circuit

We propose the following hypothetical model to explain our observations (Figure 2). If the feed-forward projections of the cortical areas are considered to be excitatory [55], the feedback circuits would probably modify the properties of the receptive field through the excitatory and inhibitory neurons present in the intrinsic circuits. The most common effect observed during the 10 min after GABA injection into area MT, V4 or pulvinar was a decrease in the spontaneous and the driven activity in the V2 neurons. We propose that pyramidal neurons within direction selective modules in area MT, V4 and pulvinar containing $GABA_A$ receptors [30] are inhibited by the GABA injection. A decrease in neurotransmitter release to the superficial and deep layers of area MT, V4 and pulvinar would then ensue. As a result, the excitatory caudally directed synapses become inhibited, causing a decrease in the spontaneous and driven activity of the V2 neurons. The injections affect each direction-selective column, resulting in a decrease in the spontaneous and driven activity of the neurons for all directions.

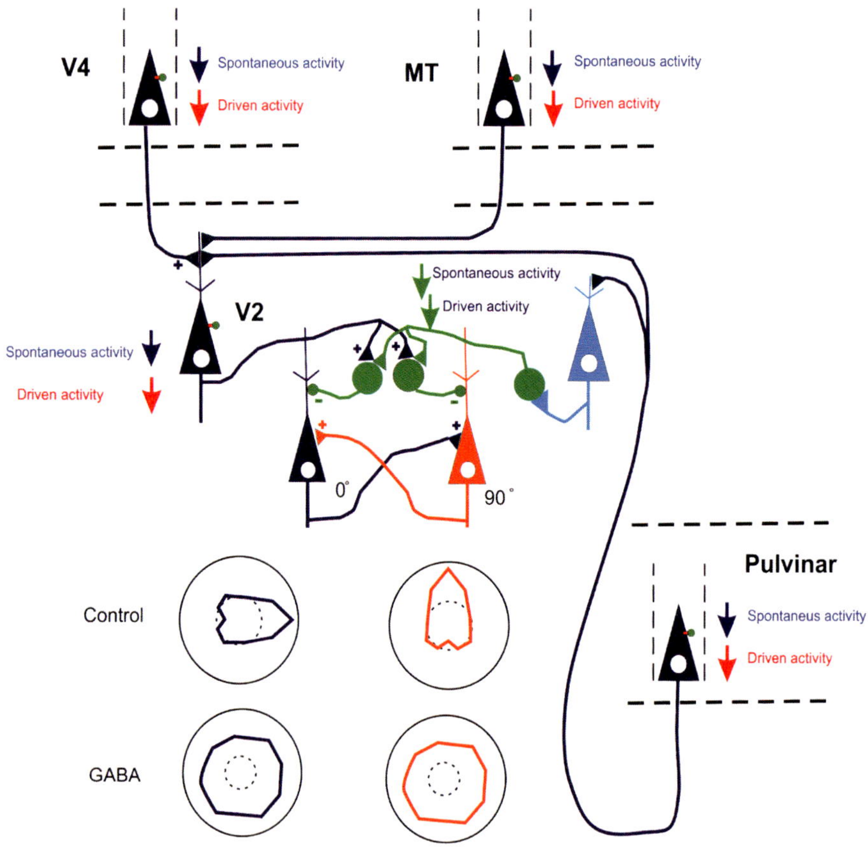

Figure 2. Hypothetical circuit of the GABA effect. Schematic diagram of cortical cells (blue triangles) and the pulvinar showing a circuit that generates loss of direction selectivity in V2 neurons after injection into MT, V4 or pulvinar. In these circuit direction selective pyramidal neurons in target areas, containing $GABA_A$ receptors capture the GABA injected, resulting in decrease of the firing rate activity of these neurons. The arborization neurons project back to the superficial and deep layers of V2. Neurons in MT, V4 or pulvinar decreased neurotransmitter release, and the frequency of firing rate in excitatory synapses result in a decrease of the spontaneous activity of neurons in V2.

A loss of selectivity was the most frequent receptive field alteration in the V2 neurons after GABA inactivation of the topographically corresponding portions of area MT, V4 or pulvinar. We hypothesize the existence of a circuit involving projections from deep and superficial layers of area MT (probably pyramidal neurons) containing $GABA_A$ receptors. The excitability of these neurons would decrease after the activation of GABA receptors. This decrease in excitability would influence the pyramidal neurons in V2 that receive these projections and would also influence intrinsic inhibitory neurons. Intrinsic inhibitory interneurons decrease the influence of neuronal afferents to neighboring columns and cause a loss of direction selectivity for the majority of neurons. The directionality of the remaining 10% of the neurons in our population became selective after the GABA injection. Therefore, we propose that the inactivation of area MT, V4 or pulvinar have partial and asymmetrical effects, causing some direction columns to remain active whereas others are suppressed. This asymmetrical inhibition would generate direction selectivity in neurons that were pan-directional before the injection.

4.4. Other interpretations

These results of GABA inactivation challenge the notion that serial hierarchical processing and lateral projections are the only responsible for the construction of receptive-field properties in early cortical visual areas. We propose that larger recurrent networks may also contribute to the construction of response properties of single cells and those properties are established after several cycles of feed-forward and feedback information.

The paradigm used in this study does not allow the distinction between an intrinsic change in direction/orientation selectivity and a change in the shape of the receptive fields or their surround. For instance, if GABA or lidocaine caused the RFs to become smaller, this would presumably show up as a decrease in responsiveness. Likewise if they became asymmetrical, this would be evident as a change in orientation selectivity. A superficial analysis of changes in receptive field structure of V2 neurons with GABA injections in MT did not revealed however any systematic effect. Future experiments with a selected sample of cells are necessary to further exam the spatial structure of the intersection maps before and after GABA or lidocaine inactivation.

5. Contribution of feedback projections to illusory motion processing in V2

Neurons in the secondary visual cortex (V2) are capable of responding to illusory contours [56]. A classic illusion to which V2 neurons are responsive is the Kanizsa triangle. In this visual phenomenon we can see an illusory well defined triangle, apparently having higher luminance than the background. Single neurons in V2 respond to the illusory contour of the Kanizsa triangle in a similar manner as to the presentation of a real triangle.

Visual illusions have been defined as misperceptions of the real world. This interpretation is a contradiction to the traditional feed-forward concept of visual information processing, inasmuch as the visual signal is not physically presented. Therefore, how do V2 neurons respond to something that does not exist? How does a non stimulated area of the retina generate action potentials in cortical neurons? To answer these questions we need to look into high hierarchical areas in the brain. As we go from early to advanced stages of the visual processing, the size and the structure of the visual receptive fields go from small and simple [1,48] to large and complex [22,26]. Based on these data, one should think that early visual areas have limited capacity for complex visual phenomena processing, unless they receive visual clues from visual higher-order brain areas, where neurons could integrate information from the global visual scene and send it back to neurons to the early visual stages.

A paradigm to test the functional influence of feedback projections to V2 neurons is to induce visual motion processing in a large area, with apparent motion (AM) stimuli. V2 has motion detector neurons, which are tuned to the direction of the movement. This means that the displacement of a stimulus in a preferred direction increases the firing rate of the neuron, while displacement in the opposite direction (null direction) decreases the firing rate. Visual motion processing implicates that neurons must integrate information from a defined area of the visual field, covering the distance of the motion trace. Neurons with large receptive fields, as those in higher visual areas, could integrate the information about large spatial locations in space, while neurons in the early stages would be spatially restricted due to their small receptive field sizes. The spatial distance of the motion trace can be manipulated in a monitor display by using the paradigm of apparent motion illusion. This illusion was formally described by Wertheimer in 1912 [57] and a classic representation is two static stimuli presented transiently and alternately at two different locations in the visual field. The brain interprets the two static stimuli as a single moving stimulus. The use of the apparent motion paradigm allows controlling spatial and temporal variables of the motion information. By keeping constant the temporal interval, different spatial intervals can be used to determine the exact range of the spatial integration carried out by neurons with small receptive fields. If the maximal spatial range is much greater than the receptive field size of these neurons, one could suggest that information from higher visual areas with large receptive fields is being added to the neuronal computation perfomed by the lower visual area neurons. The maximal spatial range can be determined by increasing the separation of the stimuli until suppression of the directional neuronal response. In this case, neurons could not discriminate the direction of the illusory motion, inasmuch as the static stimuli far from the receptive field could not be 'seen', or information sent by higher visual areas would not be enough to produce a response.

It is not yet understood how feedback signals influence the spatial integration of visual signals by V2 neurons. In regard to apparent motion processing, strong evidences show that the visual middle temporal area (MT) of nonhuman primate is a critical area for the perception of apparent motion [58], inasmuch as its specialized motion detector neurons and the large receptive fields can cover a large area of the visual field. Also in humans, activation of an area analogous to area MT in primates, the human complex hMT/V5, is directly associated with the AM perception [59].

We indirectly investigated the feedback contribution in V2 neuronal response by using an apparent motion paradigm. We delineated an experiment where short and long-range apparent motion stimuli were generated to adequately stimulate both V2 and MT, although only V2 activity was recorded. We determined the spacing (ΔS) for consecutive (directional) visual stimuli and we looked for the responses to the stimuli that fell in the center of the receptive field. A methodology for precisely mapping the receptive fields was required so that the spatial distribution of the stimuli could be correctly arranged when the illusion of apparent motion was induced at the cellular level. Extracellular multi-unit recordings were made in the secondary visual cortex of an anesthetized and paralyzed adult *Cebus* monkey (*Cebus apella*)

http://dx.doi.org/10.5772/56497

and single-units were studied by comparing the neural activity response to AM conditions versus a smooth motion condition. The neuronal activity acquired was classified as to belong to individual neurons by'spike sorting' software. The apparent motion condition was generated by a white bar presented at 30 Hz with different spatial intervals (gaps) producing apparent speeds from 15°/s to 135°/s. The smooth motion condition was given by the same stimulus presented in a 60 Hz refresh rate monitor and moving at 15°/s. To infer that neurons were detecting motion, the neuronal response was quantified by calculating a directional selectivity index which takes into account responses for the best and null directions of the stimulus. The presence of direction selective neurons would suggest that V2 is able to process AM in that particular space and time intervals. However, we found directional V2 single-units that stopped to discriminate directions of motion with stimuli spatially separated that exceeded the receptive field size of the neuron, suggesting that these neurons would not process long-range apparent motion. Figure 3 shows a single-unit example of such a neuron.

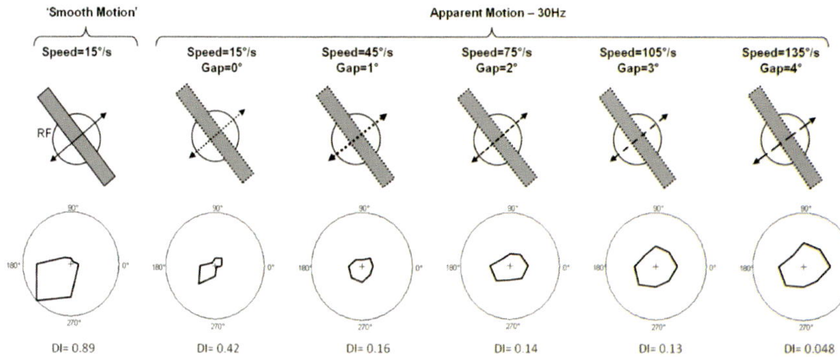

Figure 3. Representation of single-unit responses of a V2 neuron to a smooth motion stimuli and to apparent motion stimuli. Direction selective responses are represented by polargrams and quantified in directional indexes (DI) values. Each condition (column) generates a directional response when the stimulus crossed the center of the receptive field (RF). The same bar stimulus (in gray) was presented in smooth motion (bar in continuous line) and in 30 Hz apparent motion (dotted line). Apparent speeds were produced by increasing the distance (gap in degrees). Increasing the distance of the flashed bars increased the speed of apparent motion. The directional response was extracted by the bar in smooth motion (left column). In this particular example, it is possible to see by polargram and by the directional index (DI=0.89) that the neuron is unidirectional (from 45° to 215°). However, when the bar was presented in apparent motion condition the directional response (DI=0.42) was maintained just at the first condition (no gap between the bars). By increasing the distance between the bars the neuron loses its directional selectivity.

To study the range of spatial integration in V2, and to indirectly illustrate the role of feedback or intrinsic circuitry in apparent motion processing in V2, new experiments will be needed to analyze directional response to apparent motion of different spatial and time intervals. The exact functional role of feedback contribution to V2 neuronal response to illusory motion remains a topic of current research.

6. Conclusion

The inactivation of feedback connections from MT or V4 to area V2 produces a general decrease in the excitability of the V2 neurons, which included an increase in spontaneous activity, a decrease of the stimulus-activity, and sometimes changes in directional selectivity. These changes in selectivity were toward an increase in directional selectivity and a decrease in orientation selectivity. The effects of inactivation of the cortical visual area V4 are different from those of inactivation of visual area MT or from the inactivation of subcortical nuclei, such as the pulvinar. Inactivation of the feedback connections of V4 and MT promote inhibitory modulations in V2, while inhibition of the pulvinar produces both excitatory and inhibitory modulations on the target cells in V2. GABA inactivation of areas MT and V4 produced an early and short decrease in both spontaneous activity and responsiveness, followed by a transitory increase of spontaneous activity and change in V2 neuronal direction and orientation selectivity. GABA inactivation of the pulvinar induces both excitatory and inhibitory changes in V2 neuronal activity and produces a decrease in orientation selectivity. The effects of inactivation of the visual area MT are quantitatively different from those of inactivation of area V4. While inactivation of MT, on average, decreases DI, the inactivation of V4 increases DI [51,53]. In addition, inactivation of MT, on average, increases OI, while inactivation of V4 or pulvinar decreases OI [51,54].

We also attempted to study the role of feedback from higher visual areas to V2 by designing a study in which spatial integration was accessed by using an apparent motion paradigm. Preliminary results suggest a minor contribution of the feedback projections to the apparent motion processing in V2.

Acknowledgements

The scientific studies described here were supported by Brazilian government grants (CNPq, FAPERJ, FUJB, PRONEX, FINEP, CEPG).

Author details

Ana Karla Jansen-Amorim[1*], Cecilia Ceriatte[2], Bruss Lima[2], Juliana Soares[2], Mario Fiorani[2] and Ricardo Gattass[2]

*Address all correspondence to: anajansenamorim@gmail.com

1 Institute of Biological Sciences, Federal University of Pará, Belém, PA, Brazil

2 Institute of Biophysics Carlos Chagas Filho, Federal University of Rio de Janeiro, Rio de Janeiro, RJ, Brazil

http://dx.doi.org/10.5772/56497

References

[1] Hubel DH, Wiesel TN. Receptive fields and functional architecture of monkey striate cortex. J Physiol 1968;195(1):215-43.

[2] McGuire BA, Gilbert CD, Rivlin PK, Wiesel TN. Targets of horizontal connections in macaque primary visual cortex. J Comp Neurol 1991;305(3):370-92.

[3] Johnson RR, Burkhalter A. Microcircuitry of forward and feedback connections within rat visual cortex. J Comp Neurol 1996;368(3):383-98.

[4] Lamme VA, Super H, Spekreijse H. Feedforward, horizontal, and feedback processing in the visual cortex. Curr Opin Neurobiol 1998;8(4):529-35.

[5] Sincich LC, Park KF, Wohlgemuth MJ, Horton JC. Bypassing V1: a direct geniculate input to area MT. Nat Neurosci 2004;7(10):1123-8.

[6] Ponce CR, Lomber SG, Born RT. Integrating motion and depth via parallel pathways. Nat Neurosci 2008;11(2):216-23.

[7] Ponce CR, Hunter JN, Pack CC, Lomber SG, Born RT. Contributions of indirect pathways to visual response properties in macaque middle temporal area MT. J Neurosci 2011;31(10):3894-903.

[8] Hupe JM, James AC, Payne BR, Lomber SG, Girard P, Bullier J. Cortical feedback improves discrimination between figure and background by V1, V2 and V3 neurons. Nature 1998;394(6695):784-7.

[9] Bullier J. Feedback connections and conscious vision. Trends Cogn Sci 2001;5(9): 369-370.

[10] Angelucci A, Levitt JB, Walton EJ, Hupe JM, Bullier J, Lund JS. Circuits for local and global signal integration in primary visual cortex. J Neurosci 2002;22(19):8633-46.

[11] Borra E, Rockland KS. Projections to early visual areas v1 and v2 in the calcarine fissure from parietal association areas in the macaque. Front Neuroanat 2011;5:35.

[12] Mignard M, Malpeli JG. Paths of information flow through visual cortex. Science 1991;251(4998):1249-51.

[13] Alonso JM, Cudeiro J, Perez R, Gonzalez F, Acuna C. Influence of layer V of area 18 of the cat visual cortex on responses of cells in layer V of area 17 to stimuli of high velocity. Exp Brain Res 1993;93(2):363-6.

[14] Rockland KS, Knutson T. Feedback connections from area MT of the squirrel monkey to areas V1 and V2. J Comp Neurol 2000;425(3):345-68.

[15] Wang C, Waleszczyk WJ, Burke W, Dreher B. Modulatory influence of feedback projections from area 21a on neuronal activities in striate cortex of the cat. Cereb Cortex 2000;10(12):1217-32.

[16] Galuske RA, Schmidt KE, Goebel R, Lomber SG, Payne BR. The role of feedback in shaping neural representations in cat visual cortex. Proc Natl Acad Sci U S A 2002;99(26):17083-8.

[17] Huang L, Chen X, Shou T. Spatial frequency-dependent feedback of visual cortical area 21a modulating functional orientation column maps in areas 17 and 18 of the cat. Brain Res 2004;998(2):194-201.

[18] Sandell JH, Schiller PH. Effect of cooling area 18 on striate cortex cells in the squirrel monkey. J Neurophysiol 1982;48(1):38-48.

[19] Hupe JM, James AC, Girard P, Bullier J. Response modulations by static texture surround in area V1 of the macaque monkey do not depend on feedback connections from V2. J Neurophysiol 2001;85(1):146-63.

[20] Rosa MG, Sousa AP, Gattass R. Representation of the visual field in the second visual area in the Cebus monkey. J Comp Neurol 1988;275(3):326-45.

[21] Kaas JH, Collins CE. The organization of sensory cortex. Curr Opin Neurobiol 2001; 11(4):498-504.

[22] Fiorani M, Jr., Gattass R, Rosa MG, Sousa AP. Visual area MT in the Cebus monkey: location, visuotopic organization, and variability. J Comp Neurol 1989;287(1):98-118.

[23] Hubel DH, Livingstone MS. Segregation of form, color, and stereopsis in primate area 18. J Neurosci (1987)7(11):3378-3415.

[24] Tanigawa H, Lu HD, Roe AW. Functional organization for color and orientation in macaque V4. Nat Neurosci 2010;13(12):1542-8.

[25] Gattass R, Sousa AP, Gross CG. Visuotopic organization and extent of V3 and V4 of the macaque. J Neurosci 1988;8(6):1831-45.

[26] Pinon MC, Gattass R, Sousa AP. Area V4 in Cebus monkey: extent and visuotopic organization. Cereb Cortex 1998;8(8):685-701.

[27] Seghier M, Dojat M, Delon-Martin C, Rubin C, Warnking J, Segebarth C, et al. Moving illusory contours activate primary visual cortex: an fMRI study. Cereb Cortex 2000;10(7):663-70.

[28] Sterzer P, Haynes JD, Rees G. Primary visual cortex activation on the path of apparent motion is mediated by feedback from hMT+/V5. Neuroimage 2006;32(3):1308-16.

[29] Wibral M, Bledowski C, Kohler A, Singer W, Muckli L. The timing of feedback to early visual cortex in the perception of long-range apparent motion. Cereb Cortex 2009;19(7): 1567-82

[30] Sato H, Katsuyama N, Tamura H, Hata Y, Tsumoto T. Mechanisms underlying orientation selectivity of neurons in the primary visual cortex of the macaque. J Physiol 1996;494 (Pt 3):757-71.

[31] Crook JM, Kisvarday ZF, Eysel UT. Evidence for a contribution of lateral inhibition to orientation tuning and direction selectivity in cat visual cortex: reversible inactivation of functionally characterized sites combined with neuroanatomical tracing techniques. Eur J Neurosci 1998;10(6):2056-75.

[32] Sillito AM. The contribution of inhibitory mechanisms to the receptive field properties of neurones in the striate cortex of the cat. J Physiol 1975;250(2):305-29.

[33] Sillito AM. The effectiveness of bicuculline as an antagonist of GABA and visually evoked inhibition in the cat's striate cortex. J Physiol 1975;250(2):287-304.

[34] Crook JM, Kisvarday ZF, Eysel UT. GABA-induced inactivation of functionally characterized sites in cat visual cortex (area 18): effects on direction selectivity. J Neurophysiol 1996;75(5):2071-88.

[35] Crook JM, Kisvarday ZF, Eysel UT. GABA-induced inactivation of functionally characterized sites in cat striate cortex: effects on orientation tuning and direction selectivity. Vis Neurosci 1997;14(1):141-58.

[36] Sato H, Katsuyama N, Tamura H, Hata Y, Tsumoto T. Mechanisms underlying direction selectivity of neurons in the primary visual cortex of the macaque. J Neurophysiol 1995;74(4):1382-94.

[37] Andrade da Costa BL, Hokoc JN.. Photoreceptor topography of the retina in the New World monkey Cebus apella. Vision Research 2000; 48: 2395-2409.

[38] Silveira LC, Picanço-Diniz CW, Sampaio LF, Oswaldo-Cruz E. Retinal ganglion cell distribution in the cebus monkey: a comparison with the cortical magnification factors. Vision Research 1989;11: 1471-83.

[39] Gattass R, Oswaldo-Cruz E, Sousa AP. Visuotopic organization of the cebus pulvinar: a double representation the contralateral hemifield. Brain Res 1978;152(1):1-16.

[40] Gattass R, Sousa AP, Oswaldo-Cruz E. Single unit response types in the pulvinar of the Cebus monkey to multisensory stimulation. Brain Res 1978;158(1):75-87.

[41] Gattass R, Oswaldo-Cruz E, Sousa AP. Visual receptive fields of units in the pulvinar of cebus monkey. Brain Res 1979;160(3):413-30.

[42] Silveira LC, Yamada ES, Perry VH, Picanço-Diniz CW. M and P retinal ganglion cells of diurnal and nocturnal New-World monkeys. Neuroreport 1994; 16: 2077-81.

[43] Yamada ES, Silveira LC, Perry VH. Morphology, dendritic field size, somal size, density, and coverage of M and P retinal ganglion cells of dichromatic Cebus monkeys. Visual Neuroscience 1996; 6:1011-29.

[44] Lee BB, Silveira LC, Yamada ES, Hunt DM, Kremers J, Martin PR, Troy JB, da Silva-Filho M. Visual responses of ganglion cells of a New-World primate, the capuchin monkey, Cebus apella. Journal of Physiology 2000; 528: 573-90.

[45] Amorim AK, Picanço-Diniz CW. Intrinsic projections of Cebus-monkey area 17: cell morphology and axon terminals. Rev Bras Biol. 1996; Sup 1 2:209-19.

[46] Amorim AK, Picanco-Diniz CW. Morphometric analysis of intrinsic axon terminals of Cebus monkey area 17. Braz J Med Biol Res 1996; 29(10):1363-8.

[47] Amorim AK, Picanco-Diniz CW. Horizontal projections of area 17 in Cebus monkeys: metric features, and modular and laminar distribution. Braz J Med Biol Res 1997;30(12): 1489-501.

[48] Gattass R, Sousa AP, Rosa MG. Visual topography of V1 in the Cebus monkey. J Comp Neurol 1987;259(4):529-48.

[49] Gattass R, Nascimento-Silva S, Soares JG, Lima B, Jansen AK, Diogo AC, et al. Cortical visual areas in monkeys: location, topography, connections, columns, plasticity and cortical dynamics. Philos Trans R Soc Lond B Biol Sci 2005;360(1456):709-31.

[50] Gattass R, Gross CG. Visual topography of striate projection zone (MT) in posterior superior temporal sulcus of the macaque. J Neurophysiol 1981;46(3):621-38.

[51] Jansen-Amorim AK, Lima B, Fiorani M, Gattass R. GABA inactivation of visual area MT modifies the responsiveness and direction selectivity of V2 neurons in Cebus monkeys. Vis Neurosci 2011;28(6):513-27.

[52] Hupe JM, Chouvet G, Bullier J. Spatial and temporal parameters of cortical inactivation by GABA. J Neurosci Methods 1999;86(2):129-43.

[53] Jansen-Amorim AK, Lima B, Fiorani M, Gattass R. GABA inactivation of area V4 changes receptive-field properties of V2 neurons in Cebus monkeys. Vis Neurosci 2012;28(6):513-27.

[54] Soares JG, Diogo AC, Fiorani M, Souza AP, Gattass R. Effects of inactivation of the lateral pulvinar on response properties of second visual area cells in Cebus monkeys. Clin Exp Pharmacol Physiol 2004;31(9):580-90.

[55] Salin PA, Bullier J. Corticocortical connections in the visual system: structure and function. Physiol Rev 1995;75(1):107-54.

[56] von der Heydt R, Peterhans E, Baumgartner G. Illusory contours and cortical neuron responses. Science 1984;224(4654):1260-2.

[57] Sarris V. Max Wertheimer on seen motion: theory and evidence. Psychol Res 1989;51(2): 58-68.

[58] Newsome WT, Mikami A, Wurtz RH. Motion selectivity in macaque visual cortex. III. Psychophysics and physiology of apparent motion. J Neurophysiol 1986;55(6):1340-51.

[59] Muckli L, Kriegeskorte N, Lanfermann H, Zanella FE, Singer W, Goebel R. Apparent motion: event-related functional magnetic resonance imaging of perceptual switches and States. J Neurosci 2002;22(9):RC219.

Chapter 14

Ceasing Thoughts and Brain Activity: MEG Data Analysis

Takaaki Aoki, Michiyo Inagawa,
Kazuo Nishimura and Yoshikazu Tobinaga

Additional information is available at the end of the chapter

http://dx.doi.org/10.5772/56502

1. Introduction

Theory of mind refers to the cognitive capacity to understand and interpret the mental states of other persons in terms of their roles as intentional agents (for example, see [1]). This concept has been extensively studied in developing children and patients with autism or other developmental disorders (see [2]). It must also be researched in normal, healthy individuals, however, as this population must develop strategic communication skills for building effective interpersonal relationships. Such skills include the ability to understand other people's characters and emotions, as well as to accurately guess their thoughts, because people have different personality traits and can often behave differently even in the same situation.

The strategic communication principles mentioned above also apply to what economists call game theory (refer to [3] and other publications for further details on this concept). According to game theory, the player maximizes the payoff, basing his or her action (strategy) on knowledge of the other player's strategy. Players of the game, admitting possible differences in personality traits and behaviors, will collect information on other players' character and behavior patterns. They will also try to categorize opponents' personalities and preferences over time by analyzing their interactions with them.

While the importance of addressing interindividual differences in character traits and behavior patterns has been well recognized, only limited research has investigated this issue in the context of economics. We believe that research on thought patterns and decision-making processes will lay a new foundation for the study of consumer and investor selection decisions regarding economic and financial matters. In light of this background, we explored the factors underlying differences in interpersonal choice and the brain functions associated with them.

Nishimura et al. [7] investigated the relationship between strategy choices in dilemma games and the ability to cease thoughts. Their results demonstrated that the group of subjects without thought-stopping ability were more inclined to choose cooperative behavior than those who had the ability, and that brain activity was more pronounced in the occipital region in the latter group than in the former. This magnetoencephalography (MEG) study showed that the ability to cease thoughts is significantly correlated with specific regions of the brain.

The mental ability to intentionally cease thoughts is possibly reflected in cognitive models of thought suppression and neural models of executive control. Particularly thought suppression is the mental process of deliberately attempting to prevent a particular thought or string of thoughts, a form of restricting free thought (see [4–6]). According to Mitchell and colleagues [6], regulation of thoughts involves two control processes: sustained, proactive cognitive suppression, and transient and additional control associated with intrusion of unwanted thoughts. The former process is modulated by the prefrontal cortex and the latter by the anterior cingulate cortex.

However, there exist interpersonal variations in the ability to intentionally suppress thoughts, and the roles that such variations may play in the pursuit of economic and social opportunities have wide-ranging implications.

This article presents our recent MEG findings [7–10], together with the results of new spectrum analysis. It concludes by discussing the implications of these results and perspectives on future research directions.

Specifically, this paper covers the topics described below. Chapter 2 explains the principles and protocol for the current dipole estimation method applied to MEG measurements using the superconducting quantum interface device (SQUID). It also explains the procedure for mapping the transition of activated areas near the cerebral cortex in subjects performing thought cessation tasks. In this procedure, raw magnetic data acquired from each SQUID sensor are subjected to short-term Fourier transformation. In addition, the details of the assigned tasks are described. Chapter 3 provides the measurement results. In Chapter 4, the neuroscientific implications of the results and current methodological limitations, as well as future prospects for spatial filtering and functional magnetic resonance imaging (fMRI) techniques, are discussed.

2. Method

Our test involved tasks that were closely related to daily activities, in order to evaluate brain-specific functions in as natural a state as possible. In addition, such tasks can reduce distractions associated with the discomfort of being tested (for example, see [13]).

To evaluate individuals' characteristics with as much objectivity as possible, it is important to conduct physical experiments to obtain numerical measures. We therefore used a neuromagnetometer, the SQUID. Since this brain scanner is highly sensitive and completely non-invasive, and it allows us to detect cortical current directly and to monitor brain activities with the highest precision available today, we presume this device is ideal for measuring subjects in normal health. The measurement procedure using SQUID is called MEG (see [11, 12, 14]).

The MEG experiment used a helmet-type neuromagnetometer with 64 channels (CTF LTD, made in Canada) and was conducted at the Tsukuba Research Center of the National Institute of Advanced Industrial Science and Technology, Japan.

2.1. Experimental protocol

Prior to the experiment, we asked the subjects if they could prevent themselves from thinking or not. Three subjects, AI (female, age: 30), AK (female, age: 24), and HT (male, age: 35), replied that they could, while one subject, MT (female, age: 35), stated that she could not.

Our test protocol asked subjects to 1) visualize an image of Kiyomizudera Temple, 2) visualize an image of the National Diet Building, 3) recall the 12 horary signs in Chinese astrology, 4) recall a conversation they had earlier that day, 5) completely stop themselves from thinking, and finally 6) again not think at all. Figure 1 shows the picture of the National Diet in Japan. See Table 1 for task contents. Tasks 1–6 lasted for 10 sec each, and there were no breaks between them. Data acquisition began when a beep sounded at the start of each task, but the data actually used was only that acquired during a 1.6-sec period beginning 0.5 sec after the beep. Thus we sampled spontaneous activities of the brain and not the auditory evoked response just after the beep. Data samples were obtained every 50 msec.

The goals of each of the above tasks were as follows: Tasks 1 and 2 stimulated image visualization through recall of a familiar place. Tasks 3 and 4 tested subjects' ability to recall words.

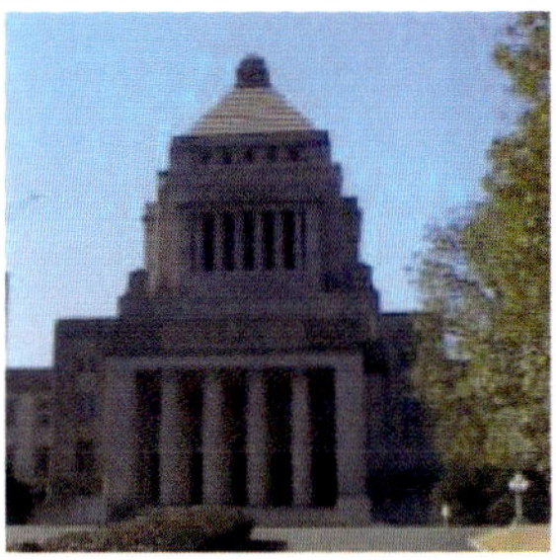

Picture of the Diet Building

Figure 1. The National Diet in Japan

Tasks 1–4 were assumed to measure neural activities during spontaneous thinking. In contrast, "non-thinking" Tasks 5 and 6 were intended to examine each subject's ability to completely suspend their thinking, and were sensitive to personal differences in this ability. We sought to ascertain whether or not SQUID measurements could detect differences in the brain activities elicited by Tasks 1–4 and those induced by Tasks 5–6.

Directions: Proceed from Task 1 to Task 6. Change to the next task at the beep. After you finish Task 6, start again with Task 1. (Each task lasts for 10 sec.)
Picture the following images:
1. Kiyomizudera Temple
2. The Diet Building
Recall the following:
3. The 12 horary signs in Chinese astrology (Mouse, Cow, Tiger, Rabbit...)
4. A conversation you had today.
Sit still and relax, trying not to think at all. If your mind is totally free of conscious thoughts, maintain this state; otherwise let your thinking proceed naturally.
5. Do not think at all.
6. Do not think at all.

Table 1. Tasks

The measured analog data were digitalized by an analog-to-digital converter with a sampling frequency of 1250 Hz, and recorded by each of the SQUID sensor channels. One session consisted of 2 continuous repetitions of the set of 6 tasks described above, and subjects completed a total of 2 sessions each.

2.2. MEG measurement and data analysis

The 64-channel neuromagnetometer used in this study measures each value of the first differentiation of magnetic field Bz (along the z-axis), that is $(\partial Bz/\partial z)_{ij}$ at time i in each SQUID sensor j equipped on the helmet. The dimension of this physical value is $fT/cm(Hz)^{1/2}$. Thus the data matrix $(\partial Bz/\partial z)_{ij}$ (i=1,2,...,64, j=1,2,...,t) is obtained.

2.2.1. Current dipole estimation

The conventional method for current dipole estimation assumes a single or multiple equivalent microcurrent dipole(s) as signal sources in the brain. However, as is clear from findings regarding contemporary brain physiology, nerve activity is too complex to be explained only by the existence of such localized dipoles. This is especially true when the brain is activated throughout the entire neural portion and the equivalent nerve current is presumed to spread out with a wide spatial distribution.

This study required subjects to actively recollect photographic images or remember the names of 12 zodiacal signs, and was therefore unlike those that observe neural activity evoked in synchronization with outside stimuli. As a matter of fact, our experimental data indicated that the measured magnetic distribution did not necessarily correspond to the typical contour patterns on the scalp surface that are expected to give rise to simple current dipoles. Therefore, we took a technical position in which we observed the change in the magnetic field on the scalp surface in both temporal and spatial terms, and sequentially counted the appearance of equivalent current dipoles, inversely derived from temporary fluctuating patterns on the magnetic field contour map.

See Figure 2 for a set of extremes and sinks on the contour map, observed from a point directly superior to the vertex. Three pairs of extremes and sinks were aligned in such a way that their circular contour lines were adjacent to each other. Between each extreme–sink pair, the cerebral cortical current is presumed to exist in accordance with the Biot-Savart Law, one of the fundamental concepts in electromagnetics. This method contrasting the extreme and sink states is only an approximation when compared with pattern recognition analysis, for example, but is still precise enough and is able to significantly reduce computation time. It is therefore practical and appropriate for screening spontaneous brain activities (for example, see [15, 16]).

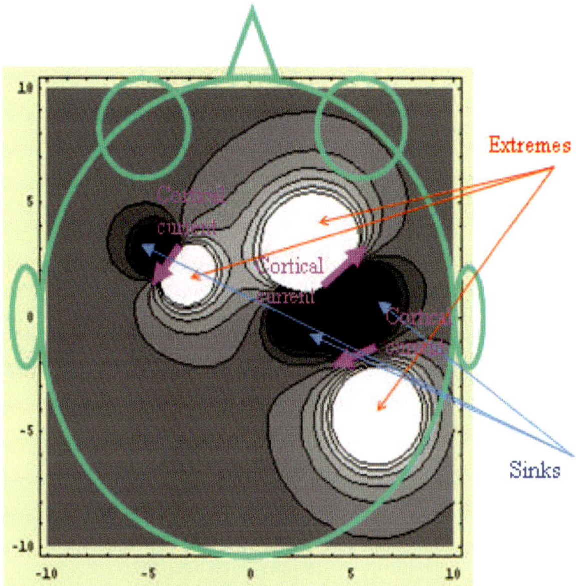

Figure 2. Magnetic field contour map with three cortical currents visible. The dipole currents (brain activity currents) are observed in the area between extreme and sink.

2.2.2. *Spectrum analysis*

The final step in our method was spectrum analysis (for example, see [17, 18]). We performed short-term Fourier transformation on the raw magnetic field data acquired from each SQUID sensor. The sampling frequency was 1250 Hz and the data used was that obtained for 1.6 sec beginning 0.5 sec after the beep that indicated the start of each task. The time window of the

Fourier transformation was 0.25 sec, and a total of 18 measurements was performed, one each 1/12 sec. We calculate the estimated spectrum densities for the following frequency bands: θ wave, 4–8 Hz; α wave, 8–12 Hz; β wave, 12–24 Hz; and γ wave, 24–36 Hz and 36–48 Hz. Then by taking the ratio of the average spectrum density in thinking Tasks 1–4 to that in non-thinking Tasks 5 and 6 for each subject, we offset the interindividual variance in shape of each subject's brain, and plotted the ratio, converted to color, on a 2-dimensional plane representing the brain surface. Thus it was possible to ascertain the global phase of neural activities near the cerebral cortex, and the transition of activated areas between the thinking and not-thinking modes, and to test them for statistical significance.

3. Results

3.1. Current dipole estimation

As already explained, in Tasks 1 and 2 the subjects were asked to recollect photographic images of Kiyomizudera Temple and the National Diet, respectively, both of which are representative and popular buildings in Japan. Next, in Tasks 3 and 4, they were asked to recall the names of 12 zodiacal signs and to remember a conversation they had had earlier that day. In Tasks 5 and 6, subjects were asked to stop their thoughts. Every 10 sec, the sound of a beep notified subjects that they should proceed to the next task. During this entire period, the magnetic fields arising from subjects' spontaneous neural activities were measured.

Four subjects, AI (female, age 30), AK (female, age 24), HT (male, age 35), and MT (female, age 35) were selected for measurement. Figure 3 shows the results of current dipole estimation as represented by distribution charts of signal sources on the scalp surface. The data for the thinking mode were obtained by averaging the data from Tasks 1–4, while those for non-thinking were derived using the average of data from Tasks 5 and 6.

The transition patterns of AI, AK, and HT, who could cease their thoughts, clearly differed between thinking and non-thinking modes. To be more specific, the cluster of estimated current dipoles, designating the activated areas of neural activity, was centered in the pre-frontal lobe in the thinking state, while shifting posteriorly across the parietal lobe into the occipital lobe region in the non-thinking state. In contrast, the activation areas of MT did not shift posteriorly so much between the 2 modes. In fact, she belonged to the type that found it difficult to spontaneously suspend thoughts. A correlation therefore seems to exist between the ability to cease thoughts and the global transition of the activated area. These results were also entirely consistent with those obtained by directly questioning the subjects prior to the experiment.

3.2. Spectrum analysis and global transition

Our results thus far support those reported in [8-10]. In this section, we verify the above implications using spectrum analysis. We initially evaluated 2 of the 4 subjects, one who was able to cease thoughts (HT) and one who could not (MT). For each of these subjects,

http://dx.doi.org/10.5772/56502

and for each frequency band and SQUID sensor, Figure 4 plots the ratio of the average spectrum density in thinking tasks to that in non-thinking tasks. Red indicates values greater than 1, while blue signifies those less than 1. This analysis verifies that in HT (able to cease thoughts), the activated region shifted posteriorly from the parietal lobe to the area near the visual cortex in the occipital lobe. This tendency is consistent with the findings reported in Section 3.1, and was particularly remarkable for the upper frequency bands (β wave, 12–24 Hz; γ wave, 24–36 Hz and 36–48 Hz) as opposed to the lower frequency bands (θ wave, 4–8 Hz; α wave, 8–12 Hz).

Subject	Thinking Tasks 1～4	Non-thinking Tasks 5～6	Direction of shift
AI Female Age: 30	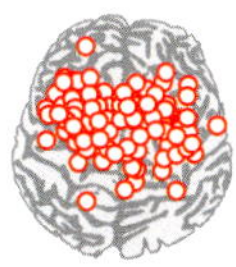	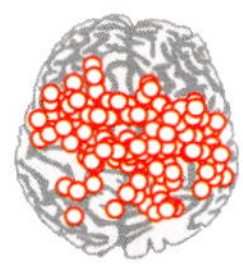	Posteriorly
AK Female Age: 24	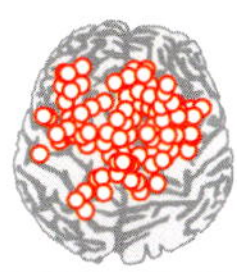	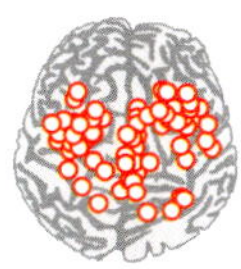	Posteriorly
HT Male Age: 35	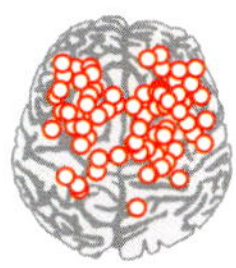	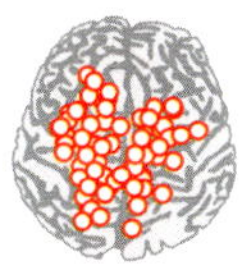	Posteriorly
MT Female Age: 35	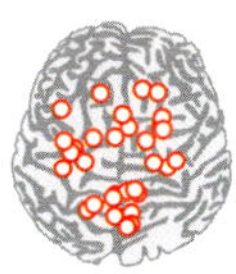	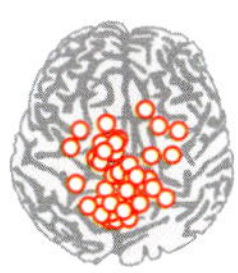	No change

Figure 3. Mapping of estimated current dipoles onto brain surface

For the cluster of sensors near the visual cortex (sensor numbers: SL17, 18, 27, 28, 46; SR17, 18), Figure 5 is a spectrogram of HT (able to stop thinking) that plots, again by color, the ratios for thinking and non-thinking tasks, both normalized by the average density in thinking tasks. The activation in non-thinking tasks is clear, especially at the β wave band, 12–24 Hz.

Finally, we tested the statistical significance of the difference between a subject who could cease thoughts and the one who could not. Figure 6 plots the spectrum density ratio of each subject in non-thinking tasks, normalized by the average density in thinking ones, as a function

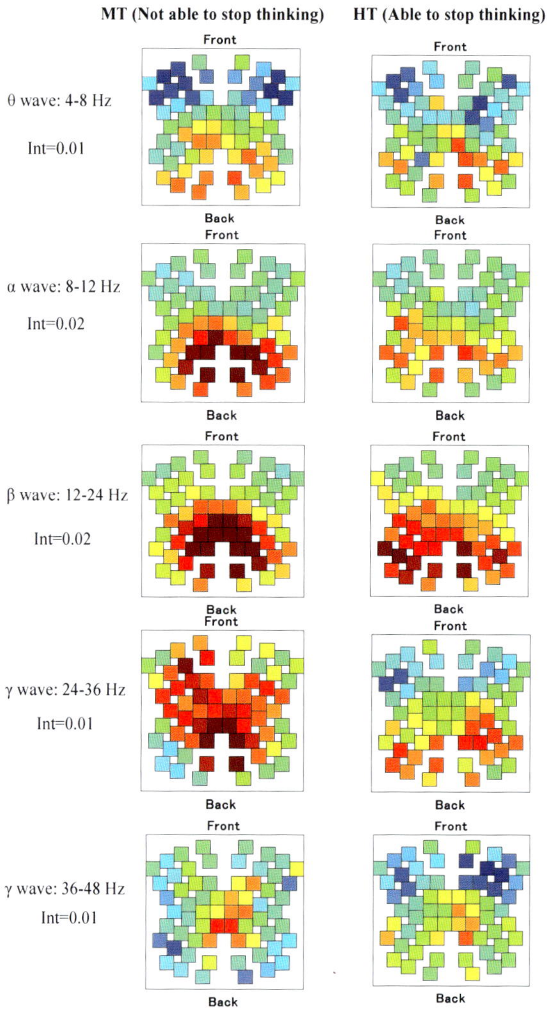

Figure 4. Mapping of estimated spectrum density ratio onto brain surface

of passed time, both near the visual cortex and the parietal lobe (sensor numbers: SL15, 16; SR15, 16). In MT, the ratio in the parietal lobe (blue line) was higher than that in the visual cortex (green line), while in HT, the ratio in the visual cortex was higher than that in the parietal lobe. To sum up, in an individual who could cease thoughts, activation during the non-thinking mode was greater in the visual cortex than in the parietal lobe in both the β and γ wave bands, while the opposite was true for individuals who could not cease thoughts.

http://dx.doi.org/10.5772/56502

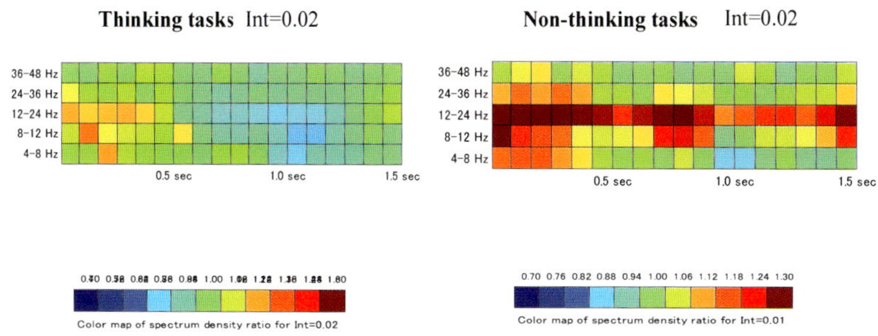

Figure 5. Spectrogram of HT (able to stop thinking) near visual cortex

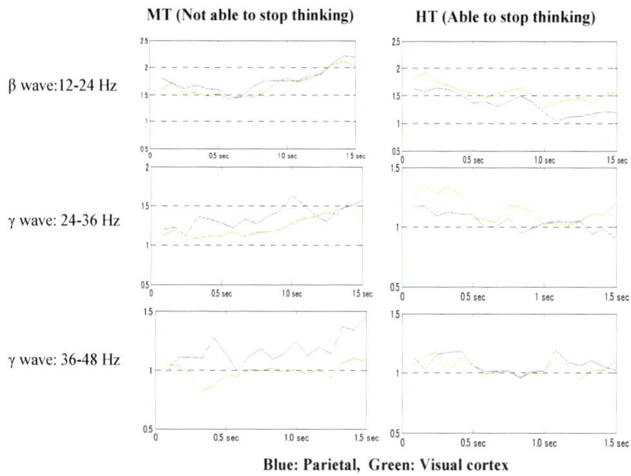

Figure 6. Spectrum density ratio as a function of time

We used the data in Figure 6 to test for the null hypothesis, namely that differences in the above spectrum density ratio between the visual cortex region (SL17, 18, 27, 28, 46; SR17, 18) and that of the parietal lobe (SL15, 16; SR15, 16), plotted as a function of time, would not be higher in HT than in MT. This hypothesis was rejected with one-sided t-statistics of $t = 5.6851$ for the β wave band at 12–24 Hz, $t = 3.2266$ for the γ wave band at 24–36 Hz, and $t = 3.0912$ for the γ wave band at 36–48 Hz; $P<0.001$ for each case. This supports at a significant level the premise that the activation area of individuals who can cease thoughts shifts posteriorly while suspending thought.

The above results suggest that we can objectively evaluate individual differences in higher brain function, including spontaneous thinking activities.

4. Conclusion

The experiment described above illustrates our methodology for analyzing interindividual differences in decision-making processes and in the involvement of specific brain areas. One of our goals is to use a neuroscientific viewpoint to elucidate how humans make economic decisions, particularly based on the relationships between decision-making styles and modes of thinking (patterns and characteristics).

It has been far more difficult to measure spontaneous neural activities (e.g., during mental imagery and self-reflection) than the neural responses evoked by external audiovisual stimuli such as light or sound. However, in this study we successfully monitored spontaneous brain activities during thought cessation by applying special data processing procedures to highly sensitive, noninvasive SQUID magnetometer measurements.

Firstly by applying multiple dipoles estimation method to MEG data, we demonstrated that interindividual differences in the ability of ceasing thoughts can be identified using neuro-scientific approaches. Secondly we showed statistically significant differences in task-related brain activation areas between 2 groups of subjects, divided according to the self-reported presence and absence of the ability to intentionally stop thoughts.

Because of the SQUID sensor characteristics, the MEG data presented in this article were primarily related to the neural activities of the cerebral cortex, and were insufficient for precise analysis of the deeper parts of the brain, such as the limbic system, basal ganglia and nucleus accumbens. For these purposes, spatial filtering of MEG signals and fMRI techniques are useful (see [19-21]). We are planning to report the results of work utilizing these techniques in the near future.

Acknowledgements

We acknowledge the financial support of the Grant-in-Aid for Scientific Research, JSPS (#23000001, #23330063).

Author details

Takaaki Aoki[1], Michiyo Inagawa[2], Kazuo Nishimura[1*] and Yoshikazu Tobinaga[3]

*Address all correspondence to: nishimura@kier.kyoto-u.ac.jp

1 Institute of Economic Research, Kyoto University, Japan

2 Graduate School of Education, Kyoto University, Japan

3 Elegaphy, Inc., Japan

References

[1] Premack D, Woodruff G. Does the chimpanzee have a theory of mind? Behavioral and Brain Science 1978; 1(4), 515-526.

[2] Baron-Cohen S, Leslie, AM, Frith U. Does the autistic child have a "thory of mind"? Cognition 1985; 21(1), 37-46.

[3] Nash, JF. Non-cooperative Games. Annals of Mathematics 1951; 54, 286-295.

[4] Wyland CL, Kelly WM, Macrae CN, Gordon HL, Heatherton TF. Neural Correlates of Thought Suppression. Neuropsychologia 2003; 41, 1863-1867.

[5] Wenzlaff RM, Wegner DM. Thought Suppression. Annual Review of Psychology 2000; 51, 59-91.

[6] Mitchell JP, Heatherton TF, Kelley WM, Wyland CL, Wegner DM, Macrae CN. Separating Sustained from Transient Aspects of Cognitive Control During Thought Suppression. Psychological Science 2007; 18, 292-297.

[7] Nishimura K, Okada A, Inagawa M, Tobinaga Y. Thinking Patterns, Brain Activities and Strategy Choice. Journal of Physics 2012; Conf. Ser. 344 012004.

[8] Tonoike M, Nishimura K, Tobinaga Y. Detection of Thinking in Human by Magnetoencephalography. World Congress of Medical Physics and Biomedical Engineering 2006; 14, 2617-20.

[9] Nishimura K, Tobinaga Y. Working of the Brain and Rationality in Economic Behavior. International Joint Conference on Neural Networks 2003; 7, 133-146.

[10] Nishimura K., Tobinaga Y, Tonoike M. Detection of Neural Activity Associated with Thinking in Frontal Lobe by Magnetoencephalograpy. Progress of Theoretical Physics 2008; Supplement Number 173, 332-341.

[11] Hämäläonen M, Hari R, Ilmoniemi RJ, Knuutila J, Lounasma OV. Magnetoencephalography- theory, instrumentation, and applications to noninvasive studies of the working human brain. Review of Modern Physics 1993; 65, 2, 413-497.

[12] Uutela K, Hämäläonen M, Somersalo E. Visualization of Magnetoencephalographic Data Using Minimum Current Estimates, Neuroimage 1999; 10, 173-180.

[13] Nicholls J, Martin R, Wallace B. From Neuron to Brain, Third Edition, Sinauer Associates Inc. Publishers, Sunderland, Mass; 1992.

[14] Williamson S, Kaufman L. Biomagnetism. Journal of Magnetism and Magnetic Materials 1981; 22, 129.

[15] Hari R, Haukoranta E. Neuromagnetic Studies of the Somatosensory System: Principle and Examples, Progress in Neurobiology 1985; 24, 233.

[16] Fehr T, Achtziger A, Hinrichs H, Hermann M. Interindividual Differences in Oscillatory Brain Activity in Higher Cognitive Functions- Methodological Approached in Analyzing Continuous MEG Data. In: Reinvang, I., Greenlee, M.W. and Hermann, M. (Eds.) The Cognitive Neuroscience of Individual Differences. Oldenburg: bis-publishers; 2003..

[17] De Pasquale F, Penna SD, Snyder AZ, Lewis C, Mantini D, Marzetti L, Belardinelli P, Ciancetta L, Pizzella V, Romani GL, Corbetta M. Temporal Dynamics of Spontaneous MEG Activity in Brain Networks. Proceedings of the National Academy of Sciences of the United States of America 2010; 107, 6040-6045.

[18] He BJ, Zempel JM, Snyder AZ, and Raichle ME. The Temporal Structures and Functional Significance of Scale-free Brain Activity. Neuron 2010; 66, 353-369.

[19] Buckner RL, Andrews-Hanna JR, Schacter DL. The Brain's Default Network: Anatomy, Function, and Relevance to Disease. Annals of The New York Academy of Science 2008; 1124,1-38.

[20] Andrews-Hanna JR, Reidler JS, Sepulcre J, Poulin R, and Buckner RL. Functional-Anatomic Fractionation of the Brain's Default Network. Neuron 2010; 65, 550-562.

[21] Mason MF, Norton MI, Van Horn JD, Wegner DM, Grafton ST, Macrae CN. Wandering Minds: The Default Network and Stimulus-Independent Thought. Science 2007; 315, 393-395.

Brain Imaging and the Prediction of Treatment Outcomes in Mood and Anxiety Disorders

Leah M. Jappe, Bonnie Klimes-Dougan and
Kathryn R. Cullen

Additional information is available at the end of the chapter

http://dx.doi.org/10.5772/55446

1. Introduction

1.1. Neuroimaging for treatment prediction: An advance in personalized medicine

In addition to elucidating the mechanisms of disease, neuroimaging holds another great promise for the mental health field: the ability to predict treatment outcomes. Evidence-based treatments are available for many mental health disorders. However, not all individuals benefit from every treatment. Psychiatric research has begun to focus on the neurobiological factors that predict who will benefit from an intervention by experiencing symptom improvement. This application of neuroimaging is still very much in development, but it has the potential to facilitate a major advance in psychiatry, namely that of personalized care. Personalization of treatment for mental health disorders has been identified as a public health priority [1]. The idea is to select the best therapy for a patient at the beginning of treatment based on a set of patient characteristics that have been shown to be associated with positive outcomes with a given intervention. Those who are well matched for a particular treatment are more likely to stay engaged in the treatment, which will lead to better outcomes [2]. Given the scarcity and expense of available mental health resources, treatment should be conserved so that sufficient resources are available for those who would benefit from a specific type of treatment [3]. Optimally, these efforts will serve to guide treatment development and planning, improve overall response rates, decrease treatment costs, and eventually improve the prognosis of those who suffer from mental illness. In this chapter we review recent advances in application of neuroimaging tools to predict treatment response in patients with internalizing psychological disorders. Following the core themes of *Brain Mapping,* this chapter focuses on describing the brain structures and functions that have been associated with clinically significant response to psychological and pharmacological treatments in internalizing disorders in addition to the underling research methodology used to investigate such relationships.

2. Internalizing disorders: The focus on mood and anxiety disorders

It is critically important to direct attention towards the study of internalizing problems. Internalizing disorders are associated with significant impairment and distress and they often lead to the development and reoccurrence of debilitating psychiatric illness [4,5]. Based on empirically derived classification models, internalizing disorders are characterized by maladjustment primarily expressed inwardly, as compared to externalizing patterns of behavior where maladjustment is expressed outwardly [6,7]. Although internalizing behavior is increasingly conceptualized as a dimensional construct, treatment research has typically focused on extreme conditions, tending to examine questions regarding internalizing behavior through the lens of discrete psychiatric disorders. Some internalizing disorders, such as Major Depressive Disorder (MDD) and Generalized Anxiety Disorder (GAD), involve negative affect characterized by anxious misery and distress. Other internalizing disorders, including Social Phobia, Specific Phobia, Agoraphobia, and Panic Disorder, involve negative affect associated with activation of the fear system. Obsessive Compulsive Disorder (OCD) has also been characterized as an internalizing disorder [8]. Grouping mental illnesses more broadly along an internalizing dimension is advantageous in a number of ways. Namely, this approach accounts for the high rates of comorbidity between internalizing disorders and it groups problems that share commonalities in pathophysiology and genetic variance [7]. For example, internalizing problems are centrally implicated in the threat response system and involve abnormalities in fronto-limbic brain circuitry. This chapter focuses on the most commonly exhibited internalized disorders, namely MDD and Anxiety Disorders [9].

3. Available treatments for major depressive disorder and anxiety disorders

The past two decades have shown significant advances in the development and refinement of treatments available to those who suffer from internalizing problems. Validated, evidence-based treatments (EBTs) are now available for treating the classes of internalizing problems discussed here, including specific mood and anxiety disorders. The commonalities in the EBTs for these classes of problems are considerable. Validated treatments include medication and/or psychotherapy [10-12].

In MDD, first-line treatments that are currently offered include antidepressant medications and psychotherapy. Regarding antidepressants, the first options are typically those that impact the monoamine neurotransmitters, such as the selective serotonin reuptake inhibitors (SSRIs). Second-line medication treatments impact other neurotransmitters such as dopamine or norepinephrine, and some impact serotonin by alternate mechanisms. Regarding psychotherapies, empirically validated interventions include cognitive behavioral therapy (CBT) and interpersonal therapy (IPT). For patients that do not respond to either or a combination of these treatments, additional options are considered including electroconvulsive therapy (ECT) and transcranial magnetic stimulation (TMS).

Similarly for anxiety disorders, antidepressant medications and behavioral therapies, including CBT, are frequently the treatments of choice. While CBT in MDD primarily aims to change behavior by altering distorted cognitions, forms of CBT in the context of anxiety disorders employ the use of exposure techniques, where individuals face feared stimuli until their fear response naturally declines. Anxiolytics (e.g., benzodiazepines) are also used to mitigate acute symptoms of anxiety and are employed for short-term treatment of anxiety in more extreme cases [13].

Unfortunately, even when treatments are delivered under ideal circumstances, 30-60% patients with depressive and anxiety disorders who are treated are not likely to achieve remission with their first treatment [14-17]. Therefore, there is a great need for the identification of biological markers that predict which interventions would work and for whom, thus helping guide clinicians in selecting a treatment with the greatest potential to provide effective symptom management.

4. Brain mapping methodologies employed to assess structural and functional predictors of treatment response

Several different types of neuroimaging techniques have been developed and increasingly employed in the context of psychiatric research. Research studies that have investigated neurobiological predictors of treatment response have relied on the use of structural and functional brain imaging technologies. In structural magnetic resonance imaging (MRI), a non-invasive imaging technique, both whole brain and individual structure volumes are examined. Researchers use this methodology to examine anatomical detail, localize individual brain regions and to identify brain pathology. Functional MRI (fMRI) methodology provides useful temporal information about brain function by measuring the blood-oxygen-level-dependent (BOLD) contrast, where changes in energy between oxygenated and deoxygenated blood within the brain across time are examined to assess neural functioning within specific task constraints. Additional functional imaging methods employed in the context of treatment prediction research include positron emission tomography (PET) and single-photon emission computed tomography (SPECT). These procedures are considered invasive procedures in that they use radioactive substances in order to generate contrasts that assess brain blood flow, blood perfusion, and glucose metabolism as an indirect measure of neural activity. This wide array of brain imaging techniques has been used to assess which brain structures and functions prior to treatment predict treatment response in individuals diagnosed with Major Depressive Disorder and Anxiety Disorders.

5. Major depressive disorder

Major Depressive Disorder is a prevalent and debilitating disorder that is a leading cause of disability worldwide [18]. MDD often starts in adolescence and places youth at risk for morbidity and mortality across the lifespan. The negative outcomes associated with MDD affect all aspects of life: personal, social, and academic functioning, and may result in chronic suffering and early death. The prognosis for depression is particularly poor when the problems are evident early on in development [19-21]. While a broader array of mood disorders (e.g., Dsythymic Disorder) may be relevant to include here, this chapter focuses on MDD because most of the predictive literature has focused on adults diagnosed with this disorder. fMRI, PET, SPECT and volumetric imaging have been used to examine predictive biomarkers of treatment response in MDD. Since a majority of findings have implicated subregions of the anterior cingulate cortex (ACC), we begin by reviewing these regions and then extend to other parts of the brain that have been implicated through various modalities as predictive of treatment response.

5.1. The anterior cingulate cortex

Many imaging studies have now implicated the pregenual ACC as a key area differentiating responders from nonresponders for a variety of psychiatric treatments. For the most part, as suggested in a meta-analysis of 23 studies of adults with MDD using various modalities and treatments [22], elevated activity or metabolism in the pregenual ACC at baseline is generally predictive of a positive response to treatment. For example, Fu and colleagues [23] reported that at baseline, increased activity in the ACC was associated with a positive treatment response to CBT. Similarly, elevated resting activity of the pregenual ACC "confers better treatment outcomes by fostering adaptive self-referential processing and by helping to recalibrate cingulate regions implicated in cognitive control" [22].

Careful attention should be paid to the problem of inconsistencies across studies. For instance, as Pizagalli [22] noted, four of the studies in his meta-analysis showed that pregenual ACC predicted non-response to paroxetine [24], venlafaxine, CBT [25], and ECT [26] as measured by PET and non-response to repetitive transcranial magnetic stimulation (rTMS) as measured by SPECT [27]. Part of the inconsistency may be due to error in the assessment. Specifically, low resolution in fMRI acquisition may interfere with the ability to pinpoint exactly which areas predict treatment response versus non-response. For example, a PET study showed that pretreatment hypermetabolism at the interface between pregenual and subgenual ACC was notable in non-responders in comparison to responders [25]. Indeed, in contrast to pregenual ACC findings, it appears that the subgenual region of the ACC is associated with the opposite pattern, where some studies have suggested that increased resting metabolism or activation predicts treatment resistance [25,28,29]. In an fMRI study, hyperactivity of the subgenual ACC in response to emotional stimuli was associated with poor response to 16 sessions of CBT in 14 adults with MDD [28]. This group replicated their finding in a second, larger sample of 49 patients with MDD, finding that individuals with the lowest pretreatment sustained subgenual ACC reactivity in response to negative words displayed the most improvement after cognitive therapy [29]. Such work focusing on the subgenual ACC has contributed to current models in which this region has become one of the targets of deep-brain stimulation for patients with treatment-refractory MDD [30]. Figure 1 provides an illustration of various divisions within the ACC, including pregenual and subgenual regions.

http://dx.doi.org/10.5772/55446

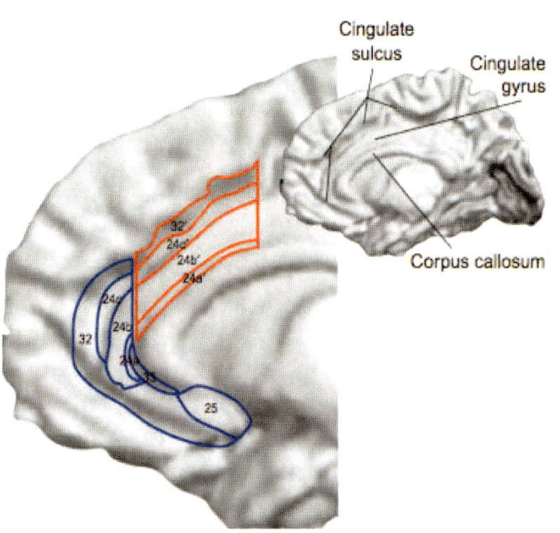

Figure 1. This figure illustrates the anatomical locations of divisions within the anterior cingulate cortex (ACC). A reconstructed MRI of the medial surface of the right hemisphere of the brain depicts the ACC (sulcus and gyrus) in relation to the underlying corpus callosum (upper right). Cytoarchitecture and functional differences have distinguished cognitive (red) and affective (blue) divisions of the ACC (left; 31). Better treatment response to pharmacological and psychological therapies in MDD has been associated with activity within the affective division of the ACC, namely increased pre-treatment activity in the pregenual ACC (includes Brodmann Area BA32 and inferior portions of BA24] and decreased activity in the subgenual ACC (BA25 and caudal portions of BA32 and BA 24). The subgenual ACC has been identified as a target for deep-brain stimulation in patients with treatment resistant MDD [30]. Reprinted and adapted from *Trends in Cognitive Sciences*, volume 4[6], Bush, G., Luu, P., & Posner, M.I., Cognitive and emotional influences in anterior cingulate cortex, pages 215-222, Copyright (2000), with permission from Elsevier [32].

5.2. Broader fronto-limbic brain regions

Not all imaging studies have pointed only to the pregenual and subgenual ACC as an important predictor of treatment response in MDD. Using a variety of methodological approaches, a growing number of studies have implicated a range of brain regions that are broadly associated with fronto-limbic circuitry. One fMRI study using an emotion-processing task before treatment with antidepressant medications (mirtazapine or venlafaxine) showed that at baseline, patients had higher activation in the dorsal/medial prefrontal cortex (PFC), posterior cingulate cortex and superior frontal gyrus. Furthermore, pre-treatment activations in caudate and insula were associated with successful treatment [33]. In an fMRI study that focused on anhedonia [34], patients with lower ventral/lateral PFC activation during cognitive reappraisal (suppression) of positive emotion at baseline had greater rates of improvement in anhedonia after 8 weeks of treatment with an antidepressant, specifically venlafaxine extended release or fluoxetine. Another study employing fMRI reported that with treatment using various antidepressants, greater right visual cortex and right subgenual ACC responses to sad stimuli, but not happy stimuli, were associated with a good clinical outcome in the early stages of treatment [35]. Similar to the findings reported by Light and colleagues [34], greater ventral/lateral PFC responses to either happy or sad faces were associated with a relatively poor outcome [35]. A recent rTMS study found that greater symptom improvement was significantly correlated with smaller deactivations at baseline in the ACC, the left medial orbitofrontal and the right middle frontal cortices, but larger activations in the putamen [36]. Using SPECT, responders to rTMS had greater perfusions in the left medial and bilateral superior frontal cortices (BA10), the left uncus/parahippocampal cortex (BA20/BA35] and the right thalamus [37]. In a PET study in adults with late-onset MDD, 34 patients remitted and 13 did not after treatment with antidepressants for 12 weeks. Left anterior fronto-cerebellar perfusion ratio had a global predictive power of 87% [38]. Analyzing this variable together with the baseline variables age of onset and duration of index episode, the predictive power of the model rose to 94% [38].

A few studies have reported on anatomical differences that have predicted MDD treatment response in broader front-limbic brain regions. Chen and colleagues [39] found that increased grey matter volumes in ACC, insula, and right tempro-parietal cortex was associated with faster rates of symptom improvement with fluoxetine. A recent study found that smaller left hippocampal volumes predicted better treatment response to six weeks of daily rTMS in adults with treatment-refractory depression; however, the significance for this prediction was only a trend [40]. If volumetric predictors could be established, these would be useful in comparison to other imaging techniques (e.g., PET, SPECT), as this type of imaging acquisition is relatively easy, safe and is consistent in analysis across sites. Like other modalities, however, the extant data are from cross-sectional studies, so it is unclear whether any differences relate to pre-existing processes or to scarring from disease exposure.

5.3. Serotonin systems

Since most medication treatments focus on serotonin, a reasonable approach is to examine how either serotonin binding or brain regions associated with serotonin production might be relevant to treatment response. A SPECT study that examined serotonin binding availability found that higher pretreatment diencephalic serotonin availability significantly predicted better treatment response to 4 weeks of paroxetine [41]. Miller and colleagues [42] used PET to assess serotonin transporter (5-HTT) binding in 19 currently depressed subjects with MDD who received naturalistic antidepressant treatment for one year. They found that non-remitters had lower 5-HTT binding than controls in midbrain, amygdala, and ACC (sub-region not specified). Remitters did not differ significantly from controls or non-remitters in 5-HTT binding. Assessment of baseline 5-HTT binding as a predictor of remission status was suggestive but not significant. In a PET study of adults with MDD who received community-based monoaminergic anti-depressant treatments by their physician, Milak and colleagues [43] reported that treatment remitters had lower activity in the region of the midbrain where monoaminergic nuclei are located prior to treatment, and that degree of improvement correlated with pretreatment midbrain activity.

5.4. Major depressive disorder summary

Studies investigating neurobiological predictors of treatment response in MDD have primarily focused on adults with the illness. The most replicated findings implicate regions within the

http://dx.doi.org/10.5772/55446

ACC as being particularly salient indicators of treatment outcome. Specifically, increased activity in areas within the ACC, namely the pregenual ACC, may be particularly predictive of improved outcome following both psychological and pharmacological intervention whereas hyperactivity in the subgenual ACC may be associated with poorer treatment response. In addition, pre-treatment serotonergic binding appears predict response to antidepressant therapy in adults with MDD. Other studies have linked structural and functional differences to pharmacological and psychological treatment response, but findings differ significantly as a function of the type of imaging modality employed (e.g., fMRI task based paradigm, PET). See Figure 2.

Cognitive Behavioral Therapy
Increased pregenual ACC activity *Decreased* subgenual ACC activity
Anti-depressant Medications
Increased: • ACC, insula, and right tempro-parietal cortex grey matter volumes • pregenual ACC activity and metabolism • dorsal/medial PFC, posterior cingulate cortex, superior frontal gyrus, caudate, and insula activity in response to emotional stimuli • diencephalic serotonin availability *Decreased* • ventral/lateral PFC activity when viewing happy and sad faces
Repetitive Transcranial Magnetic Stimulation
Increased: • putamen activity • perfusion in left medial frontal cortex, superior frontal cortex, left uncus/parahippocampal cortex, and right thalamus *Decreased:* • activity in ACC regions, left-medial OFC, and right middle frontal cortex

Figure 2. Summary of pre-treatment neuroimaging findings that have been associated with positive responses to Cognitive-Behavioral Therapy (CBT), repetitive transcranial magnetic stimulation (rTMS), and various anti-depressant medication treatments in MDD.

6. Anxiety disorders

Several distinct types of anxiety disorders have been recognized in the field of psychiatry and delineated within the Diagnostic and Statistical Manual of Mental Disorders (DSM-IV-TR). Three will be discussed here, namely Obsessive Compulsive Disorder (OCD), General Anxiety Disorder (GAD), and Social Anxiety Disorder (SAD). Some initial headway is being made using neuroimaging to attempt to identify who will respond to which type of intervention for these disorders.

6.1. Obsessive compulsive disorder

OCD is a significantly impairing mental illness associated with debilitating cycles of persistent anxiety-provoking thoughts, impulses or images that are accompanied by repetitive behaviors aimed at counteracting anxiety [44]. For example, an individual may have constant and intrusive thoughts that surfaces that he or she comes in contact with are dirty or have germs. These thoughts are experienced as extremely distressing to the individual, who as a result, engages in compulsive behavior (e.g., repetitive hand washing) to prevent or alleviate fear associated with the content of obsessive thoughts (e.g., contamination).

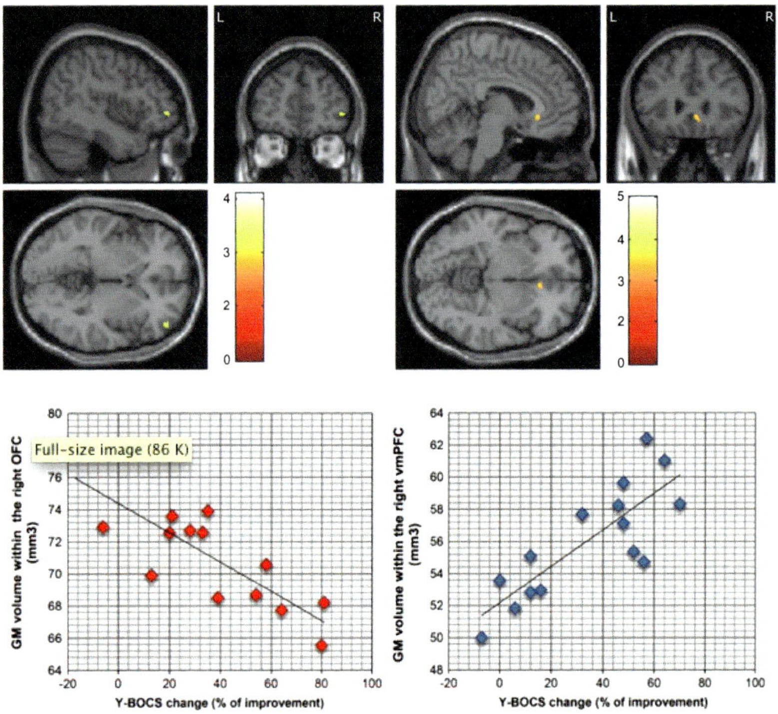

Figure 3. *Top:* Loci of significant correlations between pretreatment gray matter volume and subsequent response to Fluoxetine (top left) and CBT (top right). *Bottom left:* negative statistically significant correlation between pretreatment gray matter volume within the right middle lateral orbitofrontal cortex and improvements in OCD severity (measured by the Yale-Brown Obsessive Compulsive Scale: Y–BOCS) following treatment with fluoxetine. *Bottom right:* positive statistically significant correlation between pretreatment gray matter volume within the right medial prefrontal cortex, (subgenual anterior cingulate cortex) and Y–BOCS improvement following treatment with CBT. Reprinted and adapted from *European Neuropsychopharmacology*, published online, Hoexter et al., Differential prefrontal gray matter correlates of treatment response to fluoxetine or cognitive-behavioral therapy in obsessive–compulsive disorder, pages 1-12, Copyright (2012), with permission from Elsevier [45].

One study to date has investigated structural predictors of treatment response in OCD. Hoexter and colleagues [45] recruited thirty-eight treatment naive individuals with a primary diagnosis of OCD and randomized them to receive either 12 weeks of treatment with fluoxetine or 12 weekly sessions of group CBT. Specifically interested in structural prognostic indicators of treatment response, Hoexter et al. [45] found that smaller grey matter volumes prior to treatment initiation in the right middle lateral orbital frontal cortex (OFC) predicted a decrease in OCD symptoms following pharmacological intervention whereas greater grey matter volumes in the medial prefrontal cortex predicted better response following CBT (Figure 3). This study suggests that improvement via pharmacologic and psychological approaches in OCD may occur via different mechanisms.

Numerous functional imaging studies, primarily using PET imaging, have also investigated biological prognostic indicators in OCD. Brody and colleagues [46] showed that decreased metabolic activity in the orbitofrontal cortex (OFC) was associated with better outcomes with fluoxetine treatment whereas as increased metabolism in the same region predicted improvement following cognitive behavioral therapy (CBT). However, it is important to note that, unlike the Hoexter et al. [45] study above, treatment designation in this study was not randomized. Similar to Brody et al. [46], Saxena et al. [47] found an inverse relationship between OFC glucose metabolism using PET and response to 8-12 weeks of SSRI (paroxetine) treatment in 20 OCD outpatients. These negative correlations between regional OFC glucose metabolism and treatment response appear to be present in adults with childhood onset OCD [48]. In a symptoms provocation study, where individuals with contamination-related OCD were exposed to neutral and contamination specific stimuli, lower regional cerebral flood flow (rCBF) measured by PET in the OFC and higher pre-treatment rCBF in the bilateral posterior cinglate cortex (PCC) predicted better symptom reduction after a 12-week open trial of fluvoxamine [49]. The relationship between rCBF and treatment outcome was present in response to both OCD-related and neutral stimuli, suggesting that activity in the OFC and PCC exist independent of OCD-salient cues. Using a functional MRI paradigm that evoked OCD symptoms by displaying salient illness-related words, BOLD response in the right cerebellum and left superior temporal gyrus (STG) positively correlated with improvements in OCD symptoms following 12 weeks of SSRI (fluvoxamine) pharmacotherapy [50].

Given that SSRI medications have been shown to be effective in both OCD and MDD, Saxena et al. [47] examined whether pretreatment brain activity would differentially predict response to pharmacotherapy in these two different patient groups. 27 individuals with OCD and 27 with MDD underwent PET to measure cerebral glucose metabolism prior to paroxetine treatment. These researchers concluded that OCD symptom improvement was related to increased pretreatment metabolism in the right caudate nucleus whereas decreased depression symptoms were predicted by low amygdala and thalamus but increased medial prefrontal and ACC metabolism prior to treatment. This study, in particular, suggests that treatment with SRIs may improve OCD and MDD pathology by its impact at different brain sites.

Using SPECT imaging, investigators have examined neurochemical transporters as predictors of response to medication treatments in OCD. Specifically, Zitteral et al. [51] found that serotonin transporter (SERT) availability in thalamic and hypothalamic brain regions predicted better treatment outcomes following 14 weeks of sertraline (an SSRI) administration in a homogenous sample of OCD patients with behavioral checking compulsions. It is important to note that SERT availability has been associated with OCD symptom severity in previous studies [51,52], suggesting that individuals with higher transporter availability may be more likely to respond favorably to SSRIs as their serotonin system is less impaired prior to beginning intervention. Another SPECT study prior to 12 weeks of treatment with Inositol, a chemical precursor of second messengers in critical brain signaling pathways, found that higher blood perfusion in the left medial prefrontal regions differentiated OCD responders from nonresponders [53] and regional cerebral blood flow (rCBF) in cerebellar regions in addition to whole brain tracer uptake has also been shown to be elevated in OCD responders compared to nonresponders prior to beginning an open label trial of fluvoxamine [54].

6.2. Generalized anxiety disorder

GAD is a chronic and prevalent disorder characterized by frequent and excessive worry that is difficult to control [55]. This worry lasts for a minimum of six months and is associated with somatic and cognitive difficulties (e.g., fatigue, concentration problems), significant role impairment [44] and suicide [56].

To date, two known studies have investigated predictors of treatment response and non-response in GAD, both involving the use of fMRI methodology. Nitschke et al. [57] looked at brain reactivity to anticipatory cues of neutral and adverse stimuli (e.g., attack scenes vs. household items) in adults with GAD and examined how individual responses to these cues predicted outcome following an 8-week open label trial of venlafaxine, a type of selective serotonin and norepinephrine reuptake inhibitor (SNRI). Reminiscent of what has been found in the depression literature as discussed above, Nitschke et al. [57] found that activity in the pregenual ACC in response to anticipatory aversive and neutral cues predicted better outcomes. Specifically, individuals with hyperresponsivity in the pregenual ACC showed greater response to treatment measured by decreases in self-reported anxiety symptoms. The pregenual ACC is thought to play a role in the detection and resolution of emotional conflict [58] and thus Nitschke et al. [57] have proposed that individuals with greater pretreatment activity in this area may be better able to engage top-down control and regulate emotions when given treatment.

In the same participant pool, Whalen et al. [59] examined whether response to an emotional faces task could predict response following venlafaxine treatment in GAD. They specifically examined reactivity in the amygdala and rostral region of the ACC, as these areas have been found to be functionally related and relevant to the study of visually presented expressions of emotions [60]. Results from this study showed that increased reactivity in the rostral ACC and decreased reactivity in the amygdala when viewing fearful faces was related to improved outcomes after the 8-week medication trial (similarly measured by self-reported anxiety symptoms).

Since all participants were free from comorbid diagnoses, findings in these two studies cannot be accounted for by any other axis I disorder. In addition, results persisted after controlling for current depressive symptoms, further strengthening the conclusion that activity in these brain areas specifically predict GAD treatment outcome. However, the overlap in findings observed between studies in GAD and MDD, where activity in the pregenual ACC is implicated as a predictor of treatment response, may highlight the commonality in the underlying mechanisms of these disorders, which are commonly co-morbid. Future studies employing randomized, placebo controlled designs will need to be conducted in order to ensure that findings described above predict improvement with venlafaxine, not simply improvement in general.

6.3. Social anxiety disorder

SAD is characterized by intense fear of being in social situations in which judgment or embarrassment may occur. Age of onset in SAD is typically during mid-teen years, where symptoms tend to follow a long, protracted course of illness that often goes untreated [61].

Two known studies have investigated neuroimaging predictors of treatment outcome in SAD following psychotherapy interventions. Nine patients diagnosed with SAD underwent PET imaging using dopamine agonist ligands to examine dopamine function prior to 15 weeks of CBT [62]. The study found that reduced dopamine D2 receptor binding in the medial prefrontal cortex and the hippocampus prior to treatment predicted greater changes in self-reported social anxiety symptoms after CBT.

Employing fMRI methodology, Doehrmann et al. [63] investigated functional brain activity in response to emotional faces and scenes. Using whole-brain regression analyses, Doehrmann and colleagues found that BOLD response to angry vs. neutral faces in right occiptotemporal brain areas predicted better response to CBT, especially in initially more severe patients. This was true even when accounting for possible confounding effects of depressive co-morbidity. Researchers purport that predictive activity to faces over emotional non-face scenes is consistent with the social nature of SAD. While connectivity between higher-order visual and emotion processing areas has been shown to be altered in SAD, the authors note that further research is needed to elucidate the how the relationship between pretreatment activity in occiptotemporal brains relates to altered activity in limbic brain regions identified in other areas of research.

6.4. Anxiety disorder summary

Within the class of anxiety disorders, neuroimaging outcome prediction studies have, thus far, focused mostly on OCD. Findings implicate the OFC as being especially important in regards to predicting outcomes following pharmacological and psychological interventions in this disorder; however, areas of the PFC, ACC, caudate, cerebellum and STG in addition to serotonin system functioning may be salient predictors of treatment response in OCD as well. Research in GAD and SAD is still in its infancy; however, initial studies suggest that activity in the ACC may differentiate individual response to medication treatment in GAD whereas D2 receptor binding in the prefrontal cortex and hippocampus can be used to predict better social anxiety outcomes following psychological intervention. (Figure 4).

Obsessive-Compulsive Disorder

Cognitive Behavioral Therapy:
- larger grey matter volumes in medial PFC
- increased metabolism in OFC

Pharmacotherapy:
- smaller grey matter volumes in right middle lateral OFC
- decreased metabolic activity in OFC
- increased right caudate nucleus metabolism
- SERT availability in thalamic and hypothalamic brain regions
- lower regional cerebral flood flow in OFC and higher regional cerebral flood flow in bilateral posterior cinglate cortex in response to symptom provocation
- increased right cerebellum and left STG activity to illness-related words

Generalized Anxiety Disorder

Pharmacotherapy:
- hyperactivity in the pregenual ACC in response to anticipation of aversive and neutral stimuli
- increased activity in the rostral ACC and decreased amygdala activity when viewing fearful faces

Social Anxiety Disorder

Cognitive Behavioral Therapy:
- reduced dopamine D2 receptor binding in medial PFC and hippocampus
- increased activity in right occiptotemporal brain areas in response to response to angry vs. neutral faces

Figure 4. Summary of pre-treatment neuroimaging findings that have been associated with positive responses to either Cognitive-Behavioral Therapy or anti-depressant medication treatments in anxiety disorders. *(PFC=prefrontal cortex, OFC=orbitalfrontal cortex, SERT=serotonin transporter, STG=superior temporal gyrus, ACC=anterior cingulate cortex).*

7. Conclusions and future clinical applications

Internalizing disorders are serious and often debilitating problems associated with significant impairment and individual suffering. While pharmacological and psychological interventions show some efficacy in the treatment of MDD and anxiety disorders, more precise personalized care is needed in order to improve overall treatment outcomes and to reduce the cost of psychiatric interventions. While this avenue of research is in its infancy, the use of imaging methods to identify neurobiological markers that predict treatment outcome holds the potential to further advance the field of personalized psychiatry and may eventually help guide clinicians towards the selection of treatments that have the highest likelihood of improving individuals patients' symptoms.

Advanced technologies have greatly facilitated efforts to examine anomalies in neural structure and function over the past decade. The findings in MDD show that regions of the anterior cingulate cortex have most reliably been identified as areas differentiating treatment responders from non-responders. Studies aimed at examining predictors of treatment outcome in anxiety disorders have primarily focused on OCD, most frequently implicating the orbital frontal cortex. Treatment predication research in other anxiety disorders, such as GAD and SAD is beginning to receive more attention.

While the research reviewed above provides an initial foundation for future research to advance personalized psychiatric care, several points need to be highlighted when considering these treatment studies. Most of the studies to date have reported results on small samples with uncontrolled treatment delivery, assessing imaging in the context of either a naturalistic and community-based treatment, or in the setting of a trial that compared different treatments but then examined effects after treatment arms were collapsed. While the field is currently limited in that large-scale treatment studies that involve comprehensive neurobiological assessments are highly labor intensive and are rarely feasible (for a noted exception see Dunlop et al. [64], next steps will require larger, more diverse samples and controlled treatment delivery to more accurately and reliably assess prediction across interventions.

Most research to date has been conducted in adult samples with little research examining biological predictors of treatment response in younger populations. It will be particularly important for future research to identify predictors of treatment response for children and adolescents suffering from anxiety and depression given that neurobiological factors associated with treatment outcomes may differ across development, early onset is a negative prognostic indicator of future problems and plasticity in key neural networks may be amenable to alteration during this period in development [20,65]. Furthermore, with the exception of symptom severity [20,66,67], younger age [67] and positive family history [68], few psychosocial indexes have consistently identified who responds favorably to an intervention [69], and very little is known as to which variables differentially predict response across types of interventions. Recent work has taken initial steps towards using brain imaging methods to identify biological markers for use in tailoring treatment for adolescent depression. In the only study to date that has published data on predictive imaging for adolescent depression, Forbes et al. [70] examined reward-related brain functioning in adolescent MDD before treatment with either CBT (n=7) or CBT plus a selective serotonin reuptake inhibitor (n=6). Due to the small number, the treatment arms were combined. Greater striatal activity during reward outcome predicted higher general severity after treatment, whereas greater striatal activation during reward anticipation predicted lower anxiety after treatment.

Inclusion of broader populations characterized as suffering from internalizing disorders may provide additional insights into relevant brain mechanisms for prevention. As previously mentioned, internalizing disorders have high rates of co-morbidity with one another, and although research to date has focused on depression and anxiety disorders, future research may be needed to delineate the biological underpinnings that account for such overlap. This work may help us refine particular psychological and pharmacological treatments. Similarly, expanding prediction studies to include internalizing problems outside of those classified as mood or anxiety disorders are also needed. Particularly, Eating Disorders have been characterized as belonging to the internalizing construct [71]; however, while imaging research has begun to characterize the neurobiological underpinnings of Eating Disorders [72-75], research has yet to examine neurobiological predictors of treatment response in this population.

While research reviewed above employed the use of fMRI, PET, and SPECT imaging techniques, the study of predictive biomarkers of treatment outcome should be expanded with the use of other neuroimaging methods. For example, the use of spectroscopy would provide evidence of pretreatment chemical and metabolite profiles predictive of treatment outcome. Similarly, resting state fMRI methods might be particularly useful, potentially elucidating our understanding of how different patterns of functional connectivity within and between neural circuits relate to treatment outcome or treatment resistance. In addition, it is expected that future research will increasingly employ the use of multi-modal approaches in predictive treatment research, helping to identify other biological markers not capable of being assessed via neuroimaging techniques. For example, current efforts are underway to more definitively assess biological markers for treatment response across treatments in adults with MDD (CBT, duloxetine, escitalopram) using multi-modal techniques including resting fMRI, neuroendocrine assessments, immune markers and measures of gene expression [64]. Additionally, neurobiological predictors of treatment response that have been identified thus far are not sufficiently strong enough nor have they been sufficiently replicated to warrant changes in clinical decision making at this juncture. Perhaps and understanding of broader brain networks will be enhanced by profiling numerous brain functions and structures that, in compilation, will more aptly predict treatment response.

An exciting advance that has the potential to improve personalized care is recent work incorporating machine-learning approaches to classify groups—disease versus no disease, or responders versus non-responders. Machine learning approaches are "brain reading" or "brain decoding" methods. Instead of analyzing the brain voxel by voxel, data from groups of voxels are used to train a computer program to distinguish different classes of data (e.g., treatment responders from treatment non-responders) and provide maps which indicate the levels by which different brain regions are accurately involved in the classification [76]. In a study that analyzed grey and white matter volumes, using a support vector machine (SVM) approach, Gong and colleagues [77] showed they were able to predict response versus non-response based on gray matter with 70% accuracy and based on white matter with 65% accuracy. Another study that used SVM measured responses to sad faces with fMRI before CBT in 16 unmedicated depressed adults. Brain regions implicated in clinical remission included ACC, superior and middle frontal cortices, paracentral cortex, superior parietal cortex, precuneus, and cerebellum, with 71% sensitivity and 86% specificity of response prediction [78]. A third SVM study found that the pattern of brain activity during sad facial processing correctly classified patients' clinical response at baseline, prior to the initiation of treatment, at trend levels of significance [23]. SVM approaches are still new in the field and the value of such non-traditional statistical approaches still needs to be weighed.

Practical constraints must be considered as future efforts aim to translate knowledge of neurobiological predictors of treatment response into clinical practice. In addition to providing reliable data with high sensitivity and specificity, ideally a biomarker would be low in cost, easy to collect and simple to analyze [79]. It is possible that these approaches could be mechanized sufficiently to reduce costs and increase feasibility so that one day, routine clinical assessment will include the collection of data via neuroimaging technology [80]. For example, if activity in the ACC remains

http://dx.doi.org/10.5772/55446

a robust predictor of treatment response in larger controlled studies, one potential implication of this type of research could be that individual patients presenting with MDD may undergo an MRI to measure pregenual and subgenual ACC activity, which could in turn be used to guide whether the individual is referred for Cognitive Behavioral Therapy or pharmacotherapy. Currently, such an approach is likely cost prohibitive and may not be sufficiently feasible given the constraints of data acquisition, preprocessing and analysis. Alternatively, once neuroimaging markers that predict treatment outcome are well established, neuroimaging technology used to identify brain regions and functions associated with treatment outcome may be used to aid in the development or refinement of proxy biomarkers, such as neuropsychological functioning or serum markers, that could feasibly measure prediction and be disseminated for wide-spread application of personalized psychiatric care.

Here we have focused on neurobiological factors that can be measured at baseline to predict treatment. However, increased understanding of what aspects of neurobiological factors change over the course of treatment may also serve to enhance our understanding of the pathophysiology of internalizing problems and aid in identifying neurobiological factors that are likely to predict treatment outcomes. A recent review of the literature on changes with treatment concludes that a functional normalization of the fear network occurs with recovery across treatments [81]. Specifically, evidence suggests that both psychotherapy and psychopharmacology each in specific ways result in normalization of activity in the target structures (respectively, "top-down" and "bottom-up" effects). Methodologies that capitalize on considering both prediction of and change associated with treatment outcomes are needed.

Advanced techniques, such as those used in neuroimaging research, offer tremendous benefit to our society in that they provide the capability to improve our understanding of the pathophysiology underlying internalizing problems and may eventually offer guidance in regards to treatment selection, allowing providers to choose only those treatments that are most likely to be maximally effective for a given individual. This area of research is still developing. The concept of neural network medicine envisions a time to come when treatments will be used to target a neural network rather than simply components within the network. While personalized medicine in psychiatry is still at an early stage, "it has a very promising future" (Costa e Silva, in press).

Author details

Leah M. Jappe[1*], Bonnie Klimes-Dougan[2] and Kathryn R. Cullen[3]

*Address all correspondence to: japp0005@umn.edu

1 Department of Psychology, University of Minnesota, Minneapolis, Minnesota, USA

2 Department of Psychology, University of Minnesota, Minneapolis, Minnesota, USA

3 Department of Psychiatry, University of Minnesota, Minneapolis, Minnesota, USA

References

[1] Insel TR. Translating scientific opportunity into public health impact: a strategic plan for research on mental illness. Arch Gen Psychiatry 2009 Feb;66(2):128-133.

[2] National Committee for Quality Assurance. The state of Health Care Quality. 2007;20-21.

[3] Kakuma R, Minas H, van Ginneken N, Dal Poz MR, Desiraju K, Morris JE, et al. Human resources for mental health care: current situation and strategies for action. Lancet 2011 Nov 5;378(9803):1654-1663.

[4] Kessler RC, Avenevoli S, Costello EJ, Georgiades K, Green JG, Gruber MJ, et al. Prevalence, persistence, and sociodemographic correlates of DSM-IV disorders in the National Comorbidity Survey Replication Adolescent Supplement. Arch Gen Psychiatry 2012 Apr;69(4):372-380.

[5] Lopez AD, Mathers CD, Ezzati M, Jamison DT, Murray CJL. Measuring the Global Burden of Disease and Risk Factors, 1990-2001. In: Lopez AD, Mathers CD, Ezzati M, Jamison DT, Murray CJL, editors. Global Burden of Disease and Risk Factors Washington (DC): The International Bank for Reconstruction and Development/The World Bank Group; 2006.

[6] Achenbach T editor. Manual for the Child Behavior Checklist/2-3 and 1992 Profile. Burlington: University of Vermont, Department of Psychiatry; 1992.

[7] Krueger RF. The structure of common mental disorders. Arch Gen Psychiatry 1999 Oct;56(10):921-926.

[8] Kramer MD, Krueger RF, Hicks BM. The role of internalizing and externalizing liability factors in accounting for gender differences in the prevalence of common psychopathological syndromes. Psychol Med 2008 Jan;38(1):51-61.

[9] Kessler RC, Berglund P, Demler O, Jin R, Merikangas KR, Walters EE. Lifetime prevalence and age-of-onset distributions of DSM-IV disorders in the National Comorbidity Survey Replication. Arch Gen Psychiatry 2005 Jun;62(6):593-602.

[10] Craighead, W.E., Sheets, E.S., Bosse, A.L., Ilardi, S.S. Psychosocial treatments for major depressive disorder. In: Nathan, P.E., Gorman, J.M., editor. A Guide to Treatments that Work. 3rd ed. New York: Oxford University Press; 2007. p. 289-307.

[11] Chambless DL, Hollon SD. Defining empirically supported therapies. J Consult Clin Psychol 1998 Feb;66(1):7-18.

[12] Nemeroff, C.B., Schatzberg, A.F. Pharmacological treatments for unipolar depression. In: Nathan, P.E., Gorman, J.M., editor. A Guide to Treatments that Work. 3rd ed. New York: Oxford University Press; 2007. p. 271-289.

[13] McGrandles A, Duffy T. Assessment and treatment of patients with anxiety. Nurs Stand 2012 May 2-8;26(35):48-56; quiz 58.

[14] Mancebo MC, Eisen JL, Pinto A, Greenberg BD, Dyck IR, Rasmussen SA. The brown longitudinal obsessive compulsive study: treatments received and patient impressions of improvement. J Clin Psychiatry 2006 Nov;67(11):1713-1720.

[15] Goodman WK, McDougle CJ, Barr LC, Aronson SC, Price LH. Biological approaches to treatment-resistant obsessive compulsive disorder. J Clin Psychiatry 1993 Jun;54 Suppl:16-26.

[16] Trivedi MH, Rush AJ, Wisniewski SR, Warden D, McKinney W, Downing M, et al. Factors associated with health-related quality of life among outpatients with major depressive disorder: a STAR*D report. J Clin Psychiatry 2006 Feb;67(2):185-195.

[17] TADS Team. Fluoxetine, cognitive–behavioral therapy, and their combination for adolescents with depression: Treatment for Adolescents with Depression Study (TADS) randomized controlled trial Journal of the American Medical Association 2004;292:807-820.

[18] World Health Organization (WHO). The global burden of disease update. 2008.

[19] Zisook S, Lesser I, Stewart JW, Wisniewski SR, Balasubramani GK, Fava M, et al. Effect of age at onset on the course of major depressive disorder. Am J Psychiatry 2007 Oct;164(10):1539-1546.

[20] Brent DA, Kolko DJ, Birmaher B, Baugher M, Bridge J, Roth C, et al. Predictors of treatment efficacy in a clinical trial of three psychosocial treatments for adolescent depression. J Am Acad Child Adolesc Psychiatry 1998 Sep;37(9):906-914.

[21] Gollan J, Raffety B, Gortner E, Dobson K. Course profiles of early- and adult-onset depression. J Affect Disord 2005 May;86(1):81-86.

[22] Pizzagalli DA. Frontocingulate dysfunction in depression: toward biomarkers of treatment response. Neuropsychopharmacology 2011 Jan;36(1):183-206.

[23] Fu CH, Mourao-Miranda J, Costafreda SG, Khanna A, Marquand AF, Williams SC, et al. Pattern classification of sad facial processing: toward the development of neurobiological markers in depression. Biol Psychiatry 2008 Apr 1;63(7):656-662.

[24] Brody AL, Saxena S, Silverman DH, Alborzian S, Fairbanks LA, Phelps ME, et al. Brain metabolic changes in major depressive disorder from pre- to post-treatment with paroxetine. Psychiatry Res 1999 Oct 11;91(3):127-139.

[25] Konarski JZ, Kennedy SH, Segal ZV, Lau MA, Bieling PJ, McIntyre RS, et al. Predictors of nonresponse to cognitive behavioural therapy or venlafaxine using glucose metabolism in major depressive disorder. J Psychiatry Neurosci 2009 May;34(3): 175-180.

[26] McCormick LM, Boles Ponto LL, Pierson RK, Johnson HJ, Magnotta V, Brumm MC. Metabolic correlates of antidepressant and antipsychotic response in patients with

psychotic depression undergoing electroconvulsive therapy. J ECT 2007 Dec;23(4): 265-273.

[27] Mottaghy FM, Keller CE, Gangitano M, Ly J, Thall M, Parker JA, et al. Correlation of cerebral blood flow and treatment effects of repetitive transcranial magnetic stimulation in depressed patients. Psychiatry Res 2002 Aug 20;115(1-2):1-14.

[28] Siegle GJ, Carter CS, Thase ME. Use of FMRI to predict recovery from unipolar depression with cognitive behavior therapy. Am J Psychiatry 2006 Apr;163(4):735-738.

[29] Siegle GJ, Thompson WK, Collier A, Berman SR, Feldmiller J, Thase ME, et al. Toward clinically useful neuroimaging in depression treatment: prognostic utility of subgenual cingulate activity for determining depression outcome in cognitive therapy across studies, scanners, and patient characteristics. Arch Gen Psychiatry 2012 Sep 1;69(9):913-924.

[30] Mayberg HS, Lozano AM, Voon V, McNeely HE, Seminowicz D, Hamani C, et al. Deep brain stimulation for treatment-resistant depression. Neuron 2005 Mar 3;45(5): 651-660.

[31] Vogt BA, Nimchinsky EA, Vogt LJ, Hof PR. Human cingulate cortex: surface features, flat maps, and cytoarchitecture. J Comp Neurol 1995 Aug 28;359(3):490-506.

[32] Bush G, Luu P, Posner MI. Cognitive and emotional influences in anterior cingulate cortex. Trends Cogn Sci 2000 Jun;4(6):215-222.

[33] Samson AC, Meisenzahl E, Scheuerecker J, Rose E, Schoepf V, Wiesmann M, et al. Brain activation predicts treatment improvement in patients with major depressive disorder. J Psychiatr Res 2011 Sep;45(9):1214-1222.

[34] Light SN, Heller AS, Johnstone T, Kolden GG, Peterson MJ, Kalin NH, et al. Reduced right ventrolateral prefrontal cortex activity while inhibiting positive affect is associated with improvement in hedonic capacity after 8 weeks of antidepressant treatment in major depressive disorder. Biol Psychiatry 2011 Nov 15;70(10):962-968.

[35] Keedwell PA, Drapier D, Surguladze S, Giampietro V, Brammer M, Phillips M. Subgenual cingulate and visual cortex responses to sad faces predict clinical outcome during antidepressant treatment for depression. J Affect Disord 2010 Jan;120(1-3): 120-125.

[36] Hernandez-Ribas R, Deus J, Pujol J, Segalas C, Vallejo J, Menchon JM, et al. Identifying brain imaging correlates of clinical response to repetitive transcranial magnetic stimulation (rTMS) in major depression. Brain Stimul 2012 Feb 22.

[37] Richieri R, Boyer L, Farisse J, Colavolpe C, Mundler O, Lancon C, et al. Predictive value of brain perfusion SPECT for rTMS response in pharmacoresistant depression. Eur J Nucl Med Mol Imaging 2011 Sep;38(9):1715-1722.

[38] Navarro V, Gasto C, Lomena F, Torres X, Mateos JJ, Portella MJ, et al. Prognostic value of frontal functional neuroimaging in late-onset severe major depression. Br J Psychiatry 2004 Apr;184:306-311.

[39] Chen CH, Ridler K, Suckling J, Williams S, Fu CH, Merlo-Pich E, et al. Brain imaging correlates of depressive symptom severity and predictors of symptom improvement after antidepressant treatment. Biol Psychiatry 2007 Sep 1;62(5):407-414.

[40] Furtado CP, Hoy KE, Maller JJ, Savage G, Daskalakis ZJ, Fitzgerald PB. Cognitive and volumetric predictors of response to repetitive transcranial magnetic stimulation (rTMS) - a prospective follow-up study. Psychiatry Res 2012 Apr 30;202(1):12-19.

[41] Kugaya A, Sanacora G, Staley JK, Malison RT, Bozkurt A, Khan S, et al. Brain serotonin transporter availability predicts treatment response to selective serotonin reuptake inhibitors. Biol Psychiatry 2004 Oct 1;56(7):497-502.

[42] Miller JM, Oquendo MA, Ogden RT, Mann JJ, Parsey RV. Serotonin transporter binding as a possible predictor of one-year remission in major depressive disorder. J Psychiatr Res 2008 Oct;42(14):1137-1144.

[43] Milak MS, Parsey RV, Lee L, Oquendo MA, Olvet DM, Eipper F, et al. Pretreatment regional brain glucose uptake in the midbrain on PET may predict remission from a major depressive episode after three months of treatment. Psychiatry Res 2009 Jul 15;173(1):63-70.

[44] American Psychiatric Association. Diagnostic and Statistical Manual of Mental Disorders. Fourth Edition, Text Revision (DSM-IV-TR) ed. Arlington, VA; 2000.

[45] Hoexter MQ, Dougherty DD, Shavitt RG, D'Alcante CC, Duran FL, Lopes AC, et al. Differential prefrontal gray matter correlates of treatment response to fluoxetine or cognitive-behavioral therapy in obsessive-compulsive disorder. Eur Neuropsychopharmacol 2012 Jul 26.

[46] Brody AL, Saxena S, Schwartz JM, Stoessel PW, Maidment K, Phelps ME, et al. FDG-PET predictors of response to behavioral therapy and pharmacotherapy in obsessive compulsive disorder. Psychiatry Res 1998 Nov 9;84(1):1-6.

[47] Saxena S, Brody AL, Ho ML, Zohrabi N, Maidment KM, Baxter LR,Jr. Differential brain metabolic predictors of response to paroxetine in obsessive-compulsive disorder versus major depression. Am J Psychiatry 2003 Mar;160(3):522-532.

[48] Swedo SE, Pietrini P, Leonard HL, Schapiro MB, Rettew DC, Goldberger EL, et al. Cerebral glucose metabolism in childhood-onset obsessive-compulsive disorder. Revisualization during pharmacotherapy. Arch Gen Psychiatry 1992 Sep;49(9):690-694.

[49] Rauch SL, Shin LM, Dougherty DD, Alpert NM, Fischman AJ, Jenike MA. Predictors of fluvoxamine response in contamination-related obsessive compulsive disorder: a PET symptom provocation study. Neuropsychopharmacology 2002 Nov;27(5): 782-791.

[50] Sanematsu H, Nakao T, Yoshiura T, Nabeyama M, Togao O, Tomita M, et al. Predictors of treatment response to fluvoxamine in obsessive-compulsive disorder: an fMRI study. J Psychiatr Res 2010 Mar;44(4):193-200.

[51] Zitterl W, Stompe T, Aigner M, Zitterl-Eglseer K, Ritter K, Zettinig G, et al. Diencephalic serotonin transporter availability predicts both transporter occupancy and treatment response to sertraline in obsessive-compulsive checkers. Biol Psychiatry 2009 Dec 15;66(12):1115-1122.

[52] Hesse S, Muller U, Lincke T, Barthel H, Villmann T, Angermeyer MC, et al. Serotonin and dopamine transporter imaging in patients with obsessive-compulsive disorder. Psychiatry Res 2005 Oct 30;140(1):63-72.

[53] Carey PD, Warwick J, Harvey BH, Stein DJ, Seedat S. Single photon emission computed tomography (SPECT) in obsessive-compulsive disorder before and after treatment with inositol. Metab Brain Dis 2004 Jun;19(1-2):125-134.

[54] Ho Pian KL, van Megen HJ, Ramsey NF, Mandl R, van Rijk PP, Wynne HJ, et al. Decreased thalamic blood flow in obsessive-compulsive disorder patients responding to fluvoxamine. Psychiatry Res 2005 Feb 28;138(2):89-97.

[55] Grant BF, Hasin DS, Stinson FS, Dawson DA, June Ruan W, Goldstein RB, et al. Prevalence, correlates, co-morbidity, and comparative disability of DSM-IV generalized anxiety disorder in the USA: results from the National Epidemiologic Survey on Alcohol and Related Conditions. Psychol Med 2005 Dec;35(12):1747-1759.

[56] Weisberg RB. Overview of generalized anxiety disorder: epidemiology, presentation, and course. J Clin Psychiatry 2009;70 Suppl 2:4-9.

[57] Nitschke JB, Sarinopoulos I, Oathes DJ, Johnstone T, Whalen PJ, Davidson RJ, et al. Anticipatory activation in the amygdala and anterior cingulate in generalized anxiety disorder and prediction of treatment response. Am J Psychiatry 2009 Mar;166(3): 302-310.

[58] Etkin A, Pittenger C, Polan HJ, Kandel ER. Toward a neurobiology of psychotherapy: basic science and clinical applications. J Neuropsychiatry Clin Neurosci 2005 Spring; 17(2):145-158.

[59] Whalen PJ, Johnstone T, Somerville LH, Nitschke JB, Polis S, Alexander AL, et al. A functional magnetic resonance imaging predictor of treatment response to venlafaxine in generalized anxiety disorder. Biol Psychiatry 2008 May 1;63(9):858-863.

[60] Amaral DG, Price JL, Pitkänen A, Carmichael ST. Anatomical organization of the primate amygdaloid complex. In: Aggleton JP, editor. The Amygdala: Neurobiological Aspects of Emotion, Memory and Mental Dysfunction. New York: Wiley-Liss; 1992. p. 1-66.

[61] Grant BF, Hasin DS, Blanco C, Stinson FS, Chou SP, Goldstein RB, et al. The epidemiology of social anxiety disorder in the United States: results from the National Epide-

miologic Survey on Alcohol and Related Conditions. J Clin Psychiatry 2005 Nov; 66(11):1351-1361.

[62] Cervenka S, Hedman E, Ikoma Y, Djurfeldt DR, Ruck C, Halldin C, et al. Changes in dopamine D2-receptor binding are associated to symptom reduction after psychotherapy in social anxiety disorder. Transl Psychiatry 2012 May 22;2:e120.

[63] Doehrmann O, Ghosh SS, Polli FE, Reynolds GO, Horn F, Keshavan A, et al. Predicting Treatment Response in Social Anxiety Disorder From Functional Magnetic Resonance Imaging. Arch Gen Psychiatry 2012 Sep 3:1-11.

[64] Dunlop BW, Binder EB, Cubells JF, Goodman MG, Kelley ME, Kinkead B, et al. Predictors of Remission in Depression to Individual and Combined Treatments (PReDICT): Study Protocol for a Randomized Controlled Trial. Trials 2012 Jul 9;13(1):106.

[65] Lenroot RK, Giedd JN. Brain development in children and adolescents: insights from anatomical magnetic resonance imaging. Neurosci Biobehav Rev 2006;30(6):718-729.

[66] Asarnow JR, Emslie G, Clarke G, Wagner KD, Spirito A, Vitiello B, et al. Treatment of selective serotonin reuptake inhibitor-resistant depression in adolescents: predictors and moderators of treatment response. J Am Acad Child Adolesc Psychiatry 2009 Mar;48(3):330-339.

[67] Curry J, Rohde P, Simons A, Silva S, Vitiello B, Kratochvil C, et al. Predictors and moderators of acute outcome in the Treatment for Adolescents with Depression Study (TADS). J Am Acad Child Adolesc Psychiatry 2006 Dec;45(12):1427-1439.

[68] Tao R, Emslie G, Mayes T, Nakonezny P, Kennard B, Hughes C. Early prediction of acute antidepressant treatment response and remission in pediatric major depressive disorder. J Am Acad Child Adolesc Psychiatry 2009 Jan;48(1):71-78.

[69] Kowatch RA, Carmody TJ, Emslie GJ, Rintelmann JW, Hughes CW, Rush AJ. Prediction of response to fluoxetine and placebo in children and adolescents with major depression: a hypothesis generating study. J Affect Disord 1999 Aug;54(3):269-276.

[70] Forbes EE, Olino TM, Ryan ND, Birmaher B, Axelson D, Moyles DL, et al. Reward-related brain function as a predictor of treatment response in adolescents with major depressive disorder. Cogn Affect Behav Neurosci 2010 Mar;10(1):107-118.

[71] Forbush KT, South SC, Krueger RF, Iacono WG, Clark LA, Keel PK, et al. Locating eating pathology within an empirical diagnostic taxonomy: evidence from a community-based sample. J Abnorm Psychol 2010 May;119(2):282-292.

[72] Kaye W. Neurobiology of anorexia and bulimia nervosa. Physiol Behav 2008 Apr 22;94(1):121-135.

[73] Frank GK, Kaye WH. Positron emission tomography studies in eating disorders: multireceptor brain imaging, correlates with behavior and implications for pharmacotherapy. Nucl Med Biol 2005 Oct;32(7):755-761.

[74] Frank GK, Bailer UF, Henry S, Wagner A, Kaye WH. Neuroimaging studies in eating disorders. CNS Spectr 2004 Jul;9(7):539-548.

[75] Kaye WH, Frank GK, Bailer UF, Henry SE. Neurobiology of anorexia nervosa: clinical implications of alterations of the function of serotonin and other neuronal systems. Int J Eat Disord 2005;37 Suppl:S15-9; discussion S20-1.

[76] Brammer M. The role of neuroimaging in diagnosis and personalized medicine – current position and likely future directions. Dialogues in Clinical Neuroscience 2009;11:389-396.

[77] Gong Q, Wu Q, Scarpazza C, Lui S, Jia Z, Marquand A, et al. Prognostic prediction of therapeutic response in depression using high-field MR imaging. Neuroimage 2011 Apr 15;55(4):1497-1503.

[78] Costafreda SG, Khanna A, Mourao-Miranda J, Fu CH. Neural correlates of sad faces predict clinical remission to cognitive behavioural therapy in depression. Neuroreport 2009 May 6;20(7):637-641.

[79] Macaluso M, Drevets WC, Preskorn SH. How biomarkers will change psychiatry. Part II: Biomarker selection and potential inflammatory markers of depression. J Psychiatr Pract 2012 Jul;18(4):281-286.

[80] Carrig MM, Kolden GG, Strauman TJ. Using functional magnetic resonance imaging in psychotherapy research: a brief introduction to concepts, methods, and task selection. Psychother Res 2009 Jul;19(4-5):409-417.

[81] Quide Y, Witteveen AB, El-Hage W, Veltman DJ, Olff M. Differences between effects of psychological versus pharmacological treatments on functional and morphological brain alterations in anxiety disorders and major depressive disorder: a systematic review. Neurosci Biobehav Rev 2012 Jan;36(1):626-644.

Chapter 16

Mental Function and Obesity

Nobuko Yamada-Goto, Goro Katsuura and
Kazuwa Nakao

Additional information is available at the end of the chapter

http://dx.doi.org/10.5772/56228

1. Introduction

Obesity is defined as a high body mass index (BMI) with a large amount of adiposity. A chronic excess energy intake above energy expenditure leads to abnormal or excessive fat accumulation. Normally, humans and other mammals have an extraordinary ability to match food intake to energy expenditure over long periods so that body weight and adiposity are maintained at near-constant levels. The precise mechanism of the natural course of obesity is yet unclear. After findings on the hypothalamus as the center of energy regulation in 1940's, the central nervous system came to the forefront of attention in the pathophysiology of obesity. Recent global epidemic of obesity is one of the largest health problems in the world. Clinical studies have revealed that obesity is comorbid with several forms of mental disorder [3-5]. Epidemiological studies show that obesity is strongly related to cognitive impairment, including Alzheimer's disease and mood disorder [6, 7]. Obesity is also positively correlated with several other forms of mental disorder in general population samples. These findings suggest that obesity can affect mental function and change neural plasticity. Also, such mental disorder might cause further progression of obesity. Moreover, there is the possibility that mental disorder acts as a trigger of the development of obesity. Understanding the bidirectional interaction of obesity and mental disorder should help prevent and treat obesity. This review is aimed at highlighting the mental functions related to obesity, from basic research including our recent works to clinical findings.

2. Definition of obesity

2.1. Definition of obesity in the world

The International Association for the study of Obesity (IASO)/International Obesity Taskforce (IOTF) analysis (2010) estimates that approximately 1.0 billion adults are currently overweight, and a further 475 million are obese in the world today [8].

Being overweight or obesity are defined as having abnormal or excessive fat accumulation that presents a risk to health. The World Health Organization (WHO) defines obesity for adults based on overweight and obesity ranges determined by body mass index (BMI), a person's weight (in kilograms) divided by the square of height (in meters). An adult with a BMI under 18.5 kg/m^2 is considered underweight. An adult with a BMI between 18.5 kg/m^2 and 24.9 kg/m^2 is considered to be in the normal range. An adult with a BMI between 25 kg/m^2 and 29.9 kg/m^2 is considered overweight. An adult with a BMI of 30 kg/m^2 or higher is considered obese. Among the obese, an adult with a BMI between 30kg/m^2 and 34.9 kg/m^2 is considered to be obese class I, between 35kg/m^2 and 39.9 kg/m^2 to be obese class II, and an adult with a BMI of 40 kg/m^2 or higher to be obese class III [9]. BMI provides the most useful population-level measure of being overweight and obesity as it is the same for both sexes and for all ages of adults. However, WHO points out that it should be considered as a rough guide because it may not correspond to the same degree of fatness in different individuals. Moreover, it is well known that there is ethnic diversity in the physiology of obesity. The appropriateness of WHO criteria in non-Caucasian populations has been questioned. It was reported that South Asian, East Asian, and African-American developed diabetes at a higher rate, at an earlier age, and at lower ranges of BMI than their white counterparts [10]. In 2000, *The Asia-Pacific Perspective: Redefining Obesity and Its Treatment* recommended different ranges for the Asia-Pacific regions based on risk factors and morbidities. They suggested that in Asians, the cut-offs for being overweight should be 23 kg/m^2 and obesity 25 kg/m^2, which are lower than the WHO criteria [11].

2.2. Definition of obesity in East Asia

Substantial differences in national and local environments with genetic variances produce the wide variation in obesity prevalence in the world. The prevalence of obesity in adults is lower in East Asia including Japan compared with the USA [12]. In East Asia, China, Japan, South Korea and Taiwan have their own criteria of overweight and obesity. In Japan, according to the Japan Society for the Study of Obesity 2011 (JASSO), the BMI values considered as being underweight or in the normal range are the same as the WHO criteria [13]. However, an adult with a BMI of 25 kg/m^2 or higher is considered obese in Japan. Among the obese, an adult with a BMI between 25 kg/m^2 and 29.9 kg/m^2 is considered to be obese grade 1, between 30kg/m^2 and 34.9 kg/m^2 to be obese grade 2, between 35kg/m^2 and 39.9 kg/m^2 to be obese grade 3, and a BMI of 40 kg/m^2 or higher to be obese grade 4 in Japan. An adult with a BMI of 35 kg/m^2 or higher is considered to have morbid obesity in Japan. In China, an adult with a BMI of 24 kg/m^2 or higher is considered to be overweight, and an adult with a BMI of 28 kg/m^2 or higher is considered to be obese [14]. In South Korea, an adult with a BMI of 25 kg/m^2 or higher is considered to be obese [15]. In Taiwan, an adult with a BMI of 24 kg/m^2 or higher is considered to be overweight, and an adult with a BMI of 27 kg/m^2 or higher is considered to be obese [16].

3. Pathophysiology of obesity

3.1. Mortality and complications

The BMI classification scheme for weight status is based on data obtained from large epidemiological studies that evaluate the relationship between BMI and mortality [17]. Epidemiological studies consistently suggested that lowest overall mortality in adults is associated with a BMI in the range of 20 to 23 kg/m^2 [18]. A very high degree of obesity (BMI $\geqq$ 35 kg/m^2) seems likely to be linked to higher mortality rates, but the relationship between more modest degrees of being overweight and mortality is unclear [4, 18-21]. On the other hand, the positive correlation between obesity and many health problems both independently and in association with other diseases are clearly observed. In adults, the health complications associated with obesity increase linearly with increasing BMI until the age of 75 years [18, 22]. Both men and women who have a BMI $\geqq$ 30 kg/m^2 are considered obese and are generally at higher risk for adverse health events than are those who are considered to be overweight. In particular, obesity is associated with the development of type 2 diabetes mellitus, coronary heart disease, an increased incidence of certain forms of cancer (colon, breast, esophageal, uterine, ovarian, kidney, and pancreatic), respiratory complications (obstructive sleep apnea), and osteoarthritis of large and small joints [23]. Also, high prevalence of cognitive impairment and mental disorder is observed in obesity [3-6, 24].

3.2. Clinical aspects related to psychiatry in obesity

From the viewpoint of the endocrinologist, obesity is often comorbid with eating disorders, especially binge-eating disorder, which is thought to be present in 20-40% of obese patients [25]. Many lines of evidence suggest that obesity and depression often comorbid and might be functionally related to each other [3, 26-30]. High rates of obesity among individuals with binge eating disorder, bipolar disorder, major depressive disorder, anxiety disorders, schizophrenia, personality disorders, and other diagnoses were also observed [3, 5, 27, 31]. The link between such mental disorder and obesity is likely to be bidirectional: obesity can lead to mental disorder and, in turn, mental disorder can be an obstacle to treatments of obesity and attaining long-term weight-loss goals, thereby contributing to weight gain [25]. Evidence also indicates that obesity negatively impacts on prognosis of many kind of illness. These relationships appear to be especially strong for women and individuals with more severe obesity (BMI $\geqq$35 kg/m^2) [5]. Associations between obesity and psychiatric illness are also documented in men but in more moderately overweight individuals [5]. Obesity is also associated with significant psychosocial impairment. Obese individuals are subject to weight-based stigmatization in a variety of settings, and generally report poorer quality of life compared with lean individuals [4, 5].

From the viewpoint of the psychiatrist, obesity is defined as eating disorder. Anorexia nervosa, bulimia nervosa, eating disorders not otherwise specified, and obesity are categorized as eating disorder according to the Diagnostic and Statistical Manual of Mental Disorders (DSM)-IV TR [32]. Most of the patients of anorexia nervosa and bulimia nervosa are women. Even with the gender specificity, eating disorders are thought to share dysregulation of common neuronal pathways with obesity [33]. Some population of obesity is characterized as mental disorder with "compulsive food consumption" similar to drug addiction and suggested to be included as a mental disorder in the DSM-V [5]. The pathophysiology of anorexia nervosa draws attention as it is thought to be the opposite phenotype of obesity [Figure 1]. Functional magnetic resonance image (fMRI) study showed that brain reward circuits are more responsive to unexpected food stimuli and more sensitive in dopamine-related pathways in anorexia nervosa, but are less responsive and less sensitive in obese women [33]. Moreover, a recent fMRI study suggested that self starvation in anorexia nervosa may be driven by inappropriately assigned desire and pleasure associated with food restriction, somehow related to dependence [34]. They might perpetuate and reinforce the desire to not eat to change persistent stress, such as low self-esteem and social rejection into a positively experienced state [35]. Bulimia nervosa is another severe eating disorder characterized by the presence of episodic binge eating followed by extreme behaviors to avoid weight gain, such as self-induced vomiting, use of laxative or excessive exercise [32]. Individuals with bulimia nervosa present with fear of gaining weight, as well as food and body weight-related preoccupations, are at normal or often high-normal weight. While they are eating, they feel pleasure and arousal followed by guilt and remorse. These abnormal eating behaviors observed in anorexia nervosa and bulimia nervosa are also difficult to treat and contain life-long risk of relapse [36].

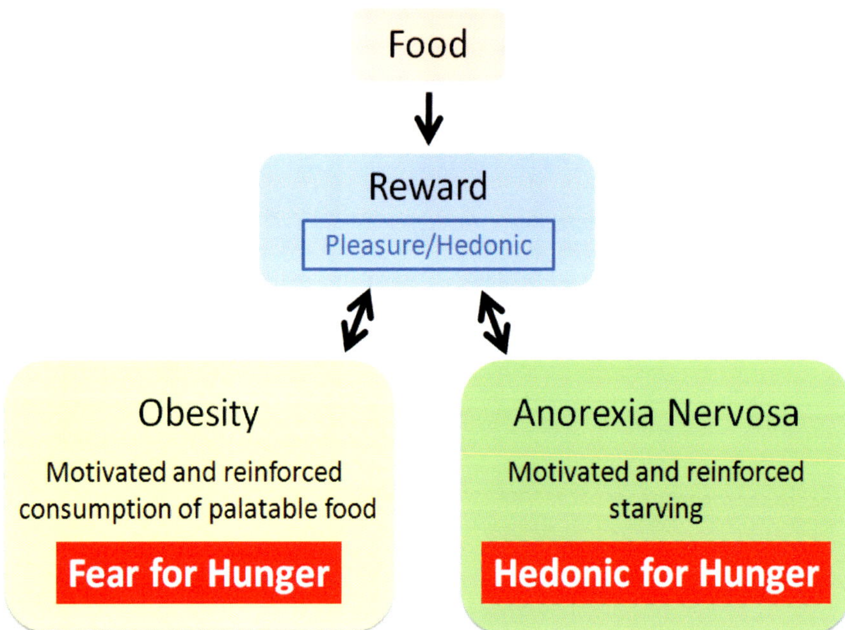

Figure 1. Postulated shared mechanisms related to reward circuits of anorexia nervosa and obesity. The sense of hunger regulated by reward circuits might be the key component of obesity and anorexia nervosa.

How about the personality of obesity? Psychological processes contribute to an individual's body shape. Body weight reflects our behaviors and lifestyle and contributes to the way we perceive ourselves and others. Personality traits are defined by cognitive, emotional, and behavioral patterns that are likely to contribute to unhealthy weight and difficulties with weight management. It is quite difficult to clarify personal traits, but there are many clinical studies on the personality of obesity using certain questionnaires [37-41]. Overweight individuals are prone to depressive state, have a poor body image, are evaluated negatively by others, and are ascribed traits based on their body size [42-45]. From the Baltimore Longitudinal Study of Aging (BLSA), which is a longitudinal study of more than 50 years on a large number of people (n = 1,988), high neuroticism and low conscientiousness, which are related to difficulty with impulse control, were associated with weight fluctuations [40]. Low agreeableness and impulsivity-related traits predicted a greater increase in BMI across the adult life span in the same study [40]. Personality traits are reported to be a useful tool for predicting diet-induced weight loss and management, which may offer ways to achieve appropriate weight loss and management strategies for individuals [46-47].

To date, however, there is no evidence to support a direct interaction between obesity and these personality traits. It is not clear that how these mental disorders and personality traits are related to the natural course of obesity.

3.3. Brain inflammation and obesity

Adiposity causes chronic low-grade systemic inflammation, which in conjunction with a high calorie diet may contribute to diseases associated with obesity [48-49]. A growing body of evidence implicates immune cell-mediated tissue inflammation as an important mechanism linking obesity to insulin resistance in metabolically active organs, such as the liver, skeletal muscle, and adipose tissue [48-49]. Peripheral inflammation passes through or bypasses the blood-brain barrier [50-51], and stimulation of neural afferents at the site of local peripheral inflammation induces an inflammatory reaction within the central nervous system [52-53]. The saturated free fatty acids, palmitic acids and lauric acid, have been shown to trigger inflammation in cultured macrophages [54]. Saturated long-chain fatty acids were demonstrated to activate inflammatory signaling in astrocytes [55]. Microglia, macrophage-like cells of the central nervous system that are activated by pro-inflammatory signals causing local production of specific interleukins and cytokines, play a pivotal role in brain inflammation [48-49, 53, 55-57]. Experimental studies in animals have confirmed neurologic vulnerability to obesity and a high-fat diet and further demonstrated that diet-induced metabolic dysfunction leads to increased brain inflammation, reactive gliosis, and vulnerability to injury, especially in the hypothalamus [49, 56, 58-59]. Hypothalamic inflammation contributes to obesity pathogenesis through the development of central leptin resistance [49, 56]. Leptin resistance is a physiological condition in which high concentrations of leptin neither reduce food intake nor increase energy expenditure, as observed in obese humans and a rodent model of diet-induced obesity (DIO) [60]. Leptin resistance is considered to be a central dogma for obesity [61]. Immune-related molecules, including proinflammatory cytokines, IL-1β, TNF-α, and IL-6, altered expression levels of many genes in the hypothalamus [49, 56, 58]. Activation of both Jnk and the inhibitor of nuclear factor kappa-B kinase subunit β(IKKβ)/ nuclear factor-κB (NF-κB) pathway as well as induction of endoplasmic reticulum stress underlie these responses and parallel the onset of reduced hypothalamic leptin sensitivity in rodent models of DIO [56, 58]. High-fat feeding increases suppressor of cytokine signaling 3 (SOCS3) and protein tyrosine phosphatase-1B (PTP1B) in the rodent hypothalamus [56, 58, 62]. Up-regulation of SOCS3, a member of a protein family originally characterized as negative feedback regulators of inflammation, inhibits insulin and leptin signaling by direct binding to their cognate receptors and targeting insulin receptor substrate (IRS) proteins for proteasomal degaradation [58]. The PTP1B is a signal termination molecule that inhibits both leptin and insulin signaling, also thought to be involved in leptin resistance [58, 62]. Diet-induced PTP1B overexpression in multiple tissues including the hypothalamus in obesity is regulated by inflammation [62]. Recent studies with animals and humans have shown that other brain structures, such as the hippocampus and orbitofrontal cortex, are also affected [53, 57, 63-64]. These inflammatory changes induced by obesity and high-fat diet might be reversible from the results of animal studies. Resveratrol, an adenosine monophosphate-activated protein kinase (AMPK) activator and potent anti-inflammatory agent, attenuated peripheral and central inflammation in the hippocampus and improved memory deficit in mice fed a high-fat diet [57]. In another study, moderate and regular treadmill running exercise markedly decreased hypothalamic inflammation in high-fat diet fed mice [59]. Evidence of brain inflammation in human obesity has been accumulating based on biologic data and imaging studies by using MRI [46, 56].

4. Mental disorders of obesity

4.1. Depression and other mood disorders

Obesity is associated with an increased risk of developing depression and a higher likelihood of current depression [3, 27-30]. Most obese individuals tend to have higher scores in depression, the projected increase in the rates of being overweight and obesity in future years could generate a parallel increase in obesity-related depression. According to the DSM-IV, an episode of major depressive disorder can be classified clinically as depression with melancholic features and depression with atypical features. Unlike melancholic depression, which is characterized by a loss of appetite or weight, atypical depression and seasonal depression are characterized by decreased activity and increased appetite and weight. Obesity among these groups is sometimes a result of the ingestion of "palatable food", which contains high amounts of fat and sugar [65]. Also, major depression in female adolescence is linked with an increased risk of obesity in adulthood [66]. To explain this mutual relationship between obesity and depression, the focus of research has been on hormones and neuropeptides, which have been implicated in both energy regulation and cognition/mood [67]. Among them, the involvement of leptin has been the subject of much attention as it has been implicated in depression associated with obesity [1]. Leptin is reported to induce an antidepressant-like activity in the hippocampus, which is considered to be an important region for regulation of the depressive state, but not in the hypothalamus of rats [68]. Decreased plasma or CSF leptin levels were observed in major depressive disorder patient group compared with controls independent of BMI [69-70]. These findings suggested that impairment of leptin action might contribute the physiology of depression. In obese rodents and humans, a high concentration of plasma leptin is observed with a blunted effect of leptin in suppressing food intake and increasing energy expenditure, which is termed "leptin resistance" [61]. Based on these observations, we postulated that the development of depression associated with obesity might be due in part to impaired leptin activity in the hippocampus.

Here we review our recent study on the central leptin action in depression associated with obesity [1]. The forced swimming test (FST) is widely accepted as a task that induces depressive behavior in depression research and has good reliability and high predictive validity for assessment of the depressive state and the detection of potential antidepressant-like activity in experimental animals. In this test, animals display "despair" behavior as observed as immobility and escape-oriented behaviors, in particular, by swimming [71-72]. Normal mice fed a control diet (CD) displayed such immobility and stress-induced despair in the FST. Subcutaneous administration of leptin significantly decreased the immobility time compared with saline treatment [Figure 2(A); 1]. Icv injection of leptin significantly decreased the immobility time of CD mice in the FST [Figure 2(B); 1]. DIO mice fed a 60% high-fat diet (HFD) for 16 weeks exhibited more depressive behavior compared with CD mice without exaggerated response of plasma corticosterone levels [Figure 2(C); 1]. Subcutaneous administration of leptin did not decrease the prolonged immobility time in DIO mice [Figure 2(D); 1]. Icv injection of leptin did not decrease the immobility time of DIO mice in the FST [1]. Moreover, in response to leptin, DIO mice did not exhibit an increase in the number of c-Fos-immunoreactive cells in the hippocampus, whereas leptin administration in CD mice has a significantly increased number of c-Fos immunoreactive cells in the hippocampus [1]. To examine whether the increased immobility time of DIO mice in the FST can be restored by diet substitution from HFD to CD, the diet of the DIO mice was changed from HFD to CD for the next 3 weeks. This led to significant reductions in body weight and fat weight and to the normalization of plasma levels of glucose, insulin, and leptin [1]. The immobility time in the FST in mice now given CD was significantly decreased and identical to that of the CD mice [1]. Moreover, subcutaneous administration of leptin significantly decreased the immobility time of FST in mice switched to CD [1]. These results are compatible with a previous report that diet substitution from HFD to CD in DIO mice restores leptin sensitivity as an anorexigenic action [73]. Brain-derived neurotrophic factor (BDNF) in the hippocampus is considered to play an important role in control of the depressive state. Injection of BDNF into the hippocampus in experimental animals has antidepressant effects in the FST, and this antidepressant effect induced by BDNF is inhibited by K252a, an inhibitor of the BDNF receptor tyrosine kinase B (TrkB) [74]. Low BDNF levels are reported in the hippocampus of humans with depression [75]. These findings support the hypothesis that decreased BDNF/TrkB signaling may induce depression. In our study, the hippocampal BDNF concentrations in DIO mice were significantly decreased compared with those of CD mice [Figure 2(E); 1]. Subcutaneous administration of leptin significantly increased BDNF concentrations in the hippocampus of CD mice but not in DIO mice [Figure 2(E); 1]. In summary, as shown in Figure 2F, in the lean state, leptin helps maintain normal body weight by acting on the arcuate nucleus of the hypothalamus (ARC), and provides an antidepressant-like action via hippocampal BDNF, whereas in the obese state, impaired leptin action even with a high concentration in plasma, may lead to rodent and human obesity occurring together with depression [Figure 2(F); 1].

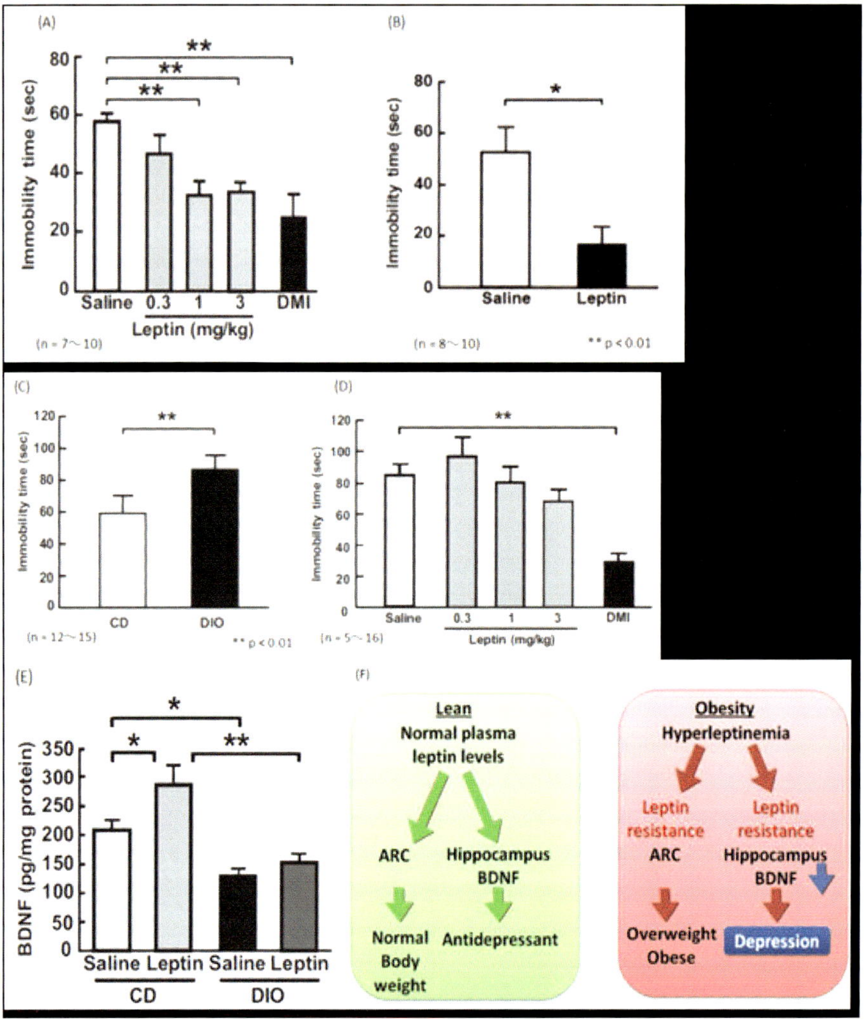

Figure 2. Central leptin action in depression associated with obesity (A) Effect of subcutaneous administration of leptin (0.3, 1, 3 mg/kg) and desipramine (DMI) (7.5 mg/kg) in CD mice on immobility time in the FST. (B) Effect of intracerebroventricular administration of leptin (1 μg/2 μl per mouse) on immobility time in CD mice in the FST. (C) Depressive behavior in DIO mice in the FST. (D) Antidepressant effects of subcutaneous administration of leptin (0.3, 1, 3 mg/kg) and DMI (7.5 mg/kg) in DIO mice. (E) Effect of subcutaneous administration of leptin (3 mg/kg) in CD and DIO mice on the hippocampal BDNF concentrations. (F) The schematic diagram of normal body weight regulation and antidepressant-like effect of leptin in lean, and overweight/obese and depression resulting in leptin resistance in obesity. Data points represent the mean ± SEM. Significantly different: *$p < 0.05$, **$p < 0.01$. CD mice: control mice given CE-2 as a control diet (CLEA Japan, Inc., Tokyo, Japan), DIO mice: diet-induced obese mice given a high-fat diet (HFD) (no. D12492; Research Diets, Inc., New Brunswick, NJ) containing 60% fat of total calories, predominantly in the form of lard.

Given the high comorbidity of metabolic disorders, such as diabetes and obesity, with depression, several lines of evidence suggest that insulin signaling in the brain is also an important regulator. Clinical investigations show the relationship between insulin resistance and depression, but the underlying mechanisms are still unclear [76-77]. Ghrelin is also play a potential role in defense against the consequences of stress, including stress-induced depression and anxiety and prevent their manifestation in experimental animals [82]. These findings suggest that both leptin and ghrelin involve in mood regulation and might have antidepressant-like effect. The target differences being treated by leptin or ghrelin in human depression are not known, yet.

What kind of treatment is effective on depression associated with obesity? One clinical study demonstrated the efficacy of a treatment combining behavioral weight management and cognitive behavioral therapy for obese adults with depression [81]. According to systematic review and meta-analysis on intentional weight loss and changes in symptoms of depression, obese individuals in weight loss trials experienced reduction in depression symptoms [80]. This finding is compatible with our experimental data [1].

4.2. Cognitive impairment and Alzheimer's disease

Epidemiologic studies have demonstrated that the incidence of cognitive impairment is higher in obese individuals than in individuals with normal body weight [6, 24]. From the study of Anstey et al., risks of cognitive impairment appeared to be highest for those with underweight and obese BMI in midlife [81]. Increasing evidence suggests that obesity is associated with impairment of certain cognitive functions, such as executive function, attention, visuomotor skills, and memory [6, 82]. A higher prevalence of attention deficit hyperactivity disorder, Alzheimer's disease and other cognitive impairment, cortical atrophy, and white matter disease is observed in obese individuals [83-84]. The mechanisms by which obesity results in cognitive impairment, however, are uncertain. Postulated mechanisms include the effects of hyperglycemia, hyperinsulinemia, poor sleep with obstructive sleep apnea, and vascular damage to the central nervous system [7, 85]. Moreover, adiposity is thought to have a direct effect on neuronal degradation [24]. C reactive protein, as well as inflammatory markers, is increased in subjects with greater adiposity and is associated with later-life cognitive impairment [86]. White matter lesions and cerebral atrophy are more common in adults with a high BMI, and midlife measures of central obesity predict poor performance on tests measuring executive function and visuomotor skills [83-84, 87. In animal studies, chronic dietary fat intake, especially saturated fatty acid intake, contributes to deficits in hippocampus- and amygdala-dependent learning and memory in rodents with diet-induced obesity by changes in neuronal plasticity [2, 88]. Neural plasticity, long-term structural alterations of synapses, are regulated by several synaptic molecules including neurotrophic factors, such as BDNF, and have been demonstrated to be essential for hippocampal functions [89].

In our recent study, cognitive behaviors in DIO mice in fear-conditioning test including both contextual and cued elements that preferentially depend on the hippocampus and amygdala, respectively, was significantly impaired [Figure 3(A); 2]. Fear-conditioning test is the method which assesses memory and learing by freezing behavior induced by electric foot shock.

Freezing was defined as the absence of all movement except for respiration. BDNF content in the cerebral cortex and hippocampus of DIO mice was significantly lower than that in CD mice [Figure 3(B); 2]. Its receptor, full-length TrkB in the amygdala of DIO mice was significantly decreased compared to that in CD mice, although not in the cerebral cortex, hippocampus and hypothalamus [Figure 3(C); 2]. By contrast, neurotrophin-3 (NT-3), which is reported to act in the opposite direction to BDNF on neurite outgrowth and neural activities, was present at significantly higher levels in the hippocampus, amygdala and hypothalamus of DIO mice than that in CD mice [90-91, Figure 3(B); 2]. Its receptor, full-length TrkC, was not significantly different between CD and DIO mice [Figure 3(C); 2].

Several lines of electrophysiological and behavioral evidence demonstrate that leptin and insulin enhance hippocampal synaptic plasticity and improve learning and memory [7, 92]. Electrophysiological studies in genetically obese Zucker rats with leptin-receptor deficiency demonstrated that long-term potentiation (LTP) of the hippocampal CA1 region, which is closely related to learning and the formation of memory and is regulated by *N*-methyl-D-aspartate (NMDA) and 2-amino-3-(3-hydroxy-5-methyl-isoxazol-4-yl)propanoic acid (AMPA) receptors, is markedly impaired compared to that of lean rats [93]. Streptozotocin-treated insulin deficient rats are reported to exhibit impaired cognition in the water maze test, which is dependent on the hippocampus [94]. Therefore, it is likely that impairment of the actions of leptin or insulin might be attributable to cognitive deficits in obesity and diabetes mellitus [61, 95].

5. Dysregulation of hunger in obesity

5.1. Metabolic hunger

Food intake and energy expenditure are controlled by complex, redundant, and distributed neural systems that reflect the fundamental biologic importance of an adequate nutrient supply and energy balance. Metabolic hunger is regulated by a homeostatic metabolic status designed to preserve energy balance and maintain minimal levels of adiposity. The hypothalamus and caudal brainstem play crucial roles in this homeostatic function. The hypothalamus serves to integrate nutrition and information from orexigenic and anorexigenic peptides that are sensitive to circulating leptin and other hormones [96-97]. The role of the hypothalamus in regulating food intake and body weight was established in 1940 by the classic experiments of Hetherington and Ranson [98]. Their destruction experiments demonstrated that the ventromedial hypothalamus resulted in hyperphagia and obesity [98]. Anand and Brobeck, in 1951, demonstrated that lesions of the lateral hypothalamus caused loss of feeding, inanition, and even death by starvation [99]. Thus, the concept arose of the lateral hypothalamic are serving as a "feeding center" and the ventromedial nucleus as a "satiety center" [100].

After more than 60 years since the Hetherington and Ranson experiments, much more precise mechanisms and the network between peripheral signals and the brain have been elucidated [97, 101]. Input signals such as sight, smell and taste allow the brain to decide whether or not it should engage in ingestive behavior. Once put into the mouth, foods elicit taste and mechanical sensations that send neural signals via mainly vagal afferents to the

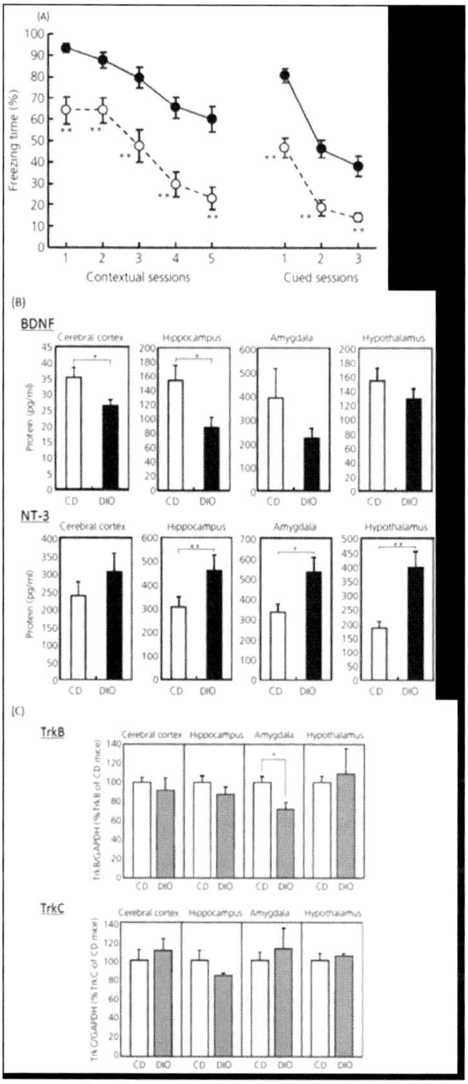

Figure 3. Impairment of fear-conditioning responses and changes of brain neurotrophic factors in diet-induced obese mice. (A) Fear-conditioning responses in CD (closed circles) and DIO (open circles) mice. Freezing percentages of CD and DIO mice in the contextual conditioning test were measured every minute for 5 min. Freezing percentages of CD and DIO mice in the cued conditioning test were measured every minute for 3 min. (B) Content of brain-derived neurotrophic factor (BDNF) and neurotrophin-3 (NT-3) in the cerebral cortex, hippocampus, amygdala and hypothalamus in CD and DIO mice. (C) Expression of full-length TrkB and TrkC in the cerebral cortex, hippocampus, amygdala and hypothalamus in CD and DIO mice. Data points represent the mean ± SEM. Significantly different from CD mice: * $p < 0.05$, ** $p < 0.01$. GAPDH: glyceraldehyde3-phosphate dehydrogenase.

brainstem and/or hormonal signals through the bloodstream to the brain [97]. Gut-to-brain communication is increasingly recognized as playing an important role not just in the determination of meal size but also in overall food intake [97]. Once absorbed, macronutrients are partitioned into either storage or immediate metabolism in various tissues [97]. The information from peripheral tissue including the gastric tract is relayed to the brain, especially to the hypothalamus and the brainstem by hormones [leptin, insulin, amylin, peptide YY (PYY), ghrelin, glucagon-like peptide-1 (GLP-1), and cholecystokinin (CCK)] and nutrient signals [glucose, free fatty acid, and amino acid] [97, 101]. Leptin, insulin and amylin deliver long-term afferent signals, PYY, GLP-1, and CCK deliver short-term meal related afferent signals and work for satiation, and ghrelin stimulate feeding. Vagal afferent neurons, whose cell bodies lie in the nodose ganglia, relay information from enteroendocrine cells of the intestinal epithelium and the enteric nervous system directly to the nucleus of the solitary tract in the brainstem [102]. During periods of hunger, the hypothalamus regulates the activity of the autonomic nervous system to promote fat release from white adipose tissue and trigger glucogenesis in the liver. These changes in peripheral nutrient levels lead to a decrease in the levels of thyroid hormones, insulin and leptin, and to an increase in the level of ghrelin and corticosteroids, which increase food-seeking behavior through their effect on the brain [101]. Through these pathways, an almost stable body weight can be maintained even under unpredictable and unstable environments.

The ARC in the hypothalamus is the gateway of above hormones and signals in the brain [97, 101, 103]. From the ARC, the first-order neuronal network was observed of anorexigenic neuropeptides, proopiomelanocortin (POMC) and cocaine-amphetamine rerated transcript (CART), orexigenic neuropeptide, NPY and Agouti-related protein (AgRP) to other nuclei in the hypothalamus, the paraventricular hypothalamus (PVN), lateral hypothalamus (LH), and ventromedial hypothalamus (VMH) [97, 103]. These nuclei have a second-order neuronal network of output projection to other sites of the brain which regulate endocrine responses, autonomic responses, cognitive processing response plan, procurement actions, reward memory, aversive memory, social screen, competing behaviors, oro-and locomotor control, and autonomic control of peripheral tissue [97, 103]. Among these nucleus in the hypothalamus, LH works as a relaying point, connecting the hypothalamus with mesolimbic dopamine system and higher brain functions. Melanin-concentrating hormone in the LH projects to the Nucleus accumbense (NAc) and many other brain areas including the amygdala, hippocampus, and cerebral cortex, and orexin in the LH project to the ventral tegmental area (VTA) and many other brain areas including the amygdala, hippocampus, and cerebral cortex [104]. From recent studies, first order neurons, which receive peripheral information and regulate food intake, are suspected to be present in other regions of the hypothalamus and extra-hypothalamus [1, 97, 105, 106]. Many hormones and neuropeptides, which were previously thought to energy regulator, have turned to regulate other higher brain functions, too.

In human obesity, genetic predisposition is expressed mainly on the central melanocortin system. Downstream targets of the central melanocortin system are implicated in food intake, meal choice, satiety and energy expenditure [107]. POMC is a large precursor protein that is processed into a variety of smaller products, including alpha melanocyte stimulating hormone (α-MSH), is an endogenous ligand of melanocortin 3 receptor (MC3R) and melanocortin 4 receptor (MC4R) in the brain [108]. AgRP is an inverse agonist of the brain MC3R and MC4R, completely dependent on the melanocortin receptors for its action, has an orexigenic effect on food intake and decreases energy expenditure [109]. Mutations in the MC4R in humans, the most commonly known monogenic cause of human obesity, have been associated with obesity, hyperphagia, tall -stature and hyperinsulinemia [110-113]. Common variants near MC4R were reported to influence fat mass, weight and obesity risk at the population level from genome-wide association data from people of European descent [114]. Mutations in MC3R have been associated with obesity, hyper leptinemia and relative hypephagia [115]. Mutations in POMC and AgRP have been also reported in human obesity [116-118]. Mutation of leptin, which target is thought to be mainly the melanocortin circuitry in the brain, leptin receptor, and prohormone convertase-I were also reported in humans with severe early-onset obesity and intense hyperphagia [118-121]. The findings that HFD altered levels of POMC, AgRP and MC4R mRNA expression in the hypothalamus and changed the response to melanocortin agonist in experimental animals [122-123], speculate that dysregulation of melanocortin system may also happen in human obesity.

5.2. Hedonic hunger

Several lines of evidence have indicated that energy regulations are also modulated by extra-hypothalamic brain areas originally related to regulation of emotion and cognition, such as the NAc, amygdala, hippocampus and cerebral cortex [124]. These findings suggest that maintaining energy homeostasis and regulating emotion and cognition share common brain regions, as well as bidirectional interaction between energy regulation and emotional/cognitive functions. The regulation of food intake by the hypothalamus interacts with reward and motivational neurocircuity to modify eating behavior. Such a cognitive-hedonic pathway permits us to adjust our feeding behavior to environment & lifestyle, palatability, liking/wanting/emotion, cues, availability, physical activity, and fuel availability [97]. Reward circuitry, which is mainly regulated by the midbrain dopamine system from the VTA to the NAc, is the main pathway of hedonic hunger. This system is the main pathway in drug addiction and part of the motivational system that regulates responses to natural reinforcers such as drink, sex, social interaction and food [125]. This dopamine neuron express κopioid receptors and receive projection of γ-aminobutyric acid (GABA) and dynorphin from the NAc [125]. Dopamine signaling within mesolimbic neurons mediates the willingness to engage in rewarding behaviors or "wanting", whereas the pleasure associated with a particular reward or "liking" is attributed to mesolimbic opioid action [126]. Memory and learning, mood, Top/Down inhibition, interoception, gustatory integration, and salience attribution interact with the reward circuitry [Figure 4; 105]. Top/Down inhibition of feeding depends heavily on the prefrontal cortex, including orbitofrontal cortex and cingulate gyrus [105]. The amygdala ascribes emotional attributes including fear, together with memory and learning circuitry, and generates conditioned responses [2]. The hippocampus is also involved in emotion, memory and learning circuitry [2, 105].

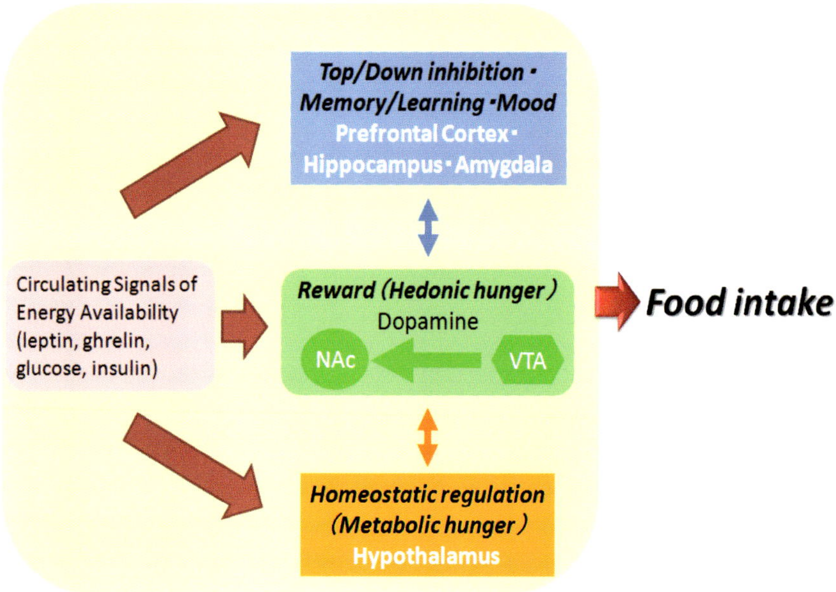

Figure 4. Schematic diagram potential interactions between metabolic hunger and hedonic hunger which regulate food intake. Food intake is controlled by complex neural system that reflects the fundamental biological importance of adequate nutrient supply and balance. Metabolic hunger regulated by homeostatic metabolic status designed to preserve energy balance and protect minimal levels adiposity. The hypothalamus plays crucial roles in the metabolic hunger. Reward circuit which is mainly regulated by the midbrain dopamine system from the VTA to NAc, is the main pathway of hedonic hunger. Memory and learning and mood interact with reward circuits. Circulating signals of energy availability, leptin, ghrelin, glucose, and insulin are thought to regulate food intake mainly via the hypothalamus, but recent studies show that they also regulate food intake via many extra-hypothalamic regions. VTA: ventral tegmental area, NAc: nucleus accumbense.

Chronic excessive consumption of palatable foods predisposes some individuals to obesity via an increased likelihood and reinforcement of overeating. Excessive activity of hedonic hunger in obesity might lead to the ingestion of more food, independent of metabolic hunger. Several recent models have emphasized the role of the dysregulation of hedonic hunger in the development and maintenance of obesity. Such "compulsive food consumption" was recently explained by an analogy to drug addiction as previously described [Figure 5]. Drug addiction is defined as the loss of control over drug use, or the compulsive seeking and taking of drugs despite adverse consequences [125]. Once formed, an addiction can be a life-long condition in which individuals show intense drug craving and increased risk for relapse after years and even decades of abstinence [125]. This means that addiction involves extremely stable changes in the brain that are responsible for these long-lived behavioral abnormalities [125]. The hypothesis of obesity treating as an analogy of drug addiction is supported by evidence for a food addiction diagnosis according to the Yale Food Addiction Scales [127-129] and fMRI in humans [92]. There are several questionnaires for the assessment of food addiction. Such

http://dx.doi.org/10.5772/56228

questionnaires include the "3Cs" of addiction, compulsive use, attempts to cut down, continued use despite consequences, among others [127]. The most common symptoms were (1) persistent desire or repeated unsuccessful attempts to cut down, (2) continued use despite problems, and (3) much time spent to obtain food, eat, or recover from eating [127]. Meule et al reported that prevalence of food addiction diagnoses differed between weight classes such that overweight and obese participants had higher prevalence than normal weight participants [Figure 6; 128]. These "compulsive food consumption" is difficult to modify, and even if weight loss is achieved, the neural plasticity "fixed" by palatable food leads individuals to crave palatable food and thus substantially regain weight. "Fear of hunger" which accelerates "hedonic eating of palatable food" might cause compulsive food consumption in obesity [35]. Moreover, a weakened Top/Down inhibition signal for food cravings and inadequate sensing of ingested nutrients resulting in hyperphagia of obesity has been detected in fMRI studies [105]. Also, from the finding that obese patients have been shown to have decreased D2 receptor level in striatum by positron emission tomography (PET) imaging, obesity has been described as a reward deficiency syndrome, where deficiency of dopamine signaling results in compensatory over eating [105, 125]. fMRI studies demonstrated that obese patients have an increased "motivation" or "wanting" for food intake, actual food intake is associated with decreased "liking" [130]. It is not known that these functional changes are the results of obesity or the cause of obesity.

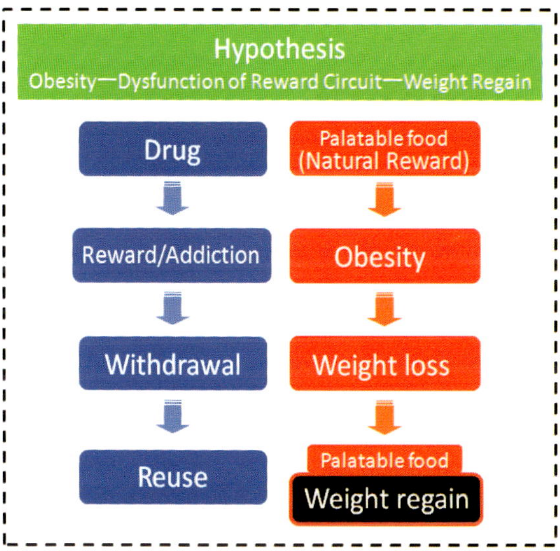

Figure 5. Hypothesis of obesity as an analogy of drug addiction. Addictive drugs are both rewarding and reinforcing. Repeated use of addictive drugs produces multiple changes in the brain that may lead to addiction. Withdrawal occurs when drug-taking stops. Withdrawal symptoms drive one to reuse the drug. Excessive consumption of hyper-palatable foods might parallel to drug addiction. Repeated taking of palatable food produces multiple changes in the brain that may lead to obesity. After weight loss was achieved in obese patients, they usually regain their weight.

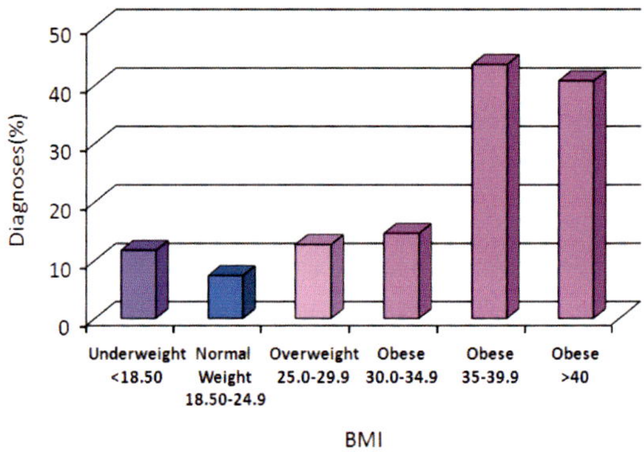

Figure 6. Percentage of food addiction diagnosis according to the Yale Food Addiction Scale as a function of weight category. This graph is made from the data of Table 1. (Meule, A., Medical Hypotheses, 2012;79(4):508-511) [128]. These are aggregated data from three studies done by Meule, A. et al, in which the Yale Food Addiction Scale was used and BMI was assessed. Participants were classified in weight categories according to the guidelines of WHO. The prevalence of food addiction diagnosis was significantly increased in overweight/obese individuals compared with normal weight individuals.

Stress is reported to modulate the reward circuit. Stress affects feeding behavior in humans in both directions, with some individuals increasing their food intake while others eat less [131]. An overall increased consumption of caloric dense and highly palatable foods following stress compared to non-stressed controls is reported, independent of stress-induced hyperphagia or hypephagia [131]. Susceptibility to stress and stress-induced hyperphagia are observed in obese individuals [132]. Depression, other mood disorders, and cognitive impairment also affect the feeding behavior of obese individuals. Direct interaction between stress-mediated mood and reward circuits in rodent was reported by Vialou et al [133].

5.3. Hormones and neurotransmitter in metabolic hunger and hedonic hunger

5.3.1. Leptin

Leptin is one of the most important adipocyte-derived hormones and circulate in proportion to body fat mass, enter the brain, and act on neurocircuit that govern food intake and energy expenditure [124]. The long form of the leptin receptor (Ob-Rb) expresses in numerous regions including the hypothalamus, VTA, and NAc. Through both direct and indirect actions, leptin diminishes perception of food reward (the palatability of food) while enhancing the response to satiety signals generated during food consumption that inhibit feeding and lead to meal termination [124]. Administrations of leptin in the VTA directly regulate mesolimbic dopamine system [134-135]. Centrally administered leptin diminishes both sucrose preference and the effect of fasting to increase the rewarding properties of electrical pleasure-center stimulation [136-137]. The effect of weight loss to lower leptin levels and hence to reduce leptin signaling increases rewarding properties of food while diminishing satiety, a combination that potently increases food intake [124].

5.3.2. *Ghrelin*

Ghrelin is recognized as the only known orexigenic peptide hormone and synthesized mainly by a distinct group of endocrine cells located within the gastric oxyntic mucosa [136]. The mechanisms by which ghrelin promotes food intake are multifaceted and include not only stimulating intake of food via homeostatic mechanisms but also enhancing the rewarding properties of pleasurable food [139-140]. Ghrelin shifts food preference toward palatable sweet and fatty food [139]. Ghrelin can directly affect dopaminergic VTA neuronal activity and increase motivational aspect of reward [139]. Intra-VTA administration of ghrelin modulates intake of freely available regular chow, food preference, motivated food reward behavior, and increases body weight [139]. Orexin signaling is required in these ghrelin's action on food reward [140]. Ghrelin also reported to mediates stress-induced food-reward behavior in mice [141].

5.3.3. *Insulin*

Insulin is produced by pancreatic β-cells, controls plasma glucose levels, increases in proportion to fat mass, consequently relay information about peripheral fat stores to central effectors in the hypothalamus to modify food intake and energy expenditure. Neurons in the ARC of the hypothalamus express insulin receptors and regulate energy homeostasis. The receptors for insulin are also present in brain reward circuitry, which are thought to be projected from LH in the hypothalamus [126, 142-143]. Insulin works as satiety hormone similar to leptin, and also attenuates food reward similar to leptin, substantially suppresses food intake [126, 144]. Insulin signaling and dopamine signaling via dopamine 2 receptor (D2R) work in tandem to regulate dopamine transporter plasma membrane expression and function [145]. Brain insulin resistance which is often accompanied with obesity also exists in brain regions regulating appetite and reward [146]. Dysregulation of brain insulin signaling might alter dopamine reward pathways resulting in changing motivation for food since these pathways are insulin sensitive [145]. Jastreboff et al demonstrated a fMRI study that in obese individuals, food craving, insulin, and HOMA-IR levels correlated positively with neural activity in corticolimbic-striatal brain regions including the striatum, insula, and thalamus during favorite-food and stress cues [147]. These findings strongly suggest that the relationship between insulin resistance and food craving in obese individuals mediated by activity in motivation-reward regions [147]. Centrally administered insulin also diminishes both sucrose preference and the effect of fasting to increase the rewarding properties of electrical pleasure-center stimulation similar to leptin [136-137].

5.3.4. *GLP-1*

GLP-1 is secreted from the L cells of intestinal tract in response to nutrients. GLP-1 is also produced in the NTS of the brainstem, resulting in the activation of GLP-1receptor (GLP-1R) expressed on both dendritic terminals of vagal afferent fibers innervating the organs of the peritoneal cavity, as well as the pancreaticβ-cells [148-149]. Activation of the GLP-1R promotes glucose dependent insulin secretion, slowing of gastric emptying, and glucose-dependent inhibition of glucagon secretion, together facilitating the rapid clearance, storage, and normalization of blood glucose [149]. GLP-1 has anorectic effects, and regulation of short and long-term food intake and body weight [148]. GLP-1Rs are expressed especially in the NTS and in the hypothalamic nuclei [155]. GLP-1 neurons in the NTS are characterized to project to the PVN and the DMH in the hypothalamus [150]. Peripheral GLP-1 regulates long-term energy balance interacting with leptin [150]. Central GLP-1 is a critical downstream mediator of leptin action [155]. Cells in both the VTA and the NAc clearly express the GLP-1R [147-148]. They receive GLP-1-positive fibers which are likely coming from the NTS and potentially contribute to the regulation of reward behavior [151-152]. Peripheral and central administration of a long-acting GLP-1 receptor agonists, liraglutide and Exendin-4, suppress food reward and motivation in rats, resulting in reduce appetite and body weight [148].

5.4. Weight management strategy in obesity

On the basis of the observation that a 10% loss of body weight frequently produces substantial beneficial change in health risk factors, even in the very obese, a 10% weight loss has been offered as a clinical definition of weight loss success [153]. Long-term success in voluntary weight loss is clearly possible but quite difficult. Lifestyle modification sometimes with cognitive behavioral therapy (CBT) is essential part of the strategy of weight management in obesity. Medications and bariatric surgery are supportive therapy. Recent new findings from successful bariatric surgery might help us to get new strategy.

5.4.1. Lifestyle modification

The health and psychosocial benefits of sustained weight loss are well established, even tough, these natural incentives are not sufficient to motivate long-term behavior change [153]. There is a lifestyle patterns associated with lean or obese population. From the study done by University of Minnesota, 5 meaningful lifestyle and weight control behavioral factors were identified [154]. Current lesser BMI and greater % weight loss are associated with good habits: regularity of meals, not watching television with meal or snuck, having intentional strategies for weight control, not eating away from home, greater fruit and vegetable intake [154]. These results strongly suggested that lifestyle modification is essential for weight loss and weight control. Lifestyle modification includes 3 primary components: diet, exercise, and behavior therapy. About dietary interventions, there are 4 well-known diets: low-carbohydrate, low-fat (including balanced calorie-restricted), Mediterranean, and low-glycemic load regimens [155]. Numerous trials have examined these diets. In summary, caloric restriction rather than macronutrient composition is the key determinant of weight loss [155]. The optimal dietary macronutrient composition for improving specific comorbid complication will be determined by further researches. About exercise, physical activity is associated with improvements in body composition and metabolic conditions independent of weight loss. For weight loss, physical activity alone is of limited benefit and much better with diet restrictions. However, physical activity appears to be critical for long-term weight loss and prevention of weight regain [156]. Moderate-intensity physical activity between 150 and 250 min/week alone will provide only modest weight loss and prevent weight gain. Greater amount of physical activity over 250 min/week have been associated with clinically significant weight loss [156]. Resistance training increase fat-free mass and increase loss of fat mass but does not enhance weight loss [156]. For weight control, multiple short bouts of activity, as brief as 10 min, throughout the day are as effective as 1 long bout (>40 min) [157]. Behavior therapy is a set of principles and techniques for helping obese individuals modify eating, activity, and thinking habits that contribute to their excess weight [156, 158]. Setting specific goal and self-monitoring are the most important components of behavioral treatment [156]. Self-monitoring contains, daily monitoring of food intake and physical activity by use of paper or electronic diaries, weekly monitoring of weight, structured curriculum of behavior change, and regular feedback from an interventionist [156]. Frequent self-monitoring is a consistent predictor of both short- and long-term weight losses [159]. Frequency and duration of treatment contact is another important component of lifestyle modification [156]. Among many lifestyle modification programs, the LEARN program developed by Dr. Kelly Brownell of Yale University, is often recommended by health professionals in the USA and UK. It is designed to produce permanent change in five areas of life (lifestyle, exercise, attitudes, relationships and nutrition) for living and maintaining a healthy body weight. It also includes a master list of various lifestyle techniques, personal charts and forms, a fast food guide, calorie guide, a Weight Loss Readiness Test, and a comprehensive index [153, 158].

5.4.2. Cognitive behavioral therapy

Cooper et al developed a new CBT for obese women based on the evidence of their CBT for bulimia nervosa [112]. It targets patients' overeating, low level of activity, and focuses on processes hypothesized to hinder successful weight maintenance [160]. CBT was successful at achieving change in participants' acceptance of body shape. The great majority of the participants lost weight while taking CBT but within the observation period regain it. It seems that sustained behavior change in people with obesity is remarkably difficult to achieve, unlike the situation with people with eating disorders. However, CBT is still valuable for its validity and safety and there is still room for improvement.

5.4.3. Medication

After Orlistat (pancreatic lipase inhibitor) was approved 13 years ago, on 1999, safety concerns or lack of efficacy have doomed past applications. Fenfluramine, serotonin re-uptake inhibitor and increases the release of serotonin, is withdrawn by US Food and Drug Administration (FDA) with side effects of hallucinations, valvulopathy, pulmonary hypertension. Sibutramine, noradrenalin and serotonin re-uptake inhibitor is withdrawn by FDA with side effects of increased risk of heart attack and stroke in patients with high risk of cardiovascular disorders. Rimonabant (SR141716; CB_1 receptor antagonist/inverse agonist) is withdrawn by European Medicines Agency with side effects of risk of suicide [101]. In this year, Belviq (lorcaserin; selective 5-HT_{2C} receptor agonist, [161-163]) and Qsymia (a combination drug of phentermine; a sympathomimetic amine anorectic, and topiramate extended-release; an antiepileptic drug, [164-166]) were approved by FDA as new weight-loss drugs. Contrave, a combination of two well-established drugs, naltrexone and bupropion, in a sustained release formulation (SR), is also under-consideration [167]. The average body weight loss is around 10%, which is not so large even with instructed diet and exercise, and they are effective only while taking them. Orlistat 30-360 mg/day can reduce nearly 10% of body weight from baseline compared with 5–6% of those in the placebo-treated groups [168]. Belviq in conjunction with a lifestyle modification program can reduce body weight from baseline, –2.7%, –4.6%, –5.6% for placebo, 10mg BID, and 10 mg QD, respectively [161]. Qsymia, controlled-release phentermine/topiramate, in conjunction with a lifestyle modification program reduced body weight from baseline, –1.8%, –9.3%, and –10.5% for placebo, 7.5 mg phentermine/46 mg controlled release topiramate, and 15 mg phentermine/92 mg controlled release topiramate, respectively [164]. Contrave can reduce body weight from baseline, –1.3%, –5.0%, and –6.1% for placebo, 16 mg naltrexone plus 360 mg bupropion, and 32 mg naltrexone plus 360 mg bupropion, respectively [167].

Besides Orlistat, most pharmacotherapies for obesity have been to target pathways that promote satiety. Dietrich and Horvath raised the interesting hypothesis that hunger promotes a healthier and longer life, and compounds that target satiety pathways will ultimately promote the homeostatic mechanisms that are related to metabolic overload and therefore chronic disorders [101]. Also, it seems almost impossible to alter only feeding behavior and energy expenditure without affecting on many other brain functions. New targets of anti-obesity drugs are needed with much safety and efficacy. Recently, from the observation of type 2 diabetes treated by GLP-1 analogs, liraglutide and Exendin-4, which reduce appetite and body weight, has drawn attention as anti-obesity drug. A randomised, double-blind, placebo-controlled study of liraglutide showed that treatment with liraglutide, in addition to an energy-deficit diet and exercise program, led to a sustained, clinically relevant, dose-dependent weight loss that was significantly greater than that with placebo and orlistat [169]. In this study, 76% of individuals treated with high-dose liraglutide, 3.0 mg/day, lost more than 5% weight, and almost 30% of individuals treated with liraglutide 3.0 mg/day lost more than 10% weight after 20 weeks of treatment [169]. Further study on the same patients group done by the same group, high-dose liraglutide (2.4/3.0 mg/day) with a diet and exercise program was successfully sustained weight loss for 2 years [170]. Moreover, Simmons et al reported that Exendin-4 resulted in considerable reduction of body weight in a patient with severe hypothalamic obesity from hypothalamic germ cell tumor [171]

5.4.4. Surgery

On the other hand, use of bariatric surgery for severe obesity has increased dramatically. The most common operations are adjustable gastric banding, Roux-en-Y gastric bypass and sleevegastrectomy. Bariatric surgery demonstrated significant and durable weight loss as well as improvement in obesity-related comorbities [172]. Although, there is no large, adequately powered, long-term randomized controlled trials of clinical efficacy and safety of bariatric surgery compared with standard care, diet and exercise, yet. The American Association of Clinical Endocrinologists (AACE)/ The Obesity Society (TOS)/ the American Society for

Metabolic & Bariatric Surgery (ASMBS) Guidelines reported weight loss as percentage of excess body weight after bariatric surgery are, gastric banding; 29-87% for 1-2 follow-up years, 45-72% for 3-6 follow-up years, 14-60% for 7-10 follow-up years, Roux-en gastric bypass; 48-85% for 1-2 follow-up years, 53-77% for 3-6 follow-up years, 25-68% for 7-10 follow-up years, sleeve gastrectomy; 33-58% for 1-2 follow-up years, 66% for 3-6 follow-up years [173]. Selected criteria for bariatric surgery are certified by AACE/TOS/ASMBS Guidelines [173]. Patients with uncontrolled, severe psychiatric illness are excluded. As already discussed above, psychiatric and personality disorders are frequent in obese patients, particularly in morbidly obese patients before bariatric surgery. The procedure needs comprehension of risks, benefits, expected outcomes, alternatives, and lifestyle changes required with bariatric surgery. A psychological assessment is surely required before proposing such intervention. Literature reviews and numerous empirical studies have described significant improvements in psychosocial functioning after bariatric surgery [174-178]. Patients typically report decreases in symptoms of anxiety and depression and significant improvements in health-related quality of life [179-183]. Patients also typically report improvements in body image as well as marital and sexual functioning [184-186]. On the other hand, a negative psychological response to bariatric surgery also has been reported [29, 187-188]. For some patients, improvements in psychosocial status dissipate 2-3 years postoperatively [196, 197]. Other studies have documented suicides postoperatively [189-190]. Postoperative eating behavior is also documented. Some patients struggle to adhere to the recommended postoperative eating plan [173]. Among psychological factors improving after surgery, eating disorders have inconsistently been reported to disappear or not, consecutively to bariatric surgery [178, 192-194]. Bariatric surgery may lead to a physical impossibility of consuming unusually large amounts of food as required by binge eating disorders diagnosis criteria. However, loss of control on eating or grazing (frequently eating relatively small amounts of food) can appear or re-appear after surgery [178]. For that reason, eating behavior should not only be screened before, but also periodically after surgery [195]. Psychological factors assessed in patients before surgery did not have an impact on weight loss 2 years after surgery [178]. Increased caloric consumption above patients' postoperative caloric demands may contribute to suboptimal weight loss or even weight regain, which may begin as early as the second postoperative year [187, 190, 196-197]. To maintain long-term weight reduction after surgery, combination of the programs focusing on lifestyle modification as for non-bariatric obese patients is important [178, 195]. The changes in energy intake and energy expenditure after bariatric surgery may be affected by alternations in gut and adipocyte hormones [130, 198]. The reduced appetite seen after bariatric surgery has been attributed to changes in gut hormones, such as PYY, ghrelin, and GLP-1 [130]. But it is not clear how these hormonal changes affecting on mental status and the substantial outcome of weight control. A decrease in preference for both of sweet taste and high calorie foods has been demonstrated in animal models. The effect of bariatric surgery on the hedonic system in humans has been consistent with decreased activation of the hedonic system being demonstrated by fMRI and decreased preference for intake of high energy foods also being observed post-surgery [130]. The effect of bariatric surgery on dopamine signaling, which is involved in the hedonic system, is still not clear. Various studies utilizing questionnaires have demonstrated increased satiety and decreased hunger after bariatric surgery [130]. Understanding of the precise physiology of bariatric surgery could pave the way for the design of newer therapies to combat the epidemic of obesity [199].

6. Conclusion and future perspectives

Mental disorder is a critical dimension of obesity. It causes obesity, affects the development of obesity, and results of obesity. It varies among individuals, and does not simply parallel BMI. Evidence suggests a pathophysiologic relevance between obesity and mental disorder. We hypothesize that there is also common vulnerability towards metabolic dysregulation and mental disorder [Figure 7]. Although clinical findings continue to be accumulated, the precise mechanisms remain unclear. A better understanding of how mental function is modulated in the development of obesity, weight reduction, and weight regain should contribute to the development of effective treatments for obesity. In our laboratory, we are going to obtain new findings of "hunger" from animal experiments, which will promote new strategy for treatment of obesity and mental disorder complicated with obesity.

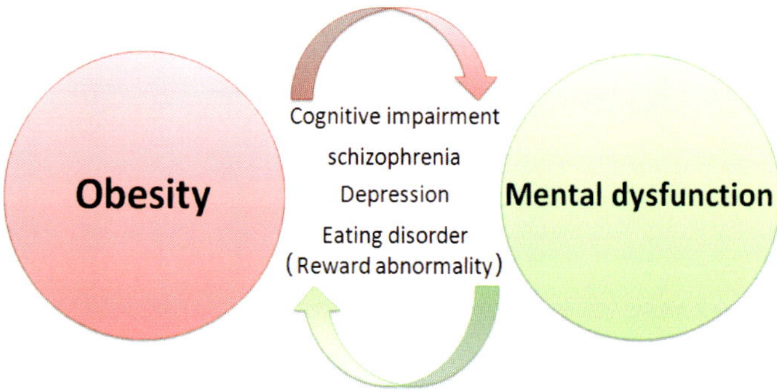

Figure 7. Schematic mutual interaction of obesity and mental disorder. The prevalence of cognitive impairment, schizophrenia, depression, and eating disorder increases in obesity. The prevalence of metabolic dysregulation, such as insulin resistance, hypertension, and dyslipidemia, in other words, metabolic syndrome and obesity are often co-morbid in mental disorder. These findings speculate that there are mutual interaction between obesity and mental disorder, common vulnerability and treatment possibility towards obesity and mental disorder.

Author details

Nobuko Yamada-Goto*, Goro Katsuura and Kazuwa Nakao

*Address all correspondence to: nobukito@kuhp.kyoto-u.ac.jp

Department of Medicine and Clinical Science, Kyoto University Graduate School of Medicine, Shogoin Kawahara-cho, Sakyo-ku, Kyoto, Japan

References

[1] Yamada N, Katsuura G, Ochi Y, Ebihara K, Kusakabe T, Hosoda K, Nakao K. Impaired CNS leptin action is implicated in depression associated with obesity. Endocrinology. 2011;152(7):2634-2643. http://dx.doi.org/10.1210/en.2011-0004.

[2] Yamada-Goto N, Katsuura G, Ochi Y, Ebihara K, Kusakabe T, Hosoda K, Nakao K. Impairment of fear-conditioning responses and changes of brain neurotrophic factors in diet-induced obese mice. J Neuroendocrinol. 2012;24(8):1120-1125. http://dx.doi.org/10.1111/j.1365-2826.2012.02327.x.

[3] Simon GE, Von Korff M, Saunders K, Miglioretti DL, Crane PK, van Belle G, Kessler RC. Association between obesity and psychiatric disorders in the US adult population. Arch Gen Psychiatry. 2006;63(7):824-830. http://dx.doi.org/10.1001/archpsyc.63.7.824.

[4] Malnick SD, Knobler H. The medical complications of obesity. QJM. 2006;99(9):565-579. http://dx.doi.org/10.1093/qjmed/hcl085.

[5] Marcus MD, Wildes JE. Obesity: is it a mental disorder? Int J Eat Disord. 2009;42(8):739-753. http://dx.doi.org/10.1002/eat.20725.

[6] Elias MF, Elias PK, Sullivan LM, Wolf PA, D'Agostino RB. Lower cognitive function in the presence of obesity and hypertension: the Framingham heart study. Int J Obes Relat Metab Disord. 2003;27(2):260-268. http://dx.doi.org/10.1038/sj.ijo.802225.

[7] Farr SA, Yamada KA, Butterfield DA, Abdul HM, Xu L, Miller NE, Banks WA, Morley JE. Obesity and hypertriglyceridemia produce cognitive impairment. Endocrinology. 2008;149(5):2628-2636. http://dx.doi.org/10.1210/en.2007-1722.

[8] International Obesity Taskforce. IOTF: The Global Epidemic: IASO/IOTF analysis 2010. http://www.iaso.org/iotf/obesity/obesitytheglobalepidemic/ (accessed 19 September 2012).

[9] World Health Organization. WHO: Obesity and overweight: http://www.who.int/mediacentre/factsheets/fs311/en/index.html (accessed 19 September 2012).

[10] Chiu M, Austin PC, Manuel DG, Shah BR, Tu JV. Deriving ethnic-specific BMI cutoff points for assessing diabetes risk. Diabetes Care. 2011;34(8):1741-1748. http://dx.doi.org/10.2337/dc10-2300.

[11] World Health Organization Western Pacific Region, International Association for the Study of Obesity, International Obesity Task Force. The Asia-Pacific perspective: Redefining obesity and its treatment. February 2000. http://www.wpro.who.int/nutrition/documents/Redefining_obesity/en/index.html (accessed 19 September 2012).

[12] Swinburn BA, Sacks G, Hall KD, McPherson K, Finegood DT, Moodie ML, Gortmaker SL. The global obesity pandemic: shaped by global drivers and local environ-

ments. Lancet. 2011;378(9793):804-814. http://dx.doi.org/10.1016/S0140-6736(11)60813-1.

[13] Japan Society for the Study of Obesity. JASSO: The Diagnostic Criteria of Obesity 2011 (in Japanese) Journal of Japan Society for the Study of Obesity. 2011;50(17):1-2. http://www.jasso.or.jp/(accessed 19 September 2012).

[14] Bao Y, Lu J, Wang C, Yang M, Li H, Zhang X, Zhu J, Lu H, Jia W, Xiang K. Optimal waist circumference cutoffs for abdominal obesity in Chinese. Atherosclerosis. 2008;201(2):378-384. http://dx.doi.org/10.1016/j.atherosclerosis.2008.03.001.

[15] Kim JA, Choi CJ, Yum KS. Cut-off values of visceral fat area and waist circumference: diagnostic criteria for abdominal obesity in a Korean population. J Korean Med Sci. 2006;21(6):1048-1053. http://dx.doi.org/10.3346/jkms.2006.21.6.1048

[16] Pan WH, Lee MS, Chuang SY, Lin YC, Fu ML. Obesity pandemic, correlated factors and guidelines to define, screen and manage obesity in Taiwan. Obes Rev. 2008;9 Suppl 1:22-31. http://dx.doi.org/10.1111/j.1467-789X.2007.00434.x.

[17] Calle EE, Thun MJ, Petrelli JM, Rodriguez C, Heath CW Jr. Body-mass index and mortality in a prospective cohort of U.S. adults. N Engl J Med. 1999;341(15): 1097-1105. http://dx.doi.org/10.1056/NEJM199910073411501

[18] Klein S, Wadden T, Sugerman HJ. AGA technical review on obesity. Gastroenterology. 2002;123(3):882-932. http://dx.doi.org/ 10.1053/gast.2002.35514.

[19] Flegal KM, Graubard BI, Williamson DF, GailMH. Excess deaths associated with underweight, overweight, and obesity. JAMA. 2005;293(15):1861-1867. http://dx.doi.org/10.1001/jama.293.15.1861

[20] Adams KF, Schatzkin A, Harris TB, Kipnis V, Mouw T, Ballard-Barbash R, Hollenbeck A, Leitzmann MF. Overweight, obesity, and mortality in a large prospective cohort of persons 50 to 71 years old. N Engl J Med. 2006;355(8):763-778. http://dx.doi.org/10.1056/NEJMoa055643

[21] Wang YC, McPherson K, Marsh T, Gortmaker SL, Brown M. Health and economi c burden of the projected obesity trends in the USA and the UK. Lancet. 2011;378(9793):815-825. http://dx.doi.org/10.1016/S0140-6736(11)60814-3.

[22] Stevens J, Cai J, Pamuk ER, Williamson DF, Thun MJ, Wood JL. The effect of age on the association between body-mass index and mortality. N Engl J Med. 1998;338(1): 1-7. http://dx.doi.org/10.1056/NEJM199801013380101

[23] Kopelman PG. Obesity as a medical problem. Nature. 2000;404(6778):635-643. http://dx.doi.org/10.1038/35007508.

[24] Whitmer RA, Gunderson EP, Barrett-Connor E, Quesenberry CP Jr, Yaffe K. Obesity in middle age and future risk of dementia: a 27 year longitudinal population based study. BMJ. 2005330(7504):1360. http://dx.doi.org/10.1136/bmj.38446.466238.E0.

[25] Pagoto S, Bodenlos JS, Kantor L, Gitkind M, Curtin C, Ma Y. Association of major depression and binge eating disorder with weight loss in a clinical setting. Obesity (Silver Spring). 2007;15(11):2557-2259. http://dx.doi.org/10.1038/oby.2007.307.

[26] Stunkard AJ, Faith MS, Allison KC. Depression and obesity. Biol Psychiatry. 2003;54(3):330-337. http://dx.doi.org/10.1016/S0006-3223(03)00608-5

[27] Scott KM, Bruffaerts R, Simon GE, Alonso J, Angermeyer M, de Girolamo G, Demyttenaere K, Gasquet I, Haro JM, Karam E, Kessler RC, Levinson D, Medina Mora ME, Oakley Browne MA, Ormel J, Villa JP, Uda H, Von Korff M. Obesity and mental disorders in the general population: results from the world mental health surveys. Int J Obes (Lond). 2008;32(1):192-200. http://dx.doi.org/10.1038/sj.ijo.0803701.

[28] Gariepy G, Wang J, Lesage AD, Schmitz N. The longitudinal association from obesity to depression: results from the 12-year National Population Health Survey. Obesity (Silver Spring). 2010;18(5):1033-1038. http://dx.doi.org/10.1038/oby.2009.333.

[29] Zhao G, Ford ES, Dhingra S, Li C, Strine TW, Mokdad AH. Depression and anxiety among US adults: associations with body mass index. Int J Obes (Lond). 2009;33(2): 257-266. http://dx.doi.org/10.1038/ijo.2008.268.

[30] de Wit L, Luppino F, van Straten A, Penninx B, Zitman F, Cuijpers P. Depression and obesity: a meta-analysis of community-based studies. Psychiatry Res. 2010;178(2): 230-235. http://dx.doi.org/10.1016/j.psychres.2009.04.015.

[31] Petry NM, Barry D, Pietrzak RH, Wagner JA. Overweight and obesity are associated with psychiatric disorders: results from the National Epidemiologic Survey on Alcohol and Related Conditions. Psychosom Med. 2008;70(3):288-297. http://dx.doi.org/10.1097/PSY.0b013e3181651651.

[32] American Psychiatric Association (2000): Diagnostic and Statistical Manual of Mental Disorders: DSM-IV-TR. 4th ed. Washington, DC: American Psychiatric Association.

[33] Frank GK, Reynolds JR, Shott ME, Jappe L, Yang TT, Tregellas JR, O'Reilly RC. Anorexia nervosa and obesity are associated with opposite brain reward response. Neuropsychopharmacology. 2012;37(9):2031-2046. http://dx.doi.org/10.1038/npp.2012.51.

[34] Fladung AK, Grön G, Grammer K, Herrnberger B, Schilly E, Grasteit S, Wolf RC, Walter H, von Wietersheim J. A neural signature of anorexia nervosa in the ventral striatal reward system. Am J Psychiatry. 2010;167(2):206-212. http://dx.doi.org/10.1176/appi.ajp.2009.09010071.

[35] Zink CF, Weinberger DR. Cracking the moody brain: the rewards of self starvation. Nat Med. 2010;16(12):1382-1383. http://dx.doi.org/10.1038/nm1210-1382.

[36] Holsen LM, Lawson EA, Blum J, Ko E, Makris N, Fazeli PK, Klibanski A, Goldstein JM. Food motivation circuitry hypoactivation related to hedonic and nonhedonic aspects of hunger and satiety in women with active anorexia nervosa and weight-re-

stored women with anorexia nervosa. J Psychiatry Neurosci. 2012;37(5):322-332. http://dx.doi.org/10.1503/jpn.110156.

[37] Elfhag K, Rossner S, Lindgren T, Andersson I, Carlsson AM. Rorschach personality predictors of weight loss with behavior modification in obesity treatment. J Pers Assess. 2004;83(3):293-305. http://dx.doi.org/10.1207/s15327752jpa8303_11.

[38] Provencher V, Bégin C, Gagnon-Girouard MP, Tremblay A, Boivin S, Lemieux S. Personality traits in overweight and obese women: associations with BMI and eating behaviors. Eat Behav. 2008;9(3):294-302. http://dx.doi.org/10.1016/j.eatbeh.2007.10.004.

[39] Terracciano A, Sutin AR, McCrae RR, Deiana B, Ferrucci L, Schlessinger D, Uda M, Costa PT Jr. Facets of personality linked to underweight and overweight. Psychosom Med. 2009;71(6):682-689. http://dx.doi.org/10.1097/PSY.0b013e3181a2925b.

[40] Sutin AR, Ferrucci L, Zonderman AB, Terracciano A. Personality and obesity across the adult life span.J PersSoc Psychol. 2011;101(3):579-592. http://dx.doi.org/10.1037/a0024286.

[41] Munro IA, Bore MR, Munro D, Garg ML. Using personality as a predictor of diet induced weight loss and weight management. Int J Behav Nutr Phys Act. 2011;8:129. http://dx.doi.org/10.1186/1479-5868-8-129.

[42] Luppino FS, de Wit LM, Bouvy PF, Stijnen T, Cuijpers P, Penninx BW, Zitman FG. Overweight, obesity, and depression: a systematic review and meta-analysis of longitudinal studies. Arch Gen Psychiatry. 2010;67(3):220-229. http://dx.doi.org/10.1001/archgenpsychiatry.2010.2.

[43] Puhl RM, Moss-Racusin CA, Schwartz MB, Brownell KD. Weight stigmatization and bias reduction: perspectives of overweight and obese adults. Health Educ Res. 2008;23(2):347-358. http://dx.doi.org/10.1093/her/cym052.

[44] Crandall CS. Prejudice against fat people: ideology and self-interest. J PersSoc Psychol. 1994;66(5):882-894. http://dx.doi.org/10.1037/0022-3514.66.5.882.

[45] Roehling MV, RoehlingPV, Odland LM. Investigating the validity of stereotypes about overweight employees: the relationship between body weight and normal personality traits. Group and Organization Management. 2008;33(4):392-424. http://dx.doi.org/10.1177/1059601108321518.

[46] Cazettes F, Cohen JI, Yau PL, Talbot H, Convit A. Obesity-mediated inflammation may damage the brain circuit that regulates food intake. Brain Res. 2011;1373:101-109. http://dx.doi.org/10.1016/j.brainres.2010.12.008.

[47] Yoshida S, Murano S, Saito Y, Inadera H, Tashiro J, Kobayashi J,Tadokoro N,Kanzaki T, Shinomiya M, Morisaki N, OhonoK, Ishikawa Y, Shirai K, Azuma Y, Kodama K. Treatment of obesity by personality classification-oriented program. Obes Res. 1995;3 Suppl 2:205s-209s. http://dx.doi.org/10.1002/j.1550-8528.1995.tb00465.x

[48] Lumeng CN, Saltiel AR. Inflammatory links between obesity and metabolic disease. J Clin Invest. 2011;121(6):2111-2117. http://dx.doi.org/10.1172/JCI57132.

[49] Gregor MF, Hotamisligil GS. Inflammatory mechanisms in obesity. Annu Rev Immunol. 2011;29:415-445. http://dx.doi.org/10.1146/annurev-immunol-031210-101322.

[50] Banks WA, Ortiz L, Plotkin SR, Kastin AJ. Human interleukin (IL) 1 alpha, murine IL-1 alpha and murine IL-1 beta are transported from blood to brain in the mouse by a shared saturable mechanism. J Pharmacol Exp Ther. 1991;259(3):988-996.

[51] Pan W, Kastin AJ. TNFalpha transport across the blood-brain barrier is abolished in receptor knockout mice. Exp Neurol. 2002;174(2):193-200. http://dx.doi.org/10.1006/exnr.2002.7871.

[52] Goehler LE, Gaykema RP, Opitz N, Reddaway R, Badr N, Lyte M. Activation in vagal afferents and central autonomic pathways: early responses to intestinal infection with Campylobacter jejuni. Brain Behav Immun. 2005;19(4):334-344. http://dx.doi.org/10.1016/j.bbi.2004.09.002.

[53] Fung A, Vizcaychipi M, Lloyd D, Wan Y, Ma D. Central nervous system inflammation in disease related conditions: mechanistic prospects. Brain Res. 2012;1446:144-155. http://dx.doi.org/10.1016/j.brainres.2012.01.061.

[54] Laine PS, Schwartz EA, Wang Y, Zhang WY, Karnik SK, Musi N, Reaven PD. Palmitic acid induces IP-10 expression in human macrophages via NF-kappaB activation. Biochem Biophys Res Commun. 2007;358(1):150-155. http://dx.doi.org/10.1016/j.bbrc.2007.04.092,

[55] Gupta S, Knight AG, Gupta S, Keller JN, Bruce-Keller AJ. Saturated long-chain fatty acids activate inflammatory signaling in astrocytes. J Neurochem. 2012;120(6):1060-1071. http://dx.doi.org/10.1111/j.1471-4159.2012.07660.x.

[56] Thaler JP, Yi CX, Schur EA, Guyenet SJ, Hwang BH, Dietrich MO, Zhao X, Sarruf DA, Izgur V, Maravilla KR, Nguyen HT, Fischer JD, Matsen ME, Wisse BE, Morton GJ, Horvath TL, Baskin DG, Tschöp MH, Schwartz MW. Obesity is associated with hypothalamic injury in rodents and humans. J Clin Invest. 2012;122(1):153-162. http://dx.doi.org/10.1172/JCI59660.

[57] Jeon BT, Jeong EA, Shin HJ, Lee Y, Lee DH, Kim HJ, Kang SS, Cho GJ, Choi WS, Roh GS. Resveratrol attenuates obesity-associated peripheral and central inflammation and improves memory deficit in mice fed a high-fat diet. Diabetes. 2012;61(6):1444-1454. http://dx.doi.org/10.2337/db11-1498.

[58] Thaler JP, Schwartz MW. Minireview: Inflammation and obesity pathogenesis: the hypothalamus heats up. Endocrinology. 2010;151(9):4109-4115. http://dx.doi.org/10.1210/en.2010-0336.

[59] Yi CX, Al-Massadi O, Donelan E, Lehti M, Weber J, Ress C, Trivedi C, Müller TD, Woods SC, Hofmann SM. Exercise protects against high-fat diet-induced hypothala-

mic inflammation. Physiol Behav. 2012;106(4):485-490. http://dx.doi.org/10.1016/j.physbeh.2012.03.021.

[60] Schwartz MW, Peskind E, Raskind M, Boyko EJ, Porter Jr D. Cerebrospinal fluid leptin levels: relationship to plasma levels and to adiposity in humans. Nat Med. 1996;2(5):589-93. http://dx.doi.org/10.1038/nm0596-589.

[61] Myers MG, Cowley MA, Münzberg H. Mechanisms of leptin action and leptin resistance. Annu Rev Physiol. 2008;70:537-556. http://dx.doi.org/10.1146/annurev.physiol.70.113006.100707.

[62] Zabolotny JM, Kim YB, Welsh LA, Kershaw EE, Neel BG, Kahn BB. Protein-tyrosine phosphatase 1B expression is induced by inflammation in vivo. J Biol Chem. 2008;283(21):14230-14241. http://dx.doi.org/10.1074/jbc.M800061200.

[63] White CL, Pistell PJ, Purpera MN, Gupta S, Fernandez-Kim SO, Hise TL, Keller JN, Ingram DK, Morrison CD, Bruce-Keller AJ. Effects of high fat diet on Morris maze performance, oxidative stress, and inflammation in rats: contributions of maternal diet. Neurobiol Dis. 2009;35(1):3-13. http://dx.doi.org/10.1016/j.nbd.2009.04.002.

[64] Pistell PJ, Morrison CD, Gupta S, Knight AG, Keller JN, Ingram DK, Bruce-Keller AJ. Cognitive impairment following high fat diet consumption is associated with brain inflammation. J Neuroimmunol. 2010;219(1-2):25-32. http://dx.doi.org/10.1016/j.jneuroim.2009.11.010.

[65] Cizza G, Ronsaville DS, Kleitz H, Eskandari F, Mistry S, Torvik S, Sonbolian N, Reynolds JC, Blackman MR, Gold PW, Martinez PE; P.O.W.E.R. (Premenopausal, Osteopenia/Osteoporosis, Women, Alendronate, Depression) Study Group. Clinical subtypes of depression are associated with specific metabolic parameters and circadian endocrine profiles in women: the power study. PLoS One. 2012;7(1):e28912. http://dx.doi.org/10.1371/journal.pone.0028912.

[66] Richardson LP, Davis R, Poulton R, McCauley E, Moffitt TE, Caspi A, Connell F. A longitudinal evaluation of adolescent depression and adult obesity. Arch Pediatr Adolesc Med. 2003;157(8):739-745. http://dx.doi.org/10.1001/archpedi.157.8.739.

[67] Krishnan V, Nestler EJ. The molecular neurobiology of depression. Nature. 2008;455(7215):894-902. http://dx.doi.org/10.1038/nature07455.

[68] Lu XY, Kim CS, Frazer A, Zhang W. Leptin: a potential novel antidepressant. ProcNatlAcadSci U S A. 2006;103(5):1593-1598. http://dx.doi.org/10.1073/pnas.0508901103

[69] Kraus T, Haack M, Schuld A, Hinze-Selch D, Pollmächer T. Low leptin levels but normal body mass indices in patients with depression or schizophrenia. Neuroendocrinology. 2001;73(4):243-247. http://dx.doi.org/10.1159/000054641.

[70] Westling S, Ahrén B, Träskman-Bendz L, Westrin A. Low CSF leptin in female suicide attempters with major depression. J Affect Disord. 2004;81(1):41-48. http://dx.doi.org/10.1016/j.jad.2003.07.002.

[71] Porsolt RD, Bertin A, Jalfre M. Behavioral despair in mice: a primary screening test for antidepressants. Arch Int Pharmacodyn Ther. 1977;229(2):327-336.

[72] Lucki I. The forced swimming test as a model for core and component behavioral effects of antidepressant drugs. Behav Pharmacol. 1997;8(6-7):523-532. http://dx.doi.org/10.1097/00008877-199711000-00010.

[73] Enriori PJ, Evans AE, Sinnayah P, Jobst EE, Tonelli-Lemos L, Billes SK, Glavas MM, Grayson BE, Perello M, Nillni EA, Grove KL, Cowley MA. Diet-induced obesity causes severe but reversible leptin resistance in arcuate melanocortin neurons. Cell Metab. 2007;5(3):181-194. http://dx.doi.org/10.1016/j.cmet.2007.02.004.

[74] Shirayama Y, Chen AC, Nakagawa S, Russell DS, Duman RS. Brain-derived neurotrophic factor produces antidepressant effects in behavioral models of depression. J Neurosci. 2002;22(8):3251-3261. http://dx.doi.org/10.3410/f.1005737.68355

[75] Karege F, Vaudan G, Schwald M, Perroud N, La Harpe R. Neurotrophin levels in postmortem brains of suicide victims and the effects of antemortem diagnosis and psychotropic drugs. Brain Res Mol Brain Res. 2005;136(1-2):29-37. http://dx.doi.org/10.1016/j.molbrainres.2004.12.020.

[76] Pearson S, Schmidt M, Patton G, Dwyer T, Blizzard L, Otahal P, Venn A. Depression and insulin resistance: cross-sectional associations in young adults. Diabetes Care. 2010;33(5):1128-1133. http://dx.doi.org/10.2337/dc09-1940.

[77] Ahola AJ, Thorn LM, Saraheimo M, Forsblom C, Groop PH; Finndiane Study Group. Depression is associated with the metabolic syndrome among patients with type 1 diabetes. Ann Med. 2010;42(7):495-501. http://dx.doi.org/10.3109/07853890.2010.503660.

[78] Lutter M, Sakata I, Osborne-Lawrence S, Rovinsky SA, Anderson JG, Jung S, Birnbaum S, Yanagisawa M, Elmquist JK, Nestler EJ, Zigman JM. The orexigenic hormone ghrelin defends against depressive symptoms of chronic stress. Nat Neurosci. 2008;11(7):752-753. http://dx.doi.org/10.1038/nn.2139.

[79] Faulconbridge LF, Wadden TA, Berkowitz RI, Pulcini ME, Treadwell T. Treatment of Comorbid Obesity and Major Depressive Disorder: A Prospective Pilot Study for their Combined Treatment. J Obes. 2011;2011:870385. http://dx.doi.org/10.1155/2011/870385.

[80] Fabricatore AN, Wadden TA, Higginbotham AJ, Faulconbridge LF, Nguyen AM, Heymsfield SB, Faith MS. Intentional weight loss and changes in symptoms of depression: a systematic review and meta-analysis. Int J Obes (Lond). 2011;35(11):1363-1376. http://dx.doi.org/10.1038/ijo.2011.2.

[81] Anstey KJ, Cherbuin N, Budge M, Young J. Body mass index in midlife and late-life as a risk factor for dementia: a meta-analysis of prospective studies. Obes Rev. 2011;12(5):e426-437. http://dx.doi.org/10.1111/j.1467-789X.2010.00825.x.

[82] Levine ME, Crimmins EM. Sarcopenic obesity and cognitive functioning: the mediating roles of insulin resistance and inflammation? Curr Gerontol Geriatr Res. 2012;2012:826398. http://dx.doi.org/10.1155/2012/826398.

[83] Gustafson D, Lissner L, Bengtsson C, Björkelund C, Skoog I. A 24-year follow-up of body mass index and cerebral atrophy. Neurology. 2004;63(10):1876-1881. http://dx.doi.org/10.1212/01.WNL.0000141850.47773.5F.

[84] Gustafson DR, Steen B, Skoog I. Body mass index and white matter lesions in elderly women. An 18-year longitudinal study. Int Psychogeriatr. 2004;16(3):327-336. http://dx.doi.org/10.1017/S1041610204000353.

[85] Hannon TS, Rofey DL, Ryan CM, Clapper DA, Chakravorty S, Arslanian SA. Relationships among obstructive sleep apnea, anthropometric measures, and neurocognitive functioning in adolescents with severe obesity. J Pediatr. 2012;160(5):732-735. http://dx.doi.org/10.1016/j.jpeds.2011.10.029.

[86] Schmidt R, Schmidt H, Curb JD, Masaki K, White LR, Launer LJ. Early inflammation and dementia: a 25-year follow-up of the Honolulu-Asia Aging Study. Ann Neurol. 2002;52(2):168-174.http://dx.doi.org/10.1002/ana.10265.

[87] Wolf PA, Beiser A, Elias MF, Au R, Vasan RS, Seshadri S. Relation of obesity to cognitive function: importance of central obesity and synergistic influence of concomitant hypertension. The Framingham Heart Study. Curr Alzheimer Res. 2007;4(2): 111-116. http://dx.doi.org/10.2174/156720507780362263.

[88] Lindqvist A, Mohapel P, Bouter B, Frielingsdorf H, Pizzo D, Brundin P, Erlanson-Albertsson C. High-fat diet impairs hippocampal neurogenesis in male rats. Eur J Neurol. 2006;13(12):1385-1388. http://dx.doi.org/10.1111/j.1468-1331.2006.01500.x

[89] Korte M, Carroll P, Wolf E, Brem G, Thoenen H, Bonhoeffer T. Hippocampal long-term potentiation is impaired in mice lacking brain-derived neurotrophic factor. ProcNatlAcadSci U S A. 1995;92(19):8856-8860. http://dx.doi.org/10.1073/pnas.92.19.8856.

[90] McAllister AK, Katz LC, Lo DC. Opposing roles for endogenous BDNF and NT-3 in regulating cortical dendritic growth. Neuron. 1997;18(5):767-778. http://dx.doi.org/10.1016/S0896-6273(00)80316-5.

[91] Adamson CL, Reid MA, Davis RL. Opposite actions of brain-derived neurotrophic factor and neurotrophin-3 on firing features and ion channel composition of murine spiral ganglion neurons. J Neurosci. 2002;22(4):1385-1396.

[92] Wickelgren I. Tracking insulin to the mind. Science. 1998;280(5363):517-519. http://dx.doi.org/10.1126/science.280.5363.517

[93] Gerges NZ, AleisaAM, Alkadhi KA. Impaired long-term potentiation in obese zucker rats: possible involvement of presynaptic mechanism. Neuroscience. 2003;120(2): 535-539. http://dx.doi.org/10.1016/S0306-4522(03)00297-5.

[94] Gispen WH, Biessels GJ. Cognition and synaptic plasticity in diabetes mellitus. Trends Neurosci. 2000;23(11):542-549. http://dx.doi.org/10.1016/S0166-2236(00)01656-8.

[95] Greenwood CE, Winocur G. High-fat diets, insulin resistance and declining cognitive function. Neurobiol Aging. 2005;26 Suppl 1:42-45. http://dx.doi.org/10.1016/j.neurobiolaging.2005.08.017.

[96] Matias I, Di Marzo V. Endocannabinoids and the control of energy balance. Trends Endocrinol Metab. 2007;18(1):27-37. http://dx.doi.org/10.1038/ijo.2009.67.

[97] Berthoud HR, Morrison C. The brain, appetite, and obesity. Annu Rev Psychol. 2008;59:55-92. http://dx.doi.org/10.1146/annurev.psych.59.103006.093551.

[98] Hetherington AW, Ranson SW. Hypothalamic lesions and adiposity in rats. Anat Rec (Hoboken). 1940;78:149-172.

[99] Anand BK, Brobeck JR. Localization of a "feeding center" in the hypothalamus of the rat. Proc Soc Exp Biol Med. 1951;77(2):323-324. http://dx.doi.org/10.3181/00379727-77-18766.

[100] Elmquist JK, Elias CF, Saper CB. From lesions to leptin: hypothalamic control of food intake and body weight. Neuron. 1999;22(2):221-232. http://dx.doi.org/10.1016/S0896-6273(00)81084-3.

[101] Dietrich MO, Horvath TL. Limitations in anti-obesity drug development: the critical role of hunger-promoting neurons. Nat Rev Drug Discov. 2012;11(9):675-691. http://dx.doi.org/10.1038/nrd3739.

[102] Cluny NL, Reimer RA, Sharkey KA. Cannabinoid signalling regulates inflammation and energy balance: the importance of the brain-gut axis. Brain Behav Immun. 2012;26(5):691-698. http://dx.doi.org/10.1016/j.bbi.2012.01.004.

[103] Schwartz MW, Gelling RW. Rats lighten up with MCH antagonist. Nat Med. 2002;8(8):779-781. http://dx.doi.org/10.1038/nm0802-779.

[104] Kilduff TS, de Lecea L. Mapping of the mRNAs for the hypocretin/orexin and melanin-concentrating hormone receptors: networks of overlapping peptide systems. J Comp Neurol. 2001;435(1):1-5. http://dx.doi.org/10.1002/cne.1189.

[105] Volkow ND, Wang GJ, Baler RD. Reward, dopamine and the control of food intake: implications for obesity. Trends Cogn Sci. 2011;15(1):37-46. http://dx.doi.org/10.1016/j.tics.2010.11.001.

[106] Kanoski SE, Hayes MR, Greenwald HS, Fortin SM, Gianessi CA, Gilbert JR, Grill HJ. Hippocampal leptin signaling reduces food intake and modulates food-related memory processing. Neuropsychopharmacology. 2011;36(9):1859-1870. http://dx.doi.org/10.1038/npp.2011.70.

[107] Tao YX. The melanocortin-4 receptor: physiology, pharmacology, and pathophysiology. Endocr Rev. 2010;31(4):506-543. http://dx.doi.org/10.1210/er.2009-0037.

[108] Wardlaw SL. Hypothalamic proopiomelanocortin processing and the regulation of energy balance. Eur J Pharmacol. 2011;660(1):213-219. http://dx.doi.org/10.1016/j.ejphar.2010.10.107.

[109] Haskell-Luevano C, Monck EK. Agouti-related protein functions as an inverse agonist at a constitutively active brain melanocortin-4 receptor. Regul Pept. 2001;99(1):1-7. http://dx.doi.org/10.1016/S0167-0115(01)00234-8.

[110] Yeo GS, Farooqi IS, Aminian S, Halsall DJ, Stanhope RG, O'Rahilly S. A frameshift mutation in MC4R associated with dominantly inherited human obesity. Nat Genet. 1998;20(2):111-112. http://dx.doi.org/10.1038/2404.

[111] Farooqi IS, Yeo GS, Keogh JM, Aminian S, Jebb SA, Butler G, Cheetham T, O'Rahilly S. Dominant and recessive inheritance of morbid obesity associated with melanocortin 4 receptor deficiency. J Clin Invest. 2000;106(2):271-279. http://dx.doi.org/10.1172/JCI9397.

[112] Govaerts C, Srinivasan S, Shapiro A, Zhang S, Picard F, Clement K, Lubrano-Berthelier C, Vaisse C. Obesity-associated mutations in the melanocortin 4 receptor provide novel insights into its function. Peptides. 2005;26(10):1909-1919. http://dx.doi.org/10.1016/j.peptides.2004.11.042.

[113] Pandit R, de Jong JW, Vanderschuren LJ, Adan RA. Neurobiology of overeating and obesity: the role of melanocortins and beyond. Eur J Pharmacol. 2011;660(1):28-42. http://dx.doi.org/10.1016/j.ejphar.2011.01.034.

[114] Loos RJ, Lindgren CM, Li S, Wheeler E, Zhao JH, Prokopenko I, Inouye M, Freathy RM, Attwood AP, Beckmann JS, Berndt SI; Prostate, Lung, Colorectal, and Ovarian (PLCO) Cancer Screening Trial, Jacobs KB, Chanock SJ, Hayes RB, Bergmann S, Bennett AJ, Bingham SA, Bochud M, Brown M, Cauchi S, Connell JM, Cooper C, Smith GD, Day I, Dina C, De S, Dermitzakis ET, Doney AS, Elliott KS, Elliott P, Evans DM, Sadaf Farooqi I, Froguel P, Ghori J, Groves CJ, Gwilliam R, Hadley D, Hall AS, Hattersley AT, Hebebrand J, Heid IM; KORA, Lamina C, Gieger C, Illig T, Meitinger T, Wichmann HE, Herrera B, Hinney A, Hunt SE, Jarvelin MR, Johnson T, Jolley JD, Karpe F, Keniry A, Khaw KT, Luben RN, Mangino M, Marchini J, McArdle WL, McGinnis R, Meyre D, Munroe PB, Morris AD, Ness AR, Neville MJ, Nica AC, Ong KK, O'Rahilly S, Owen KR, Palmer CN, Papadakis K, Potter S, Pouta A, Qi L; Nurses' Health Study, Randall JC, Rayner NW, Ring SM, Sandhu MS, Scherag A, Sims MA, Song K, Soranzo N, Speliotes EK; Diabetes Genetics Initiative, Syddall HE, Teichmann SA, Timpson NJ, Tobias JH, Uda M; SardiNIA Study, Vogel CI, Wallace C, Waterworth DM, Weedon MN; Wellcome Trust Case Control Consortium, Willer CJ; FUSION, Wraight, Yuan X, Zeggini E, Hirschhorn JN, Strachan DP, Ouwehand WH, Caulfield MJ, Samani NJ, Frayling TM, Vollenweider P, Waeber G, Mooser V, Deloukas P, McCarthy MI, Wareham NJ, Barroso I, Jacobs KB, Chanock SJ, Hayes RB, Lam-

ina C, Gieger C, Illig T, Meitinger T, Wichmann HE, Kraft P, Hankinson SE, Hunter DJ, Hu FB, Lyon HN, Voight BF, Ridderstrale M, Groop L, Scheet P, Sanna S, Abecasis GR, Albai G, Nagaraja R, Schlessinger D, Jackson AU, Tuomilehto J, Collins FS, Boehnke M, Mohlke KL. Common variants near MC4R are associated with fat mass, weight and risk of obesity. Nat Genet. 2008;40(6):768-775. http://dx.doi.org/10.1038/ng.140.

[115] Chen AS, Marsh DJ, Trumbauer ME, Frazier EG, Guan XM, Yu H, Rosenblum CI, Vongs A, Feng Y, Cao L, Metzger JM, Strack AM, Camacho RE, Mellin TN, Nunes CN, Min W, Fisher J, Gopal-Truter S, MacIntyre DE, Chen HY, Van der Ploeg LH. Inactivation of the mouse melanocortin-3 receptor results in increased fat mass and reduced lean body mass. Nat Genet. 2000;26(1):97-102. http://dx.doi.org/10.1038/79254.

[116] Krude H, Biebermann H, Luck W, Horn R, Brabant G, Grüters A. Severe early-onset obesity, adrenal insufficiency and red hair pigmentation caused by POMC mutations in humans. Nat Genet. 1998;19(2):155-157. http://dx.doi.org/10.1038/509.

[117] Argyropoulos G, Rankinen T, Neufeld DR, Rice T, Province MA, Leon AS, Skinner JS, Wilmore JH, Rao DC, Bouchard C. A Polymorphism in the Human Agouti-Related Protein Is Associated with Late-Onset Obesity. J Clin Endocrinol Metab. 2002;87(9):4198-4202. http://dx.doi.org/10.1210/jc.2002-011834.

[118] Farooqi IS. Genetic aspects of severe childhood obesity. Pediatr Endocrinol Rev. 2006;3 Suppl 4:528-536.

[119] Montague CT, Farooqi IS, Whitehead JP, Soos MA, Rau H, Wareham NJ, Sewter CP, Digby JE, Mohammed SN, Hurst JA, Cheetham CH, Earley AR, Barnett AH, Prins JB, O'Rahilly S. Congenital leptin deficiency is associated with severe early-onset obesity in humans. Nature. 1997;387(6636):903-908. http://dx.doi.org/10.1038/43185.

[120] Clément K, Vaisse C, Lahlou N, Cabrol S, Pelloux V, Cassuto D, Gourmelen M, Dina C, Chambaz J, Lacorte JM, Basdevant A, Bougnères P, Lebouc Y, Froguel P, Guy-Grand B. A mutation in the human leptin receptor gene causes obesity and pituitary dysfunction. Nature. 1998;392(6674):398-401. http://dx.doi.org/10.1038/32911

[121] Jackson RS, Creemers JW, Ohagi S, Raffin-Sanson ML, Sanders L, Montague CT, Hutton JC, O'Rahilly S. Obesity and impaired prohormone processing associated with mutations in the human prohormone convertase 1 gene. Nat Genet. 1997;16(3): 303-306. http://dx.doi.org/10.1038/ng0797-303

[122] Huang XF, Han M, South T, Storlien L. Altered levels of POMC, AgRP and MC4 R mRNA expression in the hypothalamus and other parts of the limbic system of mice prone or resistant to chronic high-energy diet-induced obesity. Brain Res. 2003;992(1):9-19. http://dx.doi.org/10.1016/j.brainres.2003.08.019.

[123] Chandler PC, Viana JB, Oswald KD, Wauford PK, Boggiano MM. Feeding response to melanocortin agonist predicts preference for and obesity from a high-fat diet. Physiol Behav. 2005;85(2):221-230. http://dx.doi.org/10.1016/j.physbeh.2005.04.011

[124] Morton GJ, Cummings DE, Baskin DG, Barsh GS, Schwartz MW. Central nervous system control of food intake and body weight. Nature. 2006;443(7109):289-295. http://dx.doi.org/10.1038/nature05026.

[125] Wang GJ, Volkow ND, Logan J, Pappas NR, Wong CT, Zhu W, Netusil N, Fowler JS. Brain dopamine and obesity. Lancet. 2001;357(9253):354-357. http://dx.doi.org/10.1016/S0140-6736(00)03643-6.

[126] Davis JF, Choi DL, Benoit SC. Insulin, leptin and reward. Trends Endocrinol Metab. 2010;21(2):68-74. http://dx.doi.org/10.1016/j.tem.2009.08.004.

[127] Meule A. How Prevalent is "Food Addiction"? Front Psychiatry. 2011;2:61. http://dx.doi.org/10.3389/fpsyt.2011.00061.

[128] Meule A. Food addiction and body-mass-index: a non-linear relationship. Med Hypotheses. 2012;79(4):508-511. http://dx.doi.org/10.1016/j.mehy.2012.07.005.

[129] Gearhardt AN, Corbin WR, Brownell KD. Preliminary validation of the Yale Food Addiction Scale. Appetite. 2009;52(2):430-436. http://dx.doi.org/10.1016/j.appet.2008.12.003.

[130] Rao RS. Bariatric surgery and the central nervous system. Obes Surg. 2012;22(6): 967-978. http://dx.doi.org/10.1007/s11695-012-0649-5.

[131] Dallman MF. Stress-induced obesity and the emotional nervous system. Trends Endocrinol Metab. 2010;21(3):159-165. http://dx.doi.org/10.1016/j.tem.2009.10.004.

[132] Adam TC, Epel ES. Stress, eating and the reward system. Physiol Behav. 2007;91(4): 449-458. http://dx.doi.org/10.1016/j.physbeh.2007.04.011.

[133] Vialou V, Robison AJ, Laplant QC, Covington HE 3rd, Dietz DM, Ohnishi YN, Mouzon E, Rush AJ 3rd, Watts EL, Wallace DL, Iñiguez SD, Ohnishi YH, Steiner MA, Warren BL, Krishnan V, Bolaños CA, Neve RL, Ghose S, Berton O, Tamminga CA, Nestler EJ. ΔFosB in brain reward circuits mediates resilience to stress and antidepressant responses. Nat Neurosci. 2010;13(6):745-752. http://dx.doi.org/10.1038/nn.2551.

[134] Leinninger GM, Jo YH, Leshan RL, Louis GW, Yang H, Barrera JG, Wilson H, Opland DM, Faouzi MA, Gong Y, Jones JC, Rhodes CJ, Chua S Jr, Diano S, Horvath TL, Seeley RJ, Becker JB, Münzberg H, Myers MG Jr. Leptin acts via leptin receptor-expressing lateral hypothalamic neurons to modulate the mesolimbic dopamine system and suppress feeding. Cell Metab. 2009;10(2):89-98. http://dx.doi.org/10.1016/j.cmet.2009.06.011.

[135] Hommel JD, Trinko R, Sears RM, Georgescu D, Liu ZW, Gao XB, Thurmon JJ, Marinelli M, DiLeone RJ. Leptin receptor signaling in midbrain dopamine neurons regu-

lates feeding. Neuron. 2006;51(6):801-810. http://dx.doi.org/10.1016/j.neuron.2006.08.023

[136] Fulton S, Woodside B, Shizgal P. Modulation of brain reward circuitry by leptin. Science. 2000 ;287(5450):125-128. http://dx.doi.org/10.1126/science.287.5450.125

[137] Figlewicz DP, Bennett J, Evans SB, Kaiyala K, Sipols AJ, Benoit SC. Intraventricular insulin and leptin reverse place preference conditioned with high-fat diet in rats. Behav Neurosci. 2004 ;118(3):479-487. http://dx.doi.org/10.1037/0735-7044.118.3.479

[138] Cummings DE. Ghrelin and the short- and long-term regulation of appetite and body weight. Physiol Behav. 2006;89(1):71-84. http://dx.doi.org/10.1016/j.physbeh.2006.05.022.

[139] Perelló M, Zigman JM. The role of ghrelin in reward-based eating. Biol Psychiatry. 2012;72(5):347-353. http://dx.doi.org/10.1016/j.biopsych.2012.02.016.

[140] Perello M, Sakata I, Birnbaum S, Chuang JC, Osborne-Lawrence S, Rovinsky SA, Woloszyn J, Yanagisawa M, Lutter M, Zigman JM. Ghrelin increases the rewarding value of high-fat diet in an orexin-dependent manner. Biol Psychiatry. 2010;67(9):880-886. http://dx.doi.org/10.1016/j.biopsych.2009.10.030.

[141] Chuang JC, Perello M, Sakata I, Osborne-Lawrence S, Savitt JM, Lutter M, Zigman JM. Ghrelin mediates stress-induced food-reward behavior in mice. J Clin Invest. 2011;121(7):2684-2692. http://dx.doi.org/10.1172/JCI57660.

[142] Figlewicz DP, Bennett JL, Aliakbari S, Zavosh A, Sipols AJ. Insulin acts at different CNS sites to decrease acute sucrose intake and sucrose self-administration in rats. Am J Physiol Regul Integr Comp Physiol. 2008;295(2):R388-94. http://dx.doi.org/10.1152/ajpregu.90334.2008.

[143] Figlewicz DP, Evans SB, Murphy J, Hoen M, Baskin DG. Expression of receptors for insulin and leptin in the ventral tegmental area/substantia nigra (VTA/SN) of the rat. Brain Res. 2003;964(1):107-115. http://dx.doi.org/10.1016/S0006-8993(02)04087-8.

[144] Figlewicz DP, Benoit SC. Insulin, leptin, and food reward: update 2008. Am J Physiol Regul Integr Comp Physiol. 2009;296(1):R9-R19. http://dx.doi.org/10.1152/ajpregu.90725.2008.

[145] Daws LC, Avison MJ, Robertson SD, Niswender KD, Galli A, Saunders C. Insulin signaling and addiction. Neuropharmacology. 2011;61(7):1123-1128. http://dx.doi.org/10.1016/j.neuropharm.2011.02.028.

[146] Anthony K, Reed LJ, Dunn JT, Bingham E, Hopkins D, Marsden PK, Amiel SA. Attenuation of insulin-evoked responses in brain networks controlling appetite and reward in insulin resistance: the cerebral basis for impaired control of food intake in metabolic syndrome? Diabetes. 2006;55(11):2986-2992. http://dx.doi.org/10.2337/db06-0376.

[147] Jastreboff AM, Sinha R, Lacadie C, Small DM, Sherwin RS, Potenza MN. Neural Correlates of Stress- and Food- Cue-Induced Food Craving In Obesity: Association with insulin levels. Diabetes Care. 2013;36(2):394-402. http://dx.doi.org/10.2337/dc12-1112.

[148] Dickson SL, Shirazi RH, Hansson C, Bergquist F, Nissbrandt H, Skibicka KP. The glucagon-like peptide 1 (GLP-1) analogue, exendin-4, decreases the rewarding value of food: a new role for mesolimbic GLP-1 receptors. J Neurosci. 2012;32(14): 4812-4820. http://dx.doi.org/10.1523/JNEUROSCI.6326-11.2012.

[149] Hayes MR, Kanoski SE, Alhadeff AL, Grill HJ. Comparative effects of the long-acting GLP-1 receptor ligands, liraglutide and exendin-4, on food intake and body weight suppression in rats. Obesity (Silver Spring). 2011;19(7):1342-1349. http://dx.doi.org/10.1038/oby.2011.50.

[150] Barrera JG, Sandoval DA, D'Alessio DA, Seeley RJ. GLP-1 and energy balance: an integrated moel of short-term and long-term control. Nat Rev Endocrinol. 2011;7(9): 507-516. http://dx.doi.org/10.1038/nrendo.2011.77.

[151] Dossat AM, Lilly N, Kay K, Williams DL. Glucagon-like peptide 1 receptors in nucleus accumbens affect food intake. J Neurosci. 2011;31(41):14453-14457. http://dx.doi.org/10.1523/JNEUROSCI.3262-11.2011.

[152] Alhadeff AL, Rupprecht LE, Hayes MR. GLP-1 neurons in the nucleus of the solitary tract project directly to the ventral tegmental area and nucleus accumbens to control for food intake. Endocrinology. 2012;153(2):647-658. http://dx.doi.org/10.1210/en.2011-1443.

[153] Jeffery RW, Drewnowski A, Epstein LH, Stunkard AJ, Wilson GT, Wing RR, Hill DR. Long-term maintenance of weight loss: current status. Health Psychol. 2000;19(1 Suppl):5-16. http://dx.doi.org/10.1037/0278-6133.19.Suppl1.5.

[154] Fuglestad PT, Jeffery RW, Sherwood NE. Lifestyle patterns associated with diet, physical activity, body mass index and amount of recent weight loss in a sample of successful weight losers. Int J Behav Nutr Phys Act. 2012;9(1):79. http://dx.doi.org/10.1186/1479-5868-9-79.

[155] Wadden TA, Webb VL, Moran CH, Bailer BA. Lifestyle modification for obesity: new developments in diet, physical activity, and behavior therapy. Circulation. 2012;125(9):1157-1170. http://dx.doi.org/10.1161/CIRCULATIONAHA.111.039453.

[156] Donnelly JE, Blair SN, Jakicic JM, Manore MM, Rankin JW, Smith BK; American College of Sports Medicine. American College of Sports Medicine Position Stand. Appropriate physical activity intervention strategies for weight loss and prevention of weight regain for adults. Med Sci Sports Exerc. 2009;41(2):459-471. http://dx.doi.org/10.1249/MSS.0b013e3181949333.

[157] Murphy MH, Blair SN, Murtagh EM. Accumulated versus continuous exercise for health benefit: a review of empirical studies. Sports Med. 2009;39(1):29-43. http://dx.doi.org/10.2165/00007256-200939010-00003.

[158] Kelly D. Brownell, Thomas A. Wadden, LEARN Education Center. The LEARN program for weight control: lifestyle, exercise, attitudes, relationships, nutrition. Dallas: American Health Publishing Company; 1997.

[159] Helsel DL, Jakicic JM, Otto AD. Comparison of techniques for self-monitoring eating and exercise behaviors on weight loss in a correspondence-based intervention. J Am Diet Assoc. 2007;107(10):1807-1810. http://dx.doi.org/10.1016/j.jada.2007.07.014.

[160] Cooper Z, Doll HA, Hawker DM, Byrne S, Bonner G, Eeley E, O'Connor ME, Fairburn CG. Testing a new cognitive behavioural treatment for obesity: A randomized controlled trial with three-year follow-up. Behav Res Ther. 2010;48(8):706-713. http://dx.doi.org/10.1016/j.brat.2010.03.008.

[161] Fidler MC, Sanchez M, Raether B, Weissman NJ, Smith SR, Shanahan WR, Anderson CM; BLOSSOM Clinical Trial Group. A one-year randomized trial of lorcaserin for weight loss in obese and overweight adults: the BLOSSOM trial. J Clin Endocrinol Metab. 2011;96(10):3067-3077. http://dx.doi.org/10.1210/jc.2011-1256.

[162] Smith SR, Weissman NJ, Anderson CM, Sanchez M, Chuang E, Stubbe S, Bays H, Shanahan WR; Behavioral Modification and Lorcaserin for Overweight and Obesity Management (BLOOM) Study Group. Multicenter, placebo-controlled trial of lorcaserin for weight management. N Engl J Med. 2010;363(3):245-256. http://dx.doi.org/10.1056/NEJMoa0909809.

[163] O'Neil PM, Smith SR, Weissman NJ, Fidler MC, Sanchez M, Zhang J, Raether B, Anderson CM, Shanahan WR. Randomized Placebo-Controlled Clinical Trial of Lorcaserin for Weight Loss in Type 2 Diabetes Mellitus: The BLOOM-DM Study. Obesity (Silver Spring). 2012;20(7):1426-1436. http://dx.doi.org/10.1038/oby.2012.66.

[164] Garvey WT, Ryan DH, Look M, Gadde KM, Allison DB, Peterson CA, Schwiers M, Day WW, Bowden CH. Two-year sustained weight loss and metabolic benefits with controlled-release phentermine/topiramate in obese and overweight adults (SEQUEL): a randomized, placebo-controlled, phase 3 extension study. Am J Clin Nutr 2012;95(2):297-308. http://dx.doi.org/10.3945/ajcn.111.024927.

[165] Allison DB, Gadde KM, Garvey WT, Peterson CA, Schwiers ML, Najarian T, Tam PY, Troupin B, Day WW. Controlled-release phentermine/topiramate in severely obese adults: a randomized controlled trial (EQUIP). Obesity 2012;20(2):330-342. http://dx.doi.org/10.1038/oby.2011.330.

[166] Gadde KM, Allison DB, Ryan DH, Peterson CA, Troupin B, Schwiers ML, Day WW. Effects of low-dose, controlled-release, phentermine plus topiramate combination on weight and associated comorbidities in overweight and obese adults (CONQUER): a

randomised, placebo-controlled, phase 3 trial. Lancet 2011;377(9774):1341-1352. http://dx.doi.org/10.1016/S0140-6736(11)60205-5.

[167] Greenway FL, Fujioka K, Plodkowski RA, Mudaliar S, Guttadauria M, Erickson J, Kim DD, Dunayevich E; COR-I Study Group. Effect of naltrexone plus bupropion on weight loss in overweight and obese adults (COR-I): a multicentre, randomised, double-blind, placebo-controlled, phase 3 trial. Lancet. 2010;376(9741):595-605. http://dx.doi.org/10.1016/S0140-6736(10)60888-4.

[168] Bray GA, Greenway FL. Current and potential drugs for treatment of obesity. Endocr Rev. 1999;20(6):805-875. http://dx.doi.org/10.1210/er.20.6.805

[169] Astrup A, Rössner S, Van Gaal L, Rissanen A, Niskanen L, Al Hakim M, Madsen J, Rasmussen MF, Lean ME; NN8022-1807 Study Group. Effects of liraglutide in the treatment of obesity: a randomised, double-blind, placebo-controlled study. Lancet. 2009;374(9701):1606-1616. http://dx.doi.org/10.1016/S0140-6736(09)61375-1.

[170] Astrup A, Carraro R, Finer N, Harper A, Kunesova M, Lean ME, Niskanen L, Rasmussen MF, Rissanen A, Rössner S, Savolainen MJ, Van Gaal L; NN8022-1807 Investigators. Safety, tolerability and sustained weight loss over 2 years with the once-daily human GLP-1 analog, liraglutide. Int J Obes (Lond). 2012;36(6):843-854. http://dx.doi.org/10.1038/ijo.2011.158.

[171] Simmons JH, Shoemaker AH, Roth CL. Treatment with glucagon-like Peptide-1 agonist exendin-4 in a patient with hypothalamic obesity secondary to intracranial tumor. Horm Res Paediatr. 2012;78(1):54-58. http://dx.doi.org/10.1159/000339469.

[172] Padwal R, Klarenbach S, Wiebe N, Birch D, Karmali S, Manns B, Hazel M, Sharma AM, Tonelli M. Bariatric surgery: a systematic review and network meta-analysis of randomized trials. Obes Rev. 2011;12(8):602-621. http://dx.doi.org/10.1111/j.1467-789X.2011.00866.x.

[173] Mechanick JI, Kushner RF, Sugerman HJ, Gonzalez-Campoy JM, Collazo-Clavell ML, Spitz AF, Apovian CM, Livingston EH, Brolin R, Sarwer DB, Anderson WA, Dixon J, Guven S; American Association of Clinical Endocrinologists; Obesity Society; American Society for Metabolic & Bariatric Surgery. American Association of Clinical Endocrinologists, The Obesity Society, and American Society for Metabolic & Bariatric Surgery medical guidelines for clinical practice for the perioperative nutritional, metabolic, and nonsurgical support of the bariatric surgery patient. Obesity (Silver Spring). 2009;17 Suppl 1:S1-70, v. http://dx.doi.org/10.1038/oby.2009.28.

[174] Bocchieri LE, Meana M, Fisher BL. A review of psychosocial outcomes of surgery for morbid obesity. J Psychosom Res. 2002;52(3):155-165. http://dx.doi.org/10.1016/S0022-3999(01)00241-0

[175] Herpertz S, Kielmann R, Wolf AM, Langkafel M, Senf W, Hebebrand J. Does obesity surgery improve psychosocial functioning? A systematic review. Int J Obes Relat Metab Disord. 2003;27(11):1300-1314. http://dx.doi.org/10.1038/sj.ijo.0802410.

[176] van Hout GC, Boekestein P, Fortuin FA, Pelle AJ, van Heck GL. Psychosocial functioning following bariatric surgery. Obes Surg. 2006;16(6):787-794. http://dx.doi.org/10.1381/096089206777346808

[177] Zeller MH, Modi AC, Noll JG, Long JD, Inge TH. Psychosocial functioning improves following adolescent bariatric surgery. Obesity (Silver Spring). 2009;17(5):985-990. http://dx.doi.org/10.1038/oby.2008.644.

[178] Pataky Z, Carrard I, Golay A. Psychological factors and weight loss in bariatric surgery. Curr Opin Gastroenterol. 2011;27(2):167-173. http://dx.doi.org/10.1097/MOG.0b013e3283422482.

[179] Dixon JB, Dixon ME, O'Brien PE. Depression in association with severe obesity: changes with weight loss. Arch Intern Med. 2003;163(17):2058-2065. http://dx.doi.org/10.1001/archinte.163.17.2058.

[180] Dymek MP, le Grange D, Neven K, Alverdy J. Quality of life and psychosocial adjustment in patients after Roux-en-Y gastric bypass: a brief report. Obes Surg. 2001;11(1):32-39.

[181] van Gemert WG, Adang EM, Greve JW, Soeters PB. Quality of life assessment of morbidly obese patients: effect of weight-reducing surgery. Am J Clin Nutr. 1998;67(2):197-201.

[182] Choban PS, Onyejekwe J, Burge JC, Flancbaum L. A health status assessment of the impact of weight loss following Roux-en-Y gastric bypass for clinically severe obesity. J Am Coll Surg. 1999;188(5):491-497. http://dx.doi.org/10.1016/S1072-7515(99)00030-7.

[183] Schok M, Geenen R, van Antwerpen T, de Wit P, Brand N, van Ramshorst B. Quality of life after laparoscopic adjustable gastric banding for severe obesity: postoperative and retrospective preoperative evaluations. Obes Surg. 2000;10(6):502-508. http://dx.doi.org/10.1381/096089200321593698.

[184] Camps MA, Zervos E, Goode S, Rosemurgy AS. Impact of Bariatric Surgery on Body Image Perception and Sexuality in Morbidly Obese Patients and their Partners. Obes Surg. 1996;6(4):356-360. http://dx.doi.org/10.1381/096089296765556700.

[185] Adami GF, Meneghelli A, Bressani A, Scopinaro N. Body image in obese patients before and after stable weight reduction following bariatric surgery. J Psychosom Res. 1999;46(3):275-281. http://dx.doi.org/10.1016/S0022-3999(98)00094-4.

[186] Kinzl JF, Trefalt E, Fiala M, Hotter A, Biebl W, Aigner F. Partnership, sexuality, and sexual disorders in morbidly obese women: consequences of weight loss after gastric banding. Obes Surg. 2001;11(4):455-458. http://dx.doi.org/10.1381/096089201321209323

[187] Tindle HA, Omalu B, Courcoulas A, Marcus M, Hammers J, Kuller LH. Risk of suicide after long-term follow-up from bariatric surgery. Am J Med. 2010;123(11): 1036-1042. http://dx.doi.org/10.1016/j.amjmed.2010.06.016.

[188] Adams TD, Gress RE, Smith SC, Halverson RC, Simper SC, Rosamond WD, Lamonte MJ, Stroup AM, Hunt SC. Long-term mortality after gastric bypass surgery. N Engl J Med. 2007;357(8):753-761. http://dx.doi.org/10.1056/NEJMoa066603.

[189] Hsu LK, Sullivan SP, Benotti PN. Eating disturbances and outcome of gastric bypass surgery: a pilot study. Int J Eat Disord. 1997;21(4):385-390. http://dx.doi.org/10.1002/(SICI)1098-108X(1997)21:4<385::AID-EAT12>3.0.CO;2-Y.

[190] Hsu LK, Benotti PN, Dwyer J, Roberts SB, Saltzman E, Shikora S, Rolls BJ, Rand W. Nonsurgical factors that influence the outcome of bariatric surgery: a review. Psychosom Med. 1998;60(3):338-346.

[191] Powers PS, Rosemurgy A, Boyd F, Perez A. Outcome of gastric restriction procedures: weight, psychiatric diagnoses, and satisfaction. Obes Surg. 1997;7(6):471-477. http://dx.doi.org/10.1381/096089297765555197.

[192] Mitchell JE, Lancaster KL, Burgard MA, Howell LM, Krahn DD, Crosby RD, Wonderlich SA, Gosnell BA. Long-term follow-up of patients' status after gastric bypass. Obes Surg. 2001;11(4):464-8. http://dx.doi.org/10.1381/096089201321209341

[193] Kruseman M, Leimgruber A, Zumbach F, Golay A. Dietary, weight, and psychological changes among patients with obesity, 8 years after gastric bypass. J Am Diet Assoc. 2010;110(4):527-534. http://dx.doi.org/10.1016/j.jada.2009.12.028.

[194] Niego SH, Kofman MD, Weiss JJ, Geliebter A. Binge eating in the bariatric surgery population: a review of the literature. Int J Eat Disord. 2007;40(4):349-359. http://dx.doi.org/10.1002/eat.20376.

[195] Odom J, Zalesin KC, Washington TL, Miller WW, Hakmeh B, Zaremba DL, Altattan M, Balasubramaniam M, Gibbs DS, Krause KR, Chengelis DL, Franklin BA, McCullough PA. Behavioral predictors of weight regain after bariatric surgery. Obes Surg. 2010;20(3):349-356. http://dx.doi.org/10.1007/s11695-009-9895-6.

[196] Sjöström L, Lindroos AK, Peltonen M, Torgerson J, Bouchard C, Carlsson B, Dahlgren S, Larsson B, Narbro K, Sjöström CD, Sullivan M, Wedel H; Swedish Obese Subjects Study Scientific Group. Lifestyle, diabetes, and cardiovascular risk factors 10 years after bariatric surgery. N Engl J Med. 2004;351(26):2683-2693. http://dx.doi.org/10.1056/NEJMoa035622

[197] Myers VH, Adams CE, Barbera BL, Brantley PJ. Medical and psychosocial outcomes of laparoscopic Roux-en-Y gastric bypass: cross-sectional findings at 4-year follow-up. Obes Surg. 2012;22(2):230-239. http://dx.doi.org/10.1007/s11695-010-0324-7.

[198] Shah M, Simha V, Garg A.Review: long-term impact of bariatric surgery on body weight, comorbidities, and nutritional status. J Clin Endocrinol Metab. 2006;91(11): 4223-4231. http://dx.doi.org/10.1210/jc.2006-0557.

[199] Tam CS, Berthoud HR, Bueter M, Chakravarthy MV, Geliebter A, Hajnal A, Holst J, Kaplan L, Pories W, Raybould H, Seeley R, Strader A, Ravussin E. Could the mechanisms of bariatric surgery hold the key for novel therapies? report from a Pennington Scientific Symposium. Obes Rev. 2011;12(11):984-994. http://dx.doi.org/10.1111/j. 1467-789X.2011.00902.x.

Section 3

Experimental and Clinical Applications of Functional Neuroimaging

Chapter 17

Surgical Resection of Tumors Infiltrating Left Insula and Perisylvian Opercula — Utility of Anatomic Landmarks Implemented by Intraoperative Functional Brain Mapping

Francesco Signorelli, Domenico Chirchiglia,
Rodolfo Maduri, Giuseppe Barbagallo and
Jacques Guyotat

Additional information is available at the end of the chapter

http://dx.doi.org/10.5772/56568

1. Introduction

Tumors involving the insular lobe and perisylvian opercula of the dominant hemisphere are frequently managed conservatively regardless of their nature and clinical evolution, even if impending infiltration of nearby eloquent areas endangers their function. Our and other authors' experience (Duffau 2009, Duffau et al, 2000; 2001; 2006; 2009; Lang et al, 2001; Kim et al, 2002; Moshel et al, 2008; Saito et al, 2010; Sanai et al, 2010; Signorelli et al, 2010; 2011; Simon et al, 2009; Skrap et al, 2012; Yasargil et al, 1992; Wu et al, 2011; Zentner et al, 1996) demonstrate that wide surgical resection of these lesions are nonetheless feasible since tumor burden often displaces eloquent sites at the tumor boundaries (Duffau 2000; Duffau et al, 2000; 2001; 2006; 2009; Signorelli et al, 2010; 2011) and compensatory areas take over the lost function of infiltrated nervous tissue. However, accurate anatomic and functional knowledge of the sylvian fissure and structures located nearby is essential to perform any surgical act in this area, in order to decrease the risks of postoperative permanent deficits (Duffau 2009; Duffau et al, 2009; Moshel et al, 2009; Signorelli et al, 2010; 2011). Here we report our recent experience with tumors infiltrating left insula and perisylvian opercula and point out technical details helpful in guiding surgery through this region, with the purpose of locating and respecting neural and vascular structures and eloquent sites.

2. Patients and methods

Our series includes 5 patients harboring a high grade and 10 patients harboring a low grade tumor involving left insula and perisylvian opercula, operated on between 2007 and 2011 at two institutions: the Neurosurgical Department at the Hôpital Neurologique et Neurochirurgical "Pierre Wertheimer" in Lyon, France, and the Neurosurgical Department of the University Hospital of Catanzaro, Italy. They were 8 males and 7 females (mean age 50.1 years) who presented with phasic troubles in 8 cases and seizures in all cases. Preoperative antiepileptic treatment was effective in all patients but one, although 3 other patients presented with more than 1 seizure/month. Aphasia was completely regressive in four patients, all LGG, and partially regressive in one HGG patient after administration of antiedema therapy and seizure control, while in 3 other HGG cases it was progressive at a thorough preoperative neuropsychologic evaluation which comprised Montreal-Toulouse and Boston tests (Dordain et al, 1983) repeated at 1-month. They were nonetheless judged to be good candidates for, and keen and motivated to undergo intraoperative language mapping.

Motor deficit was a presenting symptom in two patients. Moreover, in all HGG patients there were symptoms of intracranial hypertension (ICHT). ICHT had an acute onset in one patient which presented to our department with an intratumoral hemorrhage. This last patient displayed a right sensorimotor deficit and a right homonymous hemianopia. Surgical indication was established in lesions with a MRI appearance of LGG in two cases because of clinical and/or radiological tumor progression and in the other eight cases at the time of diagnosis.. All patients were right handed according to the Edimburgh Handedness Inventory (Oldfield, 1971). Gadolinium-enhanced T1-, T2- and FLAIR-weighted images revealed in all cases the infiltration of left insula. The tumor involved also fronto-parietal and temporal opercula in 9 cases, while frontal and temporal opercula or just parietal or temporal operculum were infiltrated respectively in three, two and one case. Moreover, the tumor infiltrated other paralimbic structures (i.e. fronto-orbital and/or temporo-polar areas) in four cases and limbic structures in two cases. In order to elucidate the relationships of the tumor with the vascular tree of left middle cerebral artery (MCA), in particular with lenticulostriate arteries, left carotid angiography was obtained for two patient. The other 13 patients underwent angio-CT scan and/or MRI angiography. The most lateral lenticulostiate branch was shown in 3 out of 15 cases originating from the post-bifurcation tract of M1, no more than 6 mm distal from the major bifurcation, while in the other cases it originated before or at the level of the MCA bifurcation but never from M2, in accordance with other author's experience (Moshel et al, 2008). Particular attention was also paid to the venograms, to determine the course of the superficial sylvian veins, which can hinder a wide dissection of the sylvian fissure, although generally sylvian fissure was approached subpially.

2.1. Surgical procedure

All patients underwent awake craniotomy using electrical stimulation mapping (ESM) of sensorimotor and language pathways, whose technique was described in detail elsewhere (Signorelli et al, 2010; 2011). Briefly, we applied a bipolar cortico-subcortical stimulation by an electrode with tips 5 mm apart, which delivered biphasic square-wave pulses (1 ms per phase) with a frequency of 60 pulses per second. Cortical stimulation was started at 1 mA and the optimal current level for stimulation was set equal to that provoking segmental movements on the contralateral upper limb or face. The effective current intensity varied from 1 mA to 6 mA. Language tasks included counting, verbal and auditory naming (auditory task was used when testing anterior temporal lobe sites). Moreover, reading tasks were added when testing parietal or posterior temporal opercula. Neuronavigation was used for all patients for defining tumor boundaries and anatomic relationships with neural and vascular structures. Craniotomy was planned to include the whole perisylvian area from pars orbitalis of the third frontal gyrus to the postcentral sulcus, in order to expose the anterior (vallecula) and middle part (insular fossa) of the sylvian fissure, exposing also the superior temporal gyrus (T1). After performing ESM aimed at locating cortical language and sensorimotor areas, the superficial part of the lesion, which constantly infiltrated one or more of frontal, parietal and temporal opercula, was removed as to gain easy access to the depth of sylvian fissure, which was opened up to the postcentral sulcus with no need of retractors. In all our cases the tumor displaced M2 branches centrifugally, indicating to the surgeon the site on the insular surface where to start tumor debulking, after accomplishment of ESM in search of possible language areas. The removal of insular gyri, when not harboring language areas, was conducted medially up to the putamen, generally visible under the microscope as a gray, compact tissue with white strips located at the center of insula (Yasargyl et al, 1992), which we never found infiltrated in case of low grade tumors. However, while pushing medially tumor removal, we alternated surgical resection to subcortical stimulation starting at a distance of 2 cm laterally to the posterior limb of the internal capsule, as seen on neuronavigation, in order to identify and preserve subcortical motor pathways (Duffau 2009; Signorelli et al, 2010; 2011; Simon et al, 2009;). Subcortical stimulation is especially useful when pushing tumor resection above superior insular sulcus, where pyramidal fibers coursing through corona radiata are more superficial and anatomic landmarks to them lack. High attention was paid when pushing resection below the lenticular nucleus, at the level of the inferior limiting sulcus, where sublenticular fibers of the posterior limb of the internal capsule contain, in a forward-backward direction, the auditory and the optic radiations (Signorelli et al, 2010). At the level of the anterior part of the external capsule subcortical stimulation allowed the identification of the inferior occipito-frontal fasciculus inducing semantic paraphasias (Duffau 2009), which delimited the deep boundaries of tumor resection anteriorly. The temporal part of the same fasciculus marked the boundaries of the resection at the level of the temporal stem, preventing to open the temporal horn of the ventricle (Duffau 2009; Duffau et a, 2009). Of utmost importance is the recognition of the vascular anatomy. Short branches from MCA to the infiltrated insula can be interrupted because they supply the tumor, paying attention not to avulse them from the main vessel at the origin, which can lead to a lesion of the parent vessel wall. However, long perforators, supplying corona radiata, have to be respected to avoid ischemic injury to functional white matter (Duffau 2009; Lang et al, 2001; Moshel et al, 2008; Signorelli et al, 2010; 2011). During removal of limen insulae high attention has to be paid to lenticulostriate arteries, which originates mostly from the medial or superior aspect of MCA 6 mm or less around bifurcation and sometimes from early M1 branches (Signorelli et al 2010). Lesion or even manipulation of them can lead to ischemic damage of the internal capsule.

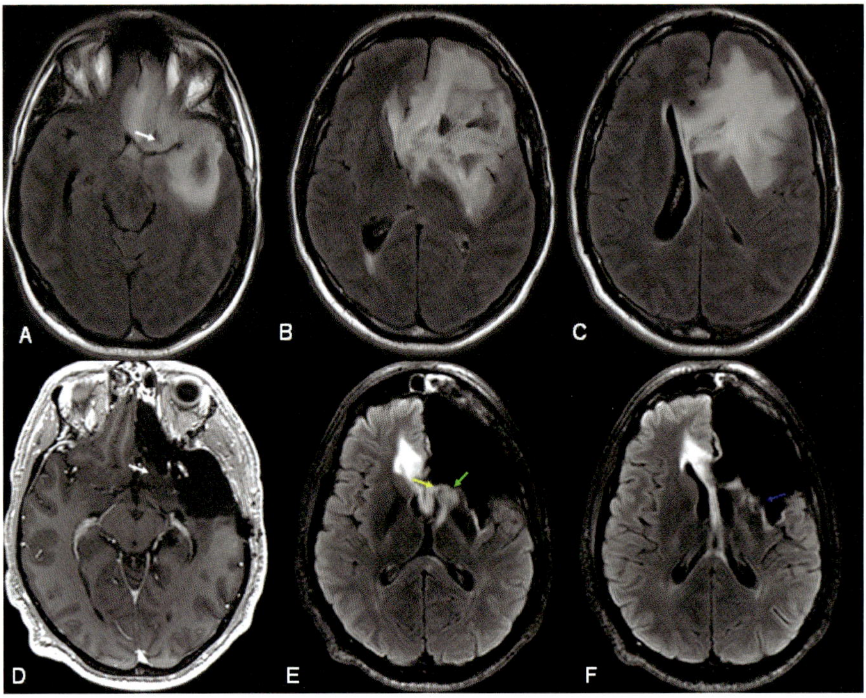

Figure 1. A, B,C: Preoperative FLAIR MR images of a low grade glioma infiltrating the left operculo-insular region and the fronto-orbital, including the perforated substance (white arrow), temporopolar and hyppocampal regions, type 5 B of Yasargil classification (Yasargil et al, 1992). **D**: Postoperative T1 gadolinium-weighted and **E,F**: Postoperative FLAIR MR images, showing the subtotal removal of the lesion. The boundaries of the resection are set based on anatomical (perforated substance, white arrow) as well as neurofunctional (subcallosal fasciculus, yellow arrow; inferior occipitofrontal fasciculus, green arrow; arcuate fasciculus, blue arrow) criteria.

3. Results

3.1. Electrophysiological results

ESM of the insular cortex surface resulted in speech arrest in 6 patients In 9 patients insula was free of language sites, as it was in all cases the cortex of opercular clefts and of superior and inferior insular clefts. For what concerns the location of eloquent sites at the level of the convexity, ESM located essential language sites on immediately perisylvian tumoral tissue in just one patient, while in the rest of cases functional areas were displaced at the periphery of grossly infiltrated nervous tissue. The insular cortical areas whose stimulation evoked abdominal sensations such as nausea, borborygmi, belching (2 patients), chewing and tongue movements without speech arrest (4 patients) were not considered eloquent sites and removed because infiltrated by tumor. In one case ESM caused intraoperative partial tonic-clonic seizures, rapidly stopped pouring cold serum on the cortex. A gross total removal was achieved in all 6 patients that did not display infiltration of perisylvian or insular functional cortex and subcortical motor or language pathways. Stimulation of uncinate fasciculus during removal of an infiltrated limen insulae was done in 8 patients and was always uneventful. In all patients stimulation of the infiltrated white matter at the anterolateral border of the frontal horn of the left lateral ventricle (i.e. the subcallosal fasciculus) triggered limited spontaneous speech and/or perseverations with preservation of normal articulation and at the level of the anterior part of the external capsule as well as at the level of the temporal stem induced semantic paraphasias, which delimited the deep boundaries of tumor resection. Moreover, ESM was used to identify motor pathways inside corona radiata above the insular superior limiting sulcus, which represented the posterosuperior limit of tumor resection.

3.2. Clinical results

Ten patients had an immediate postoperative phasic aggravation, which lasted 1 to 2 months. At an overall mean follow up of 33 months (14-56 months) 10 patients are alive and keep a good quality of life, as assessed by the EORTC QLQ-C30 (Aaronson et al, 1993). One of them presents a tumor relapse, which causes an impairment of language performances, but she is still autonomous. Seven patients keep the same functional status they had before intervention, while two patients display an improvement of their neuropsychological performance after surgery. Three of the five patients diagnosed with a HGG died after a mean survival period of 16.7 months. Two of them had a mean HQSP (high quality survival period) of 18 months, while the last patient had a postoperative nucleo-capsular infarct, due to lenticulostriate arteries damage, engendering a definitive motor and phasic aggravation. Two other HGG patients, with a follow-up of 23 and 6 months respectively, are autonomous and have a good quality of life. For what concerns seizures outcome, 9 patients were ameliorated and 6 had no variation as regards to their preoperative status. On the postoperative MRI resection was in 6 cases grossly total, in 6 cases subtotal and in three cases partial owing to tumoral infiltration of functional tissue.

4. Discussion

Several well designed controlled studies indicate that the degree of surgical resection of brain gliomas, including those in highly eloquent areas, affects survival and quality of life of patients (Duffau 2009; Ius et al, 2012; Sanai et al, 2010) and there are some good reasons to treat aggressively such tumors: cytoreduction is effective in reducing the mass effect of the lesion and it can be assumed that it reduces also the contingent of neoplastic cells that can reproduce and give origin to tumor recurrence and invasion of eloquent areas or take anaplastic transformation (Duffau 2009; Ius et al, 2012; Sanai et al, 2010). Moreover, there are evidences that aggressive removal of insular tumors can improve seizures control, which are their most frequent clinical manifestation (Taillandier et al, 2009). Authors pleading for an aggressive treatment of such tumors mostly think that it should be realized early after diagnosis to prevent clinical impairment and improve survival and recurrence free period of patients (Duffau 2009; Sanai et al, 2010).

Since the first report by Yasargil et al, other papers in the literature dealt with the surgical treatment of tumors infiltrating insular lobe (Duffau 2009, Duffau et al, 2000; 2001; 2006; 2009; Lang et al, 2001; Kim et al, 2002; Moshel et al, 2008; Saito et al, 2010; Sanai et al, 2010; Signorelli et al, 2010; 2011; Simon et al, 2009; Skrap et al, 2012; Yasargil et al, 1992; Wu et al, 2011; Zentner et al, 1996) and encompassed lesions with a variety of anatomical extensions. As a matter of fact, these series reported on purely insular tumors (type 3A of the Yasargyl's classification) as well as insulo-opercular (type 3B) and limbic-paralimbic lesions (type 5) involving both the dominant and the non-dominant hemisphere. Some authors reporting surgical removal of dominant-sided insular tumors did not find useful or did not employ awake surgery for language mapping (Hentschel et al, 2005; Lang et al, 2001; Simon et al, 2009; Yasargyl et al, 1992; Zentner et al, 1996), others demonstrated the utility of ESM mapping guided tumor resection, although seldom insula was found to harbor essential language sites (Duffau 2009; Duffau et al, 2001; 2009). In Duffau's series there were no permanent postoperative phasic deficits although he reported 10 cases of transient articulatory disorders (Duffau et al, 2000). In Hentschel and Lang's series there were 6 cases of transient speech troubles among patients with 3B tumors and in Zentner's series two of the 11 patients had a permanent postoperative aphasia (Hentschel et al, 2005; Zentner et al, 1996).

Our series, albeit small, is anatomically homogeneous in that focuses on tumors infiltrating the insular lobe of the dominant hemisphere and extended to the opercular region and, in six cases, also to adjacent deep perisylvian structures. Moreover, all patients were operated on while testing language function. The retrospective analysis restricted to these patients shows two basic findings: 6 out of 15 such patients, all harboring a LGG infiltrating the frontoparietal and temporal opercula, had speech arrest while stimulating insular cortex and these same patients did not have language sites on the opercular part invaded by the tumor. Conversely, the 9 patients for whom ESM of insular cortex did not trigger language troubles all harboured speech function on perisylvian opercula. They either had preoperative language troubles (4 cases), which did not hinder intraoperative language mapping, or a limited opercular infiltration, and no phasic deficits (5 cases).Thus, it can be speculated that for the 6 LGG patients displaying language sites on insula, this region compensated the opercular infiltration due to a plasticity phenomenon, which can be considered at least in part responsible for the preoperative regression of the phasic deficits. For the remaining patients the functional reorganization might not have occurred because of a limited opercular infiltration (1 patient) or because of a too extensive and rapid inactivation of perisylvian language sites by a high grade tumor. The compensatory role of left insula in case of infiltration of perisylvian language areas has already been pointed out as a function that must be preserved (Duffau et al, 2000). However, the compensatory potential of left insula seems to be highly variable on individual basis. There are mechanisms of cerebral plasticity taking place before the treatment of the lesion and both in an acute stage and at distance from surgical intervention. This could be explained by the fact that sensorimotor and language functions seem to be organised within multiple parallel networks. Beyond the recruitment of areas adjacent to the surgical cavity, the long term reshaping could be related to progressive involvement of regions within the hemisphere omolateral to the lesion as well as of the contralateral hemisphere (Duffau, 2006).. In these cases functional reshaping involves association areas belonging to the same functional network of the lesioned area as it is the case for dominant insula and perisilvyan language sites. However, mechanisms of compensation are limited. One of such limits is that reorganisation seems to be more effective in secondary than in primary areas, as for SMA (Duffau, 2006). Moreover, if a damaged area is compensated by another region, a lesion of this newly recruited region will induce a permanent deficit, as it could be the case for dominant insulo-opercular gliomas. Thus, surgical resection should avoid infringement of insula if there are arguments indicating that it took over, at least partially, the lost function of perisylvian opercula. Taking into account these data may guide treatment of cerebral tumors in the dominant deep perisylvian area, broadening the surgical indication and the extent of tumor removal while lessening the rate of postoperative permanent deficits, and be useful for defining prognosis and rehabilitation programs.

Abbreviations

ESM: electrical stimulation mapping; HGG: high grade gliomas; ICHT: intracranial hypertension; LGG: low grade gliomas; MCA: middle cerebral artery; MRI: magnetic resonance imaging; T1: superior temporal gyrus.

Author details

Francesco Signorelli[1,2], Domenico Chirchiglia[3], Rodolfo Maduri[1], Giuseppe Barbagallo[4] and Jacques Guyotat[1]

1 "Magna Græcia" University, Department of Experimental and Clinical Medicine "G. Salvatore", Chair of Neurosurgery, Catanzaro, Italy

2 Hospices Civils de Lyon, Hôpital Neurologique et Neurochirurgical, Department of Neurosurgery, Lyon, France

3 "Magna Græcia" University, Department of Medical and Surgical Sciences, Chair of Neurosurgery, Catanzaro, Italy

4 University of Catania, Chair of Neurosurgery, Catania, Italy

References

[1] Aaronson, N. K, Ahmedzai, S, Bergman, B, Bullinger, M, Cull, A, Duez, N. J, Filiberti, A, Flechtner, H, Fleishman, S. B, De Haes, J. C, et al. The European Organization for Research and Treatment of Cancer QLQ-C30: AQuality-of-Life Instrument for Use in International Clinical Trials in Oncology. Journal of the National Cancer Institute. (1993). , 85, 365-376.

[2] Dordain, M, Nespoulos, J. L, & Bourdeau, M. Lecours AR Verbal abilities of normal adults submitting to an aphasia linguistic protocol. Acta Neurol Belg. (1983).

[3] Duffau H, Capelle L, Lopes M, Faillot T, Sichez JP, Fohanno D. The insular lobe: physiopathological and surgical considerations. *Neurosurgery*. 2000;47:801-10.

[4] Duffau H, Bauchet L, Lehéricy S, Capelle L. Functional compensation of the left dominant insula for language. *Neuroreport*. 2001. 20;12:2159-63.

[5] Duffau H, Taillandier L, Gatignol P, Capelle L. The insular lobe and brain plasticity: Lessons from tumor surgery. *Clin Neurol Neurosurg*. 2006;108:543-8.

[6] Duffau, H. Lessons from brain mapping in surgery for low grade gliomas: study of cerebral connectivity and plasticity. In Medical Imaging and Augmented Reality. (2006). Online 978-3-54037-221-9Springer Berlin Heidelberg.

[7] Duffau H, Moritz-Gasser S, Gatignol P. Functional outcome after language mapping for insular World Health Organization Grade II gliomas in the dominant hemisphere: experience with 24 patients. *Neurosurg Focus*. 2009;27(2):E.

[8] Duffau, H. A personal consecutive series of surgically treated 51 cases of insular WHO Grade II glioma: advances and limitations. J Neurosurg. (2009). , 110, 696-708.

[9] Hentschel SJ, Lang FF. Surgical resection of intrinsic insular tumors. *Neurosurgery*. 2005;57:176-83.

[10] Ius T, Isola M, Budai R, Pauletto G, Tomasino B, Fadiga L, Skrap M. Low-grade glioma surgery in eloquent areas: volumetric analysis of extent of resection and its impact on overall survival. A single-institution experience in 190 patients: clinical article. *J Neurosurg*. 2012;117:1039-52.

[11] Kim YH, Kim CY.Current surgical management of insular gliomas. *Neurosurg Clin N Am*. 2012;23:199-206,

[12] Lang FF, Olansen NE, DeMonte F, Gokaslan ZL, Holland EC, Kalhorn C, Sawaya R. Surgical resection of intrinsic insular tumors: complication avoidance. *J Neurosurg*. 2001 Oct;95(4):638-50.

[13] Moshel YA, Marcus JD, Parker EC, Kelly PJ. Resection of insular gliomas: the importance of lenticulostriate artery position. *J Neurosurg*. 2008 Nov;109(5):825-34.

[14] Oldfield, R. C. The assessment and analysis of handedness: The Edinburgh inventory. Neuropsychologia. (1971)., 9, 97-113.

[15] Saito R, Kumabe T, Kanamori M, Sonoda Y, Tominaga T. Insulo-opercular gliomas: four different natural progression patterns and implications for surgical indications. *Neurol Med Chir (Tokyo)*. 2010;50:286-90

[16] Sanai N, Polley MY, Berger MS. Insular glioma resection: assessment of patient morbidity, survival, and tumor progression. *J Neurosurg*. 2010;112:1-9.

[17] Signorelli, F.; Guyotat, J; Elisevich, K. & Barbagallo, GM. Review of current microsurgical management of insular gliomas. *Acta Neurochirurgica.* 2010;152:19-26.

[18] Signorelli, F. Barbagallo, GM; Maduri R, Schonauer C, Guyotat, J, & Elisevich, K. Insular tumors. In Management of CNS Tumors, (2011). 978-9-53307-646-1Ed. Miklos Garami, InTech- Open Access Publisher- Rijeka, Croatia.

[19] Simon M, Neuloh G, von Lehe M, Meyer B, Schramm J. Insular gliomas: the case for surgical management. *J Neurosurg*. 2009;110:685-95.

[20] Skrap M, Mondani M, Tomasino B, Weis L, Budai R, Pauletto G, Eleopra R, Fadiga L, Ius T.Surgery of insular nonenhancing gliomas: volumetric analysis of tumoral resection, clinical outcome, and survival in a consecutive series of 66 cases. *Neurosurgery*. 2012;70:1081-93

[21] Taillandier L, Duffau H. Epilepsy and insular Grade II gliomas: an interdisciplinary point of view from a retrospective monocentric series of 46 cases. *Neurosurg Focus*. 2009 Aug;27(2):E8.

[22] Yasargil, M. G, Von Ammon, K, Cavazos, E, Doczi, T, Reeves, J. D, & Roth, P. Tumors of the limbic and paralimbic systems. Acta Neurochirurgica. (1992)., 147-149.

[23] Wu AS, Witgert ME, Lang FF, Xiao L, Bekele BN, Meyers CA, Ferson D, Wefel JS. Neurocognitive function before and after surgery for insular gliomas. *J Neurosurg*. 2011;115:1115-25.

[24] Zentner, J, Meyer, B, Stangl, A, & Schramm, J. Intrinsic tumors of the insula: a prospective surgical study of 30 patients. Journal of Neurosurg. (1996)., 85, 263-271.

Chapter 18

Optimized Signal Separation for 3D-Polarized Light Imaging

Jürgen Dammers, Lukas Breuer, Giuseppe Tabbì and Markus Axer

Additional information is available at the end of the chapter

http://dx.doi.org/10.5772/55246

1. Introduction

1.1. Anatomical connectivity mapping

"Why should we bother about connectivity in the age of functional imaging, at a time when magnets of ever increasing strength promise to detect the location of even the faintest thought? Isn't it enough to locate cortical areas engaged in deception, introspection, empathy? Do we really have to worry about their connections? The answer is "yes". In the case of the nervous system, the unit of relational architecture that allows the whole to exceed the sum of the parts is known as large-scale network. Its elucidation requires an elaborate understanding of connectivity patterns" [1]. Despite considerable advances in experimental techniques and in our understanding of animal anatomy over the last decades, the real connectivity of the human brain has essentially remained a mystery. It is the human brain's multiscale topology that poses a particular challenge to any neuroimaging technique and prevented the neuroscientists from unraveling the connectome so far.

However, it is also the brain's architecture that allows different morphological entities to be defined at different scales depending on the spatial resolution provided by the available neuroimaging techniques and the scientific objectives. Consequently, a comprehensive description of neuronal networks and their intricate fiber connections requires a multimodal approach based on complementary imaging techniques targeting different levels of organization (microscale, mesoscale, and macroscale) [2,3].

MR-based diffusion imaging is the most frequently used method to visualize fiber pathways in both the living and the postmortem human brain (for a comprehensive introduction to the field cf. [4,5]). Diffusion imaging contributes to the understanding of the macroscopic connectivity (i.e., at the millimeter scale) in the living brain, while postmortem studies already explore the upper mesoscale (i.e., the sub-millimeter scale). Hence, not surprisingly, diffusion imaging is of great appeal to neuroscientists as a method for the visualization of connectivity patterns in both clinical and basic research. However, complex fiber networks and small fiber tracts are difficult to be disentangled reliably at present. Furthermore, the termination of fields of pathways emanating from cortical areas no larger than a few millimeters in size cannot be demonstrated with the required precision.

Conversely, microscopic techniques generate data sets of impressing neuroanatomical detail, but they are limited to small sample sizes (i.e., small areas of interest in a small number of subjects) of postmortem tissue. This substantially restricts their predictive power. In the recent years, anatomical connections in the human postmortem brains were studied with dissection techniques [6,7], in myelin stained sections of adult human brains [8], or of immature brains taking advantage of heterochronic myelination of different fiber tracts during pre- and early postnatal development [9], in lesioned brains using various techniques for staining degenerating fibers [10,11], and using tract-tracing methods for discovering local connections [12,13]. These studies have enriched our knowledge about human brain fiber tracts, but all of them suffer from severe restrictions if the 3D courses of fiber pathways are to be mapped in the adult human brain. In contrast to studies in animals, the tight packing of different fiber tracts in the white substance, and the lack of specific tracers for in vitro tracking of long distance fibers made comprehensive fiber tract mapping impossible in the adult human brain [14].

1.2. 3D-polarized light imaging (3D-PLI)

Recently, a neuroimaging technique referred to as *3D-polarized light imaging (3D-PLI)* has been introduced that has opened up new avenues to study human brain regions with complex fiber architecture as well as small cortical fibers at the micrometer level [15–17]. This technique is applicable to microtome sections of postmortem brains and utilizes the optically birefringence of nerve fibers, which is induced by the optical anisotropy of the myelin sheaths surrounding axons [18–20]. 3D-PLI provides a three-dimensional description of the anatomical connectivity in form of a vector field indicating the prevailing fiber orientation per voxel. Depending on the used imaging setup and the section thickness the acquirable spatial resolution is 1.6 – 100 μm. Hence, the method bridges the microscopic and the macroscopic description of the anatomical connectivity of the human brain.

The birefringence of brain tissue is measured by passing linearly polarized light through histological brain sections and by detecting local changes in the polarization state of light using a polarimeter setup (Figure 1a-b). The polarimeter is equipped with a pair of crossed polarizers, a tilting specimen stage, a quarter-wave retarder, an LED light source (with a narrow-band green wavelength spectrum), and a charge-coupled device (CCD) camera. By rotating the optical devices simultaneously around the stationary brain section and by imaging the sample at discrete rotation angles ρ, a sinusoidal variation of the measured light intensity (i.e., the light intensity profile) is observed for each image pixel (Figure 1c). The individual course of a light intensity profile essentially depends on the locally prevailing 3D fiber orientation described by an orientation unit vector which is defined by the in-section direction angle φ and the out-of-section inclination angle α. Basic principles of optics (Snell's law and Huygens-Fresnel principle) and the Jones calculus [21] mathematically link the measured light intensity profile I to the fiber orientation via

$$I = \frac{I_0}{2} \cdot [1 + sin(2\rho - 2\varphi) \cdot sin\delta], \tag{1}$$

with $\delta \approx 2\pi \cdot \frac{d \cdot \Delta n}{\lambda} \cdot cos^2\alpha$.

The amplitude of the profile quantifies the phase retardation δ induced to the light wave by the myelin. This phase retardation is a function of the light wavelength λ, the section thickness d, the birefringence Δn of the myelin, and the inclination angle α. The transmittance I_0 denotes the intensity of the incident light modified by local extinction effects. While ρ is the azimuth angle of the transmission axis of the first polarizer, φ represents the projection of the fiber axis onto the section plane with respect to the starting angle of the polarimeter. As a consequence, the fundamental data structure gained by 3D-PLI is a 3D vector field description of fibers and fiber tract orientations – the basis for subsequent tractography and fiber modeling.

For estimating the sinusoidal profile of the 3D-PLI signal Discrete Fourier Analysis (DFA) can be used to deduce I from Equation (1):

$$I = a_0 + a_1 \cdot \sin(2\rho) + b_1 \cdot \cos(2\rho) \tag{2}$$

with $a_0 = \frac{I_0}{2}$, $a_1 = \frac{I_0}{2} \cdot \sin(\delta) \cdot \cos(2\varphi)$, $b_1 = \frac{I_0}{2} \cdot \sin(\delta) \cdot \sin(2\varphi)$.

1.3. Relevance and restoration of the light intensity profile

In 3D-PLI, the light intensity profile (cf. Figure 1) represents a crucial data set in terms of fiber orientation determination, since peak position and signal amplitude of the profile are directly related to the in-section direction and out-of-section inclination of the fiber orientation, respectively. A precise and undisturbed recording of the light intensity passing through a microtome section is therefore mandatory for the reliable reconstruction of high-resolution fiber tracts. The signal quality is however influenced by several conditions. Thermal effects and electrical noise in both the light source and the CCD-electronics deteriorate the PLI signal characteristics at each image pixel. Filter inhomogeneities of the polarizers or retarder may also manipulate the intensity profile. Therefore, a standardized image calibration technique using flat fields is usually applied to all raw images prior to analysis to compensate pixel-wise for inhomogeneities across the field-of-view [22]. Depending on the section thickness the pixel-by-pixel intensity is also influenced by the scatter properties of the investigated object. Another possible source of artifacts is dust on the polarizer. Although the polarimeter should be operated in a shielded construction to prevent for external light and dust particles, dust cannot completely be avoided. As a result of the rotation of the polarizer dust particles will deteriorate the measured light intensity only once within a half circle, if and only if they are located on the rotating system (cf. Figure 1). Hence, the measured intensity at the CCD array is a linear mixture of different light sources.

Recently, signal enhancement and restoration techniques for PLI images utilizing independent component analysis (ICA) have been introduced [22,23]. As a result, component maps corresponding to gray and white matter structures as well as noise and artifacts can be identified automatically using statistical analysis tools [23]. Remarkably, even in the presence of dust on the polarimeter ICA can effectively restore the original sinusoidal signal (Figure 2). After ICA filtering the noise and artifacts are removed and the sinusoidal nature of the PLI signal is restored (Figure 2).

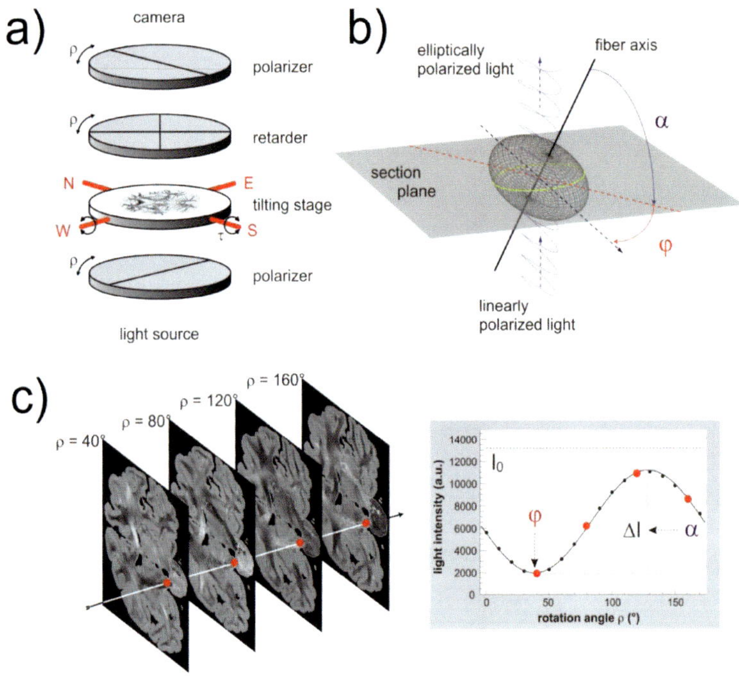

Figure 1. Polarimetry at a glance. (a) Scheme of the rotating polarimeter with tilting stage (N-North, W-West, E-East, S-South). (b) Scheme of the optical fiber model. The refractive index of a negative uniaxially birefringent medium, such as a myelinated axon, is described by an elliptically shaped oblate surface, the indicatrix (gray mesh). A beam of linearly polarized light (blue trace) interacts locally with the myelin sheath of a single axon (black line) and becomes elliptically polarized. (c) A typical 3D-PLI raw image data set consists of 18 images corresponding to equidistant rotation angles between 0° and 170°. Here, a selection of four images of a coronal section is shown, while the sketched arrow indicates one representative pixel. To obtain the fiber orientation, the measured light intensities are studied pixel-wise as a function of discrete rotation angles. The derived physical model provides a precise mathematical description of the measurement (continuous black line) and relates the sine phase to the direction angle φ and the amplitude to the inclination angle α. The highlighted data points correspond to the selected images.

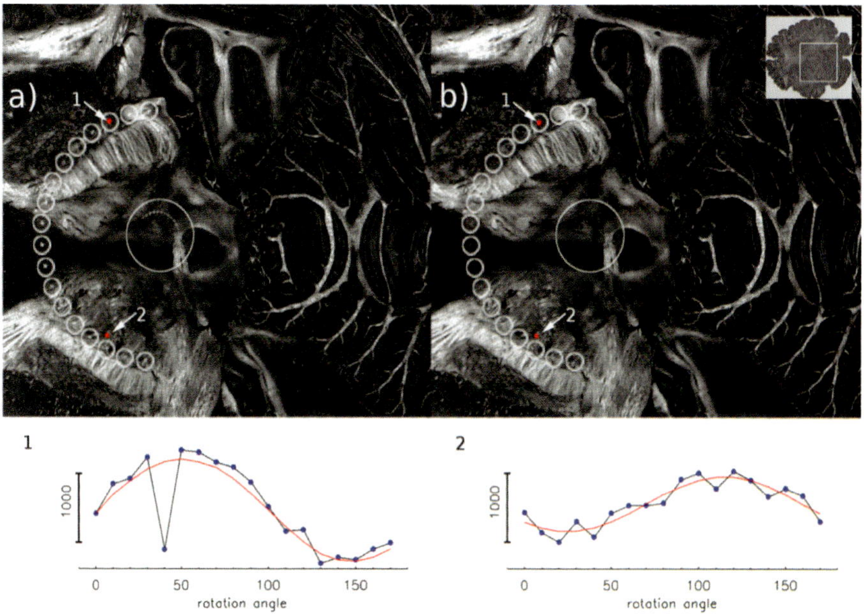

Figure 2. In (a) multiple artifacts including dust contamination are present. The trajectory of a dust particle is highlighted by the signal power inside the white circles along all rotation angles. After ICA filtering (b) the signal derogation is greatly removed. At the bottom, PLI raw signals (black) are shown together with corresponding signals after artifact rejection (red). The signals were extracted from the two locations as indicated by the red dots. In comparison to the PLI raw data ICA obviously removed the signal derogation and is capable of restoring the original sinusoidal signal in case of dust (signal #1) or noise (signal #2) contaminations.

2. A new concept for optimal signal decomposition in polarized light imaging

Although blind source separation methods are successfully applied for signal separation in all kinds of neuroimaging modalities [24–29] two major problems remain: i) the method applied must be selected carefully and the separation strategy (i.e., the internal cost function) of the applied method should be optimal for the type of data. This however, is one of the reasons why many different ICA algorithms co-exist. ii) Assuming the measured signals are adequately separated into the underlying source signals (i.e., signal of interest and non-interest), identification of the signal of interest should be performed user independently; preferably in an automatic fashion. For the latter, significant effort has to be invested in order to identify components of interest automatically from data recorded utilizing different neuroimaging techniques [29–33]. In contrast to many other ICA applications, the great advantage in PLI signal decomposition is that all profiles of the basis vectors that correspond to the signal of interest must show a sinusoidal waveform [16,22]. Since these waveforms can only vary in amplitude and phase, an automatic extraction of the signal components can be achieved utilizing this property as demonstrated in [23].

Alternatively, it has been demonstrated that by incorporating prior knowledge, i.e., by imposing temporal or spatial constraints for the source separation task, decomposition can be effectively improved [34–37]. Hesse and James [38], for example, showed that using different types of spatial constraints ICA can be trained to *i)* identify ocular artifacts automatically and *ii)* to detect and trace ictal activity. Liu and colleagues recently presented a reference based ICA concept to successfully target a specific genetic variation [36] in real and simulated data sets. For the investigation of signal detection in the imaging system of the retina in cats Barriga and colleagues introduced a constrained ICA algorithm which increases the detection of responses to visual stimuli in cats even for low levels of signal-to-noise ratio [37]. In the next section the basic principle of ICA is described shortly. For a more detailed review, we refer to [39,40].

2.1. A short introduction to independent component analysis (ICA)

For 3D-PLI a linear superposition of light at the CCD camera is assumed, where each elementary signal component refers to a distinct region in space. By applying independent component analysis (ICA) to a set of polarized light images (here a stack of 18 images at different rotation angles is used) the decomposition of the data results in spatially independent components (often called feature or basis vectors) yielding maximally (i.e., statistically) independent spatial component maps.

Let $\mathbf{X}=(X_1, X_2, \ldots, X_N)^T$ be the N-dimensional measured PLI signal mixture, where each X_i is one image mixture (flatted to a one-dimensional image vector with M pixels) detected at a corresponding rotation angle ρ. In spatial ICA $\mathbf{X}$ is considered to be a $N \times M$ matrix (as opposed to temporal ICA, where the dimension of the matrix is transposed), with M = number of pixels included in the analysis and N = number of rotation angles reflecting N different instances of the signal. The contribution of each source image varies N times over the angles ρ. Similarly, $\mathbf{S}=(S_1, S_2, \ldots, S_N)^T$ represents the N-dimensional true source signals. Hence, the linear relationship of mixed sources can be expressed as follows:

$$\mathbf{X}=\mathbf{AS} \tag{3}$$

with $\mathbf{A}$ being the unknown mixing matrix of dimension $N \times N$. The key problem in ICA is to find an unmixing matrix $\mathbf{W}$ (similar to a pseudo-inverse $\mathbf{A}^{-1}$, with $\mathbf{W} \approx \mathbf{A}^{-1}$) while imposing that the sources in $\mathbf{S}$ are statistically independent, that is:

$$\mathbf{C}=\mathbf{WX}. \tag{4}$$

Within ICA the N-dimensional data array $\mathbf{X}$ is transformed into an N-dimensional component space $\mathbf{C}$, where each of the spatial component maps carries a minimum amount of mutual information and thus is maximally independent. These independent components (or spatial maps) are stored in the rows of **C**, while in the columns of $\mathbf{W}^{-1}$ the associated spatially independent "temporal" profiles (i.e., the contrast changing function along the rotation angle, the basis vector) are stored.

Signal restoration, i.e. the cleaning process, is performed by zeroing columns in $\mathbf{W}^{-1}$ which reflect signal contributions from unwanted (e.g. artifact) sources. This is identical to zeroing rows in **C**, where the independent component maps of interest are stored in **C**'. The cleaning of measured data is performed by back transformation of **C**', which results in a new set of PLI data **X**'.

$$\mathbf{X}' = \hat{\mathbf{A}} \cdot \mathbf{C}' \qquad (5)$$

with $\mathbf{W}^{-1} = \hat{\mathbf{A}}$.

2.2. Constrained ICA for polarized light imaging (*cICAP*)

Signal separation in constrained ICA is based on incorporating prior knowledge about the underlying signals. In the study of Barriga and colleagues [37], *a priori* information is incorporated into one column of the estimated mixing matrix of the spatial decomposition via an off-on constraint, meaning that the visual response signal used in the study has to follow the stimulus signal. For this, the authors filled one column of the mixing matrix with ones for the time of the stimulation, while zero values reflect off-stimulation. Similar to the concept introduced by Barriga and colleagues in 2011, it is possible to incorporate the *a priori* information from 3D-PLI, but with the major difference that for birefringent signals an analytical expression exists to model the expected signal of interest, which only differs in amplitude and phase. Therefore, a new algorithm motivated by the results described in [23] has been developed, where signal separation and the identification of the underlying 3D-PLI source signals are combined into one method. The new algorithm (referred to as *constrained ICA for polarized light imaging, cICAP*) is based on a modified version of the Infomax principle [41] by means of incorporating prior information to the cost function of Infomax; this is similar to the work reported in [34,37]. In *cICAP* a theoretically expected function $f_i(u_\rho)$ is implemented into the Infomax cost function to control for the results of the decomposition. Recall that if the i-th column in $\hat{\mathbf{A}}$ has a sinusoidal profile, the corresponding component map in **C** represents a signal of interest (cf. Equation (4-5)). The expected function $f_i(u_\rho)$ can be derived from Equation (2), where the parameters a_0, a_1 and b_1 are fitted involving all rotation angles ρ [16].

Starting from Equation (4) the natural-gradient version in Infomax is used to update the weight matrix **W** during the ICA learning procedure [42,43]:

$$\Delta\mathbf{W} = \left[\mathbf{I} + (1 - 2\mathrm{y})\mathbf{C}^{*T}\right]\mathbf{W} \qquad (6)$$

with $\mathrm{y} = 1 / \left(1 + e^{-\mathbf{C}^*}\right)$.

In Equation (6) **I** and denote the identity matrix and the learning rate, respectively, as it is used in the standard Infomax algorithm [41]. $\mathbf{C}^*$ denotes the intermediate component matrix which is identical to **C** when the learning procedure is finished. In common with the approach of [37], the mixing matrix $\hat{\mathbf{A}}$ is estimated by $\hat{\mathbf{A}} := (\mathbf{P} \cdot \mathbf{W})^{-1}$, with **P** being the sphering matrix of the decorrelation process within Infomax. By incorporating the *a priori* information at each iteration step, $\hat{\mathbf{A}}$ is updated by:

$$\hat{\mathbf{a}}_i^* = (1 - c) \cdot \hat{\mathbf{a}}_i + c \cdot f_i(u_\rho) \tag{7}$$

where $\hat{\mathrm{a}}_i$ refers to the i-th column of the estimated mixing matrix $\hat{\mathbf{A}}$ and c is a confidence parameter ranging from 0 to 1. The confidence parameter c in Equation (7) indicates the percentage of weighting of the prior knowledge by means of the expected function $f_i(u_\rho)$. In the limit of $c \rightarrow 0$ the original Infomax weight update is used (cf. Equation (6)). It is important to note that for each iteration step only one column in $\hat{\mathbf{A}}$ is updated as expressed in Equation (7) since we do not want to influence the decomposition of the remaining components during the unmixing process. The column in $\hat{\mathbf{A}}$ which entries are most similar to the corresponding expectation function is selected and modified according to Equation (7). As a measure for similarity the kurtosis of the deviation function $d_i = \hat{a}_i - f_i(u_\rho)$ is used:

$$kurt(d_i) = \frac{1}{N} \cdot \sum_{\rho}^{N} \left(\frac{d_{i,\rho} - \bar{d}_i}{\sigma_i} \right)^4 - 3, \tag{8}$$

where $\bar{d}_i$ is the expected value of the deviation function of the i-th component. In the ideal case d_i will be zero (or close to zero); for any deviation at one or more corresponding angles ρ the measure $kurt(d_i)$ will largely be increased. For a subsequent selection of columns in $\hat{\mathbf{A}}$ the column profile with smallest kurtosis value as expressed by Equation (8) is used first. Moreover, if the mean square error (MSE) between the updated column $\hat{a}_i^*$ and the corresponding theoretically expectation function $f_i(u_\rho)$ is less than a predefined tolerance value t the entries of $\hat{a}_i^*$ are fixed. Thus, the MSE is expressed by:

$$MSE(\hat{a}_i^*, f_i(u_\rho)) = \frac{1}{N} \cdot \sum_{\rho}^{N} (\hat{a}_i^*(\rho) - f_i(u_\rho))^2. \tag{9}$$

The basic idea here is that a very small MSE (i.e., $MSE \leq t$) in Equation (9) indicates that $\hat{a}_i^*$ and $f_i(u_\rho)$ are very similar, which means that the i-th column in $\hat{\mathbf{A}}$ then represents a source of interest. This approach is repeated for the remaining columns in $\hat{\mathbf{A}}$ until no further components of interest are found. As a stopping criterion for the iteration, a predefined threshold, ε, for the

MSE (with $\varepsilon \gg t$) is used to prevent the algorithm of running into an endless loop. This differentiation of updating $\hat{a}_i^*$ is expressed in Equation (10):

$$\hat{a}_i^* = \begin{cases} (1-c)\cdot \hat{a}_i + c\cdot f_i(u_\rho) & , \text{if } kurt(d_i) < \varepsilon \wedge MSE(\hat{a}_i, f_i(u_\rho)) > t \\ \hat{a}_i & , \text{else} \end{cases} \tag{10}$$

For the weight update described in Equation (10) the choice of the confidence value c and the tolerance values t and ε should be performed in a representative but independent data set, which is described later.

2.2.1. Evaluation of the signal enhancement

For measuring the noise reduction and signal enhancement in a set of 3D-PLI data after ICA application we use the weighted reduced chi-squared statistic as introduced in [23]. The reduced chi-squared statistic χ^2 involves the variance σ^2 of the observation, where the statistical output is weighted based on the measurement error

$$\chi^2 = \frac{1}{v} \cdot \sum_{\rho}^{N} \frac{(I_\rho - f(u_\rho))^2}{\sigma_\rho^2}. \tag{11}$$

Here, I_ρ denote the intensity measured at angle ρ. The variance σ^2 used in Equation (11) was obtained from 100 flat field images, which were independently generated for the image calibration process [22]. The weighted sum over N angles is further normalized by the degrees of freedom υ. The normalization ensures a good fit when the reduced chi-square value equals one, which is achieved when the squared difference between the measurement and the expected function resemble the variance of the measurement. In order to measure the signal improvement (and the reduction of noise) through the ICA process the test statistic is determined before (χ^2_{raw}) and after (χ^2_{ICA}) ICA. Using the ratio of these values and introducing a weight factor ω that penalizes the goodness of fit, whenever a signal component is missing [23]. The weighted test statistic reads as follows:

$$wrGOF(x, y) = \frac{\chi^2_{raw}}{\omega \cdot \chi^2_{ICA}}, \tag{12}$$

with $\omega = \frac{1}{v} \cdot \sum_{\rho}^{N} \frac{(f_{raw}(u_\rho) - f_{ICA}(u_\rho))^2}{\sigma_\rho^2} \geq 1.$

The weight factor ω increases when the squared difference between the two expectation functions $f_{raw}(u_\rho)$ and $f_{ICA}(u_\rho)$ (derived from the raw and the ICA filtered PLI data sets, respectively) is large. In case of missed components of interest, the signal strength of the ICA filtered 3D-PLI signal would be largely reduced at corresponding pixel locations. Consequently the expectation function $f_{ICA}(u_\rho)$ would differ in terms of its amplitude, while the shape of the waveform may be still sinusoidal. The assumption here is that the signal power (across the rotation angles) of the signal of interest is larger compared to noise. The restriction of $\omega \geq 1$ is needed in order to not artificially improve the goodness-of-fit in cases where the two expectation functions $f_{raw}(u_\rho)$ and $f_{ICA}(u_\rho)$ are very similar (e.g., at pixel locations with low noise).

2.2.2. *Finding the optimal parameters*

The optimal parameters c, t and ε for the weight update as described above (cf. Equation (10)), should be determined using a representative but independent data set. In the test data from the same post-mortem brain were used, but from a different microtome section which is not included in the subsequent analysis. The determination of the optimal parameters for *cICAP* requires the maximization of the weighted goodness-of-fit (*wrGOF*) values across all pixel locations ($\approx 3.41 \cdot 10^5$pixels). As a control measure for this requirement the minimal *wrGOF* value was checked for all trajectories (i.e., the intensity profiles at pixel location x,y) within the brain section. In total we performed 1225 ($=35^2$) *cICAP* calculations while varying both the confidence value c and the tolerance value t accordingly to the range from 0.0 to 0.7 and 10^{-3} to 10^{-7}, respectively. Figure 3a shows the results of this benchmark run. The largest improvement (cf. blue dot in Figure 3a) was found for the confidence and tolerance values of c=0.16 and $t = 1.07 \cdot 10^{-6}$, respectively. Once both parameters c and t are fixed the stopping criterion ε, which controls the number of iterations, can be determined. For this task, we investigated the smallest and largest error found in the base functions of $\hat{\mathbf{A}}$ by means of the *MSE* value as expressed by Equation (9). As a reference for the definition of signal components, the user independent component selection tool was used, which is based on the statistically analysis of the base functions as reported in [23]. Throughout all iterations in *cICAP* the maximal *MSE* across the columns in matrix $\hat{\mathbf{A}}$ that were identified as signal components was found to be well below 0.01. Figure 3b shows that after about 35 iterations the *MSE* value converges to almost a constant for both the signal (red) and noise components (blue), where both types of components can clearly be identified by means of the corresponding *MSE* value.

In Figure 4 the progress of changes in the sinusoidal profile of one exemplary basis vector is shown for all 18 iterations (blue) within *cICAP*. The algorithm converges with a very small fit error (*MSE*) of $1.07 \cdot 10^{-6}$. The resulting sinusoidal trajectory (black) almost perfectly fits the theoretically expectation function (red).

The process of updating the weight matrix and how *a priori* knowledge is included in *cICAP* is shown in Figure 5. Once a basis vector resembles the expectation function under the criteria of $MSE(\hat{a}_i^*) < t$, this basis vector is not changed in further iterations. Note, throughout the optimization the selection of the underlying signal components is automatically included in *cICAP* and no further user interaction is required.

http://dx.doi.org/10.5772/55246

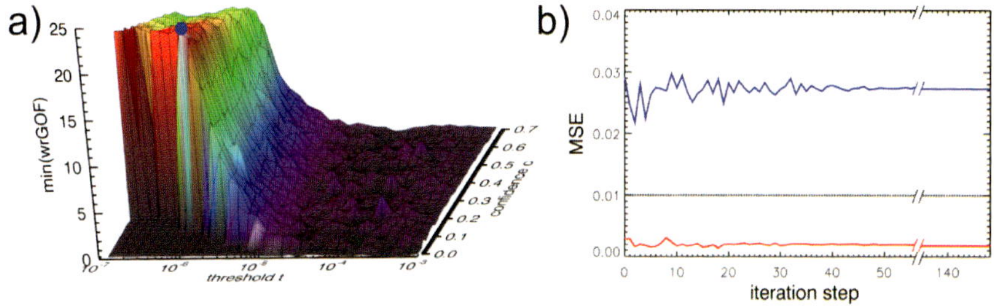

Figure 3. Parameter benchmark run. In (a) the optimal confidence value *c* and the tolerance value *t* was determined through a test run of 1225 signal decomposition steps varying both parameters *c* and *t* 35 times each through the range from 0.0 to 0.7 and 10^{-3} to 10^{-7}, respectively. As a control measure to find the best parameters, where the goodness-of-fit statistics (wrGOF) is increased at all pixel locations, the largest minimal *wrGOF* value (blue circle) is determined. The best set of parameters was found for $c=0.16$ and $t=1.07 \cdot 10^{-6}$ with a minimal wrGOF value of about 21. (b) The development of the maximal mean squared error (*MSE*) is shown for 147 iterations to determine the stopping criterion ε, which controls the number of iterations. The maximal and minimal *MSE* value is plotted for components reflecting signal of interest (red) and noise components (blue), respectively. After a few iterations the largest *MSE* value for signal components was found to be well below 1%. Therefore, setting ε to 0.01 both types of components can clearly be identified.

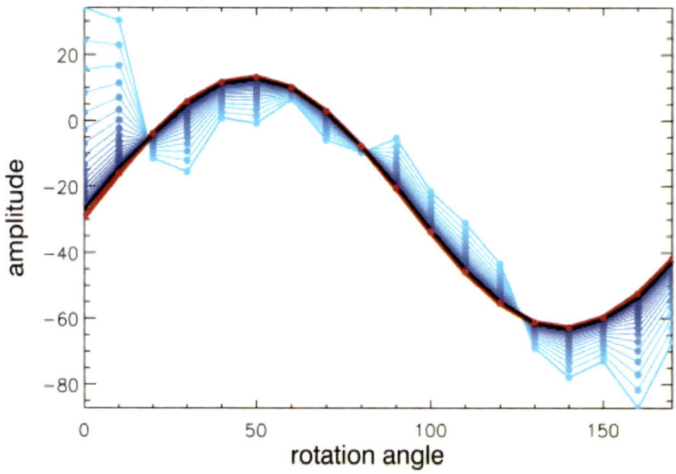

Figure 4. Stepwise changes of one exemplary basis function (changing from light blue to black). After 18 iterations using *cICAP* the algorithm converges with a very small fit error (*MSE*) of $1.07 \cdot 10^{-6}$. The resulting sinusoidal trajectory (black) almost perfectly fits the theoretically expectation function (red).

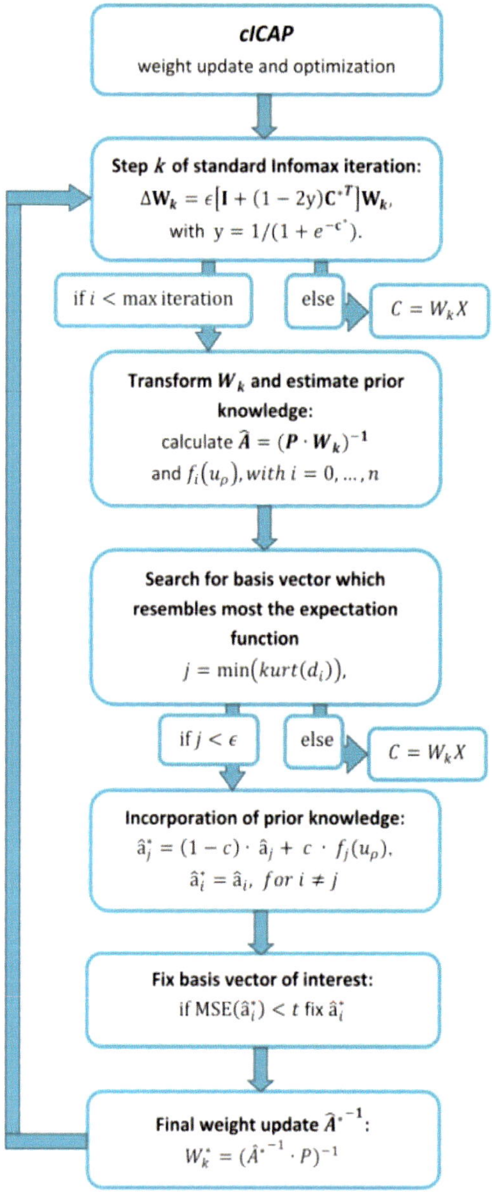

Figure 5. Scheme of the weight matrix update and optimization procedure in *cICAP*.

http://dx.doi.org/10.5772/55246

3. Signal enhancement in 3D-PLI data sets

3.1. Signal acquisition and preprocessing

The performance of *cICAP* was tested on 102 histological sections of one adult human brain acquired from the body donor program of the University of Rostock, Germany, in accordance with legal requirements. The brain was fixed in 4% formalin for 6 months, cryo-protected with glycerin and cut after freezing in a cryostat microtome (Polycut CM 3500, Leica, Germany). The brain was sectioned coronally with slice a thickness of 70 μm. The sections were mounted on glass slides with Aquatex© (Merck, Germany) and cover-slipped. Note that all preparation steps are conforming to preserve the integrity of the birefringent myelin sheaths.

The sections were digitized using the polarimeter setup described in section 1.2. Each brain section was imaged at 18 equidistant rotation angles of the polarimeter covering an angle range between 0° and 170° (Figure 1b). The acquired RGB-colored images have a size of 2776 × 2080 pixels with a pixel size of 64 μm × 64 μm. The intensities were sampled with a dynamic range of 14 bits per color channel. Since the light source of the polarimeter is composed of light-emitting diodes (LED) emitting a narrow-band green wavelength spectrum (central wavelength of 525 nm), only the green channel from the RGB color triplet was used for further analysis.

Before the images were decomposed by ICA, a standardized calibration technique using flat fields was applied, in order to compensate pixel-wise for inhomogeneities across the field of view [22]. In addition, the separation of brain tissue from the non-relevant image background was done by means of the interactive learning and segmentation toolkit (ilastik) [44]. Thus, the following calculations and statistical analyses were solely done on basis of brain tissue measurements.

3.2. Performance on signal decomposition using *cICAP*

To test the performance of the signal decomposition and signal restoration *cICAP* was applied to the data set described in section 3.1. The mean number of pixels used for ICA across the 102 brain sections was found to be $(3.32 \pm 0.95) \cdot 10^5$. The results of signal decomposition and enhancement gained by *cICAP* were compared to the automatic component selection routine, which were recently published in [23], whereas the threshold for this data set was adapted to 2.2.

After the determination of the parameters c, t and ε all values were fixed within *cICAP* and both ICA algorithms were applied to the same set of PLI data for comparison. As shown in Table 1, the identified number of signal components (on average) does not vary dramatically across both algorithms. However, the smallest variability with the fewest number of iterations needed was found in the results of *cICAP*. The number of iterations needed (on average) in *cICAP* was 192, while for the Infomax algorithm using the automatic selection routine it was found to be 406. More importantly, the goodness-of-fit criterion *wrGOF* was found to be largest using *cICAP*. It is important to note that this criterion expresses the signal enhancement (or degradation) after ICA filtering and was calculated for all trajectories (i.e., at each pixel location). If the *wrGOF* value is larger than 1, then noise and artifacts were removed (or suppressed) successfully. In cases, where the signal decomposition fails (or is not optimal) the *wrGOF* value becomes even smaller than 1 (Figure 6). To check the decomposition results for signal degradation after the application of ICA, the minimal *wrGOF* value was calculated. As illustrated in Table 1 a *wrGOF* value smaller than 1 was found in 3.57% and 0.35% of all pixels in the results from Infomax and *cICAP*, respectively.

In general both ICA algorithms produced remarkable decomposition results, where signal enhancement (*wrGOF* ≥ 1) is evident in almost all pixels. However, we found a much better signal decomposition performance in the results of *cICAP*. This is expressed by the fact that the *wrGOF* value was found to be equal or larger than 10 in about 80% of all trajectories, while for the Infomax algorithm it was 39%. For *cICAP* we still found a goodness-of-fit value of larger or equal than 100 in 56% of all pixels. In comparison to the standard Infomax this number drops down to about 15%.

	I) Infomax	**II) cICAP**
identified ICs (mean)	7.7 ± 4.75	3.8 ± 1.19
number of iterations (mean)	405.5± 32.3	191.8± 23.13
wrGOF (median)	18.8	1910.5
wrGOF < 1 (%)	3.57 %	0.35 %
wrGOF ≥ 10 (%)	38.8 %	80.0 %
wrGOF ≥ 100 (%)	15.1 %	55.6 %

Table 1. Statistical analysis of ICA decomposition results. The signal components for the ICA routine *I* were selected by means of a user independent algorithm (see text).

In Figure 6a pixel locations of a representative section is shown, where the test statistic (*wrGOF*) is larger or equal 300. In this example signal enhancement was evident at all pixel locations (i.e., *wrGOF* > 1; not shown). By focusing on larger values of the test statistic (e.g., *wrGOF* ≥ 300) the figure demonstrates that the enhancement of the optical signals is ensured in particular in the region of the neo-cortex and at the white to gray matter boundary (Figure 6a). This in general is challenging, since in such regions the 3D-PLI signal has low amplitudes and therefore the measured signal has a poor signal-to-noise ratio.

With the introduction of the weighting factor (or penalty factor) as expressed by Equation (12), the test statistic *wrGOF* is sensitive to both, changes in the signal-to-noise ratio as well as in reductions of signal strength after ICA. This in particular will be the case when one or more components of interest are not selected for signal reconstruction (e.g., when the selection is performed manually). As a result, at corresponding pixel locations the *wrGOF* value will be less than 1. The idea behind this is, that the weighted test statistic *wrGOF* accounts for missing gray and white matter components and improvements in SNR, independently to the metric used for identification of components of interest. In Figure 6b such a testing scenario is

http://dx.doi.org/10.5772/55246

demonstrated, where one component of interest was manually excluded before the 3D-PLI signal was reconstructed. For this section, 24% of all pixels have a *wrGOF* value below 1.

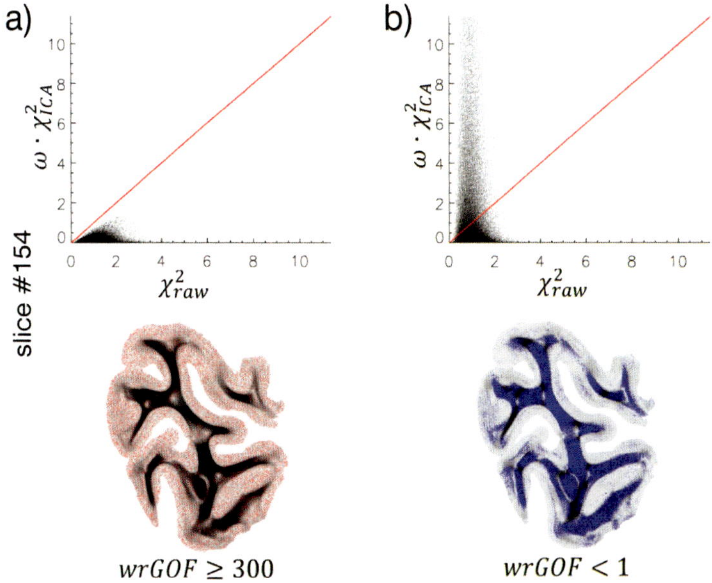

Figure 6. χ^2 ratios and pixel locations illustrating goodness-of-fit values. In a) χ^2 ratios are shown using all components identified by *cICAP*, where the goodness-of-fit statistics was larger than 1 at all pixel locations. In the coronal brain section pixels highlighted in red show locations with goodness-of-fit values larger than 300. b)To demonstrate the effect of being sensitive to missing signal of interest, one identified component was manually deselected. As a result, large areas of white matter structure do show a *wrGOF* value of less than 1 (highlighted in blue).

4. Conclusion

In recent years 3D-polarized light imaging (3D-PLI) has been shown to provide new insights into the organization of the human brain including mapping of the fiber anatomy [15,45,46]. Through advances in the experimental setup of the employed polarimeter, as well as in signal processing, this modality provides unique data sets to explore the 3D fiber architecture in the human brain at a submillimeter resolution [16,47,48]. Though the technique as described here is applicable solely to postmortem brain tissue, the comprehensive description of complex fiber orientations in distinct brain regions (e.g., prevalent fiber crossings) can be used to guide and evaluate fiber tractography algorithms based on diffusion MRI. By this means the fiber orientation maps provided by 3D-PLI might help to optimize the reliability of in-vivo diffusion MRI results. Precise information about the local individual fiber architecture of a patient is of particular interest in case of planning and performing a neurosurgical intervention, for instance.

However, in 3D-PLI the reconstruction of nerve fiber pathways strongly depends on the quality of the measured intensities represented by the so-called light intensity profiles or 3D-PLI signals, respectively. Hence, advanced signal processing tools are required to enable the precise determination of locally prevailing fiber orientations in form of unit vectors defined by the in-section direction angle φ and the out-of-section inclination angle α.

Independent component analysis (ICA) turned out to improve 3D-PLI signals significantly [22,23]. It was shown that ICA is capable of restoring the original birefringent signal by effectively removing noise and artifact components in the measured data. In addition, measures for the qualitative and quantitative evaluation of the 3D-PLI signals before and after the ICA filtering were introduced. In particular, the signal enhancement after ICA based denoising is large at the white to gray matter boundary, where the 3D-PLI signal is weak due to decreasing fiber density when approaching gray matter domains [22].

In *cICAP*, the "constrained ICA for polarized light imaging", the signal decomposition is optimized using a weight update, which incorporates the prior knowledge that the expected signal in 3D-PLI can be modeled utilizing the Jones calculus (cf. Equation (1)). This prior knowledge gives rise to a training of the unmixing procedure in *cICAP*, where the weight matrix update is optimal with respect to the sources of interest (cf. Equation (10)). Utilizing this approach the source separation and identification in *cICAP* is carried out automatically in one routine, where no further component selection tool is needed for subsequent extraction of the signal of interest.

With the introduction of *cICAP* an ICA-based source separation method is available which is optimal for the extraction of the sinusoidal trajectory along different rotation angles in a set of spatially mixed 3D-PLI images. The better quality of the source separation in *cICAP* is reflected by the increased goodness-of-fit statistic ($wrGOF$), which not only takes the improvement in the signal-to-noise ratio (SNR) into account, but also accounts for signal restoration [23].

The dedicated signal processing tool *cICAP* largely contributes to the reliability of 3D-PLI signals and, hence, the accuracy of subsequent fiber tract reconstruction. As a consequence, *cICAP* plays a key role in the 3D-PLI processing chain and helps to establish the so far missing link between the microscopic and the macroscopic characterization of the anatomical connectivity of the human brain.

Acknowledgements

We thank Prof. Dr. A. Wree, Institute for Anatomy, University of Rostock, for providing us with the postmortem human brain.

http://dx.doi.org/10.5772/55246

Author details

Jürgen Dammers[1], Lukas Breuer[1], Giuseppe Tabbì[2] and Markus Axer[2]

1 Institute of Neuroscience and Medicine, Medical Imaging Physics, INM-4, Forschungszentrum Jülich, Jülich, Germany

2 Institute of Neuroscience and Medicine, Structural and Functional Organisation of the Brain, INM-1, Forschungszentrum Jülich, Jülich, Germany

References

[1] Mesulam, M. Foreword. In: Schmahmann JD, Pandya DN, editors. Fiber pathways of the brain. Oxford University Press; (2006).

[2] Kötter, R. Handbook of brain connectivity. In: Jirsa VK, McIntosh AR, editors. Berlin New York: Springer; (2007). page , 149-1167.

[3] Sporns, O, Tononi, G, & Kötter, R. The human connectome: A structural description of the human brain. PLoS computational biology. Public Library of Science; (2005). Sep;, 1(4), 245-51.

[4] Johansen-berg, H. Behrens TEJ. Diffusion MRI: From Quantitative Measurement to In-vivo Neuroanatomy. Academic Press; (2009). page 490.

[5] Jones, D. K. Diffusion MRI: Theory, Methods, and Applications. Jones DK, editor. Oxford University Press; (2011). page 624.

[6] Türe, U, Yasargil, M. G, Friedman, A. H, & Al-mefty, O. Fiber dissection technique: lateral aspect of the brain. Neurosurgery. (2000). Aug;, 47(2), 417-27.

[7] Klingler, J. Erleichterung der makroskopischen Präparation des Gehirns durch den Gefrierprozess. Schweizer Archiv für Neurologie und Psychiatrie. (1935).

[8] Bürgel, U, Amunts, K, Hoemke, L, Mohlberg, H, Gilsbach, J. M, & Zilles, K. White matter fiber tracts of the human brain: three-dimensional mapping at microscopic resolution, topography and intersubject variability. NeuroImage. Department of Neurosurgery, RWTH Aachen University, D-52074 Aachen, Germany.; (2006). Feb 15;, 29(4), 1092-105.

[9] Flechsig, P. Developmental (myelongenetic) localisation of the cerebral cortex in the human subject. Lancet. (1901).

[10] Fink, R. P, & Heimer, L. Two methods for selective silver impregnation of degenerating axons and their synaptic endings in the central nervous system. Brain Research. (1967). Apr;, 4(4), 369-74.

[11] Clarke, S, & Miklossy, J. Occipital cortex in man: organization of callosal connections, related myelo- and cytoarchitecture, and putative boundaries of functional visual areas. J. Comp. Neurol. (1990).

[12] Burkhalter, A, Bernardo, K. L, & Charles, V. Development of local circuits in human visual cortex. The Journal of neuroscience- the official journal of the Society for Neuroscience. (1993). May;, 13(5), 1916-31.

[13] Lanciego, J, & Wouterlood, F. Neuroanatomical tract-tracing methods beyond 2000: what's now and next. Journal of Neuroscience Methods. (2000). Nov;, 103(1), 1-2.

[14] Schmahmann, J, & Pandya, D. Fiber Pathways of the Brain. Oxford University Press; (2010). page 672.

[15] Axer, M, Grässel, D, Kleiner, M, Dammers, J, Dickscheid, T, Reckfort, J, et al. High-resolution fiber tract reconstruction in the human brain by means of three-dimensional polarized light imaging. Frontiers in neuroinformatics. (2011). Jan;, 5(34), 1-13.

[16] Axer, M, Amunts, K, Grässel, D, Palm, C, Dammers, J, Axer, H, et al. A novel approach to the human connectome: ultra-high resolution mapping of fiber tracts in the brain. NeuroImage. (2011). Jan;, 54(2), 1091-101.

[17] Axer, H, Beck, S, Axer, M, Schuchardt, F, Heepe, J, Flücken, A, et al. Microstructural analysis of human white matter architecture using polarized light imaging: views from neuroanatomy. Frontiers in neuroinformatics. (2011). Jan;, 5(28), 1-12.

[18] Schmitt, F. O, & Bear, R. S. The optical properties of vertebrate nerve axons as related to fiber size. Journal of Cellular and Comparative Physiology. (1937). Feb;, 9(2), 261-73.

[19] Schmidt, W. J. Zur Doppelbrechung des Nervenmarks. Zeitschrift für wissenschaftliche Mikroskopie. (1923). , 41, 29-38.

[20] Göthlin, G. F. Die doppelbrechenden Eigenschaften des Nervengewebes. Kungliga Svenska Vetenskapsakademiens. (1913). Handlingar(51).

[21] Jones, R. C. A New Calculus for the Treatment of Optical Systems. Journal of the Optical Society of America. (1941). Jul;, 31(7), 500-3.

[22] Dammers, J, Axer, M, Grässel, D, Palm, C, Zilles, K, Amunts, K, et al. Signal enhancement in polarized light imaging by means of independent component analysis. NeuroImage. (2010). Jan;, 49(2), 1241-8.

[23] Dammers, J, Breuer, L, Axer, M, Kleiner, M, Eiben, B, Grässel, D, et al. Automatic identification of gray and white matter components in polarized light imaging. NeuroImage. (2012). Jan 16;, 59(2), 1338-47.

[24] Beckmann, C. F, & Smith, S. M. Probabilistic independent component analysis for functional magnetic resonance imaging. IEEE Transactions on Medical Imaging. (2004). Feb;, 23(2), 137-52.

[25] Cong, F, Kalyakin, I, Ahuttunen-scott, T, Li, H, Lyytinen, H, & Ristaniemi, T. Single-trial based Independent Component Analysis on Mismatch Negativity in Children. International Journal of Neural Systems. (2010).

[26] Esposito, F, Formisano, E, Seifritz, E, Goebel, R, Morrone, R, Tedeschi, G, et al. Spatial independent component analysis of functional MRI time-series: to what extent do results depend on the algorithm used? Human brain mapping. (2002). Jul;, 16(3), 146-57.

[27] Hild, K. E, & Nagarajan, S. S. Source localization of EEG/MEG data by correlating columns of ICA and lead field matrices. IEEE transactions on bio-medical engineering. (2009). Nov;, 56(11), 2619-26.

[28] Bartlett, M. S. Information maximization in face processing. Neurocomputing. (2007). Aug;70(13-15):2204-17.

[29] Dammers, J, Schiek, M, Boers, F, Silex, C, Zvyagintsev, M, Pietrzyk, U, et al. Integration of amplitude and phase statistics for complete artifact removal in independent components of neuromagnetic recordings. IEEE Trans. Biomed. Eng. (2008). Oct;, 55(10), 2353-62.

[30] Escudero, J, Hornero, R, Abásolo, D, & Fernández, A. Quantitative evaluation of artifact removal in real magnetoencephalogram signals with blind source separation. Annals of biomedical engineering. Springer Netherlands; (2011). Aug 21;, 39(8), 2274-86.

[31] Li, Y, Ma, Z, Lu, W, & Li, Y. Automatic removal of the eye blink artifact from EEG using an ICA-based template matching approach. Physiological measurement. (2006). Apr;, 27(4), 425-36.

[32] Mantini, D, Franciotti, R, Romani, G. L, & Pizzella, V. Improving MEG source localizations: an automated method for complete artifact removal based on independent component analysis. NeuroImage. (2008). Mar;, 40(1), 160-73.

[33] Nikulin, V V, Nolte, G, & Curio, G. A novel method for reliable and fast extraction of neuronal EEG/MEG oscillations on the basis of spatio-spectral decomposition. NeuroImage. (2011). Apr 15;, 55(4), 1528-35.

[34] Huang, D-S, & Mi, J-X. A New Constrained Independent Component Analysis Method. IEEE Transactions on Neural Networks. (2007). Sep;, 18(5), 1532-5.

[35] Hesse, C. W. On estimating the signal subspace dimension of high-density multichannel magnetoencephalogram measurements. Conference proceedings©: Annual International Conference of the IEEE Engineering in Medicine and Biology Society. IEEE Engineering in Medicine and Biology Society. Lyon, France. (2007). Jan;, 6228-31.

[36] Liu, J, Ghassemi, M. M, Michael, A. M, Boutte, D, Wells, W, Perrone-bizzozero, N, et al. An ICA with reference approach in identification of genetic variation and associated brain networks. Frontiers in human neuroscience. (2012). Jan;, 6(21), 1-10.

[37] Barriga, E. S, Pattichis, M, Ts, o D, Abramoff, M, Kardon, R, Kwon, Y, et al. Independent component analysis using prior information for signal detection in a functional imaging system of the retina. Medical image analysis. (2011). Feb;, 15(1), 35-44.

[38] Hesse, C. W, & James, C. J. On semi-blind source separation using spatial constraints with applications in EEG analysis. IEEE transactions on bio-medical engineering. (2006). Dec;53(12 Pt 1):2525-34.

[39] Stone, J V. Independent Component Analysis: A Tutorial Introduction. MIT Press; (2004). page 211.

[40] Hyvärinen, A, Karhunen, J, & Oja, E. Independent component analysis. John Wiley and Sons; (2001). page 481.

[41] Bell, A. J. Sejnowski T errence J. An information-maximization approach to blind separation and blind deconvolution. Neural computation. MIT Press; (1995). Nov;, 7(6), 1129-59.

[42] Brown, G. D, Yamada, S, & Sejnowski, T. J. Independent component analysis at the neural cocktail party. Trends in neurosciences. (2001). Jan;, 24(1), 54-63.

[43] Amari, S, Cichocki, A, & Yang, H. H. A new learning algorithm for blind signal separation. In: Tourezky D, Mozer M, Hazzelmo M, editors. Advances in neural information processing systems. (1996). page , 757-763.

[44] Sommer, C, Straehle, C, Kothe, U, & Hamprecht, F. A. Ilastik: Interactive learning and segmentation toolkit. 2011 IEEE International Symposium on Biomedical Imaging: From Nano to Macro. IEEE; (2011). page , 230-3.

[45] Axer, H, Klingner, C. M, & Prescher, A. Fiber anatomy of dorsal and ventral language streams. Brain and language. (2012). May 23;

[46] Larsen, L, Griffin, L. D, Grässel, D, Witte, O. W, & Axer, H. Polarized light imaging of white matter architecture. Microscopy Research and Technique. (2007). Oct;, 70(10), 851-63.

[47] Gräßel DAxer M, Palm C, Dammers J, Amunts K, Pietrzyk U, et al. Visualization of Fiber Tracts in the Postmortem Human Brain by Means of Polarized Light. NeuroImage. (2009). Jul;47(Supplement 1):142.

[48] Palm C Axer M Gräßel D, Dammers J, Lindemeyer J, Zilles K, et al. Towards Ultra-High Resolution Fibre Tract Mapping of the Human Brain- Registration of Polarised Light Images and Reorientation of Fibre Vectors. Frontiers in human neuroscience. FRONTIERS RES FOUND; (2010). Jan;, 4(9), 1-16.

Chapter 19

Causal Relationships and Network Parameters in Effective Brain Connectivity

Guiomar Niso, Ernesto Pereda, Fernando Maestú,
María Gudín, Sira Carrasco and Francisco del-Pozo

Additional information is available at the end of the chapter

http://dx.doi.org/10.5772/56499

1. Introduction

The human brain comprises approximately 10^{11} neurons, each of which makes about 10^3 synaptic connections. This huge number of connections between individual processing elements provides the fundamental scaffold for neuronal ensembles to become transiently synchronized or functionally connected [1]. A similar complex network configuration and dynamics can also be found at the macroscopic scales of systems neuroscience and brain imaging [2]. The emergence of dynamically coupled cell assemblies represents the neurophysiological substrate for cognitive function such as perception, learning, thinking [3]. Understanding the complex network organization of the brain on the basis of neuroimaging data represents one of the most impervious challenges for systems neuroscience.

Several measures to evaluate at various scales (single cells, cortical columns, or brain areas) how the different parts of the brain communicate have been recently proposed. We can classify them, according to their symmetry, into two groups: symmetric and asymmetric measures. Symmetric measures, such as correlation, coherence, phase synchronization indexes (PLV, PLI), evaluate *functional connectivity,* i.e. statistically significant relationships between signals recorded from spatially remote neurophysiological events. On the other hand, the asymmetric ones are able to detect *effective connectivity* i.e. information flow (the influence one neuronal system exerts over another) [4], and therefore they reveal the direction of the interaction. Granger Causality (GC) belongs to this latter group.

2. Granger causality

2.1. Classical approach

A notion of causality, which is relevant for the experimental study of information transfer in neural systems, is commonly attributed to Wiener. He stated that, for two simultaneously measured signals, if one can predict the first signal better by incorporating the past information from the second signal than by using only information from the first one, then the second signal can be called *causal* to the first one [5]. However, it was the Nobel Prize laureate Clive Granger who gave a mathematical formulation of this concept [6]. He argued that, if X is influencing Y, then adding past values of the first variable (X) to the regression of the second one (Y) should improve the prediction of the latter.

To quantify such influence, the most straightforward approach consists in comparing the prediction of future values of one of the variables (say, X), by using two different models. The first one is a model where these values are forecast exclusively from the past history of this variable (e.g., a purely autoregressive (AR) model of a given order). The second one incorporates instead the past history of Y as well. Then, GC is defined by comparing the forecast errors of both models (see section 4.2), and Y is said to Granger-cause X if the error of the second model is significantly lower than that of the first one.

GC has the advantage of quantifying the information flow in the data, which is important to study the direction of the relationships between different parts of the brain. GC was first introduced in the field of economics 40 years ago. However, applications to neuroscience are rather more recent, see [7] for a review on applications to neurophysiology. One of the first studies using this concept investigated the existence of directional or causal interactions by analyzing local field potentials (LFPs) from the macaque inferotemporal cortex [8]. This method was also applied to the LFP data recorded from two separate areas (primary and higher visual areas) of the cat visual cortex, to investigate the role of bottom-up and top-down interactions in a go/no-go task [9] or in a stimulus expectancy task [10]. A frequency specific Granger causality measure was utilized in LFP recordings from somatosensory and motor cortices of macaque monkeys as they performed a motor maintenance in a visual discrimination task [11]. In human, a time-variant Granger causality measure was applied to EEG signals from the standard color-word conflict Stroop task [12]. A wide study CG's advantages for neuroscience was done in [13].

3. Magnetoencephalography (MEG)

3.1. Consent

Ethical approval was granted by the local Ethics Committee. All data were analyzed anonymously. Subjects who underwent MEG recordings for research purposes had given written informed consent before participating.

Once subjects arrived at the laboratory, they got familiar with the MEG chamber in which the recording took place and were instructed about the experimental procedure. All the recordings took place during morning hours.

3.2. MEG system

MEG recordings were obtained using a 306-channel wholehead Elekta Neuromag® MEG system (Elekta Oy, Helsinki, Finland). The system has 102 magnetometers and 204 planar gradiometers in a helmet-shaped array covering the entire scalp. Subjects were seated inside a magnetically shielded room during MEG recordings (Vacuumschmelze GmbH, Hanau, Germany).

Eye movements were monitored by simultaneously recording an electrooculogram (EOG), with three Ag/Cl electrodes, two above and below the right eye and one at the right earlobe used as ground reference.

3.3. Artifact control

Participants were seated with their head in the MEG sensor helmet, which covers the entire head except the face. Four head position indicator coils (HPI) were placed on the scalp, appropriately spaced in the region covered by the MEG helmet. The locations of the nasion, two pre-auricular points, and the four HPI coils were digitized prior to each MEG study using a 3D-digitizer (FASTRACK; Polhemus, Colchester, VT) to define the subject-specific cartesian head coordinate system. 100-200 additional anatomical points were digitized on the head surface to provide a more accurate shape of the subject's head. Once a subject was comfortably positioned in the MEG machine, short electrical signals were sent to the HPI coils to localize them with respect to the MEG sensor array. The data from the HPI coils were used to correct head movement during the session.

3.4. Subjects

The data used in this study were acquired from 8 patients suffering from frontal focal epilepsy (FE), 8 patients suffering from generalized epilepsy (GE) and 8 healthy subjects (HS). Their ages range between (FE: 35.1 ± 14, GE: 23.5 ± 4, HS: 19 ± 1).

3.5. Task and parameters

MEG data was acquired at a sampling rate of 1 kHz, with on-line band-pass filter of 0.10–330 Hz. Acquisition occurred in a single 20 min session of "resting state", 10 min with eyes open looking to a cross on the screen followed by 10 min with eyes closed.

3.6. Removing artifacts

To correct the head position and the associated movement-related artifacts, a spatio-temporal signal space separation method (tSSS) with movement compensation (MC) was applied using the MaxFilter® software (Elekta Neuromag®, Elekta Oy, Helsinki, Finland). The use of tSSS is especially important for rejection of close-to-sensor artifacts.

After data reconstruction by signal space separation (referred as SSS), tSSS identifies artifacts by their correlated temporal behavior inside and outside the sensor helmet. The artifacts to be eliminated are thresholded by the quantitative level of this correlation determined by correlation limit of 0.95, and a correlation windows length of 10ms.

For each subject, artifact free epochs were then carefully selected by visual analysis Artifacts were typically due to (eye) movements, drowsiness or technical issues.

3.7. Used data

All the analysis were performed on 960 non-overlapping quasistationary segments (40 segments per subject) of 5000 ms free from eye or muscular artifacts, and epileptic activities (as, e.g., seizures or epileptic-like activity) and far (at least 20s) from recent epileptic discharges. The period of resting state with closed eyes was selected for the study. A downsampling to 500Hz was applied, thus obtaining segments of 2500 samples, as this has proven to be sufficient to detect clinically relevant differences in functional or effective connectivity in previous studies.

One important practical issue we would like to tackle here is that, in human MEG recording, not all types of magnetic sensors have the same sensitivity to deep brain sources. Magnetometers measure the overall magnitude of the magnetic field component approximately normal to the head surface; whereas planar gradiometers measure the difference of that field component at two adjacent locations. Describing MEG sensors in descending order of sensitivity to the depth of sources, magnetometers are most sensitive, followed by first-order axial gradiometers, second-order gradiometers and, finally, planar gradiometers [14]. Hence, planar gradiometers have maximum sensitivity to sources directly under them, i.e., superficial cortical sources [15], which makes them less sensitive to artifacts and distant disturbances, and therefore are suitable for studying this case, as these kinds of epilepsy have a neocortical origin. However, for the analysis, data from both the planar gradiometers and the magnetometers, was used.

4. Data analysis

4.1. Data preprocessing

In agreement with previous findings, surrogate data tests revealed that less than 4% of interdependencies between the spontaneous brain activities were nonlinear [16]. Thus, weighted brain networks were constructed by means of a definition of functional links based on Granger Causality (GC).

Application of GC requires that each time series is 'covariance stationary' (CS), i.e., that its mean and variance do not change over time. CS can be assessed in a rule-of-thumb way by examining the auto-correlation function. A non-CS time series will have an autocorrelation function that falls off slowly; a CS time series will have a sharply declining autocorrelation function. For this reason is that we take segments far enough from the spikes (at least 20s).

Prior to the causality analysis, we detrended the signals (subtracting the best-fitting line from each time series) and removed their temporal mean to provide a 'zero-mean' situation [17]. Granger causality analysis was performed to each segment of data (Anil Seth Toolbox [18]). The order of the autoregressive (AR) model was set to 4 according to the Bayesian Information Criterion (BIC) for our particular data [19].

4.2. Granger causality

As commented above, for two simultaneously measured signals, if one can predict the first signal better by incorporating the past information from the second signal than using only information from the first one, then the second signal can be called causal to the first one [5].The simplest way of quantifying this is by using univariate vs. bivariate linear regression models of a signal *x(t)*, to compare the forecast errors obtained incorporating (bivariate) or not (univariate) information from the past of *y(t)*.

For the univariate autoregressive model (AR), we have:

$$\begin{aligned} x(n) &= \sum_{k=1}^{P} a_{x,k} x(n-k) + u_x(n) \\ y(n) &= \sum_{k=1}^{P} a_{y,k} y(n-k) + u_y(n) \end{aligned} \tag{1}$$

where a_{ij} are the model parameters (coefficients usually estimated by least square method), P is the order of the AR model and u_i, are the residuals associated to the model. Here, the prediction of each signal is performed only by its own past.

$$\begin{aligned} V_{X|\overline{X}} &= \mathrm{var}(u_X) \\ V_{Y|\overline{Y}} &= \mathrm{var}(u_Y) \end{aligned} \tag{2}$$

Accordingly, for the bivariate AR:

$$\begin{aligned} x(n) &= \sum_{k=1}^{P} a_{X|X,k} x(n-k) + \sum_{k=1}^{P} a_{X|Y,k} y(n-k) + u_{XY}(n) \\ y(n) &= \sum_{k=1}^{P} a_{Y|X,k} x(n-k) + \sum_{k=1}^{P} a_{Y|Y,k} y(n-k) + u_{YX}(n) \end{aligned} \tag{3}$$

where the residuals u_{XY} and u_{YX} now depend on the past values of both signals, and their variance is:

$$\begin{aligned} V_{X|\overline{X},\overline{Y}} &= \mathrm{var}(u_{XY}) \\ V_{Y|\overline{X},\overline{Y}} &= \mathrm{var}(u_{YX}) \end{aligned} \tag{4}$$

where var(.) denote variance over time and $X \mid \overline{X}, \overline{Y}$ is the prediction of x(t) by the past samples of values of x(t) and y(t).

Therefore, Granger causality from y(t) to x(t) (predicting X from Y) is:

$$GC_{Y \to X} = \ln\left(\frac{V_{X \mid \overline{X}}}{V_{X \mid \overline{X}, \overline{Y}}}\right) \tag{5}$$

GC ranges from 0 to infinity. The lower bound indicates that the incorporating information about the past of y(t) *does not* improve the prediction of x(t): $V_{X \mid \overline{X}} \approx V_{X \mid \overline{X}, \overline{Y}}$. Accordingly, [4] is greater than 0, when the past of y(t) *does* improve the prediction of x(t): $V_{X \mid \overline{X}} > V_{X \mid \overline{X}, \overline{Y}}$ (Y G-causes X)

As indicated in the Introduction, GC belongs to the category of asymmetric connectivity indexes; therefore, it assesses effective rather than functional connectivity. However, as defined from AR models it is a linear parametric method, so it is only sensitive to linear correlations and depends on the order (P) of the autoregressive. (See [20] for an extension of the GC concept to assess nonlinear interdependencies)

4.2.1. Significance of GC values

If we calculated the GC index [5] for all possible pair of sensors of the same kind (e.g. magnetometers, planar gradiometers along one axis and planar gradiometers along the two orthogonal axis) we get three connectivity matrixes, where each element $GC_{i\to j}$ measures the degree in which the signal in the sensor *i* Granger-causes that of the sensor *j* (*i,j*=1,..,102). However, it is necessary to determine whether the value of each given index is due to real causal dependence between the corresponding two sensors or rather it is not zero due to statistical fluctuations in the estimation of variance of the forecasting. This task can be easily accomplished because it is known that time-domain GC interaction is significant if the coefficients a_{ij} are jointly significantly different from zero. This can be established via an F-test on the null hypothesis that A_{ij} are zero [6].

These have to be corrected for multiple comparisons, which we do here by applying the well-known 'false discovery rate' (FDR) method [21–23] at a desired significance threshold of 0.05. In all the cases where the (corrected) test failed to reject the null hypothesis, the corresponding GC index is set to zero.

Moreover, recent results show that correlations between magnetic fields sensors located at a distance less than 4 cm cannot distinguish between spontaneous activities of epileptic patients and control subjects [24]. To reduce the influence of these spurious correlations between MEG signals, we have excluded the nearest sensors (separated less than 4 cm) from the computation of Granger causality values.

The final effective connectivity matrixes so obtained can be interpreted as the adjacency matrix of a directed weighted network. Hence, network analysis methods derived from graph theory

[25] could be applied to assess the most significant features of the brain connectivity networks in the groups of subjects described before (i.e. GE, FE and HS), during the resting state task with closed eyes [26,27]. And from that, study their differences.

4.3. Network parameters

To characterize the network structure of brain activity of each group of subjects, we evaluated a list of measures for directed weighted graphs [28]. In this approach, MEG sensors were considered as vertices (nodes) and the GC values between sensors as edge weights (links). The edge weight represents the strength of the connection between the vertices.

Here some notation is explained (see [25] for details):

- N is the set of all nodes in the network, and n is the number of nodes.
- L is the set of all links in the network, and l is number of links.
- (i, j) is a link between nodes i and j, where $i,j \in N$.
- Links (i, j) are associated with connection weights w_{ij}.
- a_{ij} is the connection status between i and j: $a_{ij} = 1$ when link (i, j) exists (when i and j are neighbors); $a_{ij} = 0$ otherwise ($a_{ii} = 0$ for all i).
- We compute the number of links as $l = \sum_{i,j \in N} a_{ij}$ (to avoid ambiguity with directed links we count each undirected link twice, as a_{ij} and as a_{ji}).
- The sum of all weights in the network is l^w, and it is computed as $l^w = \sum_{i,j \in N} w_{ij}$. Henceforth, we assume that weights are normalized, such that $0 \leq w_{ij} \leq 1$ for all i and j.

We focused on the following global parameters, to be explained henceforth: the average degree (section 4.3.1), strength (section 4.3.2) and two measures of segregation, namely the clustering coefficient (section 4.3.3) and modularity (section 4.3.4).

4.3.1. Degree

The degree (D) of a node is the number of links connected to it. In directed weighted networks, we distinguish between the 'in degree', which is the number of links that arrive to the node, and the 'out degree', which is the number of links that go out from the node.

- (Directed) in-degree of i, $k^{in}_i = \sum_{j \in N} a_{ji}$
- (Directed) out-degree of i, $k^{out}_i = \sum_{j \in N} a_{ij}$

The global degree of a network is the average of all its nodes' degree. The mean network degree is most commonly used as a measure of density, or the total "wiring cost" of the network.

4.3.2. Strength

The weighted variant of the degree, sometimes termed the *strength*, is defined as the sum of all neighboring link weights.

4.3.3. Clustering coefficient

The clustering coefficient (C) describes the likelihood that neighbors of a vertex are also connected. It quantifies the tendency of network elements to form local clusters. We used the directed and weighted equivalent of this measure to characterize local clustering [29]:

$$C^{\rightarrow}=\frac{1}{n}\sum_{i\in N}\frac{t_i^{\rightarrow}}{\left(k_i^{out}+k_i^{in}\right)\left(k_i^{out}+k_i^{in}-1\right)-2\sum_{j\in N}a_{ij}a_{ji}} \tag{6}$$

Here and in the following equation, the arrow next to the indexes denotes that they are calculated for directed networks. However, for the sake of clarity in the text, we will omit this arrow in the name of the indexes henceforth.

4.3.4. Modularity

Modularity (Q) quantifies how a network can be optimally divided in subgroups or modules. We used a modification for directed weighted networks by [30]

$$Q^{\rightarrow}=\frac{1}{l}\sum_{i,j\in N}\left[a_{ij}-\frac{k_i^{out}k_j^{in}}{l}\right]\delta_{m_i m_j} \tag{7}$$

Roughly speaking, the greater the value of Q, the more modular a network is, i.e., the greater the density of within-cluster connections as compared to the between-cluster ones.

4.4. Statistical tests

4.4.1. Between groups comparisons

We performed a Kruskal Wallis test to compare network parameters from the three groups (FE, GE, HS). This test compares the medians of the samples in each group, and returns the p value for the rejection of the null hypothesis that all samples are drawn from the same population (or equivalently, from different populations with the same distribution). The Kruskal-Wallis test is a nonparametric version of the classical one-way ANOVA, and an extension of the Wilcoxon rank sum test to more than two groups.

If the p value is close zero, this suggests that at least one sample median is significantly different from the others. Here, we took $p<0.05$ as the critical value to determine whether the null hypothesis can be rejected.

4.4.2. Post-hoc between (two) groups comparisons

In those cases where the Kruskall-Wallis to check was significant, we further analyzed pairwise difference between any two groups by means of a two-sided rank sum test (Wilcoxon test),

test the null hypothesis that the network parameters obtained for each group of subjects are independent samples from identical continuous distributions with equal medians, against the alternative that they do not have equal medians. This test is equivalent to a Mann-Whitney U-test. Differences were again considered significant if $p<0.05$.

5. Results

Differences in the global network parameters between the three groups (FE, GE and HS):

5.1. Differences among the planar gradiometer networks

The interdependence matrixes obtained from the planar gradiometers were sparse, i.e., they presented only a few significant GC values (effective links) between the corresponding neocortical sources. Differences among groups for the planar gradiometers were found in modularity (see figure 1).

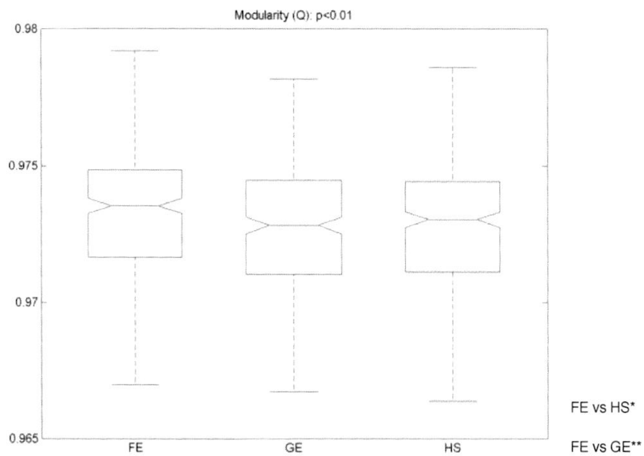

Figure 1. Modularity Q (equation (7)) of the brain networks of planar gradiometers for the healthy subjects (HS), and patients with either focal (FE) or global epilepsy (GE). The Kruskal Wallis tests for global differences among the three groups was highly significant (p<0.01]. Asterisks denote differences between any two groups; *: p<0.05; * p<0.01. The boxplots are median (red line), and the 25% and 75% percentiles (blue box), whereas the whiskers indicates the maximum and minimum of each group.

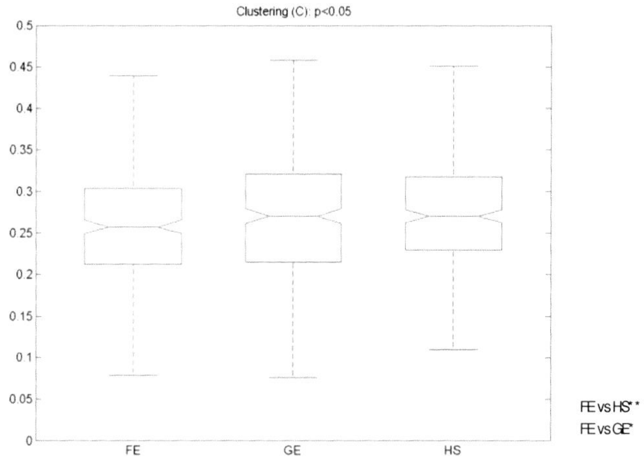

Figure 2. Clustering coefficient C (equation (6)) for the networks of magnetometers. Global differences (Kruskal Wallis test) were significant at the p<0.01 level. Group notation, boxplots, whiskers and differences between two groups as in figure 1.

Patients suffering from frontal focal epilepsy, present a higher value of Q as compared to those suffering from generalized epilepsy and healthy subjects. Differences in magnetometers

5.2. Between-group differences in brain networks recorded from magnetometers

Differences in network parameters for magnetometers were found in cluster coefficient (figure 2), degree (figure 3), strength (figure 4) and number of clusters (figure 5).

As can be seen from figure 2, the FE group presents a lower value of C than those from the GE and the HS group.

Also, for the average degree D (figure 3) patients from the FE group, present a higher value of global network degree as compared to GE patients and healthy controls.

Moreover, for the average strength S (figure 4), FE patients showed the highest values of the index as compared to GE patients and healthy controls.

Finally, for the number of clusters (figure 5) healthy subjects present a lower number of clusters as compared to both group of epileptic.

6. Discussion

The assessment of functional brain networks from multivariate fMRI, EEG or MEG data has become a very popular line of research nowadays [25,31]. This is most likely because the

http://dx.doi.org/10.5772/56499

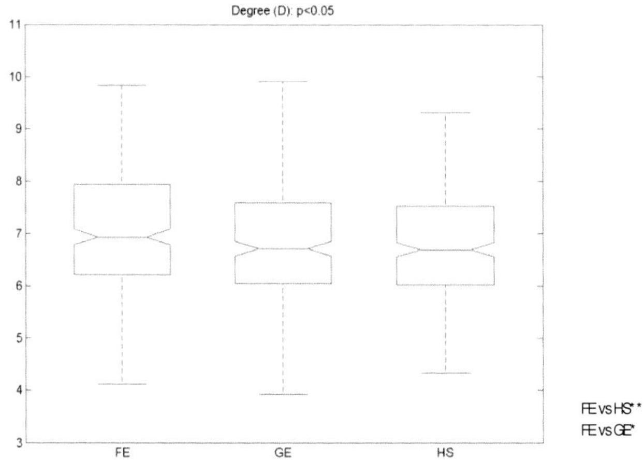

Figure 3. Average degree D for the networks of magnetometers. Global differences (Kruskal Wallis test) were significant at the p<0.05 level. Group notation, boxplots, whiskers and differences between two groups are as in previous figures.

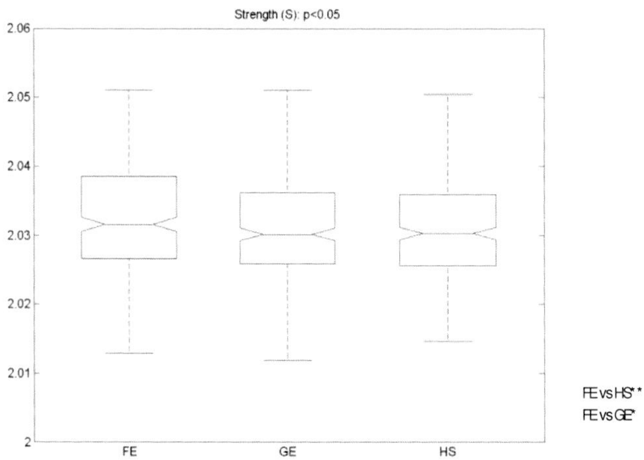

Figure 4. Average strength (S) for the networks of magnetometers. Global differences (Kruskal Wallis test) were significant at the p<0.05 level. Group notation, boxplots, whiskers and differences between two groups as in previous figures.

parameters derived from this approach are relatively easy to calculate and interpret in neurophysiological terms. In fact, one only needs, on the one hand, a measure of functional or

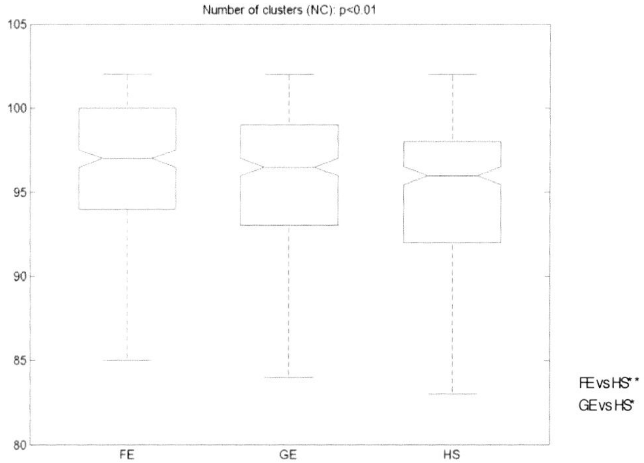

Figure 5. Average number of clusters in the networks of magnetometers. Global differences (Kruskal Wallis test) were significant at the p<0.01 level. Group notation, boxplots, whiskers and differences between two groups as in previous figures.

effective connectivity between any two signals and, on the other, a way of estimating the significance of such a measure. Once you are equipped with these two tools, the characterization of the corresponding brain network is only a few calculations ahead.

Yet even these apparently straightforward steps (e.g., estimation of bivariate connectivity index and their significance) are deceptively simple, and their careless, mechanical application may result in misleading results and/or false conclusions. Common sources of error are the misuse of a given connectivity index, failing to assess its significance in a proper way or not taking into account what the data we have recorded are actually measuring. This latter issue is specially significant when dealing with extra-cranially recorded signals (whether EEG or MEG data), in which it is well-known that signals in different sensors are often measuring the activity of the same deep brain source, this resulting in a statistically significant relationship between these signals that has very few (if any) to do with the existence of connectivity between the sensors.

This important question can be tackled in different ways. One obvious attempt consists in trying to reconstruct, from the recorded data, the neurological sources of activity before applying the network connectivity approach. But the so-called inverse problem of source reconstruction is known to be ill-posed, in the sense that it is underdetermined, as the number of sources is much larger than that of the measures, and has not a single solution. Another possibility includes the use of carefully devised indexes [32], which are robust against common source effects but which, unfortunately, are not without their own particular problems [33]. In this work, we have dealt with the question in a different way, by taking advantage of the complementary information provided by two kinds of

http://dx.doi.org/10.5772/56499

sensors (magnetometers and planar gradiometers) in a modern MEG recording device. The key idea consists in the fact that whereas magnetometers are sensitive to all sources (whether cortical or deep ones) in the direction normal to the head surface where they record, gradiometers are only sensitive to cortical sources *right behind* the recorded surface [14], and therefore unlikely to be affected by the common source problem. Thus, comparing the results from the magnetometers and the planar gradiometers recorded simultaneously from the same subject, we may get insight into the possible effect that common sources has on the functional brain network assessed by the former sensors, which are by far the most common sensors used in MEG literature.

Here, we have applied this approach to study brain networks of effective connectivity from planar gradiometers and magnetometers recorded during rest with closed eyes in three groups of subjects, one of healthy controls and two of patients suffering from different kinds of epilepsy: generalized and frontal focal. The connectivity index used was the GC index, whose significant was assessed by a careful combination of F-test estimation and FDR statistical test to deal with the multiple comparison problem. And we think we might rightly conclude that the results obtained justify our use of what we may call this *multi-sensor approach*. Indeed, thanks to it, two important questions have come out. First, if we were to analyze the data from the magnetometers alone, we would have come to the conclusions that the functional networks from the three groups are different in a number of parameters, whereas these networks, when only the cortical sources are recorded, do not present differences among the three groups in any of these parameters. Second, networks of cortical sources do present differences in modularity between healthy and epileptic groups, as well as between the two epileptic patients.

Thus, by analyzing the information provided by the combined use of both sensors, we have a greater insight into the brain networks of the three groups (and the differences among them). The information from the planar gradiometers suggests that connectivity between neocortical sources is sparse, and the corresponding networks are only weakly modular (low Q), but the intra-cluster connectivity of the epileptic groups are greater than that of healthy subjects, with the FE group in turn being significantly more modular than the GE group. This result is very interesting, as it is well-known that the greater the intra-cluster connectivity, the easier it is for a network to become fully synchronized [34]. Thus, it would indicate that in both types of epilepsy, the network of neocortical sources is more prone to become (pathologically) synchronized that in normal subjects.

When we review the information from the magnetometers, we can get information about deeper brain sources. The first interesting result is that the networks constructed from magnetometers are more densely connected that those from the gradiometers. Besides, these networks are scarcely modular in any of the groups (as the number of clusters in Figure 5 is close to the number of sensors) and present a higher number of (stronger) links (higher C, D and S as shown in figures 2, 3 and 4, respectively) in the epileptic groups as compared to healthy subjects. Unfortunately, it is difficult to interpret these results simply in terms of the corresponding connectivity between deep sources, as the possibility of the same source being recorded in different magnetometers cannot be ruled out. Yet rather than whether these results are a consequence of more active deep sources or more interconnected ones, what is really important is the fact that network theory as applied to MEG data is able to disclose changes in neurological activity of epileptic subjects as compared to healthy subjects even when no epileptogenic activity is apparent in the raw data.

6.1. Future work

The results presented above are certainly interesting, not only because of their methodological and neurological implications, but also because they pave the way for future studies in the same line. One obvious question to further investigate from these data is whether the between-groups differences found in various global parameters in both planar gradiometers and magnetometers can be explored in terms of their (possibly local) origin. Namely, whether they are due to local differences between the corresponding networks, which are detected by these global parameters but can be also characterized topologically. Indeed, it is tempting to hypothesize that the FE group, whose epilepsy has a focal origin, presents differences with both the GE and the HS group precisely in the frontal sensors. Another important question that we should elucidate is whether differences are present at all the frequencies of the signal or are rather constrained to a certain frequency band (as found in former works [26]), but detected here by the GC index, which operates on the broadband signal in the time domain. One last issue of practical interest that we are currently studying is the possible usefulness of the differences in network connectivity patterns to assist in the classification (diagnosis) of recorded subjects using machine learning algorithms. This latter application is potentially very important from the clinical point of view. Additionally, it would also allow circumventing the problem of determining if the patterns of GC index (or any other connectivity index for that matter) are due to true connectivity or are the result of volume conduction of deep brain sources, which are reflected in many sensors at the same time. As long as these patterns are different in each group, they would be useful to detect deviations from healthy condition. Here also, the fact that the information from the two type of magnetic sensors available (magnetometers and planar gradiometers) is not redundant but complementary, speaks clearly in favor of analyzing both sensors at the same time, whenever possible.

We hope that this line of research will continue to provide further insight into the pattern of connectivity networks in health and disease and its possible application as an additional tool for diagnostic purposes in different neurologic pathologies.

Acknowledgements

Guiomar Niso, Ernesto Pereda and Francisco del Pozo acknowledge the financial support of the Spanish Ministry of Economy and Competitiveness through the grants TEC2012-38453-CO4-01 and -03. Fernando Maestú, María Gudín and Sira Carrasco acknowledge the financial support of the Castilla La Mancha Sanitary System through grant PS09/00450. Guiomar Niso has also received the financial support of the Spanish Ministry of Education and Science through the FPU grant AP2008-02383.

Author details

Guiomar Niso[1*], Ernesto Pereda[2], Fernando Maestú[1], María Gudín[3], Sira Carrasco[3] and Francisco del-Pozo[1]

*Address all correspondence to: guiomar.niso@ctb.upm.es

1 Center for Biomedical Technology, Technical University of Madrid, Madrid, Spain

2 Electrical Engineering and Bioengineering Group, Dept. of Basic Physics, University of La Laguna, Tenerife, Spain

3 Ciudad Real Universitary Hospital, Ciudad Real, Spain

References

[1] Buzsaki G. Rhythms of the Brain. Oxford University Press; 2006 Oct 26;

[2] Bressler SL. Large-scale cortical networks and cognition. Brain Research. Brain Research Reviews. 1995 Mar;20(3):288–304.

[3] Varela F, Lachaux J, Rodriguez E, Martinerie J. The brainweb: phase synchronization and large-scale integration", Nature Review Neuroscience 2001, 2(4):229-39.

[4] Friston KJ. Functional and effective connectivity in neuroimaging: A synthesis. Human Brain Mapping. 1994 Oct 13;2(1-2):56–78.

[5] Wiener N. The Theory of Prediction. In: Beckenbach EF, editor. Modern mathematics for the engineer. New York: McGraw-Hill; 1956. p. 165 – 190.

[6] Granger C. Investigating causal relations by econometric models and cross-spectral methods. Econometrica: Journal of the Econometric Society. 1969;37(3):424–38.

[7] Pereda E, Quiroga RQ, Bhattacharya J, Quian Quiroga R. Nonlinear multivariate analysis of neurophysiological signals. Progress in Neurobiology. 2005;77(1-2):1–37.

[8] Freiwald W, Valdes P, Bosch J, Biscay R, Jimenez JC, Rodriguez LM, et al. Testing non-linearity and directedness of interactions between neural groups in the macaque inferotemporal cortex. Journal of Neuroscience Methods. 1999 Dec 15;94(1):105–19.

[9] Bernasconi C, Von Stein A, Chiang C, König P. Bi-directional interactions between visual areas in the awake behaving cat. Neuroreport. 2000 Mar 20;11(4):689–92.

[10] Salazar RF, König P, Kayser C. Directed interactions between visual areas and their role in processing image structure and expectancy. The European Journal of Neuroscience. 2004 Sep;20(5):1391–401.

[11] Brovelli A, Ding M, Ledberg A, Chen Y, Nakamura R, Bressler SL. Beta oscillations in a large-scale sensorimotor cortical network: directional influences revealed by Granger causality. Proceedings of the National Academy of Sciences of the United States of America. 2004 Jun 29;101(26):9849–54.

[12] Hesse W, Möller E, Arnold M, Schack B. The use of time-variant EEG Granger causality for inspecting directed interdependencies of neural assemblies. Journal of Neuroscience Methods. 2003 Mar;124(1):27–44.

[13] Bressler SL. AKS. Wiener–Granger Causality: A well established methodology. NeuroImage. 2011, 15;58(2):323-9

[14] Hansen P, Kringelbach M, Salmelin R. MEG An Introduction to methods. Oxford University Press. 2010. p. 448.

[15] Hämäläinen MS. Functional localization based on measurements with a whole-head magnetometer system. Brain Topography. Springer New York; 1995;7(4):283–9.

[16] Stam CJ, Breakspear M, Van Cappellen van Walsum A-M, Van Dijk BW. Nonlinear synchronization in EEG and whole-head MEG recordings of healthy subjects. Human Brain Mapping. 2003 Jun;19(2):63–78.

[17] Ding M, Bressler SL, Yang W, Liang H. Short-window spectral analysis of cortical event-related potentials by adaptive multivariate autoregressive modeling: data preprocessing, model validation, and variability assessment. Biological Cybernetics. Springer; 2000 Jul;83(1):35–45.

[18] Seth AK. A MATLAB toolbox for Granger causal connectivity analysis. Journal of Neuroscience Methods. Elsevier B.V.; 2010 Feb 15;186(2):262–73.

[19] Schwarz G. Estimating the dimension of a model. The Annals of Statistics. 1978;6(2): 461–4.

[20] Ancona N, Marinazzo D, Stramaglia S. Radial basis function approach to nonlinear Granger causality of time series. Physical Review E. 2004 Nov;70(5):056221.

[21] Benjamini Y, Hochberg Y. Controlling the false discovery rate: a practical and powerful approach to multiple testing. Journal of the Royal Statistical Society. Series B. 1995; 57:289-300

[22] Benjamini Y, Yekutieli D. The control of the false discovery rate in multiple testing under dependency. Annals of Statistics. 2001;29(4):1165–88.

[23] Genovese CR, Lazar N a, Nichols T. Thresholding of statistical maps in functional neuroimaging using the false discovery rate. NeuroImage. 2002 Apr;15(4):870–8.

[24] Garcia Dominguez L, Wennberg R a, Gaetz W, Cheyne D, Snead OC, Perez Velazquez JL. Enhanced synchrony in epileptiform activity? Local versus distant phase synchronization in generalized seizures. The Journal of Neuroscience. 2005 Aug 31;25(35):8077–84.

[25] Rubinov M, Sporns O. Complex network measures of brain connectivity: uses and interpretations. NeuroImage. 2010;52(3):1059–69.

[26] Chavez M, Valencia M, Navarro V, Latora V, Martinerie J. Functional Modularity of Background Activities in Normal and Epileptic Brain Networks. Physical Review Letters. 2010;104(11):1–4.

[27] Van Dellen E, Douw L, Hillebrand A, Ris-Hilgersom IHM, Schoonheim MM, Baayen JC, et al. MEG Network Differences between Low- and High-Grade Glioma Related to Epilepsy and Cognition. PloS one. 2012 Jan;7(11):e50122.

[28] Boccaletti S, Latora V, Moreno Y, Chavez M, Hwang D. Complex networks: Structure and dynamics. Physics Reports. 2006 Feb;424(4-5):175–308.

[29] Fagiolo G. Clustering in complex directed networks. Physical Review E. 2007; 76(2): 026107

[30] Leicht E, Newman M. Community structure in directed networks. Physical Review Letters. 2008;1–5.

[31] Stam CJ, Van Straaten ECW. The organization of physiological brain networks. Clinical Neurophysiology. 2012 Jun;123(6):1067–87.

[32] Stam CJ, Nolte G, Daffertshofer A. Phase lag index: assessment of functional connectivity from multi channel EEG and MEG with diminished bias from common sources. Human Brain Mapping. 2007 Nov;28(11):1178–93.

[33] Vinck M, Oostenveld R, Van Wingerden M, Battaglia F, Pennartz CM a. An improved index of phase-synchronization for electrophysiological data in the presence of volume-conduction, noise and sample-size bias. NeuroImage. 2011 Apr 15;55(4): 1548–65.

[34] Balanov A, Janson N, Postnov D, Sosnovtseva O. Synchronization: From Simple to Complex. Berlin: Springer Series in Synergetics, Springer; 2009.

Chapter 20

Neuroimaging of Epilepsy: EEG-fMRI in the Presurgical Evaluation of Focal Epilepsy

Mirko Avesani, Silvia Giacopuzzi and
Antonio Fiaschi

Additional information is available at the end of the chapter

http://dx.doi.org/10.5772/55197

1. Introduction

Epilepsies of surgical interest are focal and drug-resistant forms associated with various different conditions (malformations, stroke, tumors, infectious and/or inflammatory processes, brain injuries). There is mounting evidence that early resective surgery can achieve seizure-free status or reduce seizure frequency. The main challenge in the presurgical assessment of patients with epilepsy is to localize the area of seizure onset (the epileptogenic zone) and to distinguish it from lesional and interictal foci (the irritative zone) because it is only by treating the epileptogenic zone that seizure freedom or a reduction in events may be attained (Thorton, 2010).

This is explained by the fact that since the interictal focus is larger than the epileptogenic zone, the epileptogenic zone does not always overlap the lesional area and the epileptogenic focus is often larger than lesional area (Avesani, 2008/a; Manganotti, 2008; Thorton, 2010). In general, interictal epileptic discharges may affect brain areas well beyond the presumed region in which they are generated (Gotman, 2008). While resection of the lesional area alone is not sufficient, neither can the entire interictal focus be removed due to the high risk of cognitive, motor, sensitive or language deficits.

Presurgical evaluation involves invasive investigation by stereoelectroencephalography (SEEG) performed after other routine exams (standard EEG, video-EEG, functional neuroimaging) to identify the interictal focus within the epileptogenic zone. The lesional area, instead, is nowadays studied with advanced MRI techniques developed to better identify the interictal focus.

2. Functional imaging in epilepsy

Functional imaging refers to noninvasive methods to identify the interictal focus and the epileptogenic zone which, in a subsequent step, is studied with an invasive technique (SEEG, electrocortical mapping). The most widely used are:

- positron-emission tomography (PET)
- single-photon-emission computed tomography (SPECT)
- magnetic resonance spectroscopy (MRS)
- functional magnetic imaging (fMRI)

These techniques allow the study of a specific area of the brain, obviating the need for invasive studies of the entire brain. PET and SPECT were initially utilized for this purpose. While both provide a better knowledge of the brain's functional anatomy, they rarely allow for a precise localization of an epileptogenic focus, making them less useful for surgical planning (Marks, 1992; Henry, 1993; Newton, 1995).

The rationale for SPECT is based on its ability to reveal, in vivo, the volume distribution of a radiotracer after intravenous injection, and to evaluate, quantitatively and qualitatively, regional brain perfusion (Devous, 2005). The application of SPECT in epilepsy derives from a known association between an electrical event and brain perfusion: brain perfusion increases during the ictal phase and decreases during the interictal phase. Studies using dynamic and static SPECT have demonstrated interictal temporal hypoperfusion in 50% patients with temporal-lobe epilepsy (TLE). Nevertheless, the limitation of this technique is that 5-10% of patients demonstrate contralateral hypoperfusion, which raises the risk of false localization (Krausz, 1991). The localization power of SPECT during the interictal phase is, therefore, variable, with a sensitivity of 36% and a specificity of 95% (Engel, 1982). For this reason, SPECT is useful as a comparative study of ictal and interictal perfusion in selected patients. When applied during a seizure, it demonstrates the dynamic aspect of the seizure during its development. Unlike interictal studies, ictal SPECT, in both temporal and extratemporal epilepsy, is accurate in localizing an epileptogenic focus. During the ictal phase it can reveal, with a sensitivity of 70-95%, hyperperfusion in an area activated by seizures (Engel, 1983; Lee, 1994).

PET is a powerful imaging technique to quantify, in vivo and noninvasively, cerebral blood flow, metabolism and receptorial links. Its main application derives from the need to identify epileptogenic foci in patients with drug-resistant epilepsy, potential candidates for surgical treatment to control or abolish drug-resistant focal seizures. In up to 20-30% of such patients, who are candidates for surgical treatment, the MRI exam is negative (Duncan, 1997) because microscopic structural malformations, identifiable only by histological study, are not detectable with conventional MRI (Kuzniecky, 1991). Using [11C]flumazenil positron-emission tomography ([11C]FMZ-PET), Hammers studied 18 patients with TLE and normal MRI: 16 demonstrated abnormalities in the binding of ^{11}C-FMZ in the temporal lobe; 7 of these were concordant with clinical and standard EEG data; 3 patients underwent surgical treatment of

http://dx.doi.org/10.5772/55197

the anterior temporal lobe, with marked clinical improvement. The neuropathological data revealed microdysgenesis not detected by MRI (Hammers, 2002).

In patients with focal seizures, glucose metabolism and cerebral blood flow in a particular focal region are increased during an ictal event (Engel, 1983). In the postictal phase, hyperperfusion gradually returns to the basal level, but glucose metabolism remains elevated for 24-48 hours after seizure termination (Leiderman, 1994). In the interictal phase, PET demonstrates a decrease in glucose metabolism and cerebral blood flow in the epileptogenic focus. Studies using *18*-fluoro-2-deoxy-glucose-positron emission tomography (*18F-FDG-PET*) demonstrated hypometabolism in the temporal lobe in 60-90% of patients with interictal spikes (Duncan, 1997). Nevertheless, an area with abnormal cerebral blood flow and metabolism, as detected with PET, is larger than the real structural anomaly generating an epileptogenic focus probably because of deafferentation phenomena in the surrounding neurons in areas of seizure propagation (Duncan, 1997). Since this carries the risk of false localization, PET is regarded as being more suitable for studying lateralization than localization (Tai, 2004).

MR spectroscopy can be utilized in the noninvasive assessment of specific cerebral metabolites. In epilepsy the aim is to determine a focal change in the main metabolites deriving from focal brain dysfunction. The initial aim of the method was to delimit the epileptogenic focus and to analyze the distant repercussions of the lesion and the focus. For example, spectroscopy can reveal bilateral hippocampal abnormalities in unilateral mesial temporal sclerosis (MTS). The technique has demonstrated its utility in identifying metabolic dysfunction in patients with TLE. Nevertheless, owing to its high sensitivity, metabolic abnormalities may be revealed in regions without an epileptogenic focus, making it difficult to distinguish the causal abnormalities from their consequences (Ruben, 2005).

In patients with drug-resistant TLE, spectroscopy demonstrated a lower N-acetyl aspartate/ creatine (NAA/Cr) ratio, a reliable marker of neuronal integrity, in the ipsi- and contralateral lobes, and this finding correlated negatively with seizure duration (Bernasconi, 2002). Patients with frequent generalized seizures were noted to have a lower NAA/Cr ratio than those with rare or no seizures. Another interesting finding was the demonstration of reversible dysfunction in the cortical area after surgical treatment (Hugg, 1996). What all this suggests is that seizures may induce additional neuronal damage that will progress with the duration of epilepsy. From this point of view, spectroscopy may be useful as a metabolic marker of disease progression. In the future, it may be possible to decide whether evidence of disease progression on spectroscopy may be sufficient to suggest a change of therapy (Petroff, 2002).

Functional MRI (fMRI) provides high-resolution images using the classical principles of MRI, with the difference that signal recording exploits the paramagnetic properties of hemoglobin when its iron atom changes from Fe^{3+} (oxygenated hemoglobin) to Fe^{2+} (deoxygenated hemoglobin). Only Fe^{2+} has the ability to locally modify the magnetic state of cerebral tissues (Berns, 1999). Activation of a cerebral area causes both oxidative metabolism and local cerebral blood flow to increase, leading to greater oxygen extraction by the tissues. This results in a local increase of deoxyhemoglobin. Functional MRI reveals the activation of a cerebral area from the higher level of deoxyhemoglobin compared to the basal condition. And it does this indirectly by measuring the vascular response to activation of the cerebral area under study.

The response has a variable latency (from 3-5 to 10 seconds), which is why this kind of information is defined as "functional", and the recorded signal, related to hemoglobin oxygenation, is defined as BOLD (Blood Oxygen Level Dependent) (Ogawa, 1990; Prichard, 1994).

fMRI works by comparing the images obtained in rest condition with those acquired during a task. Whether and to what extent physiological correlates match different BOLD phases (Menon, 2001) continues to fuel debate, though studies suggest that the fMRI signal is closely related to neuronal activation (Logothetis, 2001). The method was first applied to localize areas associated with motor, sensory and cognitive functions in epileptic patients and to obtain a precise localization of these functions in the presurgical evaluation of epilepsy (Puce, 1995; Binder, 1996; Dupon, 2002).

3. EEG-fMRI

This noninvasive technique provides reliable information to localize cerebral regions generating interictal epileptic activity. It involves the simultaneous recording of EEG and fMRI. With ongoing refinement of the technology (first of all removal of magnetic field artifact on EEG), initial technical limitations have been overcome (Ives, 1993). EEG-fMRI permits the study cerebral activation and deactivation related to infra-clinical spikes by comparing EEG with spiked activity against EEG without abnormalities (Krakow, 1999 and 2001; Lazeyras 2000; Archer, 2003).

Research to date has investigated lesional epilepsy in the temporal region in particular, the most frequent cause of epilepsy of surgical interest. Up until several years ago, triggered EEG-fMRI was used. EEG was recorded during a scanning session, and fMRI acquisition was performed when a neurologist identified, on line, interictal (spikes, polyspikes, spike waves) activity on EEG. Acquisition was performed after a fixed latency (3-5 seconds) from detected interictal activity, which was decided before starting acquisition. The technique had several limitations: it was based on the concept of standardized cerebral hemodynamic activity, even if we know that such activity varies widely (from 3 up to 10 seconds); analysis had to be performed offline using, as a task, spikes with different morphology; and the temporal dynamics of hemodynamic responses could not be identified. Owing to these limitations, early studies with triggered EEG-fMRI (Krakow, 1999 and 2001) showed low sensitivity (60%) in detecting hemodynamic activation related to interictal activity.

Later studies (Lazeyras, 2001; Lemieux, 2001; Al-Asmi, 2003) demonstrated the superiority of continuous EEG-fMRI based on offline analysis after simultaneous EEG recording during a fMRI scanning session and following artifact removal. This development brought about clear advantages: since it was no longer necessary to decide beforehand which abnormal events were to be studied (and recorded) during a single acquisition, the temporal evolution of activations (after 1 to 10 seconds) could be identified and pathophysiological hypotheses about their propagation postulated. Continuous EEG-fMRI detects activation with a sensitivity of 80%.

Numerous studies have applied continuous EEG-fMRI to investigate various different epileptic syndromes (Boor, 2003; Salek-Haddadi, 2003 and 2006; Bagshaw, 2004 and 2006; Aghakhani, 2004 and 2005; Gotman, 2004 and 2005; Kobayashi, 2005 and 2006; Laufs, 2006; Di Bonaventura, 2006; Vaudano, 2009). Some studied focal epilepsies, while others examined idiopathic generalized forms underlying absence seizures.

4. EEG-fMRI in absence seizures

The application of EEG-fMRI in idiopathic generalized epilepsy (IGE), for evident technical problems, is limited to absence seizures or nonconvulsive status, to analyze the network underlying impaired consciousness related to generalized spike wave (GSW) discharges. Clinically, absences are characterized by a blank stare and impaired consciousness. Activities requiring vigilant attention have been coupled with a lesser likelihood of absences, whereas an increased frequency of seizures during relaxation is well established (Andermann, 2000; Guey, 1969). These findings suggest a causal link between changes in the level of awareness and the occurrence of GSW discharges.

Recent functional imaging studies have revealed the existence of a set of brain regions which show increased functional and metabolic activity during rest, compared to attention-demanding tasks (Raichle, 2000; Mazoyer, 2001). Involved brain areas (the posterior cingulated cortex, the precuneus, the medial prefrontal cortex, the mid-dorsolateral prefrontal and the anterior temporal cortices) have been hypothesized to constitute the so-called default mode network (DMN) (Raichle, 2000). Decreased DMN activity during cognitive tasks indicates that the network sustains spontaneous thought processes or self-oriented mental activity that characterizes the brain's resting state.

Additionally, the precuneus/posterior cingulate node has been recently demonstrated to have the highest degree of interactions (as shown by a partial correlation approach to fMRI data) with the rest of the DMN (Frasson, 2008), suggesting a pivotal role of this area within the network. This interpretation is in line with evidence from previous PET studies that this brain region, and the precuneus in particular, has the highest metabolic rate, consuming 35% more glucose than any other area of the cerebral cortex at rest (Gusnard, 2001).

The DMN shows decreased activity during both attention-demanding tasks and states of reduced vigilance and, especially in the posteromedial cortical regions, during altered states of consciousness (Laureys, 2004; Faymonville, 2006). From these observations, several authors (Cavanna, 2006 and 2007; Boly, 2008) suggested a pivotal role of the posteromedial cortical region in self-consciousness inside the DMN.

EEG-correlated functional magnetic resonance imaging (EEG-fMRI) studies have shown a common pattern of BOLD signal decrease in the precuneus and other DMN areas, together with an increase in the thalamic BOLD signal, during ictal and interictal GSW discharges (Aghakhani, 2004; Archer, 2003; Gotman, 2005; Hamandi, 2006; Laufs, 2006; Salek-Haddadi, 2003; De Tiège, 2007; Labate, 2005). Decreased cerebral blood flow consistent with a decrease in neuronal activity was demonstrated in DMN regions during GSW discharges (Hamandi, 2008). Therefore, these relative BOLD signal decreases can be interpreted as a transitory suspension of the brain's "default state" which occurs in association with an altered level of awareness observed during GSW discharges and absences, respectively (Gotman, 2005; Hamandi, 2006; Laufs, 2006; Salek-Haddadi, 2003).

The pathophysiological substrate of GSW remains enigmatic. Studies in animals and humans have tried to answer persistent questions about the putative role of the thalamus and cortex as generators. Data from invasive recordings and manipulations in well-validated genetic models of absence epilepsy have lent support to the hypothesis that absence seizures are of cortical origin (Steriade, 1998; Meeren, 2002 and 2005; Polack, 2007; Holmes, 2004; Tucker, 2007).

Following on the suggestion of the involvement of dorsal cortical regions (particularly the posterior-medial cortical regions) in GSW discharges from neuroimaging studies (Gotman, 2005; Hamandi, 2006; Laufs, 2006; Salek-Haddadi, 2003) and their role in conscious awareness (Faymonville, 2006; Boly, 2008), a recent work (Vaudano, 2009) attempted to elucidate the interaction between these areas and the (frontal)cortical-thalamic loop by means of dynamic causal modeling (DCM) to study effective connectivity based on simultaneously recorded EEG-fMRI data in 7 patients with GSW discharges.

The results of this study are consistent with the concept of the precuneus as a key region that changes its activity with altered states of vigilance, thus influencing the occurrence of generalized seizures: changes in the precuneus state (an increase or decrease in its neuronal activity), which reflects spontaneous fluctuations in awareness, act on the thalamic-(frontal) cortical network, facilitating the development of GSW. This contrasts with previous observations (Gotman, 2005; Hamandi, 2006; Laufs, 2006) that decreases in precuneal activity reflect the semiology of impaired consciousness and are a consequence of GSW.

A similar hypothesis was advanced by Archer et al. (Archer, 2003) who observed a significant posterior cingulate negative BOLD response in 5 IGE patients with interictal GSW discharges but no BOLD signal changes in the thalamus or prefrontal cortex. The authors suggested that decreases in posterior cingulate activity and associated regions may be involved in the initiation of GSW activity.

Additionally, a fMRI study showed a BOLD signal decrease in the posterior cingulate in IGE subjects following photic stimulation whether or not GSW activity occurred, while the control subjects showed no change in this region (Hill, 1999). Such changes would be consistent with a decrease in posterior cingulate activity being a precursor (or facilitator) of GSW activity rather than a secondary phenomenon. The posterior cingulate cortex is adjacent to the precuneus and some authors would define it as part of the precuneal cortical area (Frackowiak, 1997; Frasson, 2008).

Current thinking about the pathophysiology of GSW has it that the neuronal state of the precuneus, and the level of awareness, may reflect a "physiological initiator" of generalized synchronous discharges. In this connection, EEG-fMRI adds electrophysiological data to GSW generation and precuneal involvement where, besides the scant evidence for a strict consequentiality between a particular state of vigilance and the occurrence of GSW discharges, there

http://dx.doi.org/10.5772/55197

is a notable lack of studies on the possible role of cortical structures (particularly the precuneus) other than the thalamus and frontal cortex in GSW.

Unlike surface electrophysiological recordings, fMRI studies with concurrent EEG in patients with GSW discharges have shown common hemodynamic changes not only in the thalamus and frontal cortex, but also in the precuneus and other brain regions (including the fronto-parietal association cortices) of the DMN (Aghakhani, 2004; Archer, 2003; Gotman, 2005; Laufs, 2007). Moreover, fMRI's relatively homogeneous sensitivity across the brain compared to that of scalp EEG may explain why recent EEG-fMRI studies have been able to reveal precuneal involvement in epilepsies characterized by impaired consciousness and associated with GSW (Gotman, 2005; Hamandi, 2006; Laufs, 2006).

In brief, there is an active role in generalized epilepsy for the precuneus, a region previously neglected in electrophysiological studies of GSW. DCM based on EEG-fMRI data has shown that the precuneus is not only strongly connected with the frontal cortex and the thalamus but also that the neuronal activity in this area may facilitate epileptic activity within a thalamo-cortical loop, the existence of which is well established. These findings suggest that GSW may arise through the direct influence of the neuronal state of the precuneus associated with spontaneous changes in the level of awareness.

5. EEG-fMRI in focal seizures: Introduction

5.1. Interictal focal spiked activity correlated BOLD signal changes: Aims and results

EEG-fMRI provides insight into the pathophysiology of changes in the level of awareness during GSW discharges in absence seizures; however, the practical usefulness of technique resides in the study of focal epilepsy, especially if drug resistant and associated with a condition which, if amenable to removal, could achieve seizure freedom or a reduction of frequency. Numerous studies have applied EEG-fMRI to focal seizures to identify the interictal focus and the ictal onset zone (Krakow 1999 and 2001; Boor, 2003; Salek Haddadi, 2006; Bagshaw, 2004 and 2006; Aghakani, 2005; Kobayashi, 2005 and 2006). Some also applied SEEG and electrocortical mapping to study areas previously identified with EEG-fMRI and confirmed co-localization between interictal events (IEDs) and hemodynamic activation detected on fMRI (Krakow, 1999; Kobayashi, 2006; Benar, 2006).

All these studies analyzed patients with spiked activity on focal EEG (spikes, spikes and waves, polyspikes) that differed in frequency. It was then suggested that a limiting factor to obtain sufficient BOLD activation is IED frequency. Two studies (Krakow, 1999 and 2001) proposed 1 IED/minute as the minimum value to obtain sufficient activation. But because a lower frequency does not have sufficient power to stimulate an IED-correlated BOLD signal change, the sensitivity of the technique is very low. More recent studies applied EEG-fMRI to compare the location of IED-correlated BOLD signal change with the resected area and postoperative outcome (Thorton, 2010). Seven out of 10 surgically treated patients were seizure-free following surgery and the area of maximal BOLD signal change was concordant with resection in 6 out of 7 patients. In the remaining 3 patients with reduced seizure frequency post-surgically, the areas of significant IED-correlated BOLD signal change lay outside the resection, thus confirming that the epileptogenic zone (to be removed) is different from the lesional area.

5.2. Interictal focal slow wave activity correlated BOLD changes: The first case reports

Although some studies analyzed focal epilepsies (Liu, 2008), focal slow-wave activity as a marker of activation of cerebral blood flow was initially studied in only two single case reports (Laufs, 2006/a; Avesani 2008/a-b). The one additionally used SEEG to demonstrate co-localization between IEDs and fMRI activation. The second, our case report (Avesani 2008/a), involved a patient with temporal lobe epilepsy (TLE) due to a cavernoma, who had undergone surgical treatment without attaining freedom of seizures. This woman had no medical history of note until the age of 24 years (1975), when symptoms characterized by painful sensations including a lightening stabbing pain developed in the left parietal region of the head, preceded by absence attacks lasting 30 seconds. After seizures she always experienced profound weakness. Her seizures recurred at a variable rate, ranging from more than one a day to one every 10-15 days. During the seizure-free periods she remained healthy. The EEG at that time was negative for an interictal focus. In 1986, when the patient was 35 years old, the EEG disclosed an interictal focus in left temporal regions, characterized by very frequent, and polymorphous, theta-delta activity in association with sharp waves, blocked by eye opening and without contralateral diffusion. Subsequent EEG confirmed the irritative focus in the left fronto-temporal region. When the patient was 37-year-old she began therapy with phenobarbitone (PB) and carbamazepine (CBZ), benefiting from a decrease in seizure intensity (but not frequency). A computed tomographic (CT) brain scan disclosed a mild, non-homogeneous, subcortical hyperdensity on the mesial side of the left temporal lobe, containing rough calcifications with no contrast enhancement. An MRI scan revealed two small lesions in the left temporal lobe, similar to cavernomas (one anterior, in the Sylvian fissure and another posterior, in the paratrigonal region). The patient underwent surgery but the partial seizures remained unchanged. Treatment with PB and CBZ was therefore continued. Twelve years later (2002), another MRI scan revealed three small independent cavernomas in the left temporal lobe (left temporo-basal, left temporo-mesial, and in the left post-central gyrus). A year later (2003), bleeding of the large lesion (localized in the left temporo-basal region) caused the patient to be re-admitted to the neurosurgical ward to undergo a second operation. Despite repeat surgery the seizures continued so she needed further therapy. A following MRI scan (2005), confirmed the presence of the previous cavernomas without bleeding.

Using interictal focus of slow waves recorded in the left temporal region as a trigger of activation (Fig. 1), we obtained activation in the left posterior cortical region around the poro-encephalic cavity (residual of previous surgical treatment) (Fig. 2). Our findings confirmed observations by Thorton of 3 patients in whom surgical treatment failed to achieve seizure freedom: in these situations areas of significant IED correlated BOLD signal change lay outside the resection (Thorton, 2010).

http://dx.doi.org/10.5772/55197

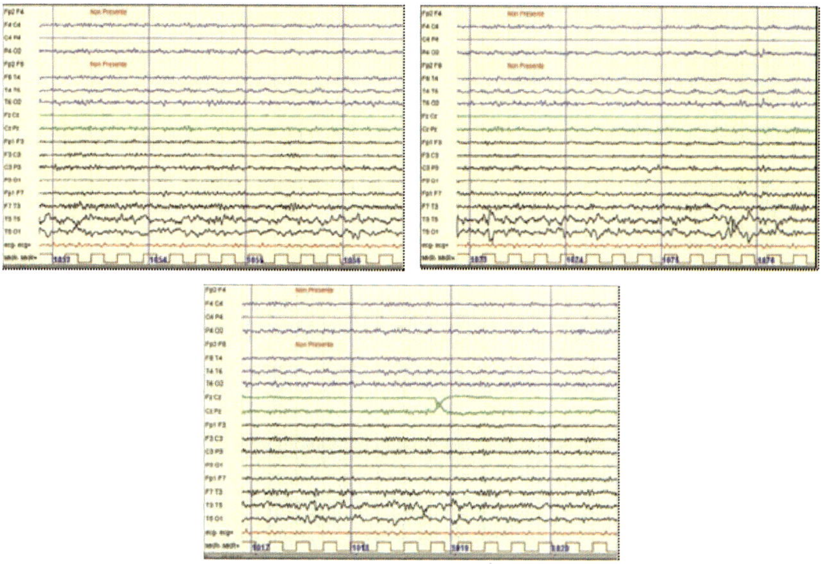

Figure 1. Interictal EEG of patient affected by cavernosa. Focal IEDs in left temporal region

6. EEG fMRI in focal seizures: The first study of interictal slow wave activity correlated bold changes

6.1. Patients enrolled in the study

In a previous study involving 8 patients with focal slow-wave interictal discharges on EEG (Manganotti, 2008), we suggested that an IED-correlated BOLD change triggered by interictal slow-wave activity could be obtained if the focal activity is frequent (about 2 IEDs/min). The study was primarily designed to verify whether the interictal slow waves originating from an EEG interictal focus were sufficient to increase cerebral blood flow in a spatially related brain area. To do so, using EEG-fMRI, we investigated BOLD responses to IEDs characterized by focal interictal slow-wave activity in patients with partial epilepsy.

We also wanted to understand whether, in patients with lesional epilepsy, fMRI-BOLD activation areas were correlated with lesions previously identified with standard MRI. We then investigated whether EEG-fMRI could document the spatial relationship between the interictal zone and the ictal onset zone in patients with interictal focal slow-wave discharges arising from a known epileptogenic lesion (i.e., the lesional area).

To obtain a homogeneous study sample, 8 patients with focal epilepsy were selected from among patients hospitalized in our epilepsy ward whose routine EEG recordings showed frequent focal IEDs manifesting as 5-6 Hz focal EEG activity (slow waves, slow spike waves, high-amplitude slow waves), over a few lateralized electrodes. Three of the 8 patients selected

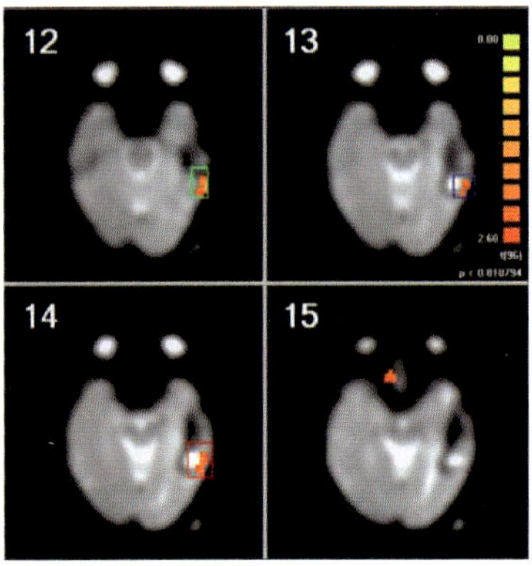

Results of data analysis in 2D reconstruction

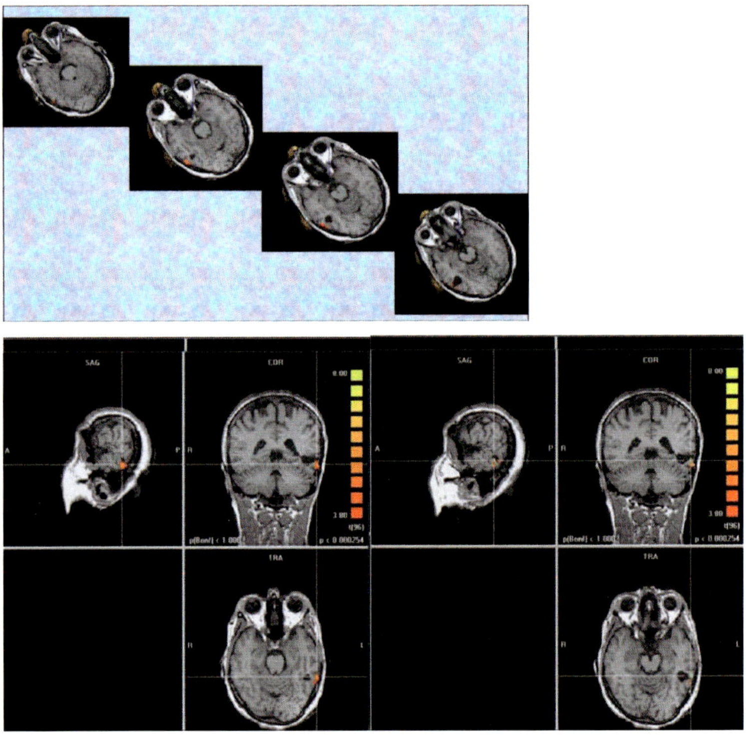

Results of data analysis in 3D recontruction

Figure 2. Interitcal focal slow wave activity correlated BOLD activation in patient affected by cavernoma: results of data analysis both in 2D and in 3D recontruction

http://dx.doi.org/10.5772/55197

for study had a structural lesion on MRI: 2 patients with hippocampal atrophy secondary to mesial temporal sclerosis (MTS) and 1 patient with a cavernous angioma. Among the remaining 5 patients, 1 patient had cryptogenic epilepsy and 4 patients had nonlesional (idiopathic) epilepsy. Routine EEG showed slow-wave activity in 1 patient with MTS (P4), the patient with cryptogenic epilepsy (P2) and the one with idiopathic epilepsy (P7); slow spike waves were observed in the patient with a cavernoma (P3) and the 2 patients with idiopathic epilepsy (P5 and P8); high-amplitude slow-waves (> 130 μV) were noted in 1 patient with idiopathic epilepsy (P6) and the second patient with MTS (P1) (Table 1).

Patients	Type of Epilepsy	Standard MRI findings	IED morphology	Irritative focus
1	Lesional	MTS	HASW	T3-T5
2	Cryptogenic	Negative	SW	T3-T5
3	Lesional	Cavernoma	SPSW	T5
4	Lesional	MTS	SW	T4-T6
5	Idiopathic	Negative	SPSW	O1
6	Idiopathic	Negative	HASW	T4-T6
7	Idiopathic	Negative	SW	F7
8	Idiopathic	Negative	HASPSW	T4-T6

MTS denotes mesial temporal sclerosis; SW slow waves; HASW high-amplitude slow waves; SPSW spiked slow waves; HASPSW high- amplitude spiked slow waves.

Table 1. Patients enrolled in the first study (Manganotti, 2008).

The good results we obtained (BOLD activations correlated to IEDs in 8/8 patients) allowed us to extend the study to 8 other patients (for a total of 16 patients), all with the same characteristics: focal epilepsy in which routine EEG recordings showed frequent focal IEDs manifesting as 5-6 Hz focal EEG activity (slow waves, slow spike waves, high-amplitude slow waves) over a few lateralized electrodes. The results did not change. MRI revealed a structural lesion in 4 patients: MTS in 2, tuberose sclerosis (TS) in 1; and hypothalamic hamartoma (HH) in 1. Three patients had cryptogenic and one nonlesional (idiopathic) epilepsy.

Standard EEG showed: focal sharp-wave activity in 1 patient (P15) with idiopathic epilepsy; high-amplitude slow-wave activity (or high-amplitude sharp waves) in 1 with TS (P12) and in 1 with HH (P14); spiked sharp waves in 1 with MTS (P10) and in 2 patients with cryptogenic epilepsy (P13 and P16); and high-amplitude spiked waves in 1 with MTS (P9) and in 1 with cryptogenic epilepsy (P11) (Table 2).

Patient	Type of epilepsy	Standard MRI findings	IED morphology	Irritative focus
9	Lesional	MTS	HASPSW	T8
10	Lesional	MTS	SPSW	F7-T3
11	Cryptogenic	Negative	HASPSW	F7-T3
12	Lesional	TS	HASW	P4
13	Cryptogenic	Negative	SPSW	T6
14	Lesional	HH	HASW	T4-T6
15	Idiopathic	Negative	SW	T3-T5
16	Cryptogenic	Negative	SPSW	F8-T4

Table 2. Characteristics of the 8 additional patients. MTS denotes mesial temporal sclerosis; TS tuberose sclerosis; HH: hypothalamic hamartoma.

6.2. Matherials and methods

6.2.1. EEG recordings and analysis

The EEG was acquired using a MR compatible EEG amplifier (SD MRI 32, Micromed, Treviso, Italy) and a cap providing 32 Ag/AgCl electrodes positioned according to a 10/20 system (impedance was kept below 10 kΩ). To remove pulse and movement artifacts during scanning two of these electrodes were used to record the electrocardiogram (ECG) and electromyogram (EMG). The EMG electrode was placed on the right abductor pollicis brevis (APB) muscle and the other (ECG) on the precordial area.

The reference was placed anterior to Fz, and the ground posterior to Fz as in other studies (Gonçalves et al. 2006; Avesani et al. 2008/a; Formaggio et al., 2008; Manganotti et al. 2008) using the same system. To ensure subjects' safety, the wires were carefully arranged to avoid loops and physical contact with the subject. To minimize the variability in the EEG artifacts due to the MR sequence and avoid wire movement caused by mechanical vibration the wires rested on foam pads.

EEG data were acquired at the rate of 1024 Hz using the software package SystemPlus (Micromed, Treviso, Italy). To avoid saturation, the EEG amplifier had a resolution of 22 bits with a range of ±25.6 mV. An anti-aliasing hardware band-pass filter was applied with a bandwidth between 0.15 and 269.5 Hz. Details of the EEG recording method are given in Bènar (Bènar et al, 2003). The EEG artifact induced by the gradient magnetic field was digitally removed off-line by an adaptive filter (Micromed). EEG artifacts associated with pulsatile blood flow were digitally removed off-line using a simple averaging procedure (Allen, 1998-2000). Subsequently a single electroencephalographer visually reviewed the filtered EEGs, and marked the time of onset and duration of each IED.

6.2.2. fMRI acquisition and analysis

Images were acquired on a 1.5 T MR scanner (Symphony, Siemens, Erlangen, Germany) equipped with EPI capability and a standard transient/receive (TR) head coil. At the start of each study, a T1-weighted anatomical MRI was acquired (192 slices; FOV = 256X256; scanning matrix 512X512; slice thickness 1 mm; sagittal slice orientation; echo time (TE) = 3ms; repetition time (TR) = 1990 ms).

All patients then underwent a 24-min fMRI recording session, after giving informed consent. BOLD fMRI data were acquired, using a standard gradient-echo (EPI) sequence, on the axial orientation, in 1 run of 8 minutes with the patient in the resting state, as described by the Kobayashi team (Kobayashi,2006) (voxel dimension 3x3x3 mm; 36 slices; matrix 64x64; TE = 50 ms, TR = 3.7 s; and slice thickness = 3 mm). At the onset of each fMRI acquisition, the scanner provided a trigger signal that was recorded by the EEG system and used as a volume marker.

For image processing and statistical analysis of the fMRI time series data we used BrainVoyager QX 1.9 software (*Brain Innovation, Maastricht, Netherlands*) running in windows VISTA enviroment. Pre-processing of the functional MRI included three-dimensional motion correction, slice scan time correction (linear interpolation), linear trend removal by temporal high-pass filtering (3 cycles in time course) and transformation into the Talairach coordinate space. Neither spatial nor temporal smoothing was used.

In each subject, activated voxels were identified with a single-subject general linear model (GLM) approach for time series data (Friston, 1995). To account for the hemodynamic delay, the boxcar waveform representing the rest and task conditions was convolved with an empirical hemodynamic response function (Friston, 1998).

A t statistic was used to determine significance on a voxel-by-voxel basis and correlation values were transformed into a normal distribution (Z statistic). The results were displayed on parametric statistical maps in which the pixel Z value is expressed on a colorimetric scale. We identified the single region of condition-associated BOLD signal changes with a statistical threshold based on the amplitude ($p<0.05$) and extent of the regions of activation. The location of voxels with maximal signal increase was expressed in terms of x, y, and z in the Talairach space, and activation volumes were expressed in terms of number of activated voxels. Positive BOLD-fMRI responses were defined as activations. Significant responses were defined as almost five contiguous voxels with $p<0.05$ over at least two contiguous slices (Krakow 1999 and 2001; Salek-Haddadi 2006) in 2D-reconstruction. The anatomic localization of BOLD responses was determined by co-registration of the anatomic data and statistical t maps.

We analyzed the extent and maximum fMRI response for each study, considering all areas with significative activations. We also determined the locations of maximum activation based on the maximum peak response (maximum t value).

6.3. Results

In all patients, EEG showed unilateral focal activity during the EEG-fMRI session. IEDs recorded inside the scanner had a localization, amplitude and morphology similar to those seen in the previous routine EEG recordings. EEG recordings showed focal high-amplitude slow waves in 4 patients (P1, P6, P12 and P14), and slow-wave discharges over the temporal electrodes in the other 3 patients (P2, P4 and P15). In 1 patient (P7) slow-wave activity was detected in the extratemporal (F7) region. In the patient with a cavernoma (P3), in 1 with MTS

(P10), and in 2 patients with cryptogenic epilepsy (P13 and P16), focal EEG activity was characterized by focal slow-spiked wave activity, reaching maximal amplitude over the left temporal electrodes (T5). In 1 patient (P5) slow-spiked waves were detected in the extratemporal region (left occipital region). The EEG tracings also showed high-amplitude spiked slow-wave activity in 3 patients (P8, P9 and P11): in the right temporal region in 2 (P8 and P9) and in the left fronto-temporal region in 1 patient (P11).

The mean frequency was 2.4 IEDs per minute (SD 0.17) for the first 8 patients and 2.495 for the second 8 patients, thus confirming sample homogeneity.

In all 8 patients from the first study and in 7/8 from the second study, fMRI analysis showed, in 2-D reconstruction, significant focal BOLD activation in a single activated area related to the EEG irritative focus (Tables 3 and 4). This activation was considered significant (Krakow, 1999) because it was identified in two contiguous MRI slices.

Patient	IEDs/24 min	IEDs/min	BOLD activation in 2D reconstruction	No. of slices
1	**61**	**2.54**	Left mesial temporal lobe	2
2	**55**	**2.29**	Left mesial temporal lobe	2
3	**54**	**2.25**	Left superior temporal lobe – neocortical region	3
4	**58**	**2.41**	Right mesial temporal lobe	2
5	**64**	**2.66**	Left occipital lobe-calcarin cortex	2
6	**51**	**2.13**	Right superior temporal lobe	2
7	**58**	**2.41**	Left frontal lobe	2
8	**62**	**2.58**	Right superior temporal lobe	2

Table 3. Number of IEDs revealed on EEG during recording and BOLD activation in 2D reconstruction of fMRI, with number of contiguous activated slices.

Patient	IEDs/24 min	IEDs/min	BOLD activation in 2D reconstruction	No. of slices
9	**57**	**2.38**	Left mesial temporal lobe	3
10	**57**	**2.38**	Left mesial temporal lobe	3
11	**59**	**2.45**	Left supplementary motor cortex	5
12	**62**	**2.59**	Right parietal lobe	3
13	**64**	**2.66**	Right mesial temporal lobe	2
14	**65**	**2.70**	Right mesial temporal lobe	2
15	**53**	**2.20**	====	0
16	**63**	**2.60**	Left mesial temporal lobe	2

Table 4. Number of IEDs revealed on EEG during recording and BOLD activation in 2D reconstruction of fMRI, with number of contiguous activated slices, in the second study of 8 patients.

This result was confirmed with analysis of 3D reconstruction of fMRI: in all 8 patients from the first study (Manganotti, 2008) and in 7/8 from the second study, fMRI BOLD activation corresponded to the irritative focus on standard EEG recordings (Tables 5 and 6).

http://dx.doi.org/10.5772/55197

Patient	No of voxels	Corresponding area in 3D reconstruction
1	177	Left cerebrum, limbic lobe, parahippocampal gyrus, **Brodmann area 34**
2	522	Left cerebrum, limbic lobe, parahippocampal gyrus, **Brodmann area 30**
3	540	Left cerebrum, temporal lobe, inferior temporal gyrus, **Brodmann area 20**
4	175	Right cerebrum, limbic lobe, parahippocampal gyrus, **Brodmann area 28**
5	1227	Left cerebrum occipital lobe, lingual gyrus, **Brodmann area 18**
6	364	Right cerebrum, temporal lobe, transverse temporal gyrus, **Brodmann area 42**
7	442	Left cerebrum, frontal lobe, precentral gyrus, **Brodmann area 6**
8	422	Right cerebrum, temporal lobe, middle temporal gyrus, **Brodmann area 21**

Table 5. Number of activated voxels, and localization, according to the Talairach system, of activated regions in 3D reconstruction, of the 8 patients from the first study (Manganotti, 2008).

Patient	No. of voxels	Activation in 3D reconstruction
9	368	1) Right cerebrum, temporal lobe, superior temporal gyrus **Brodmann area 38** 2) Right cerebrum, frontal lobe, mesial frontal region **Brodman area 10**
10	350	Left cerebrum, temporal lobe, fusiform gyrus **Brodmann area 20**
11	322	Left cerebrum, frontal lobe, supplementary motor cortex **Brodmann area 6**
12	52	Right cerebrum, parietal lobe, precuneus **Brodmann area 7**
13	256	Right cerebrum, temporal lobe, superior temporal gyrus **Brodmann area 38**
14	200	Right cerebrum, anterior cingulate, limbic lobe **Brodmann area 32**
15	0	=====
16	150	Right cerebrum, parahippocampal gyrus, limbic lobe **Brodmann area 34**

Table 6. Number of activated voxels, and localization, according to the Talairach system, of activated regions in 3D reconstruction, of the 8 patients from the second study.

6.3.1. Temporal lobe activation

Focal BOLD signal changes in 11 patients reached statistical significance in the temporal regions. In 10 patients (4 of which with MTS [P1, P4, P9, and P10]; 1 with HH [P14]; 3 with cryptogenic epilepsy [P2, P13, and P16]; in 2 of the 4 with idiopathic epilepsy [P6 and P8]), the significant BOLD changes were located in the mesial temporal lobe and in the neocortical regions (laterally and posteriorly to the resection margins) in the 1 patient with a cavernoma (P3).

An interesting case of surgically treated mesial temporal sclerosis involved P9. Of Moroccan origin, he has suffered from focal seizures since the age of 6 years, with loss of consciousness and oral and motor automatisms of the legs (pedaling) and arms, preceded by an epigastric aura, lasting 1 minute and resistant to therapy. On MRI, right mesial temporal sclerosis (MTS) was detected (fig.3). Standard EEG demonstrated an interictal focus in the right temporal region. The seizures first occurred rarely but then increased in frequency with time, eventually manifesting in "clusters" of 10-15 seizures every 1 to 2 months. Auras occurred every 2 weeks. Video-EEG demonstrated the same abnormal activity in the right temporal region, with an ictal event manifesting with the same characteristics. The hypothesis was that the seizures arose in an epileptogenic area related to the known MTS and then spread anteriorly to the right mesial frontal region (cause of motor manifestation). EEG-fMRI recording session identified an interictal slow wave activity in right temporal region (T4-T6), with a following diffusion both to contralateral region and to right frontal region (fig. 4). Two significant activations were detected (figg. 5-6): one in the right mesial temporal region (Brodmann area 38) and one in the right mesial frontal region (Brodmann area 10). Also in this case, BOLD activations were concordant with focal IEDs and with clinical syndrome. On subsequent analysis with invasive techniques (SEEG), the origin of seizure in an epileptogenic zone correlated with MTS was confirmed, with spread to the right mesial frontal region. The study also confirmed the co-localization between EEG and fMRI data. He was surgically treated and is now seizure free.

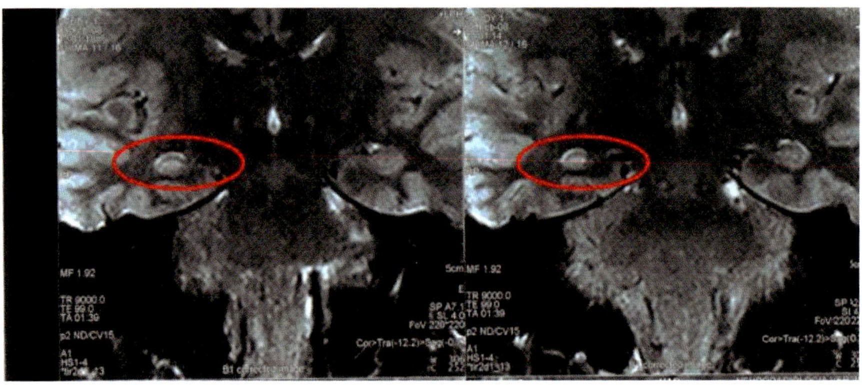

Figure 3. Right mesial temporal sclerosis (MTS) in Patient n. 9

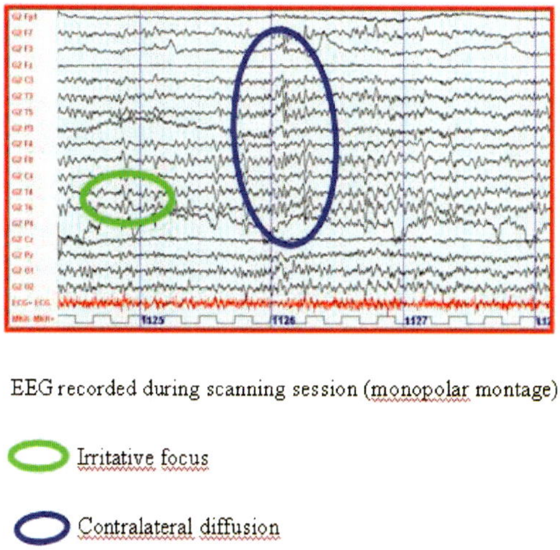

Figure 4. Patient n. 9. Focal IEDs in right temporal region, with following diffusion both to contralateral region and to right frontal region

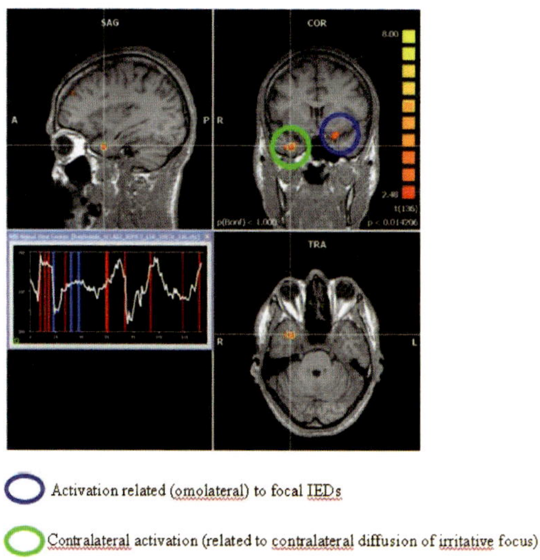

Figure 5. Patient n. 9. Focal IEDs correlated BOLD activations in mesial right temporal region, with following diffusion to contralateral region

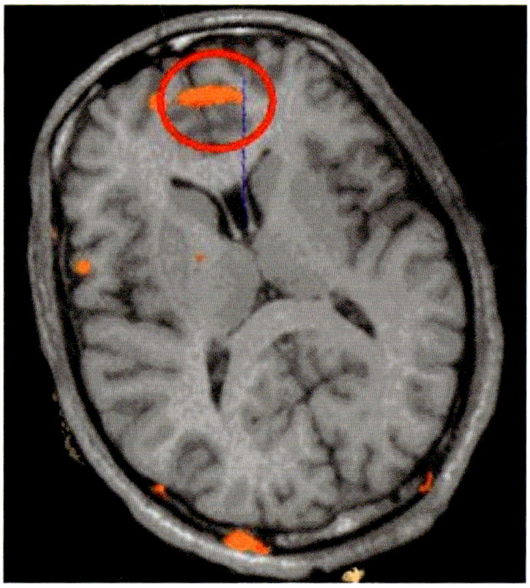

Figure 6. Patient n. 9. Focal IEDs correlated BOLD activation in right mesial frontal region

Another case involved a young man (P14) affected with gelastic seizures due to a hypothalamic hamartoma and manifesting since he was 2 years old. They were well defined: dissociated deviation of the eyes (the left eye toward the right and the right eye upwards) or associated deviation of both eyes upwards, followed by right head deviation, absent facial expression, and asymmetric smile. Often, an aura (tingling in the left temporal region) would precede the seizures, with concurrent rubor. The patient attempted to speak but was impeded by fixed smiling. The episode frequency was very high (up to 5 seizures/day). Over time, the syndrome worsened, with falls and subsequent injuries. SEEG confirmed an epileptogenic zone inside the hamartoma, with spread to the right mesial temporal region during the seizures. EEG-fMRI detected a significant BOLD activation in the limbic lobe (anterior cingulate), substantiating the anatomic-clinical correlation suggested by seizures and EEG.

This case parallels recently published findings on the networks involved in seizure generation in hypothalamic hamartoma (Kokkinos, 2012). EEG-fMRI was performed in 2 adult patients with hypothalamic hamartoma, the one with predominantly gelastic seizures and the other with complex partial but no typical gelastic seizures. Ictal and interictal analysis of the patient with gelastic seizures revealed involvement of the hypothalamic hamartoma, the cingulate gyrus, the precuneus and prefrontal cortex. The interictal analysis of the patient with complex partial seizures showed BOLD signal changes over the temporal lobes, the base of the frontal lobe, the precuneus and prefrontal cortex but not the hypothalamic hamartoma. It was presumed that the differences in the neural networks implicated may have accounted for the differences in the clinical manifestation of seizures owing to the tumor.

Other interesting cases are cryptogenic (P2, P13) and idiophatic forms (P6, P8, P15), all characterized by atypical absences and vagal symptomatology. In patient n. 2, focal IEDs (fig.

http://dx.doi.org/10.5772/55197

7) were recorded in left temporal region and focal IEDs correlated BOLD activation (fig. 8) was detected in mesial left temporal region, in limbic lobe. In patient n. 6 focal IEDs were recorded in right temporal region, with a characteristic phase reversal in T4 (fig. 9), and focal IEDs correlated BOLD activation was detected in Brodam area 42 (fig. 10). In patient n. 8, focal IEDs were recorded in right temporal region (fig. 11) and focal IEDs correlated BOLD activation was detected in Brodman area 21 (fig. 12).

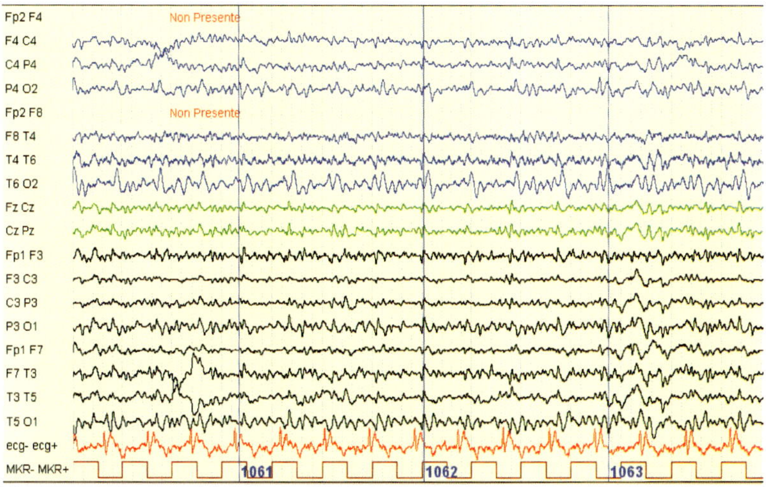

Figure 7. Patient n. 2 (cryptogenic epilepsy). Focal IEDs in left temporal region during scanning session

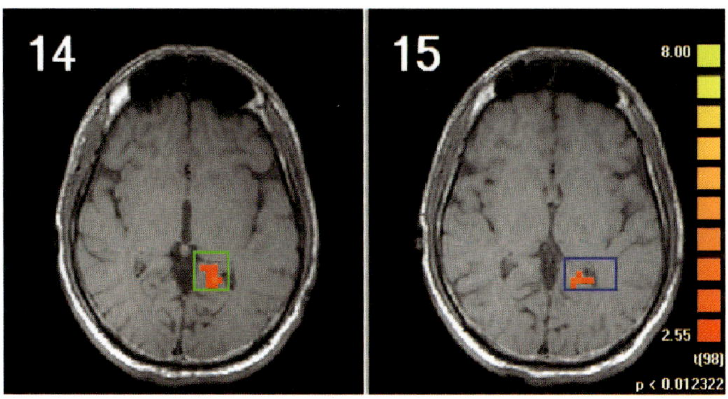

Figure 8. Patient n. 2. Focal IEDs correlated BOLD activations in left mesial temporal lobe

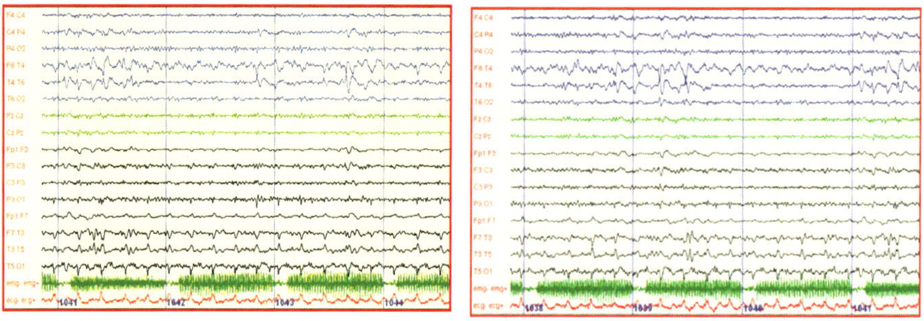

Figure 9. Patient n. 6. Focal IEDs in right temporal lobe with phase reversal in T4

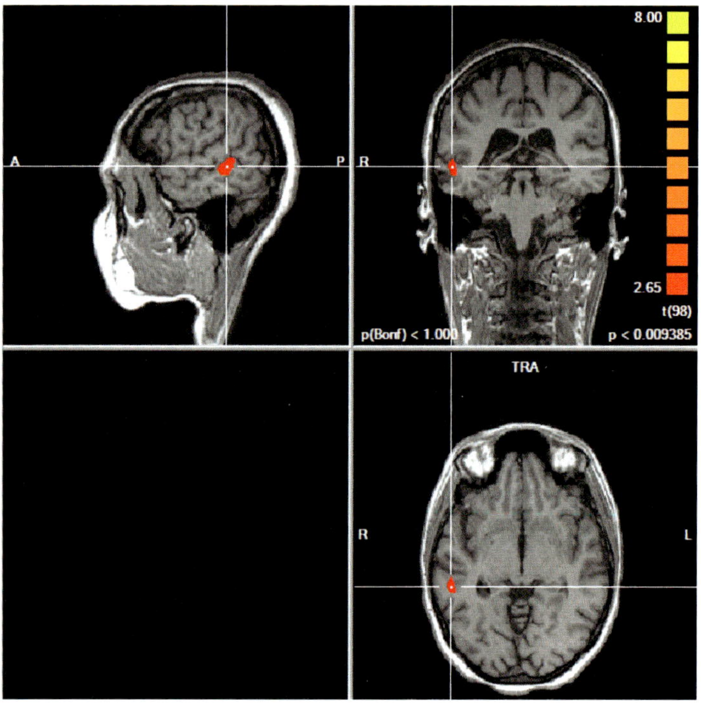

Figure 10. Patient n. 6. Focal IEDs correlated activation in transverse temporal gyrus, Brodmann area 42

http://dx.doi.org/10.5772/55197

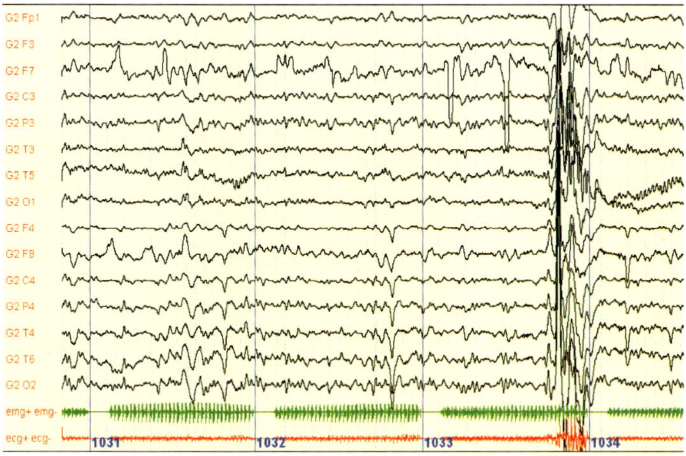

Figure 11. Patient n. 8. Focal IEDs in right temporal region

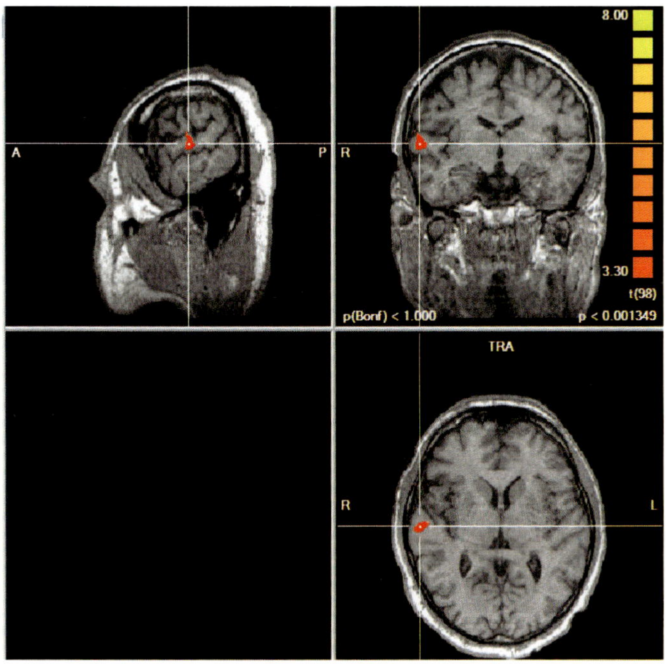

Figure 12. Patient n.8. Focal IEDs correlated BOLD activation in middle temporal gyrus, Brodmann area 21

6.3.2. Extratemporal activation

In our series, fMRI showed extratemporal activation in 4 patients: the left occipital lobe (P5); the left frontal lobe (P7); the left supplementary motor cortex (P11); and the right parietal lobe (P12). In all four cases there was a correlation between BOLD activation and IEDs and with clinical syndromes as well. This correlation is relevant to the discussion about the technique's sensitivity in revealing activation in extratemporal regions.

A rare case (P5) involved non ketotic hyperglycemia (NKH)-induced seizures occurring in the left occipital lobe studied by EEG-fMRI (Del Felice, 2009). These seizures usually occur in the frontal regions and cause motor ictal syndromes, whereas occipital seizures have been described in very rare situations. Cases of NKH presenting as hemichorea or hemianopia have also been reported. Seven such patients (Seo, 2003; Raghavendra, 2007) were studied by standard MRI transient T_2-weighted and fluid-attenuated inversion recovery (FLAIR). Subcortical hypointensity with or without abnormalities in the occipital overlying cortex or striatal nuclei was documented in occipital seizures associated with NKH. A single case investigated by Tc-99m HMPAO SPECT (Wang, 2005) showed occipital hyperperfusion during seizure recurrence and hypoperfusion during the interictal state.

Our patient (P5) was a 50-year-old woman admitted to hospital after repeated emergency room visits because of visual disturbances and left-sided headache. On clinical examination, she was obese and had a right-sided homonymous hemianopia. Her medical history was unremarkable, except for hypertension and a 15-kg weight gain during the past 12 months. She had no history of migraine, epilepsy or neurological disorders. Two days before admission she reported a short-lasting episode of visual disturbance (distortion). A few hours later, she noted diplopia when looking to the right, with image distortion in the right visual field and intermittent right-sided hemianopia, lasting several minutes, elicited by looking to the right or by fixation. The episodes were accompanied by a left-sided throbbing headache but no other autonomic symptoms (i.e., nausea or vomiting). No language disturbance was reported. She was presented to the emergency room.

On neurological examination, a right-sided homonymous hemianopia was noted. A standard computed tomography (CT) scan of the brain and an ophthalmologic exam were negative. She was discharged with a diagnosis of migraine with aura and started on antiplatelet therapy, with the recommendation to undergo out-patient visual field analysis.

Two days later, she was admitted to our ward owing to the persistence of symptoms, including a transient conjugated deviation of the eyes and the head to the right. On that occasion, which lasted less than 1 minute, the patient did not lose consciousness and referred seeing red flashing lights in her right visual field. Standard EEG performed immediately thereafter showed multiple clinical-EEG seizures during a prolonged recording, with spiked slow waves originating from the left posterior region, and with bilateral diffusion (fig. 13). Laboratory data on admission revealed hyperglycemia (14.5 mm/L to 261 mg/dL) with a serum osmolarity of 333 mmol/kg, and glycosilated hemoglobin of 10.5%. Urine analysis was negative for ketone bodies but was strongly positive for glycosuria (>1 g/dL) and microalbuminuria (up to 6 mg/24 h). A brain MRI scan with and without gadolinium, an MR angiography, and a 3T brain

http://dx.doi.org/10.5772/55197

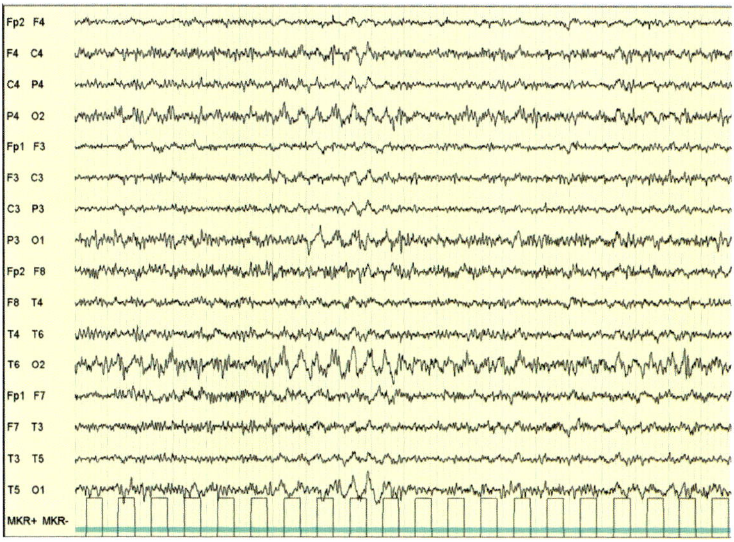

Figure 13. Patient n. 5. Standard EEG tracing during clinical seizures. Spiked slow waves on posterior regions (O1 and O2).

MRI were normal. Tc-99m hexamethylpropylene amine oxime (HMPAO) single-photon-emission computed tomography (SPECT), during which no clinical seizures were reported, showed non-significant hypocaptation over the posterior regions bilaterally.

On continuous EEG-fMRI a few days later, no clinical or EEG manifestations of ictal events occurred, but interictal spiked slow wave discharges (IEDs) with localization, amplitude and morphology similar to those previously recorded on routine EEG (fig. 13) were noted. A slow-spiked wave on the left occipital (O1) channel was detected. The mean frequency was 2.4 IEDs per minute. Functional MRI analysis showed significant focal BOLD activation in a single area related to the EEG paroxysmal activity. In a 3D reconstruction using the Talairach system (fig. 14), focal significant BOLD activation based on the EEG-related protocol was identified in Brodmann area 18 (grey matter of the left cerebrum occipital lobe and lingual gyrus). During her hospital stay, she was started on carbamazepine (200 mg/daily, up to 800 mg t. d.), with only partial benefit in frequency and intensity of symptoms. Since her glycemia was still uncontrolled (250 mg/dL), she was started on insulin therapy. Over the following 2 weeks, seizures and hyperglycemia both progressively decreased. On the basis of a possible diagnosis of NKH-induced seizures, carbamazepine was tapered, without the reappearance of symptoms. Serial EEG showed a decrease in epileptic activity (sharp waves) with persistent bilateral slowing. A few weeks later, insulin therapy was replaced with oral antidiabetics. One year later, the patient was seizure free, with a normal EEG. Following the loss of 18 kg, the oral antidiabetics were tapered, with good control of serum glucose and HbA1 values.

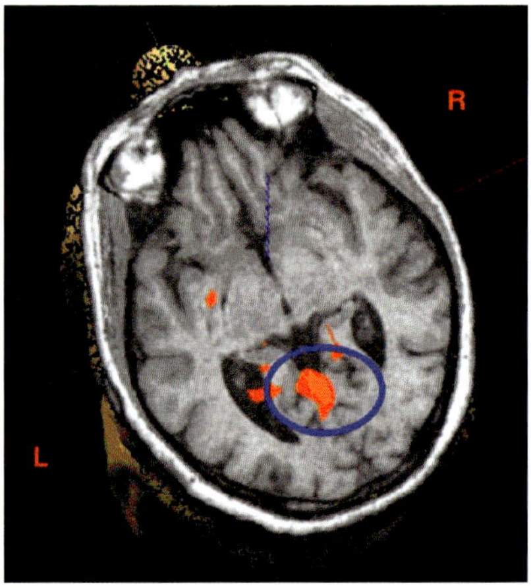

Figure 14. Patient n. 5. 3D fMRI-BOLD activation in Brodmann area 18.

A BOLD occipital activation in patients referring visual symptoms has been reported, confirming the involvement of visual functional areas in the occipital lobes: Brodmann areas 19 and 37 in reported cases of fixation sensitivity occipital spiking (Iannetti et al., 2002; Avesani, 2008/b) or the left occipital lobe in cases of cryptogenic and symptomatic (cortical malformation) occipital epilepsy (Salek-Haddadi et al., 2006). In our patient, an analogous BOLD activation was elicited by the NKH. Hyperglycemia may induce paroxysmal activity in brain areas more susceptible to metabolic changes – the occipital lobe in this case - with an analogous pattern of activation of self-sustained focal discharges. Neuroimaging, in this case fMRI-EEG co-registration, pointed to a change in blood volume in the involved posterior areas.

In the patient (P7) in whom fMRI revealed BOLD activation in the left frontal region (Brodmann area 6), standard EEG showed a left fronto-temporal irritative focus characterized by frequent slow-spiked waves. A recent polygraphic study (recorded during stage I and II non-rapid-eye-movement [NREM] sleep) showed polymorphic slow waves (theta-delta) in the left frontal regions, with phase inversion at F7 and without spread. These findings suggested that the patient was a good candidate for an EEG-fMRI study. During the EEG-fMRI sessions, we confirmed the fMRI activation area within the precentral gyrus.

Patient no. 11, a young woman, illustrates an interesting case of frontal lobe epilepsy characterized by focal seizures, with speech arrest and right arm clonus followed by generalization (Borelli, 2010), where, as reported elsewhere (So, 1998; Westmoreland, 1998), scalp EEG is often ambiguous because it is poorly sensitive to deep generators on the mesial surface of the frontal lobe. Also in this instance, EEG-fMRI effectively identified the interictal focus.

According to a detailed account by relatives, the events took the form of sudden episodes of speech arrest lasting from a few seconds up to several minutes, without any warning sensation. The patient reported she was able to move, understand and write properly during the ictal phase (sometimes writing a note to her husband that she was unable to speak). No clonic movements or orofacial automatisms were experienced at this early stage. Usually, an event did not progress any further and the patient was able to fully recollect the episode. Sometimes an episode was followed by clonic jerking over the right side of the face and arms with occasional, generalized tonic-clonic seizures. The seizure frequency was weekly despite polytherapy. The 3T MRI was normal. She reported no febrile seizures nor having sustained significant head injuries. Pregnancy, delivery and developmental milestones were unremarkable, as was the remainder of her medical history. Trials with various antiepileptic drugs (first with dintoine, then carbamazepine, and then fenobarbital) were unsuccessful. She was admitted to an intensive care unit for a status epilepticus and begun on valproate and lamotrigine.

Interictal scalp EEG showed frequent generalized high-amplitude (2 to 3 Hz) spiked slow-wave discharges. There was an inconstant, mild amplitude prevalence over the left hemisphere electrodes (F7-T3).

During a conventional scalp EEG recording, she complained of a brief episode of speech arrest associated with an EEG pattern characterized by diffuse spike and wave discharges (fig. 15). This event was witnessed by a neurologist from our ward who was aware of the patient's clinical history. He noted that the patient had a brief inability to speak (a few seconds) during which she waved her hands to attract his attention. There were no clonic movements, and after regaining speech, she accurately described the event. Three-hour video-EEG monitoring during a day of seizure clustering recorded no usual events. On the basis of these elements, a diagnosis of generalized epilepsy was also made in another hospital.

The clinical syndrome suggested involvement of the left supplementary motor area (SMA) with spread to the primary motor area. EEG -fMRI recording session confirmed the same pattern EEG identified by standard EEG (fig. 16) and following analysis showed prominent BOLD activation over the left SMA during the high-amplitude spiked slow-wave discharges compared to the rest state (Fig. 17). According to the Duncan criteria, such an activation pattern is reproducible since it was present in two contiguous slices (Duncan, 1999). The statistical significance of the activation was $p < 0.0028$ even after FDR correction. More activations were found in the contralateral SMA and homolateral motor strip as well. No significant deactivation areas or thalamic involvement (activation or deactivation) were found. The patient was referred to a level II epilepsy surgery center for presurgical work-up, including long-term video-EEG monitoring, but she refused further testing.

The speech arrest noted in this patient is an epileptic feature usually related to involvement of the supplementary motor cortex over either the dominant or the non-dominant hemisphere. A bilateral spike and wave discharge pattern (secondary bilateral synchrony) is often detected in frontal-lobe epilepsy, particularly if the generator is deep, for instance, over the mesial surface of the frontal lobe (So, 1998; Westmoreland, 1998). In the presurgical work-up for epilepsy surgery, such a scalp EEG pattern certainly raises questions about the origin of the focal epilepsy especially when conventional MRI is negative. In the latter case, more investigations are usually obtained to guide depth electrode placement for invasive EEG. Ictal SPECT and interictal PET are commonly used for this purpose, but they are expensive, difficult to interpret, and usually provide regional rather than local data. In addition, if the ictal event is

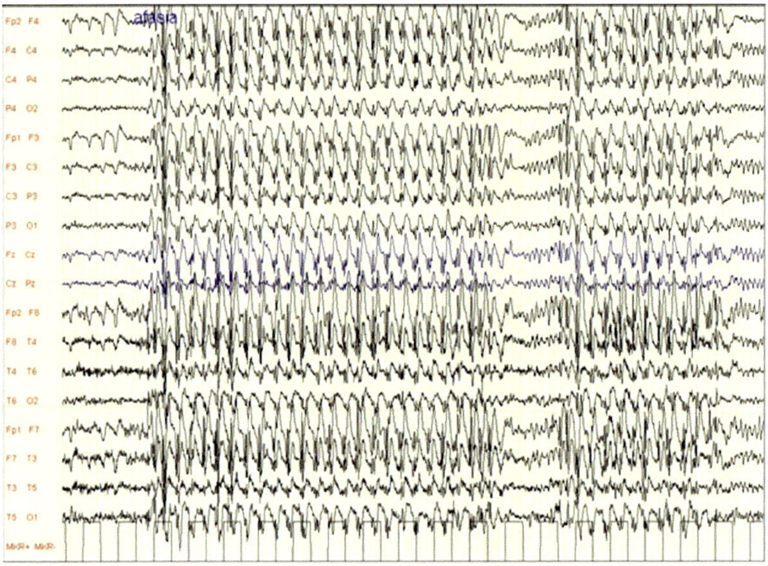

Figure 15. Patient n. 11. Ictal EEG during a brief speech arrest episode (''Afasia'' marks the beginning of the speech impairment).

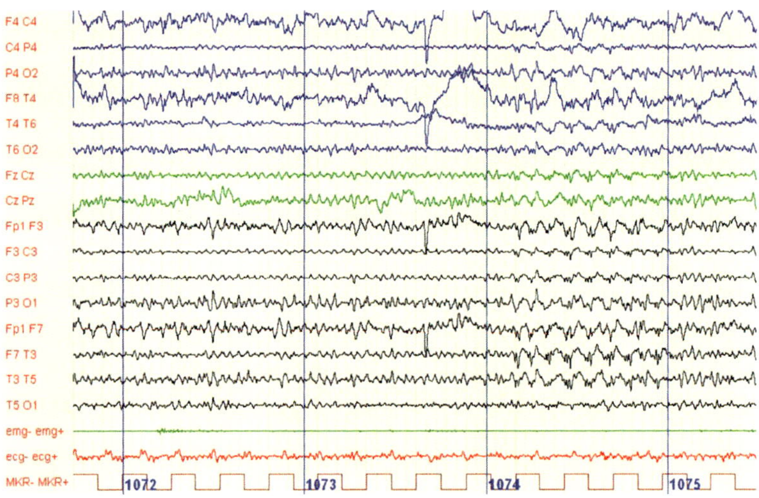

Figure 16. Patient n.11. EEG recorded during the fMRI acquisition showing generalized high amplitude spiked slow wave discharges, prevalent on left fronto-temporal regions.

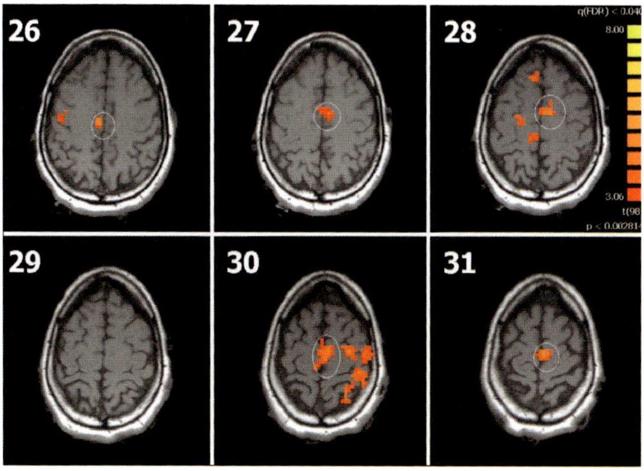

Figure 17. Patient n. 11. The EEG-fMRI shows a clear-cut activation of the left (radiological convention) Supplementary Motor Area (SMA) and on the contralateral SMA on a lesser degree. Spread over the left motor strip is also evident.

brief, SPECT may yield false negatives due to incorrect timing of the tracer injection (Salmenpera, 2005; Devous, 1998). The use of radioactive substances also raises safety issues.

A relatively new tool to obtain localizing data on the basis of EEG changes, EEG-fMRI is safe for the patient and relatively inexpensive (Al Asmi, 2003; Di Bonaventura, 2006). As our knowledge about the technique increases, it is gaining acceptance in the study of focal nonlesional epilepsy and presurgical work-up, as reported by Moeller et al. and Zijlmans et al. (Devous, 1998; Moeller, 2009). Nonetheless, few studies to date have applied EEG-fMRI in patients with secondary bilateral synchrony, except for one by Aghakhani (Aghakhani, 2006) involving 11 patients with such an EEG pattern, with a variable activation-deactivation pattern including thalamic involvement in 6 out of 11 (55%). The clinical seizure pattern and the MRI findings were variable.

In our patient, EEG-fMRI revealed the origin of the epileptiform discharges, including the spread over the homolateral motor strip, which was highly consistent with the patient's clinical features (speech arrest followed by clonic jerks over right half of the face and right arm), whereas 3T MRI and conventional interictal scalp EEG were useless in this regard. Some involvement of the contralateral SMA was also detected but its significance is less clear: it may have been the result of a transcallosal spread from the left SMA or simply an imperfect spatial resolution of the technique. In contrast with Aghakhani (Aghakhani, 2006) in our case no thalamic changes were seen.

Unfortunately, our localizing hypothesis could not be proved by invasive EEG and postsurgical outcome since the patient refused surgical treatment. Nonetheless, this patient suggests that, in the presurgical work up for epilepsy, EEG-fMRI may be considered a useful tool to generate a localizing hypothesis to be tested with invasive recording also in patients with focal epilepsy and bilateral slow spiked-wave discharges on EEG (secondary bilateral synchrony) and negative MRI. The recording of ictal EEG demonstrates that the slow waves we triggered in our study were irritative and not lesional.

7. Conclusions

The main finding in our EEG-fMRI study of patients with partial epilepsy is that the focal interictal slow-wave activity was invariably associated with increased focal fMRI-BOLD activation responses in a spatially related brain area. Our study extends current knowledge on epileptic foci localization and confirms previous reports suggesting that EEG-fMRI BOLD activation associated with modeled slow activity might have a role in localizing the epileptogenic region, even in the absence of clear interictal spikes (Laufs, 2006; Avesani, 2008/a).

All the patients with partial epilepsy we enrolled in this study had frequent interictal focal slow-wave activity on standard EEG. In all continuous EEG-fMRI recording sessions, after fMRI artifact removal, we obtained good quality EEG that allowed us to detect spontaneous IEDs and analyze the related fMRI BOLD activation. The EEG recording left the quality of the fMRI data almost undistorted, and the focal activity seen in the concurrent EEG was associated, in 15 of 16 patients enrolled, with a focal increase in the MRI signal in all patients. In their focal distribution, these BOLD activations resembled the focal IEDs seen on routine scalp EEG and EEG recorded during EEG-fMRI sessions.

An interesting finding came from the patients with lesional epilepsy. These patients, whose standard MRI documented a lesion and whose standard EEG identified an irritative focus, are ideal candidates for verifying a possible spatial relationship between the epileptogenic and the irritative focus (Ebersole, 1991; Benbadis, 1996).

In the patient who had undergone surgery to remove a cavernoma (P3), the EEG-fMRI study, by localizing the irritative focus and linking it to fMRI as an "active state", showed a significant BOLD activation signal closely related to the poro-encephalic cavity (a residual of previous treatment). Although this focal BOLD activation presumably arose from a blood vessel (residual cavernoma), it was undoubtedly obtained by a protocol study linking an active fMRI state to IEDs on EEG. To clarify the relationship, we decided to progressively test the specificity to a very high level ($p < 0.0001$), as demonstrated in the iconography. Even with these high specificity values, the BOLD activation in that site persisted.

Another new finding is the BOLD activation we detected on fMRI in the patients with MTS. In contrast to others who studied a series of patients with MTS (5 studied with continuous co-registration) (Al Asmi, 2003) and found no significant activation, we detected significant BOLD activation in 4 patients (P1, P4, P9 and P10). These results suggest a possible role of simultaneous EEG-fMRI in disclosing focal activation in the mesial temporal cortex. This cortical area is notoriously difficult to study with standard methods because the deep localization of the irritative area often makes spikes smoother and therefore harder to recognize on recordings from standard EEG scalp electrodes than in SEEG. Hence, IEDs presenting as slow-wave discharges could be useful in determining significant BOLD activation in a corresponding area, as previously suggested by Laufs et al. (Laufs, 2006).

Useful information that may help us to understand BOLD responses in various forms of epilepsy came also from studying activation in extratemporal IEDs. In the patients with extratemporal discharges (P5, P7, P11, and P12), we noted a good correlation between the clinical polygraphic data and BOLD activation during fMRI. No significant difference was found between activation in the frontal or the occipital lobe. In both regions, BOLD activation increased after focal IEDs. One patient (P11) demonstrated the usefulness of EEG-fMRI, especially when scalp EEG is ambiguous because it is poorly sensitive to detect deep generators on the mesial surface of the frontal lobe, and confirmed that the slow waves were irritative and not lesional.

The reason for such good results (15/16 activations -- significant concordance between EEG and fMRI data) is open to question. The most plausible reason is that during enrolment, to obtain the largest possible percentage of activations, patients were explicitly selected whose standard EEGs showed a high IED firing rate confirmed on EEG during the scanning session. The mean frequency of IEDs in the 15 patients was about 2/min, considerably higher than the 1 IED per minute Duncan considered as the minimum to obtain a focal BOLD activation (Krakow, 1999). Collectively, these findings confirm the importance of IED firing rates in EEG-fMRI.

Perhaps the most interesting finding in this study was that morphology seemed less important than IED firing rates in triggering EEG-fMRI-BOLD activation: 8 of the 16 patients had pure slow waves on standard EEG (4 with high amplitude and 4 with a normal voltage) and 7 had slow spike-wave discharges (4 with high amplitude and 3 with normal voltage); 1 patient (P10) had a focus of normal amplitude, sometimes pure, sometimes with spiked morphology. There were no differences in BOLD activation between the two groups.

Although these slow spike-wave discharges might have originated from a spike focus smoothed by filtering (unlikely because EEG detected the same IEDs before the patients entered the magnet room), there was no difference in the statistical significance of BOLD activation between the two groups. Specifically, slow spike-wave IEDs were no more efficient than slow-wave IEDs in eliciting significant BOLD activation. Hence, it was agreed as previously suggested (Laufs, 2006/a; Avesani, 2008/a) that slow-wave IEDs, like spikes, could elicit a significant increase in cerebral blood flow in a spatially related brain area.

The study also suggests that voltage might have a minor role in determining BOLD activation: in this small study sample there were no differences in BOLD activations between IEDs with high-amplitude (9 patients) and those with normal amplitude slow waves (7 patients).

The significant concordance between EEG and fMRI data, and the absence of multiple activation areas in particular, depended on the high specificity threshold the study design envisaged. In designing this study, only the single activation with the strongest specificity was maintained so that we could verify whether this activation, and this activation alone, coincided with the epileptic focus previously documented by standard EEG and used as a paradigm for the activation-state during the fMRI analysis.

Given the criticism raised against the use of EEG-fMRI instead of other techniques such as EEG-source analysis in the presurgical work-up (Elshoff, 2012), a possible objection to the conclusions we draw could derive from our decision to include only a well-defined sample of patients, all characterized by a focus with a high firing rate, without evidence of the same result in other patients with low firing rate foci (being the most frequent among patients affected by focal drug-resistant epilepsy of surgical interest. We reply that this study was the first approach to investigating interictal slow-wave foci. This will be addressed in a future study in order to validate the technique in patients with slow-wave interictal activity with a low firing rate focus.

At the moment, the complete EEG-fMRI concordance achieved in this study suggests that slow-wave IEDs, even without spikes, may be useful in activating fMRI BOLD responses during the presurgical, noninvasive evaluation of patients with partial drug-resistant seizures.

Acknowledgements

The authors wish to thank:

- Prof. Bernardo Dalla Bernardina, Dp of Life and Reproduction Sciences, University of Verona
- Dr. Giuseppe Moretto and Dr. Tiziano Zanoni, Dp of Neurological Sciences, Civil Hospital of Verona, Dp of Neurological Sciences, Civil Hospital of Verona
- Prof. Nicolò Rizzuto, Dp of Neurological, Neuropsychological, Morphological and Movement Sciences, University of Verona
- Dr. Paolo Manganotti, Dr. Luigi Giuseppe Bongiovanni, Dr. Paolo Borelli, Dr. Alessandra Del Felice, dott. Emanuela Formaggio, dott. Silvia Francesca Storti, Dp of Neurological, Neuropsychological, Morphological and Movement Sciences, University of Verona, Dp of Neurological, Neuropsychological, Morphological and Movement Sciences, University of Verona for their collaboration
- Prof. Roberto Pozzi Mucelli, Dr.ssa Anna Gasparini and Dr. Roberto Cerini , Dp of Radiology University of Verona

Author details

Mirko Avesani[1], Silvia Giacopuzzi[2] and Antonio Fiaschi[1]

1 University of Verona, Department of Neurological, Neuropsychological, Morphological and Movement Sciences, Italy

2 University of Verona, Department of Life and Reproduction Sciences, Italy

References

[1] Aghakhani et al. fMRI activation during spike wave discharges in idiopatic generalized epilepsy. Brain, 2004; 127: 1127-1144

[2] Aghakhani et al. The role of periventricular nodular heterotopia in epileptogenesis. Brain, 2005; 128: 641-651

[3] Aghakhani et al. Cortical and thalamic fMRI responses in partial epilepsy with focal and bilateral synchronous spikes. Clin Neurophysiol 2006;117:177–91.

[4] Archer et al. fMRI "deactivation" of the posterior cingulate during generalized spike and wave. Neuroimage. 2003;20:1915–1922.

[5] Al-Asmi et al. fMRI activation in continuous and spike-triggered EEG-fMRI studies of epileptic spikes. Epilepsia, 2003; 44: 1328-1339.

[6] Allen et al. Identification of EEG events in the MR scanner: the problem of pulse artifact and a method for its subtraction. Neuroimage, 1998; 8: 229-239.

[7] Allen et al. A method for removing imaging artefact from continuous EEG recorded during functional MRI. Neuroimage, 2000; 12:230-239.

[8] Archer et al. fMRI "deactivation" of the posterior cingulate during generalized spike and wave. Neuroimage. 2003;20:1915–1922.

[9] Archer et al. Spike-triggered fMRI in reading epilepsy: involvement of left frontal cortex working memory areas. Neurology, 2003; 60: 415-421

[10] Avesani et al. Continuous EEG-fMRI in pre surgical evaluation of a patient affected by symptomatic seizures: BOLD activation linked to interictal epileptiform discharges caused by cavernoma. The Neuroradiology Journal, 2008/a; 21: 183-191.

[11] Avesani et al. fMRI in epilepsy with spike and wave activity evoked by eye closure: different BOLD activation in a patient with idiopathic partial epilepsy with occipital spikes and a control group. Neuroradiol. J., 2008/b; 21:159—165.

[12] Bagshaw et al. EEG-fMRI of focal epileptic spikes: analysis with multiple haemodyamic functions and comparision with gadolinium-enhanced MR angiograms. Human Brain Mapping, 2004; 22: 179-192

[13] Bagshaw et al. Correspondence between EEG-fMRI and EEG dipole localization of interictal discharges in focal epilepsy. Neuroimage, 2006; 30: 417-425

[14] Benar et al. Quality of EEG in simultaneous EEG-fMRI for epilepsy. Clin Neurophysiol, 2003; 114: 569-580.

[15] Benar et al. EEG-fMRI of epileptic spikes. Concordance with EEG source localization and intracranial EEG. Neuroimage, 2006; 30: 1161-1170

[16] Berns. Functional neuroimaging. Life Sci. 1999; 65: 2531-2540.

[17] Bernasconi et al. Proton magnetic resonance spectroscopic imaging suggests progressive neuronal damage in human temporal lobe epilepsy. Prog. Brain Res, 2002; 135: 297-304

[18] Binder et al. Determination of language dominance using functional MRI: a comparision with Wada test. Neurology, 1996; 46: 978-984

[19] Boly et al. Intrinsic brain activity in altered states of consciousness: how conscious is the default mode of brain function? Ann N Y Acad Sci. 2008;1129:119–129.

[20] Boor et al. EEG-related functional MRI in beningn childhood epilepsy with centrotemporal spikes. Epilepsia, 2003; 44: 688-692

[21] Borelli et al. EEG-fMRI as an useful tool to detect epileptic foci associated with secondary

[22] bilateral synchrony. Seizure, 2010; 19:605-608.

[23] Cavanna. The precuneuos and consciousness. CNS Spectr. 2007;12:545–552.

[24] Cavanna et al . The precuneus: a review of its functional anatomy and behavioural correlates. Brain. 2006;129:564–583.

[25] David et al. Identifying neural drivers with functional MRI: an electrophysiological validation. PLoS Biol. 2008;23:2683–2697.

[26] Del Felice et al. EEG-fMRI coregistration in non ketotic hyperglicemic occipital seizures. Epilepsy Research, 2009;85(2-3):321-324

[27] De Tiège et al. Impact of interictal epileptic activity on normal brain function in epileptic encephalopathy: an EEG-fMRI study. Epilepsy Behav. 2007;11:460–465.

[28] Devous et al. SPECT brain imaging in epilepsy: a meta-analysis. J Nucl Med 1998;39:285–93.

[29] Devous et al. Single-photon emission computed tomography in neurotherapeutic. NeuroRx 2005, 2: 237-249

[30] Di Bonaventura. EEG/fMRI study of ictal and interictal epileptic activity: methodological issues and future perspectives in clinical practice. Epilepsia, 2006; 47, Suppl. 5: 52-58.

[31] Duncan et al. Imaging and epilepsy. Brain 1997; 120: 339-377

[32] Dupon et al. Bilateral hemispheric alteration of memory processes in right medial temporal lobe epilepsy. J Neurol Neurosurg Psych, 2002; 73: 478-485

[33] Elshoff et al. The value of EEG-fMRI and EEG source analysis in the presurgical setup of children with refractory focal epilepsy. Epilepsia, 2012; 53: 1597-1606.

[34] Engel et al. Comparative localization of epileptic foci in partial epilepsy by PCT and EEG. Ann Neurol 1982; 12: 529-537.

[35] Engel et al. Local cerebral metabolism during partial seizures. Neurology, 1983; 33: 400-413

[36] Faymonville et al. Functional neuroanatomy of the hypnotic state. J Physiol Paris. 2006;99:463–469.

[37] Frackowiak RSJ, Friston KJ, Frith CD, Dolan RJ, Mazziotta JC, editors. San Diego: Academic Press; 1997. Human brain function.

[38] Friston et al. Statistical parametric maps in functional imaging: a general linear approach. Hum Brain Mapp, 1995; 2: 173-181.

[39] Friston et al. Event-related fMRI: characterizing differential responses. Neuroimage, 1998; 7: 30-40

[40] Fransson et al. The precuneus/posterior cingulate cortex plays a pivotal role in the default mode network: Evidence from a partial correlation network analysis. Neuroimage. 2008;42:1178–1184.

[41] Gonçalves,et al. Correlating the alpha rhythm to BOLD using simultaneous EEG-fMRI: inter-subject variability. Neuroimage, 2006; 30: 203-213;

[42] Gotman et al. Combining EEG and fMRI in epilepsy: methodological challenges and clinical results. I Clin Neurophysiol, 2004; 21: 229-240

[43] Gotman et al. Generalized epileptic discharges show thalamocortical activation and the suspension of the default state of the brain. PNAS, 2005; 142: 15236-15240

[44] Gotman et al. Epileptic networks studied with EEG-fMRI. Epilepsia, 2008; 49 Suppl 3:42-51.

[45] Gusnard et al. Medial prefrontal cortex and self-referential mental activity: relation to a default mode of brain function. Proc Natl Acad Sci USA. 2001;98:4259–4264.

[46] Gusnard et al. Searching for a baseline: functional imaging and the resting human brain. Nat Rev Neurosci. 2001;2:685–694.

[47] Hamandi et al. EEG-fMRI of Generalized Spike-Wave Activity. Neuroimage. 2006;31:1700–1710.

[48] Hamandi et al. BOLD and perfusion changes during epileptic generalised spike wave activity. Neuroimage. 2008;39:608–618.

[49] Hammers et al. Abnormalities of grey and white matter [11C] flumazenil binding in temporal lobe epilepsy with normal MRI. Brain 2002; 125: 2257-2271

[50] Henry et al. Positron emission tomography. In: J. Engel, Jr. (Ed.), Surgical Treatment of Epilepsies, 2nd edn, Raven Press, New York, 1993: pp. 211-232

[51] Hill et al. Haemodynamic and metabolic aspects of photosensitive epilepsy revealled by functional magnetic resonance imaging and magnetic resonance spectroscopy. Epilepsia. 1999;40:912–920.

[52] Holmes et al. Are "generalized" seizures truly generalized? Evidence of localized mesial frontal and frontopolar discharges in absence. Epilepsia. 2004;45:1568–1579.

[53] Huggs et al. Normalization of controlateral metabolic function following temporal lobectomy demonstrated by 1H magnetic resonance spectroscopic imaging. Ann Neurol 1996; 40: 236-239

[54] Iannetti et al. fMRI/EEG in paroxysmal activity elicited by elimination of central vision and fixation. Neurology, 2002; 58: 976—979.

[55] Ives et al. Monitoring the patient's EEG during echo planar MRI. EEG and Clin Neurophysiol, 1993; 87: 417-420

[56] Kobayashi et al. Intrisic epileptogenicity in polymicrogyric cortex suggested by EEG-fMRI BOLD responses. Neurology, 2005; 64: 1263-1266

[57] Kobayashi et al. Grey matter heterotopia: what EEG-fMRI can tell us about epileptogenicity of neuronal migration disorder. Brain, 2006; 129: 366-374

[58] Kobayashi et al. Widespread and intense BOLD changes during brief focal electrographic seizures. Neurology, 2006; 66: 1049-1055

[59] Kobayashi et al. Negative BOLD responses to epileptic spikes. Human Brain Mapping, 2006; 27: 488-497

[60] Kobayashi et al.Temporal and extratemporal BOLD responses to temporal lobe interictal spikes. Epilepsia, 2006; 47: 343-354

[61] Kokkinos et al. "Epileptogenic networks in two patients with hypothalamic hamartoma." Brain Topogr. 2012;25(3):327-31.

[62] Krakow et al. EEG-fMRI of interictal epileptiform activity in patients with partial seizures. Brain, 1999; 122: 1679-1688

[63] Krakow et al. Spatio-temporal imaging of focal interictal epileptiform activity using EEG-triggered functional MRI. Epileptic Disord, 2001; 3: 67-74

[64] Kuzniecky et al.Cortical dysplasia in temporal lobe epilepsy: magnetic resonance imaging correlations. Ann. Neurol, 1991; 29: 293-298

[65] Krausz et al. Brain SPECT imaging in temporal lobe epilepsy. Neuroradiol 1991; 33: 274-276.

[66] Labate et al. Typical childhood absence seizures are associated with thalamic activation. Epileptic Disord. 2005;7:373–377.

[67] Laufs et al. EEG-fMRI mapping of asymmetrical delta activity in a patient with refractory epilepsy is concordant with the epileptogenic region determined by intracranial EEG. Magnetic Resonance Imaging, 2006/a; 24: 367-371

[68] Laufs et al. linking generalized spike-and wave discharges and resting state brain activity by using EEG-fMRI in a patient with absence seizures. Epilepsia, 2006; 47: 444-448

[69] Laufs et al. Linking Generalized Spike-and-Wave Discharges and Resting State Brain Activity by Using EEG-fMRI in a Patient with Absence Seizures. Epilepsia. 2006;47:444–448.

[70] Laufs et al. Electroencephalography/functional MRI in human epilepsy: what it currently can and cannot do. Curr Opin Neurol. 2007;20:417–423.

[71] Laureys et al. Brain function in coma, vegetative state, and related disorders. Lancet Neurol. 2004;3:537–546.

[72] Lazeyras et al. Functional MRI with simultaneous EEG recording: feasibility and application to motor and visual activation. J Magn Reson Imaging, 2001; 13: 943-948

[73] Lee et al. Single Photon emission computed tomography (SPECT) brain imaging using N,N,NI-trimethyl-N-(2 hydroxy-3-methyl-5-123-iodobenzyl)-1,3-propanediamine 2 HCl (HIPDM): intractable complex partial seizures. Neurology 1986; 36:1471-1477

[74] Leiderman et al. The dynamic of metabolic change following seizures ad measured by positron emission tomography with fludeoxyglucose F 18. Arch Neurol, 1994; 51: 932-936

[75] Lemieux et al. Event-related fMRI with simultaneous and continuous EEG: description of the method and initial case report. Neuroimage, 2001; 1: 780-787

[76] Liu et al. EEG-fMRI study of the interictal epileptic activity in patients with partial epilepsy. J Neurol Sci, 2008; 268: 117-123

[77] Logothetis et al. Neurophysiological investigation of the basis of the fMRI signal. Nature, 2001; 412: 150-157

[78] Manganotti et al. Continuous EEG-fMRI in patients with partial epilepsy and focal interictal slow-wave discharges on EEG. Magn Res Imaging, 2008; 26: 1089-1100.

[79] Marks et al. Localization of extra-temporal epileptic foci during single photon emission computed tomography. Ann Neurol 1992; 31:250-255

[80] Meeren et al. Cortical focus drives widespread corticothalamic networks during spontaneous absence seizures in rats. J Neurosci. 2002;22:1480–1495.

[81] Meeren et al. Evolving concepts on the pathophysiology of absence seizures: the cortical focus theory. Arch Neurol. 2005;62:371–376.

[82] Menon et al. Imaging function in the working brain with fMRI. Curr Op Neurobiol, 2001; 11:630-636.

[83] Moeller et al. EEG-fMRI: adding to standard evaluations of patients with nonlesional frontal lobe epilepsy. Neurology 2009;73:2023–30.

[84] Newton et al. SPECT in the localisation of extra-temporale and temporal seizure foci. J Neurol Neurosurg Psychiatry, 1995; 59: 26-30

[85] Ogawa et al. Brain Magnetic Resonance Imaging with contrast dependent on blood oxygenation. Proc Natl Acad Sci, 1990; 87: 9868-9872

[86] Petroff et al. GABA and glutamate in the human brain. Neuroscientist, 2002; 8: 562-573

[87] Polack et al. Deep Layer Somatosensory Cortical Neurons Initiate Spike and Wave Discharges in a Genetic Model of Absence Seizures. J Neurosci. 2007; 27:6590–6599.

[88] Prichard et al. Fuctional study of the brain by NMR. J Cereb Blood Metab, 1994; 14: 365-372

[89] Puce et al. Functional Magnetic Resonance Imaging of sensory and motor cortex: comparision with electrophysiological localisations. I Neurosurg, 1995; 83: 262-270

[90] Ruben et al. Neuroimaging of epilepsy: therapeutic implications. Neurorx, 2005; 2: 384-393

[91] Salek-Haddadi. Functional magnetic resonance imaging of human absence seizures. Ann Neurol, 2003; 53: 663-667

[92] Salek-Haddadi et al. Hemodynamic correlates of epileptiform discharges: an EEG-fMRI study of 63 patients with focal epilepsy. Brain Research, 2006; 1088: 148-166

[93] Salmenpera TM, Duncan JS. Imaging in epilepsy J. Neurol Neurosurg Psychiatry 2005;76:2–10.

[94] So. Mesial frontal epilepsy. Epilepsia, 1998; 39(Suppl 4):S49–61.

[95] Steriade et al. Spike-Wave Complexes and Fast Components of Cortically Generated Seizures. I. Role of Neocortex and Thalamus. J Neurophysiol. 1998;80:1439–1455.

[96] Tai et al. Applications of positron emission tomography (PET) in Neurology. J. Neurol Neurosurg Psych, 2004; 75: 669-676.

[97] Thorton et al. EEG correlated functional MRI and postoperative outcome in focal epilepsy. J Neurol Neurosurg Psychiatry,2010; 81:922-927.

[98] Tucker et al. Discharges in ventromedial frontal cortex during absence spells. Epilepsy Behav. 2007;11:546–557.

[99] Vaudano. Causal hierarchy within the thalamo-cortical network in spike and wave discharges. PLoS One, 2009; 4(8):e6475

http://dx.doi.org/10.5772/55197

[100] Westmoreland. The EEG findings in extratemporal seizures. Epilepsia, 1998; 39(Suppl 4):S1–8.

Chapter 21

Brain Function in Fibromyalgia: Altered Pain Processing and Cognitive Dysfunction

Francisco Mercado, Paloma Barjola,
Marisa Fernández-Sánchez, Virginia Guerra and
Francisco Gómez-Esquer

Additional information is available at the end of the chapter

http://dx.doi.org/10.5772/56495

1. Introduction

Since several decades ago chronic pain understanding has become in one of the most intriguing challenges for health professionals (rheumatologists, psychologists, physiotherapists, anaesthesiologists, pharmacologists, etc). Different reasons are behind that traditionally poor knowledge about the etiology, mechanisms and treatment of chronic pain. Pain has been very often considered as a peripheral entity in which peripheral causes, such as inflammation and structural joint damage, have been only explored. Thus, difficulties to explain painful symptomatology associated to chronic pain patients, such as the great discordance between pain complaints or severity and their supposed peripheral causes, have lead to the development of investigations to advance in the knowledge of pain mechanisms in chronic pain diseases (p.e., non-inflammatory conditions), such as it occurs in fibromyalgia (Buskila, 2009). These studies have highlighted both the important role of central pain-processing mechanisms and its evidently multifactorial status (Lee et al., 2011; Schweinhardt et al., 2008).

Fibromyalgia (FM) constitutes a chronic syndrome mainly characterized by the presence of widespread and diffuse pain (Fan, 2004). Traditionally, FM diagnosis has been only established by the presence of widespread pain during at least three months and tenderness to palpation at specific locations (the so-called 'tender points') following the American College of Rheumatology criteria (ACR, Wolfe et al., 1990). refer to 18 places symmetrically distributed at both sides of the body where patients feel pain when a weak pressure is applied on them with the thumb of the examiner (lower than 4kg/cm2, see Figure 1). Currently, this syndrome is affecting between 2-4% of population (between 80 and 90 percent of patients diagnosed with FM are women) being one of the most common causes of pain and disability. However, the biological bases for the clinical characteristics of FM remain elusive (Martínez-Lavin, 2004; Montoya et al., 2005; Vierck, 2006). Studies have focused particularly on the mechanisms underlying pain perception, and central signals processing. FM patients refer two kinds of somatic sensations: a) enhanced pain sensitivity to painful stimulation (hyperalgesia) and b) a painful response to a normally innocuous stimulus (allodynia). Central augmentation mechanisms underlying this amplified pain perception have been investigated using advanced imaging techniques that aim to localize and describe alterations in specific areas of the brain. Indeed, scientific evidence suggests that central abnormalities in the processing of pain signals seem to be responsible of such altered pain manifestations (diffuse hyperalgesia and allodynia) in FM (Staud et al., 2004; Thieme et al., 2005).

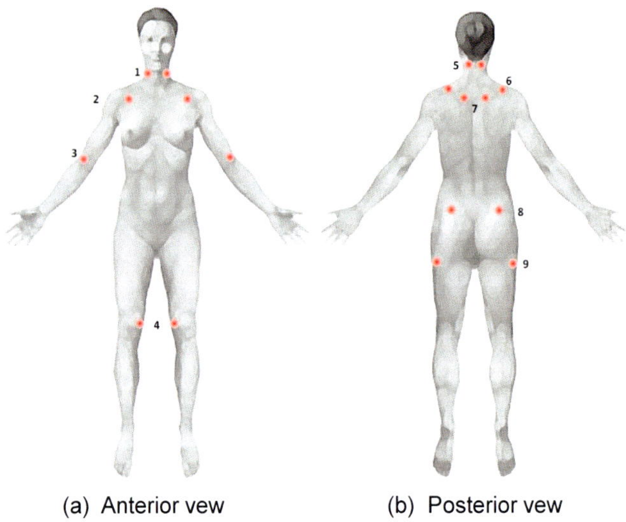

Figure 1. Bilateral tender point locations for the traditional ACR diagnosis criteria for Fibromyalgia (adapted from Wolfe et al., 1990). (a) ANTERIOR VIEW: 1. *Low cervical*: the anterior aspects of the intertransverse spaces at C5-C7, 2. *Second rib*: the second costochondral junctions, lateral to the junctions on upper surfaces, 3. *Lateral epicondyle*: 2cm distal to the epicondyles, 4. *Knee*: the medial fat pad proximal to the joint line. (b) POSTERIOR VIEW: 5. *Occiput*: the suboccipital muscle insertions, 6. *Trapezius*: the midpoint of the upper border, 7. *Supraspinatus*: above the scapula spine near the medial border, 8. *Gluteal*: upper outer quadrants of buttocks in anterior fold of muscle, 9. *Greater trochanter*: posterior to the trochanteric prominence.

Additionally, people with FM frequently experience a great amount of other accompanying symptoms apart from pain, such as physical complaints (stiffness, fatigue, sleep problems), affective disorders (anxiety or depression) and cognitive dysfunctions (failures in memory, attention and concentration). In fact, cognitive failures represent one of the most important complaints of these patients, recently denominated as *fibrofog* (Glass, 2010), leading to produce even greater functional impact than pain itself (Glass, 2009). Based on growing evidence from

http://dx.doi.org/10.5772/56495

neuropsychological and neuroimaging studies, ACR criteria have been recently modified including the cognitive dysfunction and affective disturbances, among other symptoms, as key factors for FM diagnosis (Wolfe et al., 2010). These findings, along with the lack of peripheral signs of inflammation to account for pain, support the hypothesis that FM is a syndrome characterized by an abnormal processing of information at the level of central nervous system. Therefore, psychoneurobiologic dysfunctions seem to be crucial for trying to explain this multifactorial and still not fully understood clinical condition (Lee et al., 2011; Schweinhardt et al., 2008), but also to give response, at least partially, to the appearance and maintenance of both pain-related and cognitive symptomatology. In the following review, we will try to describe what is currently known about the cerebral mechanisms in pain processing, the neural correlates of cognitive dysfunction and the pathogenesis of FM, with special attention to the genetic basis.

2. Cerebral pain processing in fibromyalgia

Fibromyalgia is considered a chronic pain syndrome which cause (still remain elusive) does not have been found in localized lesions, inflammatory processes or damage to the joints, muscles or other tissues. Experimental evidence indicates that pain processing abnormalities leading to maintenance of pain showed by these patients (e.g., hyperalgesic states) could be due to both central sensitization mechanisms and specific defects in central pain processing related to the loss of normal activity of descending pain-inhibitory (e.g., serotonin-norephi-nephrine-opioidergic) pathways (Ceko et al., 2012; Lee et al., 2011). Central sensitization related to diffuse hyperalgesia and allodynia is functionally linked to central nervous changes caused by the release of different excitatory neurotransmitters such as serotonin, substance P or glutamate, among others. Through their action on specific receptors (e.g., NMDA) those neurotransmitters might produce enhanced and amplified responses at central nervous level (Woolf, 2004). Specifically, central sensitization can also produce an augmentation of receptive fields in neurons belonging to spinal cord and peripheral fibers. Other neurophysiological indices found in FM patients have involved elevated levels of substance P and serotonin metabolites in cerebrospinal fluid compared with healthy people (Russell et al., 1994; Russell et al., 1992), along with a diminished level of neurotransmitters, which dampen pain sensitivity response (e.g., norepinephrine) suggesting again defects in central pain processing (Russell et al., 1992). Behaviourally, the phenomenon of central sensitization is characterized by lower thresholds in pain perception, pain tolerance and by an enhancement of noxious sensations as a consequence of repeated stimulation, as it occurs in temporal summation (Staud et al., 2003). Additionally, whereas the activation of NMDA receptor channels produces central sensitization, the administration of NMDA receptor antagonists such as ketamine reduces significantly pain perception and facilitates the inhibition of hyperalgesia indices (i.e., temporal summation) in FM patients (Price et al., 2002; Graven-Nielsen et al., 2000). Neuroi-maging studies have demonstrated the presence of an augmented activation pattern of pain processing involving several cortical and subcortical regions in FM (Gracely et al., 2002). This augmented pain processing pattern resulted in response to the same perceived intensity of painful stimulation compared to control participants (Gracely et al., 2002; Cook et al., 2004).

Pain descending inhibitory pathways start from different cerebral levels localized on the brainstem, bulbar region, diencephalic structures and cortical areas. These pathways constitute one of the most important mechanisms involved in the pain perception modulation of sensory information in the dorsal horn of spinal cord. Experimental evidence has described defects in those pain inhibitory pathways leading to a loss of descending endogenous analgesia and the maintenance and enhancement of painful sensations in patients with FM (Julien et al., 2005). These results have been found using different types of acute noxious stimulation. Staud and colleagues (2003) highlighted the presence of diminished pain inhibitory mechanisms in response to hot water in a sample of women with and without FM. Previous studies applying tonic thermal stimulation and by using a tourniquet to produce ischemic pain showed evidence for the defects in descending inhibitory pain activity in FM (Lautenbacher et al., 1997; Kosek et al., 1997). In the same line, diminished periaqueductal gray responses to heat stimulation have been reported in these patients when it was compared with the activity of healthy participants (Cook et al., 2004). Periaqueductal gray region (PGR) has been described as an important structure involved in both ascending and descending pain processing signals (Stahl, 2009). Descending projections from PGR to dorsolateral pontine structures act inhibiting pain signals from peripheral afferent neurons in the dorsal horn of the spinal cord through the release of noradrenaline and serotonin neurotransmitters. Thus, the observed lack of activation within PGR in FM could lead to a loss of descending analgesia enhancing chronic responses of hyperalgesia in these patients (Herrero et al., 2000). Exposed findings demonstrate the main role of abnormalities in central mechanisms as an important key to understand chronic pain in the FM syndrome (Abeles et al., 2007; Bennett, 2005; Lee et al., 2011).

2.1. Morphological brain changes associated with abnormal pain processing in fibromyalgia

Experimental evidence focused on the study of brain areas involved in the processing of painful stimulation has revealed that chronic pain patients show an abnormal activation pattern at specified brain regions (e.g., Kwiatek et al., 2000). Neuroimaging research and its application to the study of pain, has facilitated the identification of a brain network involved in pain processing that has been denominated as 'pain matrix', comprised, among others, by different cortical and subcortical regions: for example, somatosensory regions, insular areas and anterior cingulated cortices (ACC) (Bushnell et al., 2005; Tracey &Mantyh, 2007). Although recently the referred pain matrix has been functionally redefined not only as a pain processing network but also as salience detection system (Iannetti et al., 2010; Legrain et al., 2011; Tracey & Johns, 2010), the role played by somatosensory cortices and other cortical regions, such as posterior parietal cortex or prefrontal areas in the processing of nociceptive signals and in the affective/cognitive modulation processes of pain perception, has been extensively documented (Lorenz et al., 2003; Peyron et al., 2000; Rolls et al., 2003; Sawamoto et al., 2000; Singer et al., 2004; Wiech et al., 2008). For instance, attentional modulations on pain perception have been seen in the increase and/or decrease of activations within insula and ACC (Valet et al., 2004; Wiech et al., 2005).

http://dx.doi.org/10.5772/56495

Chronic pain diseases are commonly characterized by an abnormal functioning when painful events are processed and as a consequence of it, chronic pain has been understood as an altered perceptual state (Apkarian et al., 2005). Nevertheless, chronic pain is also defined as a dysfunctional condition derived from the appearance of structural brain changes that become more generalized as a function of the years suffering from pain (Baliki et al., 2011). Such changes could cause a dysfunctional neural reorganization affecting brain dynamics (Baliki et al., 2008; Tagliazucchi et al., 2010). Evidence accumulated from the last years through the use of different brain imaging methodologies supports the presence of changes in the brain of FM patients (i.e., structural and functional changes) (García-Campayo et al., 2010; Gracely et al., 2011), although such changes are heterogeneous and a unique interpretation about its clinical meaning remains still unclear. Altered brain morphology was reported by voxel-based morphometry (VBM) studies showing that FM patients had less grey matter density than healthy subjects in several brain regions including insula and ACC (Kuchinad et al., 2007). However, grey matter increase in other cerebral areas belonging to the somatosensory system, such as the Striatum or in those other ones involved in the cognitive modulation of pain (i.e., Orbitofrontal Cortex-OFC) have been seen in patients suffering from FM (Schmidt-Wilcke et al., 2007). Further findings combining diffusion-tensor imaging (DTI) and VBM methodologies have described not only a reduction in grey matter density in FM but also abnormalities in white matter microstructure within thalamus and insular cortex, being highly correlated with the intensity of main FM symptoms (Lutz et al., 2008). Specifically, patients showing higher pain intensity scores were characterized by DTI measurements indicating changes within superior frontal gyrus (SFG). Moreover, changes in SFG and ACC were positively correlated with increased fatigue and self-perceived physical impairment. Affective symptoms defined by higher scores in posttraumatic stress scales were negatively correlated with microstructural changes represented by values of fractional anisotropy (FA) in FM. In this line, Hsu and colleagues (2009) reported decreased grey matter volume in the left anterior insula for patients with FM compared to healthy control participants. This difference in grey matter volume disappeared when the presence of affective disorders in FM patients was controlled. Thus, grey matter volume within this area was inversely correlated with scores in trait anxiety, highlighting the important role of affective disturbances in the explanation of these morphological brain changes. More recent studies have documented that patients with FM syndrome show grey matter atrophy within ACC, mid-cingulate Cortex (MCC) and insular cortex, but affective symptoms like depression are not related to these grey matter changes (Robinson et al., 2011). Along with emotional symptomatology, cognitive alterations in FM have been correlated with changes in grey matter values (Luerding et al., 2008). They found that working memory performance in FM patients was highly and positively correlated with decreased grey matter values within medial prefrontal cortex (MPFC) and ACC, showing that cognitive deficits in FM are associated with changes in brain morphology.

Therefore, mentioned brain abnormalities in the traditionally denominated pain matrix regions might contribute to the alteration of pain processing in FM patients, but they could also affect other domains such as cognitive and affective symptomatology. In fact, it has been proposed that pain and cognitive impairment in FM may co-occur sharing underlying neural networks (Luerding et al., 2008), and as a consequence of it, performance derived from carrying out a cognitive task when individual is in pain might decrease due to the availability of neural resources is limited and they are invested in pain processing (Seminowicz and Davis, 2007). Additionally, the presence of chronic pain along the years might contribute to the appearance of changes in the brain leading to abnormal activation of brain regions that could exacerbate pain itself and also disturb cognitive function in FM (Kuchinad et al., 2007). Although structural neuroimaging evidence supports the association of chronic pain in FM with grey matter abnormalities, future investigations should be projected to confirm and extend these findings.

2.2. Functional brain changes associated with abnormal pain processing in fibromyalgia

Beyond morphological brain changes, functional imaging investigations have revealed abnormal activation patterns at specific cerebral regions in FM patients (e.g., Cook et al., 2004), however, these anomalies in pain processing are not always circumscribed to activation of brain areas intimately or traditionally related to pain. It has been observed during different experimental situations: in response to painful stimulation, when somatosensory (not painful) information has to be processed and even during resting-state conditions. One of the first neuroimaging studies conducted to investigate such issues demonstrated enhanced brain activation in many regions (i.e., primary and secondary somatosensory cortex, ACC, insula) for FM patients in response to similar levels of pressure stimulation to that one applied to control subjects (Gracely et al., 2002). Moreover, when subjectively painful conditions were established to be comparable (i.e., intensity of stimulation was significantly greater to healthy people than patients for provoke a similar subjective level of pain perception) similar brain activation patterns were found between both patients and control groups. These results indicate that central sensitization defects could be explaining the presence of such augmented activation pattern for painful signals in FM. More recent studies aimed to test the hypothesis of central augmentation pain processing in FM have confirmed and extended those findings (Maestú et al., 2013). Abnormal brain activation of different regions related to the affective/motivational components of pain processing was found in patients with FM during a pain situation induced by a small incision into the skin (Burgmer et al., 2009). Thus, enhanced activations were observed within frontal and cingulated cortices, along with supplementary motor areas. Such altered responses were especially prominent during the pain anticipation period. Additionally, that altered temporal BOLD-signal pattern was found as specific for FM patients when they were compared to other patients suffering from rheumatoid arthritis (Burgmer et al., 2010). It leads to think that fronto-cingulated regions could play a key role as central mechanisms of pain processing responsible to the maintenance and exacerbation of chronic pain in FM.

Previous investigations had already given data about the role of cognitive, affective and social factors on pain processing in FM. Neural responses to somatosensory stimuli can be modulated by cognitive and emotional factors (Cook et al., 2004). Specifically, the catastrophyzing thinking style has been associated with enhanced cerebral responses to pain. Cortical areas involved in pain expectancy or pain-related attention (ACC, MPFC or dorsolateral prefrontal cortex –DLPFC-) showed more intense activity in FM patients who scored high in catastrophizing (Gracely et al., 2004). Affective conditions such as comorbid depression, seem to have influence in the activation of amygdala, but not of somatosensory brain regions during pain processing information (Giesecke et al., 2005). Event-related potentials (ERP) studies have also provided data demonstrating abnormal emotional modulation of brain processing in response to somatosensory/non-painful stimuli (Montoya et al., 2005). Somatosensory components (i.e, P50) displayed largest amplitudes when FM patients were introduced within a negative emotional context created with unpleasant slides. The influence of the emotional context was also described during the processing of painful stimulation (Montoya et al., 2004). At the same time, the presence of significant others during the application of painful stimulation was found as a social factor that diminish magnetic brain responses and subjective pain in FM patients compared to control participants (Montoya et al., 2004). Other works have observed that FM patients show a significant enhancement of brain activation within regions involved in the emotional/cognitive aspects linked to pain processing as compared to control subjects, given a painful stimulation (Burgmer et al., 2009). Indeed, larger activation within CCA and anterior insula along with more persisting responses in insular cortex were found for FM patients as well (Pujol et al., 2009). It supports the hypothesis that both affective/cognitive and social factors may play a very important role for pain processing in patients with FM.

On the other hand, the role played by several neurotransmitters, such as dopamine or glutamate, which exerts their functions at the level of central neural system, has been also highlighted in the pathogenesis of FM and studied through the use of neuroimaging techniques (Harris, 2010; Stahl, 2009). Different genetic polymorphisms associated with the functional activity of those neuromodulators have been documented (Ablin et al., 2008), as it will be extensively described later. Evidence on altered levels of mentioned neurotransmitters within the brain of patients with FM has recently reported (Harris et al., 2008; 2009). Dysregulation in levels of glutamate, an excitatory neurotransmitter, has been found within the posterior insula of FM patients being such altered levels associated with experimental pain (Harris et al., 2010). Higher concentration levels of glutamate and glutamine were also detected within the amygdala (Valdés et al., 2010) and posterior insula (Fayed et al., 2010). Patients group showed diminished pain thresholds and high scores in pain and tenderness suggesting that neuronal hiperexcitability elicited by the presence of glutamate may lead to an augmented central pain processing. With respect to other neurotransmitters, different investigations have indicated an abnormal dopamine response to pain in FM (Wood et al., 2007b; Wood et al., 2009). It is known that dopamine is a neurotransmitter involved in pain modulation, but whereas general population showed an increase of dopamine release when a painful stimulus was perceived FM patients did not (Wood et al., 2007a). Thus, that deficiency in dopaminergic reactivity might have a relevant impact on the development and maintenance of chronic pain in FM. In fact, some studies have shown reduced presynaptic dopaminergic activity suggesting that such disrupted neurotransmission could prevent for natural analgesia in FM (Wood et al., 2007b). More recent findings have associated alterations in dopaminergic neurotransmission with a decrease in grey matter density within posterior cingulated cortex, ACC and parahippocampal gyri (Wood et al., 2009). Therefore, these data suggest that pharmacological approaches targeted to the specific or combinated use of glutamatergic and dopaminergic treatments may be effective and should be explored (for a review see, Smith-Wilcke & Clauw, 2010).

Finally, recent investigations postulate that FM could be characterized by an alteration of brain connectivity among different brain networks (Cifre et al., 2012; Napadow et al., 2010). It has been documented that chronic pain produces a disruption in the default mode network (DMN;

Baliki et al., 2008). Evidence coming from neuroimaging studies reported increased resting state connectivity between insula and other brain networks such as the DMN in FM patients. This connectivity pattern was highly and positively correlated with spontaneous pain (Napadow et al., 2010). In fact, when a sample of patients underwent to an acupuncture treatment aimed to diminish pain perception, the degree of connectivity between insula and DMN was also decreased leading to consider resting state connectivity as an objective marker to assess pain in FM (Napadow et al., 2012). Other studies have confirmed the presence of an altered connectivity pattern among brain regions belonging to pain processing network in FM during rest (Cifre et al., 2012). Indeed, such alteration might be due to slow temporal summation effects evoked by C-fiber pain (Craggs et al., 2012).

3. Neural correlates of cognitive dysfunction in fibromyalgia

3.1. Cognitive complaints in FM

It has been suggested that FM syndrome is characterized by an abnormal processing of information in the central nervous system (Montoya et al., 2005; Okijufi et al., 2002) affecting the response to somatosensory stimulation (e.g., painful signals) but also to information belonging to other modalities (e.g., visual, auditory, etc). Several studies indicate that apart from pain and other physical symptoms, cognitive failures are referred by these patients as one of the most important complaints (recently denominated as *fibrofog*; Glass, 2009; Williams et al., 2011), leading to produce even greater functional impact than pain itself (Arnold et al., 2008; Glass et al., 2005). Thus, the incidence rate for memory and concentration difficulties exceeds 90% in FM, being significantly higher that one ocurred in other chronic pain conditions (Arnold et al., 2008; Mease et al., 2008). Additionally, self-reports of patients support the presence of a higher number of cognitive problems than patients suffering from other chronic pain syndromes (Katz et al., 2004), affecting several cognitive domains (Williams et al., 2011). For example, memory complaints of FM patients were positively correlated with the objective perfomance obtained in tasks which set in motion memory resources (Glass et al., 2005). Moreover, these cognitive difficulties manifest persistently in many of daily activities involving the allocation of attentional control resources such as to remember that they have to call someone the next day or to inhibit thoughts that do not allow them to develop other concurrent daily tasks. Experimental evidence confirms that attention, concentration, episodic memory and verbal fluency are impaired in FM (Glass, 2009) showing that such difficulties in the processing of information constitute a very disruptive symptom for patients who have FM, worsening its quality of life and leading to consider it as an independent symptom (Schmidt-Wilcke *et al.*, 2010).

3.2. Neuropsychological and behavioural data on cognitive dysfunction in FM

Since the beginning of the past decade growing objective evidence based mainly on neuropsychological studies has shown real and significant impairments of cognitive functions in FM (Glass & Park, 2001; Park et al., 2001). First attempts to characterize dyscognition in FM reported deficits in the two declarative memory systems related to the explicit recall of information, episodic and semantic memory. Experimental data revealed poor performance on both standardized (Grace et al., 1999) and non-standarized episodic memory tests (Landro et al., 1997; Grisart et al., 2002). Semantic memory problems have also been documented. FM group showed lower ability for accessing to stored general knowledge than control group when patients were asked to report as many words as they could say starting with a given letter (for example, 'p') and belonging to a specific category (for example, 'fruits and vegetables') (Landro et al., 1997; Park et al., 2001). Along with verbal fluency difficulties, a decrease in naming speed (Leavitt et al., 2008) and speed processing (Veldhuijzen et al., 2012) was also found in FM patients. However, those results are not unequivocal since some studies failed to find differences in cognitive function between patients and healthy control participants (Suhr, 2003). This variability could be related to the lack of previous systematic and detailed research, suggesting that cognitive impairment in FM patients is not generalized; rather is specific-process dependent.

Recent data have suggested that findings on cognitive dysfunction in FM are particularly solid when patients have to deal with tasks demanding for both executive control and working memory resources (Ambrose et al., 2012; Glass, 2010). Impairments in those domains seem to be the key to explain a great part of the cognitive dysfunction in FM. Executive functions (EF) refer to those mechanisms that allow the regulation of both behaviour and other cognitive processes to achieve a specific objective (Muñoz-Céspedes and Tirapu, 2001). Within this theoretical frame, working memory is defined as the support system of those EF aimed to temporarily hold in mind and manage with a variable amount of information (Baddeley, 2000). Thus, working memory dysfunctions have also been seen in FM (Luerding et al., 2008). It has been also observed that patients perform poorly in a variety of tasks involving the allocation of executive control resources to alternate between cognitive sets (Verdejo-García et al., 2009) and to make emotional decisions (Verdejo-García et al., 2009; Walteros et al., 2011) or to face with a task-switching test (Glass, 2006). Tests commonly used to study those executive function processes are Wisconsin Card Sorting Test (WCST) and the Iowa Gambling Task (IGT). Several studies using the Paced Auditory Serial Attention Test (PASAT) have detected a diminished perfomance in FM individuals compared to controls (Leavitt & Katz, 2006; Munguía-Izquierdo et al., 2008). Other working memory components like response inhibition are also suggested to be impaired in FM (Correa et al., 2011). Very similar results have been found during the performance in those tests with a high degree of ecological validity (Test of Everyday Attention, TEA) that includes everyday attentional tasks (Dick et al., 2008). Working memory components measured by TEA were impaired in FM, especially when stimuli competition had to be solved. In this sense, the fact that attentional control difficulties become more evident during distraction (derived from a situation of stimuli competition) has lead to consider it as a key point to better understand cognitive dysfunction in FM (Leavitt & Katz, 2006). It was proposed that failures to inhibit competing stimulation might be an explanation for this difficulty; due to FM patients show hypersensitivity to process information coming from any sensorial modality (Geisser et al., 2008). Such general distractibility could be translated into an attentional orientation towards any type of task-irrelevant stimuli (González et al., 2010) leading to difficulties to focalize attention on relevant information. However, recent data derived from the use of cognitive inhibition tests indicate that patients with FM do not show a specific problem in such processes (Veldhuijzen et al., 2012).

Although the body of research on cognitive dysfunction in FM has strongly grown in recent years, there are still several unexplored issues in this field of knowledge that should be investigated such as the delimitation of the specific cognitive mechanisms that are altered in these patients. For instance, it is accepted that working memory abilities are impaired in FM, but are different components (e.g., temporal holding of information, inhibition, manage with two concurrent tasks, etc) characterizing working memory equally affected? Kim and colleagues (2012) have indicated that memory is selectively impaired in FM showing the possible existence of a memory dissociation. Data coming from neuropsychological assessments reveal that whereas visuospatial memory abilities are dysfunctional, verbal memory is quite unaffected. Following a similar reasoning, several studies postulate that cognitive dysfunction in FM is restricted to those cognitive mechanisms based on controlled processes (Grisart et al., 2002). However, the presence of a generalized hypervigilance response in FM (Carrillo de la Peña et al., 2006) seems to be under the control of automatic processes, rather than controlled ones (Crombez et al., 2005). Moreover, recent data have demonstrated a reduced performance of patients with FM during an implicit memory task (Duschek et al., 2013). It is the first direct evidence of cognitive disruption associated with processes non-dependent from conscious and controlled resources in FM. Finally, several comorbid symptoms of FM (e.g., anxiety, depression, sleep disturbances, medication, pain, etc) have been associated with a worsening of cognitive dysfunction. Although the impact of affective symptomatology (anxiety and depression) and sleep problems on the cognitive dysfunction in FM might be important, these variables do not entirely explain it (Park et al., 2001; Dick et al., 2008). However, the negative impact of both chronic and acute pain seems to be very robust. When this variable is controlled FM patients show a marked impairment in tasks involving different cognitive domains (Glass et al., 2011; Reyes del Paso et al., 2012; Verdejo-García et al., 2009). Additionally, level of self-reported pain is correlated with cognitive performance in FM (Glass et al., 2005) and it has been highlighted as a mediating variable to explain deficits in self-regulatory processes in these patients (Solberg et al., 2010). Therefore, the role of pain on cognitive disturbances is considered as quite relevant. Nevertheless, the neurocognitive mechanisms by means pain interferes on patient's cognitive function are still unknown.

3.3. Brain activity related to cognitive dysfunction in FM

As it was previously indicated, accumulated evidence supports the presence of clear objective impairments in cognitive function of patients with FM. Cognitive dysfunctional pattern associated with FM (i.e., executive control deficits, working memory failures and declarative memory difficulties) points out to the existence of an altered neural substrate, presumably at least within prefrontal regions, such as inferior prefrontal cortex (IPC), MPFC or ACC along with their connexions with temporal and parietal regions (Glass, 2010; Glass et al., 2011). Although studies focused on these neural mechanisms underlying dysfunctional cognitive processes in FM are still surprisingly scarce, new findings cast some light on the possible altered neurocognitive mechanisms. In this sense, neuroimaging investigations have repeatedly showed increased haemodynamic activity at prefrontal regions (i.e., dorsolateral prefrontal cortex –DLPFC-, ventromedial prefrontal –VMPFC- cortex and ACC) during tasks involving working memory and executive control processes (Bunge et al., 2000; Dagher et al., 1999). Moreover, Altamura and coworkers (2007) have highlighted that the right allocation of working memory resources to accomplish a given task depends on prefrontal regions.

Specific data related to FM patients, have found that working memory performance in FM patients was highly and positively correlated with grey matter values within MPFC and ACC, showing that a decrease of grey matter volume within those prefrontal regions is associated with working memory deficits in FM (Luerding et al., 2008). Additionally, recent functional neuroimaging investigations have revealed diminished activations in cortical regions belonging to the inhibition network, such as ACC, mid-cingulated cortex (MCC) and motor processing areas in patients with FM during the performance in a simple go/no-go task (Glass et al., 2011). At the same time, inefficient activations were detected within insular cortex and IFG when patients had to perform on the mentioned response motor inhibition task. It has been suggested that such effects might be explained via either a greater brain recruitment of cortical compensatory regions different from those involved in response inhibition network. Extending such findings, our research group has tried to characterize cognitive inhibition mechanisms, as part of the altered working memory functions, in patients with FM. Patients showed both enhanced P450 amplitudes and brain activations within IFG in response to an emotional Stroop task (Mercado et al., in press). More in detail, symptom-related words were the kind of stimulation that elicited both the greater frontal P450 amplitudes and the higher IFG activations as compared to rest of stimuli (i.e., general negative-arousing, positive-arousing and neutral words; see Figures 2 and 3). This abnormally enhanced brain activity suggests the presence of a specific difficulty in cognitive inhibition in FM patients (under conditions intimately linked with the core concerns of their disease). However, such supplementary recruitment of neural resources by means same cortical areas only allow them to achieve a comparable behavioural performance to healthy control group during the cognitive inhibition task. These results are in contradiction with those coming from behavioural studies indicating intact cognitive inhibition abilities in FM (Veldhuijzen et al., 2012). A tentative explanation could be related to the idea that brain activity techniques might be more sensitive to detect subtle dysfunctions than behavioural measures alone such as often occurs in FM patients (Glass et al., 2011). Other functional neuroimaging studies have showed that working memory dysfunction (measured through a n-back task) in FM are related to a reduction of neural activity not only at prefrontal regions but also within inferior parietal cortex (IPC) (Seo et al., 2012). It suggests that a different neural activation pattern of the frontoparietal memory network could be explaining, at least partially, cognitive impairments in FM. Diminished early ERP activity of FM patients during a 2-back task has been also detected at inferior parietal sites, Suggesting that problems associated with the early storage of information might be attributable to analtered functioning of parietal areas (Mercado et al.,in preparation). On the other hand, some investigations have indicated the presence of differences associated with the hippocampus activity between patients and healthy control participants (Emad et al., 2008).

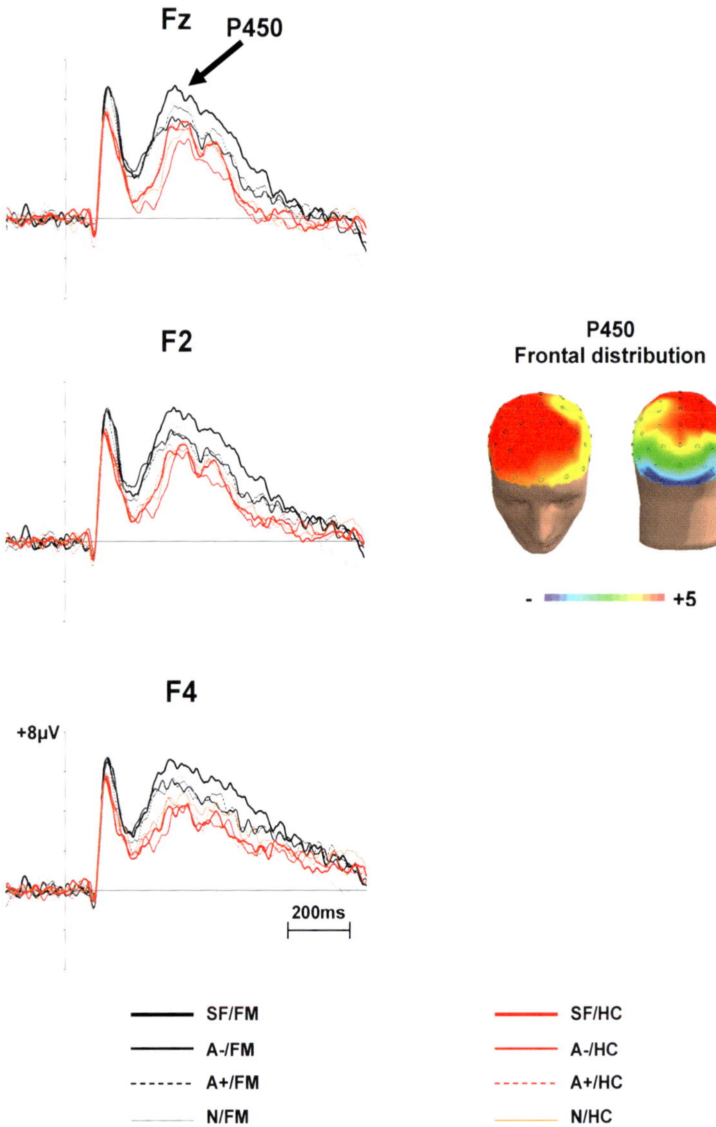

Figure 2. Grand averages of P450 component corresponding to Fibromyalgia (FM) and Healthy control (HC) participants in response to FM symptoms (SF), negative-arousing (A-), positive-arousing (A+) and neutral (N) stimuli. Scales and polarity are shown at F4. 3D maps show topographical distribution of the P450 component. Red areas reflect high activity.

http://dx.doi.org/10.5772/56495

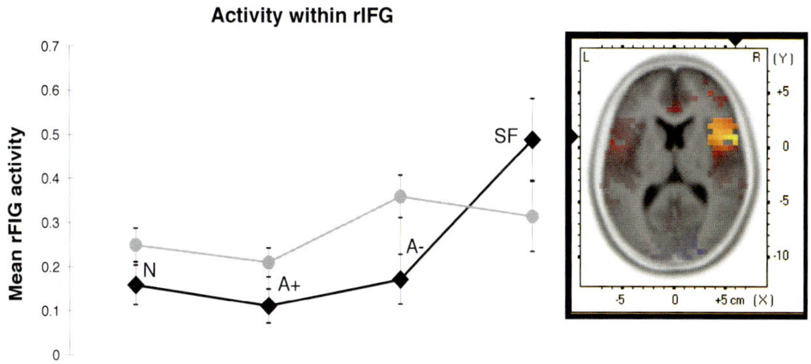

Figure 3. rIFG activity from the emotional Stroop task for patients with fibromyalgia (FM) and healthy control participants (HC). Right side shows sLORETA solutions to non-parametric randomization tests on P450 component. Coronal brain view in MNI305 template, sliced through the region of maximum activity, is illustrated. Left side shows mean rIFG activity for FM patients and HC participants across the four word categories: FM symptoms (SF), negative-arousing (A-), positive-arousing (A+) and neutral (N) stimuli. Error bars reflect standard errors. Black line represent rIFG activity for FM patients and, grey line, for HC participants.

As mentioned before, cognitive dysfunctions and pain processing may rely on partially overlapping regions in FM patients. As a consequence of this, resources taken up by pain processing may not be available for executive functioning (Glass et al., 2011). Pain level of patients might contribute to this effect over cognition. Neuroimaging techiques represent an opportunity to advance in the comprehension of FM and further studies should be done to delimitate deficits in order to develop better diagnostic and classification criteria of FM patients and to better design neuropsychological interventions oriented to increase their quality of life.

4. Genetics in fibromyalgia: Pain and cognition

Genetic predisposition is likely to be an important factor in the development of FM as suggested by several familial studies (Buskila et al., 1996, 2007; Arnold et al., 2004). These studies found that first-degree relatives of patients with FM had lower pain threshold than controls and were 8.5 times more likely to develop FM than relatives of patients with rheumatoid arthritis. The studies also indicated that the relatives of FM patients are more likely to suffer from comorbidities commonly seen in FM, such as mood disorders, irritable bowel syndrome (IBS), temporomandibular disorder (TMD) and headache (Ablin et al., 2008; Buskila et al., 1996, 2007). Identifying the genes responsible for this genetic contribution to risk should provide a better understanding of the complex mechanisms underlying FM and other chronic pain diseases. In recent years, attempts have been made to identify the genes involved in FM using candidate gene genetic association studies, which look for differences in the frequency of different polymorphisms between cases and controls, or with a quantifiable trait. The majority of such candidates have been genes involved in catecholaminergic or serotonergic neurotransmission, including receptors and transporters for dopamine, serotonin, norepinephrine, and epinephrine, as well as the catabolic enzymes catechol-O-methyltransferase (COMT).

Next we will review, in outline, the main findings made on genes associated with FM. The most widely studied gene to date is **Catechol-O-Methyltransferase (COMT)**, which degrades catecholamines such as dopamine, noradrenaline and adrenalin that are involved in various physiological functions including mood, cognition and stress response (Belfer and Segal, 2011). In particular, a single nucleotide polymorphism (SNP), (rs4680), has received a great deal of attention due its functional implications (Zubieta et al., 2003). This polymorphism causes a substitution from a valina (Val) to a methionine (Met) at amino acid position 158 (*Val158Met*), leading to a three to four fold reduced activity of the COMT enzyme (Lotta et al., 1995). In 2005, Diatchenko and colleagues described three very common haplotypes consisting of four SNPs (rs6269, rs 4633, rs4818 and rs4680-*Val158Met*) accounting for 96% of all haplotypes observed in human populations (Diatchenko et al., 2005). They identified them as low (LPS), average (APS) and high (HPS) pain sensitivity haplotypes, and they found a correlation with much more profound change in COMT activity (up to 20-fold difference).

The *met/met* genotype of the COMT *Val158Met* polymorphism has been associated with higher sensitivity in response to pain stimuli and the number of tender points in FM (Cohen et al., 2009) as well as with a high risk for the development of FM (García-Fructuoso et al., 2006; Barbosa et al., 2012). Recently, Martínez-Jauand and colleagues (2013) have shown that the HPS-APS haplotypes are more frequent in FM patients than in healthy controls and that FM patients who possess those genetic combinations displayed an increased sensitivity to experimental pain. These results are in accordance with previous reports showing a strong association between the HPS haplotype and high score on the Fibromyalgia Impact Questionnaire (Vargas-Alarcón et al., 2007). These haplotypes might be associated with increased risk of developing chronic pain disorders (Diatchenko et al., 2005). These data suggest that a decrease of COMT activity might contribute to the maintenance of pain symptoms in FM, and might play a significant role in classifying FM patients (Martínez-Jauand et al., 2013).

COMT variants moderate not only pain but also maladaptive coping processes in patients with FM. Finan and colleagues (2010 and 2011) demonstrated that Met158 allele homozygotes experience more pain in days when pain catastrophizing and pain attention scores were elevated, and a greater decline in positive affect on days when pain was elevated. These findings support the role of COMT and catecholamines in affective reactivity to pain, and in pain-related cognition pathways in patients with FM. A recent study has proposed that the Val158Met can play a relevant role in phenotypic expression of FM. They showed that women with FM and Met/Met genotype had more severe psychological and functional impact scores than those with the Val/Val genotype, although the differences were not significant (Desmeules et al., 2012). More recently, Fernández de las Peñas and colleagues (2012) have shown that FM patients with Met/Met genotype exhibit higher disability, anxiety and depression than those with Val/Val and Val/Met genotype.

As indicated above, cognitive dysfunction has been considered as one of the most disturbing symptoms, apart from pain, in patients with FM. Neuropsychological investigations have suggested that executive control and working memory impairments seem to be the key to explain a great part of this cognitive dysfunction in FM (Glass, 2010) and it points out to the existence of an altered neural substrate, presumably within prefrontal regions, such as inferior prefrontal cortex (IPFC), MPFC or ACC (Glass et al., 2011). In this context, it has been shown that more than 60% of released dopamine is metabolized by COMT in the frontal cortex (Karoum et al., 1994), and that the Val158Met polymorphism affects working memory and executive functions in healthy population (Bruder et al., 2005) and some mental disorders such as schizophrenia (Diaz-Asper et al., 2006; Hosak, 2007). Therefore, COMT may be a good candidate for the study of cognitive impairment in patients with FM.

The **endogenous serotonergic system** is comprised of the neurotransmitter serotonin (5-HT), multiple serotonin receptors (5-HT2A, 5-HT3A, 5-HT3B) and the serotonin transporter (5-HTT). This system is a key contributor to both depression and pain in FM. In fact, serotonin is decreased in FM, and selective serotonin reuptake inhibitors have some efficacy in FM (Gupta and Silman, 2004). Despite the complexity of the serotonergic pathway, research has mainly focused on a limited number of genes. Offenbaecher and colleagues (1999) analyzed the genotypes of the promoter region of the serotonin transporter gene (5-HTT) in patients with FM and healthy controls. A significantly higher frequency of the S/S genotype of the serotonin transporter promoter region was found in FM as compared to healthy participants. The S/S subgroup exhibited higher mean levels of depression and psychological distress. It was suggested that these results support the notion of an altered serotonin metabolism in at least a subgroup of patients with FM (Buskila et al., 2007). These findings were subsequently confirmed by a study analyzing Palestinian Arabs and Israeli Jews (Cohen et al., 2002). However, the study in other candidate genes within the serotonergic system failed to demonstrate a significant difference in the frequency of the polymorphism among FM patients and controls (Bondy et al., 1999; Frank et al., 2004; Matsuda et al., 2010).

The **dopaminergic system** has also been the target of extensive study in search of the genetic factors related to FM. Dopamine is a crucial neurotransmitter involved in multiple activities including pain transmission and endogenous analgesia (Wood, 2008). A single nucleotide polymorphism (Ser9Gly) in the dopamine-D3 receptor gene predicts changes in pain threshold in FM patients but not in healthy subjects (Potvin et al., 2009). In the FM group, the Ser9Gly polymorphism was a predictor of decreased thermal pain threshold and diffuse noxious inhibitory control (DNIC) efficacy (Potvin et al., 2009). Polymorphisms in the dopamine receptor 4 (DRD4) gene has also been associated with FM. Buskila and colleagues (2004) reported a significant decrease in the frequency of the 7 repeated allele in exon III of the D4 receptor gene in FM patients, who also demonstrated an association between this polymorphism and the low novelty seeking personality trait. This was considered consistent with the personality profile of FM patients, who scored high on anxiety related personality traits and low on novelty or sensation seeking. In a study of 384 subjects with DRD4 polymorphism, allele 4 was the most common, occurring in 279 of the 384 subjects (Treister et al., 2009). However, there was no change in cold tolerance, cold perception, cold pain threshold, or heat pain intensity in those subjects compared to subjects with allele 2 or allele 7 (Treister et al., 2009). Dopamine D2 receptor (DRD2) is implicated in different cognitive processes and brain disorder, and polymorphisms in this gene affect gene expression, splicing, and neuronal activity during working memory (Zhang et al., 2007). This has been demonstrated in patients with schizophrenia, whose presence relatively increased density of DRD2 (Laruelle, 1998). Curiously, it has also been observed an increased sensitivity or density of dopamine D2 receptors (DRD2) in FM patients (Malt et al., 2003). Preliminary results in our research group found a significant relationship between promoter SNP (rs12364283) in DRD2 and working memory functioning in FM patients. Specifically, we found significant differences during the performance in both Spatial Span (forward sequence) and n-back tasks. Heterozygotes (TC)-FM patients had a lower performance compared to TC-HC in both Spatial Span and n-back tasks. They also perform worse than homozygotes TT-FM patients but only in the Spatial Span task (Gómez-Esquer et al., 2012). Our results suggest that DRD2 could be playing an important role in working memory functioning in FM patients and support the implication of dopaminergic pathways in the cognitive symptoms of FM.

Another candidate gene is the **β_2-adrenergic receptor** (ADRB2). It mediates physiologic responses such as vasodilation and bronchial smooth-muscle relaxation, and represents a connection between the sympathetic nervous system and the immune system (Small et al., 2003; Catapano & Mangi, 2007). Alterations in the ADRB2 function have been implicated in several psychiatric and psychological disorders, including those associated with chronic pain (Lee et al., 2012). Vargas-Alarcón and colleagues (2009) reported that having the AC haplotype of the two SNPs (rs1042713 and rs1042714) was associated with an increased risk for suffering FM among Mexican and Spanish individuals. Recently, it has been published the first study to demonstrate ADRB2 polymorphism-related differences in intracellular cyclic Adenosine Monophosphate (cAMP) levels in FM Peripheral Blood Mononuclear Cells (PBMC), before and after ADRB2 stimulation. These findings suggest that ADRB2 polymorphisms may influence the response to a variety of β-adrenergic ligands and may help to explain some differences in responsiveness of FM subgroups to the adrenergic agonist medication currently approved for FM treatment (Xiao et al., 2011).

Finally, we will briefly discuss about **SCN9A**, a gene that encodes sodium channel in dorsal root ganglia (DRG). A consistent line of investigation suggests that autonomic nervous system dysfunction may explain the multi-system features of FM. In this context, DRG play a key role in pain perception and sodium channels located in DRG act as molecular gatekeepers of pain detection at peripheral nociceptors. Mutations in this gene have caused severe pain disorders and congenital insensitivity to pain in families, thus demonstrating a critical role in pain processing (Drenth and Waxman, 2007). In FM, Vargas Alarcón and colleagues (2012) demonstrated that, in Mexican women, the frequency of rs6754031 polymorphism of SCN9A was significantly different between FM patients and healthy controls. Interestingly, patients with

GG genotype had higher Fibromyalgia Impact Questionnaire (FIQ) scores than patients with the GT or TT genotype. These results show that there is an association between the rs6754031 polymorphism and the risk of developing FM as well as the FIQ score. This association raises the possibility that some patients with severe FM may have a DRG sodium channelopathy (Vargas-Alarcón et al., 2012). However, further investigation will be necessary in other ethnic groups with a large sample size to verify this observation.

Despite the large number of studies examining the potential contribution of the candidate gene polymorphism to FM susceptibility, many studies have produced conflicting results (Potvin et al., 2010; Frank et al., 2004; Gursoy, 2002). The explanation for these results could be that individual studies based on small sample sizes have insufficient power to detect positive associations and they are incapable of demonstrating the absence of such association. Recently, Lee and colleagues (2012) have conducted a systematic meta-analysis of seventeen candidate genes and over 35 polymorphisms were identified in studies on FM susceptibility. This meta-analysis demonstrates that the 5-HT2A receptor 102T/C polymorphism confers susceptibility to FM. In contrast, no association was found between the 5-HTTLPR S/L allele, COMT Val158Met, and susceptibility to FM. However, the authors were aware of the limitations of their meta-analysis since both the number of the studies and the number of the subjects included in such studies were too small. This may have not enough power to explore the association between the candidate gene polymorphism and FM. They could not perform the ethnic-specific meta-analysis to detect associations in ethnic groups due to limited data. They have not been able either to examine whether the candidate gene polymorphisms are associated with clinical features of FM (Lee et al., 2012). Therefore, additional research including large numbers of patients and controls is required to conclude the association of the candidate gene polymorphisms with FM. Another approach being made lately to identify genetic factors involved in FM is the use of a large-scale candidate gene approach (Smith et al., 2012). This is the largest candidate genes association study of the FM to date, analyzing 3,295 SNPs corresponding to > 350 genes involved in the biological pathways relevant to nociception, inflammation, and mood. This work observed significant differences in allele frequencies between cases and controls for several novel genes: GABRB3 (in the promoter region of the GABA-A β receptor gene), TAAR1 (trace amine-associated receptor 1), GBP1 (guanylate binding protein 1), RGS4 (regulator of G-protein signaling 4), CNR1 (CB-1 cannabinoid receptor gene), and GRIA4 (AMPA ionotropic glutamate receptor 4 subunit). Three of these genes, TAAR1, RGS4, and CNRI play roles in the modulation of analgesic pathways (Smith et al., 2012). Variation in these 4 replicated genes may serve as a basis for the development of new diagnostic approaches, and the products of these genes may contribute to the pathophysiology of FM and represent potential target for therapeutic actions.

5. Conclusions and future directions

Evidence from FM investigations indicates that psychoneurobiological dysfunctions play a relevant role in the pathophysiology of this multifactorial and still not fully understood syndrome. Specifically, it was suggested that abnormalities in central brain mechanisms are crucial in the understanding of chronic pain in FM, having little relevance the involvement of peripheral processing systems. Mechanisms of central sensitization and those involving descending inhibitory pathways, along with abnormalities in neurotransmission regulatory processes, seem to underlie patient's manifestations of hyperalgesia and allodynia, among other pain-related symptoms. Experimental findings also have demonstrated that both morphological and functional brain changes are related to widespread and diffuse pain and cognitive symptoms suffered by patients with FM.

On the other hand, patients with FM are characterized by the presence of difficulties in the processing of information reporting that it constitutes a very disruptive symptom in their everyday functioning. Cognitive disturbances are mainly related to both executive functions and working memory processes. Neuroimaging investigations have found abnormal activity within prefrontal and parietal regions when patients had to face a demanding task of executive control resources. However, many researchers are trying to answer an important question in order to advance in the knowledge on FM. Can cognitive dysfunction in FM be considered as a primary symptom like abnormal pain perception or, by contrast, is it a direct consequence of the structural or functional changes produced by pain? Based on present findings, cognitive dysfunctions and pain processing seem to share brain networks (prefrontal, supplementary motor regions and parietal cortices) and as a consequence of this, resources taken up by pain processing may not be available for executive functioning. Thus, performance in those tasks, which need a recruitment of working memory resources from the frontoparietal brain network to be correctly completed, would be very poor in FM. Neuroimaging techniques represent an opportunity to advance in the comprehension of pain and cognition interactions in FM and further studies should be done to explore such deficits and their interrelations.

Current data support the statement that FM constitutes a real syndrome characterized by the existence of multiple changes into the brain. Future investigations should be projected to extend these findings and to establish comprehensive explanations about: 1) cerebral mechanisms that provoke those changes, 2) its consequences on the functional state of patients and, 3) if brain changes constitute a reversible or permanent condition in the brain of FM patients. In this sense, different therapeutic approaches targeted to reverse such changes in the brain (e.g., pharmacological treatments, neuropsychological interventions, transcraneal magnetic stimulation, etc) may be effective and should be explored. The investigation about different genetic polymorphisms is a promising approach that may also help to improve the comprehension of the pathogenesis of this multifactorial and intriguing syndrome.

Acknowledgements

This work was supported by the grants URJC-CM-2007-1636 from the Universidad Rey Juan Carlos/ComunidadAutónoma de Madrid and PSI2009-08883 from the Ministryof Science and Innovation of Spain.

http://dx.doi.org/10.5772/56495

Author details

Francisco Mercado[1], Paloma Barjola[1], Marisa Fernández-Sánchez[1], Virginia Guerra[1] and Francisco Gómez-Esquer[2]

1 Department of Psychology, Faculty of Health Sciences, Rey Juan Carlos University, Madrid, Spain

2 Department of Anatomy and Human Embryology, Faculty of Health Sciences, Rey Juan Carlos University, Madrid, Spain

References

[1] Abeles, A., Pillinger, M., Solitar, B. and Abeles, M. (2007). Narrative Review: The Pathophysiology of Fibromyalgia. Annals of Internal Medicine 146, 726-734.

[2] Ablin, J., Neumann, L., Buskila, D. (2008). Pathogenesis of fibromyalgia – A review. Joint Bone Spine 75 (3), 273-279.

[3] Altamura, M., Elveväg, B., Blasi, G., Bertolino, A., Callicott, J.H., Weinberger D.R. et al. (2007). Dissociating the effects of Sternberg working memory demands in prefrontal cortex. Psychiatric Research 154, 103-114.

[4] Ambrose, K.R., Gracely R.H., Glass, J.M. (2012). Fibromyalgia dyscognition: concepts and issues. Rheumatismo 64 (4), 206-215.

[5] Apkarian, A.V., Bushnell, M.C., Treede, R.D., Zubieta, J.K. (2005). Human brain mechanisms of pain perception and regulation in health and disease. European Journal of Pain 9 (4), 463-484.

[6] Arnold, L.M., Crofford, L.J., Mease, P.J., Burgess, S.M., Palmer, S.C., Abetz, L., Martin, S.A. (2008). Patient perspectives on the impact of fibromyalgia. Patient Education and Counseling 73 (1), 114-120.

[7] Arnold, L.M., Hudson, J.I., Hess, E.V., Ware, A.E., Fritz, D.A., Auchenbach, M.B., Starck, L.O., Keck, P.E. Jr. (2004). Family study of fibromyalgia. Arthritis & Rheumatism 50 (3), 944-52.

[8] Baddeley, A. (2000). The episodic buffer: A new component of working memory? Trends in Cognitive Sciences 4, 417-423.

[9] Baliki, N., Schnitzer, T., Bauer, W. and Apkarian, V. (2011). Brain Morphological Signatures for Chronic Pain. Plos ONE 6 (10), 1-13.

[10] Baliki, M.N., Geha, P.Y., Apkarian, A.V., Chialvo, D.R. (2008). Beyond feeling: chronic pain hurts the brain, disrupting the default-mode network dinamics. The Journal of Neuroscience 28 (6), 1398-1403.

[11] Barbosa, F.R., Matsuda, J.B., Mazucato, M., de Castro França, S., Zingaretti, S.M., da Silva, L.M., Martinez-Rossi, N.M., Júnior, M.F., Marins, M., Fachin, A.L. (2012). Influence of catechol-O-methyltransferase (COMT) gene polymorphisms in pain sensibility of Brazilian fibromyalgia patients. Rheumatology International 32 (2), 427–430.

[12] Belfer, I., Segall, S. (2011). COMT genetic variants and pain. Drugs Today (Barc). 47 (6), 457-67.

[13] Bennett, R. (2005). Fibromyalgia: present to future. Current Rheumatology Reports 7, 371–376.

[14] Bondy, B., Spaeth, M., Offenbaecher, M., Glatzeder, K., Stratz, T., Schwarz, M., de Jonge, S., Krüger, M., Engel, R.R., Färber, L., Pongratz, D.E., Ackenheil, M. (1999). The T102C polymorphism of the 5-HT2A-receptor gene in fibromyalgia. Neurobiology of Disease 6 (5), 433-9.

[15] Bruder, G.E., Keilp, J.G., Xu, H., Shikhman, M., Schori, E., Gorman, J.M., Gilliam, T.C. (2005). Catechol-O-methyltransferase (COMT) genotypes and working memory: associations with differing cognitive operations. Biological Psychiatry 58 (11), 901-7.

[16] Bunge, S.A., Klingberg, T., Jacobsen, R.B., Gabrieli, J.D.E. (2000). A resource model of the neural basis of executive working memory. Proceedings of the National Academy of Sciences of the United States of America (PNAS) 97 (7), 3573-3578.

[17] Burgmer, M., Pogatzki-Zahn, E., Markus, G., Stüber, C., Wessoleck, E., Heuft, G., and Pfleiderer, B. (2010). Fibromyalgia unique temporal brain activation during experimental pain: a controlled fMRI Study. Journal Neural Transmission 117, 123-131.

[18] Burgmer, M., Pogatzki-Zahn, E., Gaubitz, M. Wessoleck, E., Heuft, G. Pfleiderer, B. (2009). Altered brain activity during pain processing in fibromyalgia. Neuroimage 44 (2), 502-508.

[19] Bushnell, M.C., Apkarian, A.V. (2005). Representation of pain in the brain. In: McMahon S, Koltzenburg M (eds). Textbook of pain, 5th edn. Churchill Livingstone, Philadelphia, pp. 267–289

[20] Buskila, D. (2009). Developments in the scientific and clinical understanding of fibromyalgia. Arthritis Research and Therapy 11 (5), 242-249.

[21] Buskila, D., Cohen, H., Neumann, L., Ebstein, R.P. (2004). An association between fibromyalgia and the dopamine D4 receptor exon III repeat polymorphism and relationship personality traits. Molecular Psychiatry 9 (8), 730-731.

[22] Buskila, D., Neumann, L., Hazanov, I., Carmi, R. (1996). Familial aggregation in the fibromyalgia syndrome. Seminars in Arthritis and Rheumatism 26 (3), 605-11.

[23] Buskila, D., Sarzi-Puttini, P., Ablin, J.N. (2007). The genetics of fibromyalgia syndrome. Pharmacogenomics 8 (1), 67-74.

[24] Carrillo-de-la-Peña, M.T., Vallet, M., Pérez, M.I., Gómez-Perretta, C. (2006). Intensity Dependence of Auditory-Evoked Cortical Potentials in Fibromyalgia Patients: A Test of the Generalized Hypervigilance Hypothesis. Journal of Pain 7, 480-487.

[25] Catapano, L.A., Manji, H.K. (2007). G protein-coupled receptors in major psychiatric disorders. Biochimica et Biophysica Acta 1768 (4), 976-93.

[26] Ceko, M., Bushnell, C. and Gracely, R. (2012). Neurobiology Underlying Fibromyalgia Symptoms. Pain Research and Treatment 2012, Article ID 585419, 8 pages

[27] Cifre, I., Sitges, C., Fraiman, D., Muñoz, M.A., Balenzuela, P., González-Roldán, A., Martínez-Jauand, M., Birbaumer, N., Chialvo, D.R., Montoya, P. (2012). Disrupted functional connectivity of the pain network in fibromyalgia. Psychosomatic Medicine 74 (1), 55-62.

[28] Cohen, H., Buskila, D., Neumann, L., Ebstein, R.P. (2002). Confirmation of an association between fibromyalgia and serotonin transporter promoter region (5- HTTLPR) polymorphism, and relationship to anxiety-related personality traits. Arthritis & Rheumatism 46 (3), 845-7.

[29] Cohen, H., Neumann, L., Glazer, Y., Ebstein, R.P., Buskila, D. (2009). The relationship between a common catechol-O-methyltransferase (COMT) polymorphism val(158) met and fibromyalgia. Clinical and Experimental Rheumatology 27 (5), 51-6.

[30] Cook, D.B., Lange, G., Ciccone, D.S., Liu, W.C., Steffener, J. Natelson B.H. (2004). Functional imaging of pain in patients with primary fibromyalgia. Journal of Rheumatology 31 (2), 364-378.

[31] Correa, A., Miró, E., Martínez, P., Sánchez, A. and Lupiáñez, J. (2011). Temporal preparation and inhibitory deficit in fibromyalgia síndrome. Brain and Cognition 75, 211-216.

[32] Craggs, J.G., Staud, R., Robinson, M.E., Perlstein, W.M., Price, D.D. (2012). Effective connectivity among brain regions associated with slow temporal summation of C-fiber-evoked pain in fibromyalgia patients and healthy controls. The Journal of Pain 13 (4), 390-400.

[33] Crombez, G., Van Damme, S., Eccleston, C. (2005). Hypervigilance to pain: An experimental and clinical analysis. Pain 116, 4-7.

[34] Dadabhoy, D., Crofford, L., Spaeth, M., Russell, J. and Clauw, D. (2008). Evidence-based biomarkers for fibromyalgia syndrome. Arthritis Research & Therapy 10 (211), 1-18.

[35] Dagher, A., Owen, A. M., Boecker, H., Brooks, D.J. (1999). Mapping the network for planning: A correlational PET activation study with the Tower of London task. Brain 122 (10), 1973-1987.

[36] Desmeules, J., Piguet, V., Besson, M., Chabert, J., Rapiti, E., Rebsamen, M., Rossier, M.F., Curtin, F., Dayer, P., Cedraschi, C. (2012). Psychological distress in fibromyalgia patients: A role for catechol-O-methyl-transferase Val158met polymorphism. Health Psychology 31 (2), 242-249.

[37] Diatchenko, L., Slade, G.D., Nackley, A.G., Bhalang, K., Sigurdsson, A., Belfer, I., Goldman, D., Xu, K., Shabalina, S.A., Shagin, D., Max, M.B., Makarov, S.S., Maixner, W. (2005). Genetic basis for individual variations in pain perception and the development of a chronic pain condition. Human Molecular Genetics 14 (1), 135-43.

[38] Diaz-Asper, C.M., Weinberger, D.R., Goldberg, T.E. (2006). Catechol-O-methyltransferase polymorphisms and some implications for cognitive therapeutics. NeuroRx 3 (1), 97-105.

[39] Dick, B.D., Verrier, M.J., Harker, K.T., and Rashiq, S. (2008). Disruption of cognitive function in fibromyalgia syndrome. Pain 139 (3), 610-616.

[40] Drenth, J.P., Waxman, S.G. (2007). Mutations in sodium-channel gene SCN9A cause a spectrum of human genetic pain disorders. The Journal of Clinical Investigation 117 (12), 3603–3609.

[41] Duschek, S., Werner, N.S., Winkelmann, A. Wankner, S. (2013). Implicit Memory Function in Fibromyalgia Syndrome. Behavioral Medicine 39 (1), 11-16.

[42] Emad, Y., Ragab, Y., Zeinhom, F., El-Khouly, G., Abou-Zeid, A., Rasker, J.J. (2008). Hippocampus dysfunction may explain symptoms of fibromyalgia syndrome. A study with single-voxel magnetic resonance spectroscopy. Journal of Rheumatology 35, 1371-1377.

[43] Fan, P.T. (2004). Fibromyalgia and chronic fatigue syndrome. APLAR Journal of Rheumatology 7 (3), 219-231.

[44] Fayed, N., García-Campayo, J., Magallón, R., Andrés-Bergareche, H., Luciano, JV., Andres, E., Beltrán, J. (2010). Localized 1H-NMR spectroscopy in patients with fibromyalgia: a controlled study of changes in cerebral glutamate/glutamine, inositol, choline, and N-acetylaspartate. Arthritis Research & Therapy 12 (4), R134.

[45] Fernández-de-Las-Peñas, C., Ambite-Quesada, S., Gil-Crujera, A., Cigarán-Méndez, M., Peñacoba-Puente, C. (2012). Catechol-O-methyltransferase Val158Met polymorphism influences anxiety, depression, and disability, but not pressure pain sensitivity, in women with fibromyalgia syndrome. The Journal of Pain 13 (11), 1068-74.

[46] Finan, P.H., Zautra, A.J., Davis, M.C., Lemery-Chalfant, K., Covault, J., Tennen, H. (2011). COMT moderates the relation of daily maladaptive coping and pain in fibromyalgia. Pain 152 (2), 300-307.

[47] Finan, P.H., Zautra, A.J., Davis, M.C., Lemery-Chalfant, K., Covault, J., Tennen, H. (2010). Genetic influences on the dynamics of pain and affect in fibromyalgia. Health Psychology 29 (2), 134-142.

[48] Frank, B., Niesler, B., Bondy, B., Späth, M., Pongratz, D.E., Ackenheil, M., Fischer, C., Rappold, G. (2004). Mutational analysis of serotonin receptor genes: HTR3A and HTR3B in fibromyalgia patients. Clinical Rheumatology 23 (4), 338-344.

[49] García-Campayo, J., Fayed, N., (2010). Clinical Magnetic Resonance Neuroimaging in Fibromyalgia. Neuroimaging, Cristina Marta Del-Ben (Ed.), 111-124.

[50] García-Fructuoso, F.J., Lao-Villadóniga, J.I., Beyer, K., Santos, C. (2006). Relationship between COMT gene genotypes and the severity of fibromyalgia. Reumatología Clínica 2 (4), 168–172.

[51] Geisser, M.E., Glass, J.M., Rajcevska, L.D., Clauw, D.J., Williams, D.A., Kileny, P.R., and Gracely, R.H. (2008). A Psychophysical Study of Auditory and Pressure Sensitivity in Patients With Fibromyalgia and Healthy Controls. Journal of Pain 9, 417-422.

[52] Giesecke, T., Gracely, R.H., Williams, D.A., Geisser, M.E., Petzke, F.W. (2005). The relationship between depression, clinical pain, and experimental pain in a chronic pain cohort. Arthritis and Rheumatism 52 (5), 1577-1584.

[53] Glass, J.M., Williams, D.A., Fernández-Sánchez, M.L., Kairys, A., Barjola, P., Heitzeg, M.M., Clauw, D.J., and Schmidt-Wilcke, T. (2011). Executive Function in Chronic Pain Patients and Healthy Controls: Different Cortical Activation During Response Inhibition in Fibromyalgia. The Journal of Pain 12 (12), 1219-1229.

[54] Glass, J.M. (2010). Cognitive dysfunction in fibromyalgia syndrome. Journal of Musculoskeletal Pain 18 (4), 367-372.

[55] Glass, J.M. (2009). Review of cognitive dysfunction in fibromyalgia: a convergence on working memory and attentional control impairments. Rheumatic Diseases Clinics of North America 35 (2), 299-311.

[56] Glass, J.M. (2006). Cognitive dysfunction in fibromyalgia and chronic fatigue syndrome: new trends and future directions. Current Rheumatology Reports 8 (6), 425-429.

[57] Glass, J.M., Park, D.C., Minear, M., and Crofford, L.J. (2005). Memory beliefs and function in fibromyalgia patients. Journal Psychosomatic Research 58, 263- 269.

[58] Glass, J.M., Park, D.C. (2001). Cognitive dysfunction in fibromyalgia. Current Rheumatology Reports 3 (2), 123-127.

[59] Gómez-Esquer, F., Barjola, P., Fernández-Sánchez, M., Mercado, F. (2012). Dopamine D2 receptor polymorphism influence on working memory functioning in Fibromyalgia. 14th World Congress on Pain – International Association for the Study of Pain (IASP)

[60] González, J.L., Mercado, F., Barjola, P., Carretero, I., Lopez-Lopez, A., Bullones, M.A., Fernandez-Sanchez, M., Alonso, M. (2010). Generalized hypervigilance in fibromyalgia patients: an experimental analysis with the emotional Stroop paradigm. Journal Psychosomatic Research 69, 279-287.

[61] Grace, G., Nielson, W., Hopkins, M. and Berg, M. (1999) . Concentration and Memory Deficits in Patients with Fibromyalgia Syndrome. Journal of Clinical and Experimental Neuropsychology 21 (4), 477-487.

[62] Gracely, R.H., Ambrose, K.R. (2011). Neuroimaging of fibromyalgia. Best Practice and Research: Clinical Rheumatology 25 (2), 271-284.

[63] Gracely, R.H., Geisser, M.E., Giesecke, T., Grant, M.A., Petzke, F. Williams, D.A. et al. (2004). Pain catastrophizing and neural responses to pain among persons with fibromyalgia. Brain 127 (4), 835-843.

[64] Gracely, R.H., Petzke, F., Wolf, J.M., and Clauw, D.J. (2002). Functional magnetic resonance imaging evidence of augmented pain processing in fibromyalgia. Arthritis and Rheumatism 46 (5), 1333-1343.

[65] Graven-Nielsen, T., Aspegren Kendall, S., Henriksson, K.G., Bengtsson, M., Sorensen, J., Johnson, A., Gerdle, B., Arendt-Nielsen, L. (2000). Ketamine reduces muscle pain, temporal summation, and referred pain in fibromyalgia patients. Pain 85, 483-491.

[66] Grisart, J., Van del Linden, M. and Masquelier, E. (2002). Controlled processes and automaticity in memory functioning in Fobromyalgia patienes: relation with emotional distress and hypervigilance. Journal of Clinical and Experimental Neuropsychology 24 (8), 994-1009.

[67] Gupta, A., Silman, A.J. (2004). Psychological stress and fibromyalgia: a review of the evidence suggesting a neuroendocrine link. Arthritis Research & Therapy 6 (3), 98-106.

[68] Gursoy, S. (2002). Absence of association of the serotonin transporter gene polymorphism with the mentally healthy subset of fibromyalgia patients. Clinical Rheumatology 21 (3), 194-197.

[69] Harris, R.E. (2010). Elevated excitatory neurotransmitter levels in the fibromyalgia brain. Arthritis Research & Therapy 12 (5), 141.

[70] Harris, R.E., Sundgren, P.C., Craig, A.D., Kirshenbaum, E., Sen, A., Napadow, V., Clauw, D.J. (2009). Elevated insular glutamate in fibromyalgia is associated with experimental pain. Arthritis & Rheumatism 60 (10), 3146-3152.

[71] Harris, R.E., Sundgren, P.C., Pang, Y., Hsu, M., Petrou, M., Kim, S.H., McLean, S.A., Gracely, R.H., Clauw, D.J. (2008). Dynamic levels of glutamate within the insula are associated with improvements in multiple pain domains in fibromyalgia. Arthritis & Rheumatism 58 (3), 903-907.

[72] Herrero, J.F., Laird, J.M., Lopez-García JA. (2000). Wind-up of spinal cord neurones and pain sensation: much ado about something? Progress Neurobiology 61, 169–203.

[73] Hosák, L. (2007). Role of the COMT gene Val158Met polymorphism in mental disorders: a review. European Psychiatry 22 (5), 276-281.

[74] Hsu, M.C., Harris, R.E., Sundgren, P.C., Welsh, R.C., Fernandes, C.R., Clauw, D.J., Williams, D.A. (2009). No consistent difference in gray matter volume between individuals with fibromyalgia and age-matched healthy subjects when controlling for affective disorder. Pain 143 (3), 262-267.

[75] Iannetti, G.D., Mouraux, A. (2010). From the neuromatrix to the pain matrix (and back). Experimental Brain Research 205 (1), 1-12.

[76] Julien, N., Goffaux, P., Arsenault, P., Marchand, S. (2005). Widespread pain in fibromyalgia is related to a deficit of endogenous pain inhibition. Pain 114, 295-302.

[77] Karoum, F., Chrapusta, S.J., Egan, M.F. (1994). 3-Methoxytyramine is the major metabolite of released dopamine in the rat frontal cortex. Journal of Neurochemistry 63 (3), 972-979.

[78] Katz, R.S., Heard, A.R., Mills, M., Leavitt, F. (2004). The prevalence and clinical impact of reported cognitive difficulties (fibrofog) in patients with rheumatic disease with and without fibromyalgia. Journal Clinical Rheumatology 10 (2), 53–58.

[79] Seong-Ho, K, Sang-Hyon, K, Seong-Kyu, K, Eun Jung, N, SeungWoo, H &SeungJae, L. (2012). Spatial versus verbal memoryimpairments in patientswithfibromyalgia Rheumatology Int 32, 1135-1142

[80] Kosek, E., Hansson, P. (1997). Modulatory influence on somatosensory perception from vibration and heterotopic noxious conditioning stimulation (HNCS) in fibromyalgia patients and healthy subjects. Pain 70, 41-51.

[81] Kuchinad, A., Schweinhardt, P., Seminowicz, D.A., Wood, P.B., Chizh, B.A., and Bushnell, M.C. (2007). Accelerated brain gray matter loss in fibromyalgia patients: premature aging of the brain? The Journal of Neuroscience 27 (15), 4004-4007.

[82] Kwiatek, R., Barnden, L., Tedman, R., Jarrett, R., Chew, J., Rowe, C. and Pile, K. (2000). Regional cerebral blood flow in fibromyalgia: Single-photon–emission computed tomography evidence of reduction in the pontine tegmentum and thalami. Arthritis and Rheumatism 43 (12), 2823–2833.

[83] Landro, N.I., Stiles, T.C., Sletvold, H. (1997). Memory functioning in patients with primary fibromyalgia and major depression and healthy controls. Journal Psychosomatic Research 42 (3), 297–306.

[84] Laruelle, M. (1998). Imaging dopamine transmission in schizophrenia. A review and meta-analysis. The Quarterly Journal of Nuclear Medicine 42 (3), 211-221.

[85] Lautenbacher, S., Rollman GB. (1997). Possible deficiencies of pain modulation in fibromyalgia. Clinical Journal of Pain 13, 189-196.

[86] Leavitt, F, &Katz, R.S. (2008). Speed of Mental Operations in Fibromyalgia: A SelectiveNamingSpeedDeficit Journal of Clinical Rheumatology 14 (4), 214-218

[87] Leavitt, F., Katz, R.S. (2006). Distraction as a key determinant of impaired memory in patients with fibromyalgia. The Journal of Rheumatology 33 (1), 127-132.

[88] Lee, Y.H., Choi, S.J., Ji, J.D., Song, G.G. (2012). Candidate gene studies of fibromyalgia: a systematic review and meta-analysis. Rheumatology International 32 (2), 417-426.

[89] Lee, Y.C., Nassikas, N.J., Clauw, D.J. (2011). The role of the central nervous system in the generation and maintenance of chronic pain in rheumatoid arthritis, osteoarthritis and fibromyalgia. Arthritis Research & Therapy 13 (2), 211-221.

[90] Legrain, V., Iannetti, G.D., Plaghki, L., Mouraux, A. (2011). The pain matrix reloaded: A salience detection system for the body. Progress in Neurobiology 93 (1), 111-124.

[91] Lorenz, J., Minoshima, S., Casey, K.L. (2003). Keeping pain out of mind: the role of the dorsolateral prefrontal cortex in pain modulation. Brain 126 (5), 1079-1091.

[92] Lotta, T., Vidgren, J., Tilgmann, C., Ulmanen, I., Melén, K., Julkunen, I., Taskinen, J. (1995). Kinetics of human soluble and membrane-bound catechol O-methyltransferase: a revised mechanism and description of the thermolabile variant of the enzyme. Biochemistry 34 (13), 4202-4210.

[93] Luerding, R., Weigand, T., Bogdahn, U., and Schmidt-Wilcke, T. (2008). Working memory performance is correlated with local brain morphology in the medial frontal and anterior cingulate cortex in fibromyalgia patients: structural correlates of pain–cognition interaction. Brain 131 (12), 3222-3231.

[94] Lutz, J., Jäger, L., de Quervain, D., Krauseneck, T., Padberg, F., Wichnalek, M., Beyer, A., Stahl, R., Zirngibl, B., and Morhard, D. (2008). White and gray matter abnormalities in the brain of patients with fibromyalgia: A diffusion-tensor and volumetric imaging study. Arthritis and Rheumatism 58 (12), 3960-3969.

[95] Maestú, C., Cortes, A., Vazquez, J.M., del Rio, D., Gomez-Arguelles, J.M., del Pozo, F., Nevado, A. (2013). Increased brain responses during subjectively-matched mechanical pain stimulation in fibromyalgia patients as evidenced by MEG. Clinical Neurophysiology 124 (4), 752-760.

[96] Malt, E.A., Olafsson, S., Aakvaag, A., Lund, A., Ursin, H. (2003). Altered dopamine D2 receptor function in fibromyalgia patients: a neuroendocrine study with buspirone in women with fibromyalgia compared to female population based controls. Journal of Affective Disorders 75 (1), 77-82.

[97] Martínez-Jauand, M., Sitges, C., Rodríguez, V., Picornell, A., Ramon, M., Buskila, D., Montoya, P. (2013). Pain sensitivity in fibromyalgia is associated with catechol-O-methyltransferase (COMT) gene. European Journal of Pain 17 (1), 16-27.

[98] Martínez-Lavín M. (2004). Fibromyalgia as a sympathetically maintained pain syndrome. Current Pain Headache Reports 8, 385-389.

[99] Matsuda, J.B., Barbosa, F.R., Morel, L.J., et al. (2010). Serotonin receptor (5-HT 2A) and catechol-O-methyltransferase (COMT) gene polymorphisms: triggers of fibromyalgia? Revista Brasileira de Reumatologia 50 (2), 141-149.

[100] Mease, P.J., Arnold, L.M., Crofford, L.J., Williams, D.A., Russell, I.J., Humphrey, L., Abetz, L., and Martin, S.A. (2008). Identifying the clinical domains of fibromyalgia: contributions from clinician and patient Delphi exercises. Arthritis & Rheumatism 59, 952-960.

[101] Mercado, F., Gonzalez, J.L., Barjola, P., Fernández-Sánchez, M., López-López, A., Alonso, M., and Gómez-Esquer, F. (in press). Brain correlates of cognitive inhibition in Fibromyalgia: Emotional intrusion of symptom-related words. International Journal of Psychophysiology.

[102] Mercado, F., Barjola, P., Fernández-Sánchez, M., Dragoi, D., Fresno, V., Cardoso, S., Gómez-Esquer, F. (submitted). Evidence of altered working memory processes in fibromyalgia patients: an event-related potential study. Pain

[103] Montoya, P., Sitges, C., García-Herrera, M., Izquierdo, R., Truyols, M., Blay, N., and Collado, D. (2005) Abnormal Affective Modulation of Somatosensory Brain Processing Among Patients With Fibromyalgia. Psychsomatic Medicine 67, 957-963.

[104] Montoya, P., Larbig, W., Braun, C., Preissl, H., Birbaumer, N. (2004). Influence of Social Support and Emotional Context on Pain Processing and Magnetic Brain Responses in Fibromyalgia. Arthritis & Rheumatism 50 (12), 4035-4044.

[105] Munguia-Izquierdo, D., Legaz-Arrese, A., Moliner-Urdiales, D., Reverter-Masia, J. (2008). Neuropsychological performance in patients with fibromyalgia syndrome: relation to pain and anxiety. Psicothema 20, 427-431.

[106] Muñoz-Céspedes, J.M., Tirapu-Ustárroz, J. (2001). Rehabilitación Neuropsicológica. Ed. Síntesis.

[107] Napadow, V., Kim, J., Clauw, D. and Harris, R. (2012) Decreased Intrinsic Brain Connectivity Is Associated With Reduced Clinical Pain in Fibromyalgia. Arthritis & Rheumatism, 64 (7), 2398-2403.

[108] Napadow, V., LaCount, L., Park, K., As-Sanie, S., Clauw, D.J., Harris, R.E. (2010). Intrinsic brain connectivity in fibromyalgia is associated with chronic pain intensity. Arthritis and Rheumatism 62 (8), 2545-2555.

[109] Okifuji, A., Turk, DC. (2002). Stress and psychophysiological dysregulation in patients with fibromyalgia syndrome. Applied Psychophysiology and Biofeedback 27, 129-141.

[110] Offenbaecher, M., Bondy, B., de Jong, S., Glatzeder, K., Kruger, M., Schoeps, P., Ackenheil, M. (1999). Possible association of fibromyalgia with a polymorphism in the serotonin transporter gene regulatory region. Arthritis and Rheumatism 42 (11), 2482-2488.

[111] Park, D.C., Glass, J.M., Minear, M., Crofford, L.J. (2001). Cognitive function in fibromyalgia patients. Arthritis & Rheumatism 44 (9), 2125-2133.

[112] Peyron, R., Laurent, B., García-Larrea, L. (2000). Functional imaging of brain responses to pain. A review and meta-analysis. Neurophysiologie Clinique 30 (5), 263-288.

[113] Potvin, S., Larouche, A., Normand, E., de Souza, J.B., Gaumond, I., Grignon, S., Marchand, S. (2009). DRD3 Ser9Gly polymorphism is related to thermal pain perception and modulation in chronic widespread pain patients and healthy controls. The Journal of Pain 10 (9), 969-975.

[114] Potvin, S., Larouche, A., Normand, E., de Souza, J.B., Gaumond, I., Marchand, S., Grignon, S. (2010). No relationship between the ins del polymorphism of the serotonin transporter promoter and pain perception in fibromyalgia patients and healthy controls. European Journal of Pain 14 (7), 742-746.

[115] Price, D.D., Staud, R., Robinson, M.E., Mauderli, A.P., Cannon, R., Vierck, C.J. (2002). Enhanced temporal summation of second pain and its central modulation in fibromyalgia patients. Pain 99, 49-59.

[116] Pujol, J., López-Solá, M., Ortiz, H., Vilanova, J.C., Harrison, B.J. Yücel, M., Soriano-Mas, C., Cardoner, N. Deus, J. (2009). Mapping brain response to pain in fibromyalgia patients using temporal analysis of fMRI. PLoS One 4 (4), e5224.

[117] Reyes del Paso G.A., Pulgar A., Duschek S., Garrido S. (2012). Cognitive impairment in fibromyalgia syndrome: the impact of cardiovascular regulation, pain, emotional disorders and medication. European Journal of Pain 16, 421-429.

[118] Robinson, M.E., Craggs, J.G., Price, D.D., Perlstein, W.M., Staud, R. (2011). Gray matter volumes of pain-related brain areas are decreased in fibromyalgia syndrome. The Journal of Pain 12 (4), 436-443.

[119] Rolls, E.T., O'Doherty, J., Kringelbach, M.L., Francis, S., Bowtell, R., McGlone, F. (2003). Representations of pleasant and painful touch in the human orbitofrontal and cingulate cortices. Cerebral Cortex 13 (3), 308-317.

[120] Russell, I.J., Orr, M.D., Littman, B., Vipraio, G.A., Alboukrek, D., Michalek, J.E., et al. (1994). Elevated cerebrospinal fluid levels of substance P in patients with the fibromyalgia syndrome. Arthritis and Rheumatism 37, 1593-1601.

[121] Russell, I.J., Vaeroy, H., Javors, M., Nyberg, F. (1992). Cerebrospinal fluid biogenic amine metabolites in fibromyalgia/fibrositis syndrome and rheumatoid arthritis. Arthritis and Rheumatism 35, 550-556.

[122] Sawamoto, N., Honda, M., Okada, T., Hanakawa, T., Kanda, M., Fukuyama, H., Konishi, J., Shibasaki, H. (2000). Expectation of pain enhances responses to nonpainful somatosensory stimulation in the anterior cingulate cortex and parietal operculum/posterior insula: an event-related functional magnetic resonance imaging study. The Journal of Neuroscience 20 (19), 7438-7445.

[123] Schmidt-Wilcke, T., Clauw, D.J. (2010). Pharmacotherapy in fibromyalgia (FM) – Implications for the underlying pathophysiology. Pharmacology & Therapeutics 127 (3), 283-294.

[124] Schmidt-Wilcke, T., Luerding, R., Weigand, T., Jürgens, T., Schuierer, G., Leinisch, E., Bogdahn, U. (2007). Striatal grey matter increase in patients suffering from fibromyalgia – a voxel-based morphometry study. Pain 132 (1), 109-116.

[125] Schweinhardt, P., Sauro, K.M. Bushnell, C. (2008). Fibromyalgia: a disorder of the brain? The Neuroscientist 14 (5), 415-421.

[126] Seminowicz, D.A., Davis, K.D. (2007). Pain enhances functional connectivity of a brain network evoked by performance of a cognitive task. Journal of Neurophysiology 97 (5), 3651-3659.

[127] Seo., J. Kim, S.H., Kim, Y.T., Song, H.J., Lee, J.J., Kim, S.H., Han, S.W., Nam, E.J., Kim, S.K., Lee, H.J., Lee, S.J., Chang, Y. (2012). Working memory impairment in fibromyalgia patients associated with altered frontoparietal memory network. PLoS One 7 (6), e37808.

[128] Singer, T., Seymour, B., O'Doherty, J., Kaube, H., Dolan, R.J., Frith, C.D. (2004). Empathy for pain involves the affective but not sensory components of pain. Science 303 (5661), 1157-1162.

[129] Small, K.M., McGraw, D.W., Liggett, S.B. (2003). Pharmacology and physiology of human adrenergic receptor polymorphisms. Annual Review of Pharmacology and Toxicology 43, 381-411.

[130] Smith, S.B., Maixner, D.W., Fillingim, R.B., Slade, G., Gracely, R.H., Ambrose, K., Zaykin, D.V., Hyde, C., John, S., Tan, K., Maixner, W., Diatchenko, L. (2012). Large candidate gene association study reveals genetic risk factors and therapeutic targets for fibromyalgia. Arthritis and Rheumatism 64 (2), 584-93.

[131] Solberg, L., Carlson, C., Crofford, L., Leeuw, R. and Segerstrom, S. (2010). Self-regulatory deficits in fibromyalgia and temporomandibular disorders. Pain 151, 37-44.

[132] Stahl, S.M. (2009). Fibromyalgia – pathways and neurotransmitters. Human Psychopharmacology and Clinical Experiment 24 (1), 11-17.

[133] Staud, R., Price, D.D., Robinson, M.E., Mauderli, A.P., Vierck, C.J. (2004). Maintenance of windup of second pain requires less frequent stimulation in fibromyalgia patients compared to normal controls. Pain 110 (3), 689-696.

[134] Staud, R. Cannon R.C., Mauderli, A.P., Robinson, M.E., Price, D.D., Vierck, C.J., Jr. (2003). Temporal summation of pain from mechanical stimulation of muscle tissue in normal controls and subjects with fibromyalgia syndrome. Pain 102, 87-95.

[135] Suhr, J. (2003). Neuropsychological impairment in fibromyalgia Relation to depression, fatigue, and pain. Journal of Psychsomatic Research 55, 321-329.

[136] Tagliazucchi, E., Balenzuela, P., Fraiman, D., Chialvo, D.R. (2010). Brain resting state is disrupted in chronic back pain patients. Neuroscience letters 485 (1), 26-31.

[137] Thieme, K., Spies, C., Sinha, P., Turk, D.C., Flor, H., 2005. Predictors of pain behaviors in fibromyalgia syndrome. Arthritis and Rheumatism 53, 343–350.

[138] Tracey, I., Johns, E. (2010). The pain matrix: reloaded or reborn as we image tonic pain using arterial spin labelling. Pain 148 (3), 359-360.

[139] Tracey, I., Mantyh P.W. (2007). The cerebral signature for pain perception and its modulation. Neuron 55 (3), 377-391.

[140] Treister, R., Pud, D., Ebstein, R.P., Laiba, E., Gershon, E., Haddad, M., Eisenberg, E. (2009). Associations between polymorphisms in dopamine neurotransmitter pathway genes and pain response in healthy humans. Pain 147 (1-3), 187-193.

[141] Valdés, M., Collado, A., Bargalló, N., Vázquez, M., Rami, L., Gómez, E., Salamero, M. (2010). Increased glutamate/glutamine compounds in the brains of patients with fibromyalgia: a magnetic resonance spectroscopy study. Arthritis and Rheumatism 62 (6), 1829-1836.

[142] Valet, M., Sprenger, T., Boecker, H., Willoch, F., Rummeny, E., Conrad, B., Erhard, P., Tolle, TR. (2004). Distraction modulates connectivity of the cingulo-frontal cortex and the midbrain during pain – an fMRI analysis. Pain 109 (3), 399-408.

[143] Vargas-Alarcón, G., Álvarez-León, E., Fragoso, J.M., Vargas, A., Martínez, A., Vallejo, M., Martínez-Lavín, M. (2012). A SCN9A gene-encoded dorsal root ganglia sodium channel polymorphism associated with severe fibromyalgia. BMC Musculoskeletical Disorders 20, 13-28.

[144] Vargas-Alarcón, G., Fragoso, J.M., Cruz-Robles, D., Vargas, A., Martínez, A., Lao-Villadóniga, J.I., García-Fructuoso, F., Vallejo, M., Martínez-Lavín, M. (2009). Association of adrenergic receptor gene polymorphisms with different fibromyalgia syndrome domains. Arthritis and Rheumatism 60 (7), 2169-2173.

[145] Vargas-Alarcón, G., Fragoso, J.M., Cruz-Robles, D., Vargas, A., Vargas, A., Lao-Villadóniga, J.I., García-Fructuoso, F., Ramos-Kuri, M., Hernández, F., Springall, R., Bojalil, R., Vallejo, M., Martínez-Lavín, L. (2007). Catechol-O-methyltransferase gene

haplotypes in Mexican and Spanish patients with fibromyalgia. Arthritis Research & Therapy 9 (5), R110.

[146] Veldhuijzen, D., Sondaal, S. and Oosterman, J. (2012). Intact Cognitive Inhibition in Patients With Fibromyalgia but Evidence of Declined Processing Speed. The Journal of Pain 13 (5), 507-515.

[147] Verdejo-Garcia, A., Lopez-Torrecillas, F., Calandre, E.P., Delgado-Rodriguez, A., Bechara, A. (2009). Executive function and decision-making in women with fibromyalgia. Archives of Clinical Neuropsychology 24 (1), 113-122.

[148] Vierck, C.J. (2006). Mechanisms underlying development of spatially distributed chronic pain (fibromyalgia). Pain 124 (3), 242-263.

[149] Walteros, C., Sánchez-Navarro, J.P., Muñoz, M.A., Martínez-Selva, J.M., Chialvo, D., and Montoya, P. (2011). Altered associative learning and emotional decision making in fibromyalgia. Journal of Psychosomatic Research 70 (3), 294-301.

[150] Wiech, K., Seymour, B., Kalisch, R., Stephan, K.E., Koltzenburg, M., Driver, J., Dolan, R.J. (2005). Modulation of pain processing in hyperalgesia by cognitive demand. Neuroimage 27 (1), 59-69.

[151] Wiech, K, Ploner, M, & Tracey, I. (2008). Neurocognitive aspects of pain perception. Cell 12 (8), 306-313

[152] Williams, D.A., Clauw, D.J., Glass, J. (2011). Perceived Cognitive Dysfunction in Fibromyalgia Syndrome. Journal of Musculoskeletal Pain 19 (2), 66-75.

[153] Woolf, C.J. (2004). Pain: moving from symptom control toward mechanism-specific pharmacologic management. Annual International Medicin, 140, 441-451.

[154] Wolfe, F., Clauw, D.J., Fitzcharles, M.A., Goldenberg, D.L., Katz, R.S., Mease, P., Russell, A.S., Russell, I.J., Winfield, J.B., Yunus, M.B. (2010). The American College of Rheumatology preliminary diagnostic criteria for fibromyalgia and measurement of symptom severity. Arthritis Care & Research (Hoboken) 62 (5), 600-610.

[155] Wolfe, F., Smythe, H.A., Yunus, M.B., Bennett, R.M., Bombardier, C., Goldenberg, D.L., Tugwell, P., Campbell, S.M., Abeles, M., Clark, P. (1990). The American College of Rheumatology 1990 Criteria for the Classification of Fibromyalgia. Report of the Multicenter Criteria Committee. Arthritis and Rheumatism 33 (2), 160-172.

[156] Wood, P.B., Glabus, M.F., Simpson, R., Patterson, J.C., 2nd. (2009). Changes in gray matter density in fibromyalgia: correlation with dopamine metabolism. The Journal of Pain 10 (6), 609-618.

[157] Wood, P.B. (2008). Role of central dopamine in pain and analgesia. Expert Review of Neurotherapeutics 8 (5), 781-797.

[158] Wood, P.B., Patterson, I., James, C., Sunderland, J.J., Tainter, K.H., Glabus, M.F., Lilien, D.L. (2007b). Reduced presynaptic dopamine activity in fibromyalgia syndrome

demonstrated with positron emission tomography: a pilot study. The Journal of Pain 8 (1), 51-58.

[159] Wood, P.B., Schweinhardt, P., Jaeger, E., Dagher, A., Hakyemez, H., Rabiner, E.A., Bushnell, M.C., Chizh, B.A. (2007a). Fibromyalgia patients show an abnormal dopamine response to pain. The Journal of Neuroscience 25 (12), 3576-3582.

[160] Xiao, Y., He, W., Russell, I.J. (2011). Genetic polymorphisms of the beta2-adrenergic receptor relate to guanosine protein-coupled stimulator receptor dysfunction in fibromyalgia syndrome. The Journal of Rheumatology 38 (6), 1095-1103.

[161] Zhang, Y., Bertolino, A., Fazio, L., Blasi, G., Rampino, A., Romano, R., Lee, M.L., Xiao, T., Papp, A., Wang, D., Sadée, W. (2007). Polymorphisms in human dopamine D2 receptor gene affect gene expression, splicing, and neuronal activity during working memory. Proceedings of the National Academy of Sciences of the United States of America 104 (51), 20552-20557.

[162] Zubieta, J.K., Heitzeg, M.M., Smith, Y.R., et al. (2003). COMT val158met genotype affects mu-opioid neurotransmitter responses to a pain stressor. Science 299 (5610), 1240–1243.

Chapter 22

FDG- PET Imaging in Neurodegenerative Brain Diseases

L. K. Teune, A. L. Bartels and K. L. Leenders

Additional information is available at the end of the chapter

http://dx.doi.org/10.5772/56505

1. Introduction

1.1. Cerebral glucose metabolism

Increases and decreases of synaptic activity in the brain are accompanied by proportional changes in capillary perfusion and local glucose consumption. These changes in glucose consumption are the effect of changed activity or density of the afferent nerve terminals in that region. Loss of neurons may result in decreased glucose consumption in distant brain regions by deafferentiation, while also increased regional glucose consumption by increased activation of afferent neurons can occur. The PET tracer [^{18}F]fluorodeoxyglucose (FDG) allows the measurement of glucose consumption. FDG is a glucose analog with physiological aspects almost identical to glucose. It is transported from the blood to the brain by a carrier-mediated diffusion mechanism. FDG and glucose are phosphorylated by hexokinase as the first step of the glycolytic process. FDG differs from glucose in that a hydrogen atom replaced the hydroxyl group at the second carbon atom of the molecule. Glucose is then phosphorylated to glucose-6-PO_4, and continues along the glycolytic pathway for energy production. However, FDG is phosphorylated to FDG-6-PO_4, which is not a substrate for further metabolism and trapped in tissues. As glucose is the only source of energy for the brain it reflects the neuronal integrity of underlying brain pathology. Since FDG is a competitive substrate with glucose for both transport and phosphorylation, it is important for tracer uptake to avoid high blood glucose levels during an FDG-PET scan in subjects with diabetes.

In neurodegenerative brain diseases, specific brain regions degenerate and specific patterns of metabolic brain activity develop. This happens before clear structural changes can be detected with imaging techniques.

Measurement of glucose consumption with FDG PET imaging thus allows us to identify disease-specific cerebral metabolic brain patterns in several neurodegenerative brain diseases at an early disease stage. Since the first FDG PET study in man in 1979 (Reivich, et al. 1979) regional differences in cerebral glucose metabolism have been reported in various neurodegenerative brain diseases including parkinsonian syndromes.

2. Disease-specific metabolic brain patterns: Methods

Univariate methods like voxel-based statistical parametric mapping (SPM) analyses have been used to identify group differences between patients with neurodegenerative brain diseases and controls. (Eckert, et al. 2005, Juh, et al. 2004, Yong, et al. 2007).

At the University Medical Center Groningen, The Netherlands we have performed a retrospective study (Teune, et al. 2010) selecting typical patients with 7 different neurodegenerative brain diseases who had had a clinical FDG brain scan at a time point when their diagnosis was not sure yet. These patients developed in the following years the mentioned typical disease states. Images of each of the seven patient groups were separately compared to controls using a two-sample t test. At those early scans, already typical differences between patient - and control groups were found for each disease.

However, Scaled Subprofile modelling/principal component analysis (SSM/PCA), a multivariate method, not only identifies group differences, but is also able to identify relationships in relatively increased and decreased metabolic activity between different brain regions in combined samples of patients and control scans (Eidelberg. 2009, Moeller, et al. 1987). Covariance analysis techniques are considered appropriate methods to explore network activity. In the SSM, a threshold of the whole-brain maximum can be applied to remove out-of-brain voxels, followed by a log transformation. A threshold of 35% is used by the Eidelberg research group resulting in a mask of mainly grey matter (Spetsieris and Eidelberg. 2010). After removing between-subject and between-region averages, a principal component analysis (PCA) can be applied. PCA transformes a set of correlated variables into a new set of orthogonal uncorrelated variables that are called the principal components. Voxels participating in each principal component (PC) may have either a positive or a negative loading. The loadings express the covariance structure (i.e. the strength of the interaction) between the voxels that participate in the PC. They are ordered in terms of the variability they represent. That is, the first principal components represents for a single dimension (variable) the greatest amount of variability in the original dataset. Each succeeding orthogonal component accounts for as much of the remaining variability as possible. They can be very helpful in determining how many of the components are really significant and how much the data can be reduced.

In most studies, the components that together describe at least 50% of the variance are used for further analysis, but this is an arbitrary limit. To identify a covariance pattern that best discriminates a patient group from a control group, each subject's expression of the selected principal components with the lowest AIC (Akaike information criterion) value (Akaike. 1974) are entered into a stepwise regression procedure. This regression results in a linear combination of the PCs that best discriminated the two groups and is designated as the disease-specific metabolic covariance pattern.

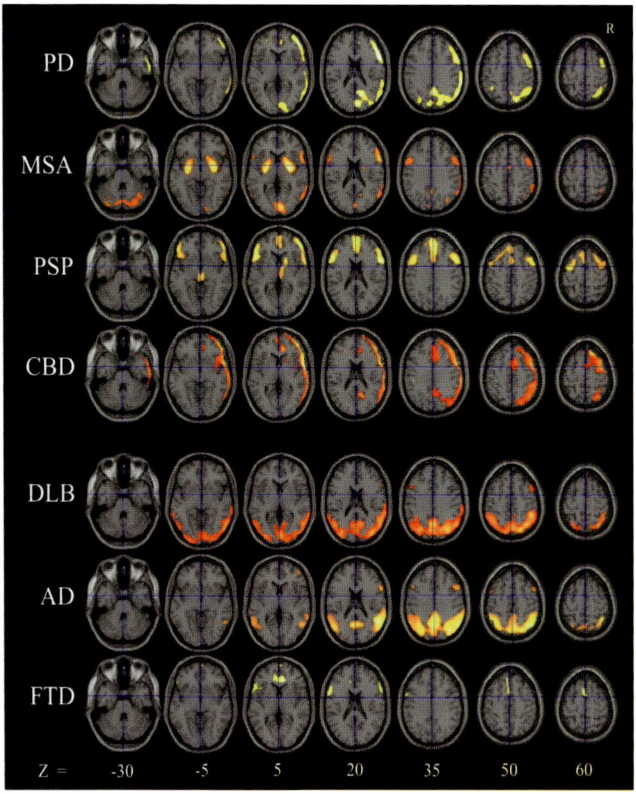

Figure 1. Typical cerebral metabolic patterns in neurodegenerative brain diseases. SPM (t) maps of decreased metabolic activity were overlaid on a T1 MR template thresholded at P< 0.001 with cluster cutoff of 20 voxels. Patient groups are indicated on the vertical axis and on the horizontal axis, seven transversal slices through the brain are shown. PD = Parkinson's disease: decreased metabolic activity in the contralateral to the most affected body side parieto-occipital and frontal regions; MSA = multiple system atrophy: decreased metabolic activity in bilateral putamen and cerebellum; PSP = progressive supranuclear palsy: decreased metabolic activity in the prefrontal cortex, caudate nucleus, thalamus and mesencephalon; CBD = corticobasal degeneration: decreased metabolic activity in the contralateral to the most affected body side cortical regions; DLB = dementia with Lewy bodies: decreased metabolic activity in the occipital and parieto-temporal regions. AD = Alzheimer's Disease: decreased metabolic activity in the angular gyrus and other parieto-temporal regions including precuneus extending to the posterior- and middle cingulate gyrus. FTD = frontotemporal dementia: decreased metabolic activity in the superior and inferior frontal gyrus, anterior cingulate gyrus, SMA, sensorimotor area and middle temporal gyrus. Adapted from: Teune et al. (2010) Typical cerebral metabolic patterns in neurodegenerative brain diseases. Movement Disorders. 2010;25:2395-404.

Important for its use in clinical practice is that this metabolic covariance pattern can then be applied to individual patients to test whether they express the pattern or not. Every voxel value in a subject scan is multiplied by the corresponding voxel weight in the covariance pattern, with a subsequent summation over the whole brain volume. The resulting subject score captures to what extent a subject expresses the covariance pattern.

3. Disease-specific metabolic brain patterns in patients with parkinsonism

3.1. Parkinson's disease

Parkinson's disease (PD) is characterized by bradykinesia, rigidity, sometimes rest tremor and postural instability. A disturbed α-synuclein protein forming so-called Lewy bodies seems to play a causal role, which was a reason to designate PD as a α-synucleinopathy. The main pathophysiological changes result from degeneration of catecholaminergic, especially dopaminergic cells in brainstem regions.

A characteristic metabolic covariance pattern has been identified in PD patients (PD-related pattern, PDRP) showing regionally relatively increased metabolism in the globus pallidus and putamen, thalamus, pons and cerebellum and relatively decreased metabolism in the lateral frontal, premotor and parietal association areas (Ma, et al. 2007) Network expression in PD patients also increases linearly with disease progression(Huang, et al. 2007b). Tang et al. tried to study network changes in the PD-related motor pattern before symptom onset by studying 15 hemiparkinsonian patients and focusing mainly on the "presymptomatic" hemisphere. They conclude that abnormal PDRP activity antecedes the appearance of motor signs by approximately 2 years (Tang, et al. 2010a). However, this needs to be proven in future research in true presymptomatic patients.

3.2. Parkinson's disease and metabolic brain patterns related to specific symptoms

In addition to motor symptoms, cognitive dysfunction is also common in PD, especially executive and visuospatial dysfunction. FDG-PET studies have been performed to study these specific symptoms and their relations with neural network pathophysiology. The Eidelberg research group has shown PD subclassifications related to specific symptoms. Network analysis with the SSM/PCA approach detected a significant covariance pattern in non-demented PD patients that correlated with memory and executive functioning tasks. The expression of this PD-related cognitive pattern (PDCP) in individual patients correlated with severity of cognitive dysfunction(Huang, et al. 2007a).

Alterations in neuropsychological test results in advanced PD were found to correlate with decreases in glucose metabolism in the dorsolateral prefrontal cortex (DLPFC), lateral orbitofrontal cortex (LOFC) ventral and dorsal cingulum (v/dACC) and in Broca area (Kalbe, et al. 2009). In the study of Kalbe et al, PD patients with deep brain stimulation in the subthalamic nucleus (STN-DBS) showed cognitive decline that correlated with decrease in glucose metabolism in these areas. In another study in STN-DBS treated patients, STN DBS was found to activate glucose metabolism in the frontal limbic and associative territory (Hilker, et al. 2004). Interestingly, cortical areas that show hypometabolism in patients with depression (Mayberg HS. 1994) are similar to the regions that show restored glucose metabolism after STN DBS. This finding agrees with the clinical observation that PD-related depression tends to improve after STN DBS.

Mure et al. identified a spatial covariance pattern associated with Parkinson tremor which was characterized by covarying increases in the cerebellum/dentate nucleus and primary cortex and to a minor degree in the caudate/putamen (Mure, et al. 2011).

Hallucinations in PD have been related to relative frontal hypermetabolism compared to PD patients without hallucinations(Nagano-Saito, et al. 2004). However, another study showed hypometabolism in occipitotemporoparietal regions in PD patients with hallucinations, sparing the occipital pole, while no significant increase in regional glucose metabolism was detected (Boecker, et al. 2007). Interestingly, in patients with dementia with Lewy bodies (DLB), who also suffer from hallucinations, glucose metabolism was also decreased in occipitoparietal regions, however without sparing of the occipital pole (see DLB section).

3.3. Multiple system atrophy

Multiple system atrophy is a sporadic neurodegenerative brain disease which affects both men and women and generally starts in the sixth decade of life. The main clinical features are parkinsonism, autonomic failure, cerebellar ataxia, and pyramidal signs in any combination. However, two major motor presentations can be distinguished. Parkinsonian features predominate in 80% of patients (MSA-P subtype) and cerebellar ataxia is the main motor feature in 20% of patients (MSA-C subtype) ((Gilman, et al. 2008, Wenning, et al. 1997)

In MSA-P the striatonigral system is the main site of pathology but less severe degeneration can be widespread and normally includes the olivopontocerebellar system. In MSA-C pathological changes are mainly seen in the olivopontocerebellar system and involvement of striatum and substantia nigra are less severe (Wenning, et al. 1997). The discovery of glial cytoplasmic inclusions in MSA brains highlighted the unique glial pathology as biological hallmark of the disease. Their distribution selectively involves basal ganglia, supplementary and primary motor cortex, the reticular formation and pontocerebellar system. Glial cytoplasmic inclusions contain besides classical cytoskeletal antigens also α-synuclein, which is a presynaptic protein present in Lewy Bodies, and this accumulation seems to play a central part not only in MSA but also in other α-synucleinopathies such as PD and DLB.

Disease-related metabolic patterns were also present in MSA consisting of hypometabolism in putamen and cerebellum in MSA (Eckert, et al. 2008). Poston et al. found that differences in expression of the MSA-related pattern correlated with clinical disability (Poston, et al. 2012).

3.4. Progressive supranuclear palsy

The clinical picture of progressive supranuclear palsy (PSP) has been first described by Steele, Richardson and Olszewski (Steele JC, Richardson J,Olszewski J. 1964) and is characterized by progressive parkinsonism, early gait and balance impairment, vertical gaze palsy and more profound frontal cognitive disturbances. PSP is one of several neurodegenerative diseases characterised by accumulation of hyperphosphorylated tau (tauopathy), forming abnormal filamentous inclusions in neurons and glia in the precentral and postcentral cortical areas but also in the thalamus, subthalamic nucleus, red nucleus and substantia nigra. Other neurodegenerative brain diseases which show disturbances in tau protein handling are corticobasal degeneration (CBD) and frontotemporal dementia (FTD) but there is also overlap in pathology with Alzheimer's disease (AD).

However the metabolic brain patterns in these tauopathies are quite different. The covariance pattern of PSP consists of decreased metabolism in the prefrontal cortex, frontal eye fields, caudate nuclei, medial thalamus and upper brainstem (Eckert, et al. 2008). Brain stem atrophy and atrophy of the medial frontal cortical regions have also been reported in histopathological studies (Hauw, et al. 1994).

3.5. Corticobasal degeneration

The most striking features of patients with corticobasal degeneration (CBD) include marked asymmetrical parkinsonism and apraxia but also postural instability, limb dystonia, cortical sensory loss, dementia and the alien limb phenomenon. CBD is one of the tauopathies and clinical diagnosis is complicated by both the variability of presentation of true CBD and the syndromes that look alike but are caused by other tauopathies with parkinsonism like PSP or FTD (Josephs, et al. 2006). However with functional neuroimaging a clear distinction can be made. In CBD a typical pattern of hypometabolism is seen in cortical regions contralateral to the affected body side, including parieto-temporal regions, prefrontal cortex and motor cortex. Furthermore, a decrease can be found in the contralateral caudate nucleus, putamen and thalamus (Eckert, et al. 2005, Teune, et al. 2010). No covariance pattern has been described using the SSM/PCA technique in CBD.

4. Disease-specific metabolic brain patterns in the differential diagnosis of individual patients with parkinsonism

Interestingly, Tang and co-workers studied the potential role of FDG PET in the individual diagnosis of 167 patients who had parkinsonian features but uncertain clinical diagnosis (Tang, et al. 2010b) After FDG PET imaging, patients were assessed by blinded movement disorders specialists for a mean of 2.6 years before a final clinical diagnosis was made (gold standard). SSM/PCA analysis can quantify the expression of an obtained covariance pattern in each subject which allows assessing the expression of a given pattern on a single case basis. Using this automated image-based classification procedure and the previously defined disease related covariance patterns in PD, MSA and PSP, individual patients were differentiated with high specificity.

However, blinded, prospective imaging studies (ideally involving multiple centers, a larger validation group, repeat imaging, and more extensive post-mortem confirmation) are needed to establish the accuracy and precision of this pattern-based categorisation procedure. These studies are currently undertaken.

For routine clinical practice, this knowledge of disease specific patterns of regional metabolic activity in neurodegenerative brain diseases can be a valuable aid in the differential diagnosis of individual patients, especially at an early disease stage.

http://dx.doi.org/10.5772/56505

5. Disease-specific metabolic brain patterns in dementia

5.1. Alzheimer's disease

Alzheimer's disease (AD) is a progressive neurodegenerative brain disease accounting for 50-60% of cases of dementia. AD is characterized by a severe decline in episodic memory together with general cognitive symptoms such as impaired judgement, decision making and orientation (McKhann, et al. 1984). A correct clinical diagnosis can be difficult, especially in early disease stages or in patients with for example comorbid depression, high education or young age (Bohnen, et al. 2012). FDG-PET imaging can be used to assist in the differential diagnosis, because for different dementia syndromes, a separate pattern of hypometabolism can be found. In Alzheimer's disease (AD), decline of FDG uptake in posterior cingulate, temporoparietal and prefrontal association cortex was related to dementia severity (Herholz, et al. 2002). Foster et al used visual interpretation of an automated three-dimensional stereotactic surface projection technique of patients with AD and FTD. They showed that visual interpretation of FDG-PET scans after training is more reliable and accurate in distinguishing FTD from AD than clinical methods alone (Foster, et al. 2007).

Although multivariate analytical techniques might identify diagnostic patterns that are not captured by univariate methods, they have rarely been used to study neural correlates of Alzheimer's Disease or cognitive impairment. Because cognitive processes are the result of integrated activity in networks rather than activity of any one area in isolation, functional connectivity can be better captured by multivariate methods. A study from Habeck et al. examined the efficacy of multivariate and univariate analytical methods and concluded that multivariate analysis might be more sensitive than univariate analysis for the diagnosis of early Alzheimer's disease (Habeck, et al. 2008).

Scarmeas et al. were the first to derive an AD related covariance pattern using $H_2{}^{15}O$ to measure brain perfusion (Scarmeas, et al. 2004). It consisted of relatively increased perfusion in the bilateral insula, lingual gyri and cuneus with bilaterally decreased flow in bilateral inferior parietal lobule and cingulate in AD patients. However, using this PET tracer they found a sensitivity of 76-94% and a specificity of 63-81% with considerable overlap in pattern expression among AD patients and controls. Therefore they concluded that the derived $H_2{}^{15}O$ pattern cannot be used as a sufficient diagnostic test in clinical settings. Specific FDG covariance patterns to distinguish early AD-related cognitive decline using multivariate methods have yet to be specified.

5.2. Frontotemporal dementia

Frontotemporal dementia (FTD) is one of the neurodegenerative diseases commonly mistaken for AD. FTD patients do not have a true amnestic syndrome but can present with either gradual and progressive changes in behaviour, or gradual and progressive language dysfunction. Gross examination of the post-mortem brain from a patient with FTD usually reveals frontal or temporal lobar atrophy or both, but the distribution or severity of brain atrophy are not specific for a particular neurodegenerative brain disease. Jeong et al. and Diehl-Schmid et al.

analysed FDG-PET scans of FTD patients on a voxel-by-voxel basis using Statistical Parametric Mapping (SPM). They found hypometabolism depending on disease stage in the frontal lobe, parietal and temporal cortices (Diehl-Schmid, et al. 2007, Jeong, et al. 2005).

5.3. Dementia with Lewy Bodies

The clinical overlap of dementia and parkinsonism is highlighted in Dementia with Lewy Bodies (DLB). These patients show besides dementia extrapyramidal motor symptoms and marked neuropsychiatric disturbances including visual hallucinations, depression, variability in arousal and attention (McKeith. 2006). Consistent observation of a metabolic reduction in the medial occipital cortex in DLB patients (Minoshima, et al. 2001, Teune, et al. 2010) using FDG-PET imaging suggests the use of FDG-PET in the differential diagnosis of AD and DLB and of PD and DLB. Minoshima et al. found that the presence of occipital hypometabolism distinguished DLB from AD with 90% sensitivity and 80% specificity when using post-mortem diagnosis as the gold standard diagnosis (Minoshima, et al. 2001).

6. Disease-specific metabolic brain patterns in hyperkinetic movement disorders

6.1. Huntington's disease

Huntington's disease (HD) is characterized by progressive dementia and chorea, starting around 30-40 years of age. HD is caused by a dominantly inherited CAG repeat expansion mutation that generates lengthening of the protein huntingtin, with size-dependent neuro-toxicity. Several PET studies have shown hypometabolism in the caudate nucleus, both in symptomatic and asymptomatic mutation carriers (Grafton, et al. 1992) (Antonini A., et al. 1996) In asymptomatic carriers, metabolic decreases were also significantly associated with the CAG repeat number (Antonini A., et al. 1996). Furthermore, it was found that FDG uptake in the caudate nucleus provided a predictive measure for time of onset of the disease, in addition to the mutation size (Ciarmiello A., et al. 2012).

Another study applied network analysis of FDG-PET scans in presymptomatic mutation carriers (Feigin, et al. 2001). They found a HD related metabolic covariance pattern (HDRP) characterized by caudate and putamenal hypometabolism, but also including mediotemporal reductions as well as relative increases in occipital regions. Disturbances of these striatotem-poral projections may underlie aspects of the psychiatric and cognitive abnormalities that occur in the earliest stages of HD, before the onset of motor signs (Cummings JL. 1995).

6.2. Dystonia

Dystonia is a movement disorder characterized by involuntary, sustained muscle contractions causing twisting movements and abnormal postures. The most common forms of primary torsion dystonia (PTD) are DYT1 and DYT6, both caused by autosomal inherited mutations with a reduced penetrance.

Functional neuroimaging techniques have been applied in different dystonic disorders including primary generalized dystonia, mainly DYT1 and DYT6 and dopa-responsive dystonia, as well as focal dystonic syndromes such as torticollis, writer's cramp and blepharospasm. A common finding is abnormality of the basal ganglia, cerebellum and associated outflow pathways to sensorimotor cortex and other regions involved with motor performance. However, controversial results have been found in imaging dystonias, partly attributed to methodological differences but also to the heterogeneity of the dystonias. Using the SSM/PCA approach a reproducible pattern of abnormal regional glucose utilization in two independent cohorts of DYT1 carriers have been found (Eidelberg D. 1998)(Trost M., et al. 2002).

This torsion-dystonia related metabolic pattern is characterized by increases in the posterior putamen/globus pallidus, cerebellum and SMA. Interestingly, also in clinically non-manifesting mutation carriers this pattern was found, suggesting a cerebral "vulnerability to develop dystonia" network change. Also in manifesting and non-manifesting DYT 6 carriers abnormal network activity has been identified. A difference between DYT1 and DYT6 metabolic patterns can be seen in the putamen, where glucose metabolism is increased in DYT1 and decreased in DYT6, possibly do to cell loss in DYT6. Furthermore, the cerebellum shows increased activity in DYT1 and normal activity in DYT6 (Carbon M., et al. 2004).

The TDRP network is not expressed in patients with Dopa-responsive dystonia (DRD) (Trost M., et al. 2002).

DRD is characterized by an early onset of dystonic symptoms and later appearance of parkinsonian symptoms. A defining feature is a marked and sustained response to low doses of levodopa, suggesting that the lesion may be functional in the presynaptic dopaminergic system rather than anatomical. The DRD related metabolic pattern is characterized by relative increases in the dorsal midbrain, cerebellar vermis,and SMA, assiocated with covarying decreases in putamen, lateral premotor and motor cortical regions (Asanuma, et al. 2005b). This DRD related pattern is not apparent in DYT 1 and 6 carriers supporting the hypothesis that the pathophysiology of DRD differs from that of other forms of dystonia. They also found that the Parkinson-related metabolic pattern is not apparent in DRD patients. Thus FDG-PET can be useful to distinguish PD related dystonia from dopa-responsive dystonia with parkinsonism (Asanuma, et al. 2005a).

6.3. Gilles de la Tourette

Tourette syndrome is characterized by the presence of chronic motor and vocal tics that develop before the age of 18. Comorbid behavioural abnormalities are common in Tourette syndrome, most notably obsessive-compulsive disorder and attention deficit/hyperactivity disorder (Lebowitz, et al. 2012). The neurophysiology remains poorly understood with varying and inconsistent neuropathological and neuroimaging findings, possibly due to the clinical heterogeneity of the disorder. Pourfar et al. identified a Tourette syndrome related pattern characterized by reduced metabolic activity of the striatum and orbitofrontal cortex associated with relatively increased metabolic activity in the premotor cortex and cerebellum. A second metabolic brain pattern was found in patients with Tourette syndrome and obsessive compulsive disorder characterized by reduced activity in the anterior cingulate and dorsolateral prefrontal cortex and relative increases in primary motor cortex and precuneus. Subject expression correlated with symptom severity. These findings suggest that the different clinical manifestations of the Tourette syndrome are associated with different abnormal brain networks (Pourfar, et al. 2011).

7. Conclusion

FDG-PET imaging is increasingly available for routine clinical practice and has remained the only available radiotracer to detect accurately and reliably the cerebral glucose metabolism. As glucose is the only source of energy for the brain it reflects the energy needs of underlying brain neuronal systems. The SSM/PCA method can identify relationships in relatively increased and decreased metabolic activity between different brain regions in combined samples of patients and controls. The expression of an obtained covariance pattern can be quantified in an individual patient and this resulting subject score captures to what extent a patient expresses the covariance patterns. The disease-related metabolic brain patterns can therefore be a valuable aid in the early differential diagnosis of individual patients with neurodegenerative brain diseases.

Author details

L. K. Teune, A. L. Bartels* and K. L. Leenders

*Address all correspondence to: a.l.bartels@umcg.nl

Department of Neurology, University Medical Center Groningen, The Netherlands

References

[1] Akaike, H. A new look at the statistical model identification. A New Look at the Statistical Model Identification (1974)., 1974, 716-23.

[2] Antonini, A, Leenders, K. L, Spiegel, R, Meier, D, Vontobel, P, Weigell-weber, M, et al. Striatal glucose metabolism and dopamine D2 receptor binding in asymptomatic gene carriers and patients with huntington's disease. (1996).

[3] Asanuma, K, Carbon-correll, M, & Eidelberg, D. Neuroimaging in human dystonia. (2005a).

[4] Asanuma, K, Ma, Y, Huang, C, Carbon-correll, M, Edwards, C, Raymond, D, et al. The metabolic pathology of dopa-responsive dystonia. (2005b).

[5] Boecker, H, Ceballos-baumann, A. O, Volk, D, Conrad, B, Forstl, H, & Haussermann, P. Metabolic alterations in patients with parkinson disease and visual hallucinations. Arch Neurol (2007). , 64, 984-8.

[6] Bohnen, N. I. Djang DSW, Herholz K, Anzai Y, Minoshima S. Effectiveness and safety of 18F-FDG PET in the evaluation of dementia: A review of the recent literature. Journal of Nuclear Medicine (2012). , 53, 59-71.

[7] Carbon, M, Trost, M, Ghilardi, M. F, & Eidelberg, D. Abnormal brain networks in primary torsion dystonia. (2004).

[8] Ciarmiello, A, Giovacchini, G, Orobello, S, Bruselli, L, Elifani, F, & Squitieri, F. F-FDG PET uptake in the pre-huntington disease caudate affects the time-to-onset independently of CAG expansion size. (2012).

[9] Cummings, J. L. Behavioral and psychiatric symptoms associated with huntington's disease. (1995).

[10] Diehl-schmid, J, Grimmer, T, Drzezga, A, Bornschein, S, Riemenschneider, M, Forstl, H, et al. Decline of cerebral glucose metabolism in frontotemporal dementia: A longitudinal 18F-FDG-PET-study. Neurobiol Aging (2007). , 28, 42-50.

[11] Eckert, T, Barnes, A, Dhawan, V, Frucht, S, Gordon, M. F, Feigin, A. S, et al. FDG PET in the differential diagnosis of parkinsonian disorders. Neuroimage (2005). , 26, 912-21.

[12] Eckert, T, Tang, C, Ma, Y, Brown, N, Lin, T, Frucht, S, et al. Abnormal metabolic networks in atypical parkinsonism. Mov Disord (2008).

[13] Eidelberg, D. Abnormal brain networks in DYT1 dystonia. (1998).

[14] Eidelberg, D. Metabolic brain networks in neurodegenerative disorders: A functional imaging approach. Trends Neurosci (2009). , 32, 548-57.

[15] Feigin, A, Leenders, K. L, Moeller, J. R, Missimer, J, Kuenig, G, Spetsieris, P, et al. Metabolic network abnormalities in early huntington's disease: An [(18)F]FDG PET study. J Nucl Med (2001). , 42, 1591-5.

[16] Foster, N. L, Heidebrink, J. L, Clark, C. M, Jagust, W. J, Arnold, S. E, Barbas, N. R, et al. FDG-PET improves accuracy in distinguishing frontotemporal dementia and alzheimer's disease. Brain (2007). , 130, 2616-35.

[17] Gilman, S, Wenning, G. K, Low, P. A, Brooks, D. J, Mathias, C. J, Trojanowski, J. Q, et al. Second consensus statement on the diagnosis of multiple system atrophy. Neurology (2008). , 71, 670-6.

[18] Grafton, S. T, Mazziotta, J. C, & Pahl, J. J. St George-Hyslop P, Haines JL, Gusella J, et al. Serial changes of cerebral glucose metabolism and caudate size in persons at risk for huntington's disease. (1992).

[19] Habeck, C, Foster, N. L, Perneczky, R, Kurz, A, Alexopoulos, P, Koeppe, R. A, et al. Multivariate and univariate neuroimaging biomarkers of alzheimer's disease. Neuroimage (2008). , 40, 1503-15.

[20] Hauw, J. J, Daniel, S. E, Dickson, D, Horoupian, D. S, Jellinger, K, Lantos, P. L, et al. Preliminary NINDS neuropathologic criteria for steele-richardson-olszewski syndrome (progressive supranuclear palsy). Neurology (1994). , 44, 2015-9.

[21] Herholz, K, Salmon, E, Perani, D, Baron, J. C, Holthoff, V, Frolich, L, et al. Discrimination between alzheimer dementia and controls by automated analysis of multicenter FDG PET. Neuroimage (2002). , 17, 302-16.

[22] Hilker, R, Voges, J, Weisenbach, S, Kalbe, E, Burghaus, L, Ghaemi, M, et al. Subthalamic nucleus stimulation restores glucose metabolism in associative and limbic cortices and in cerebellum: Evidence from a FDG-PET study in advanced parkinson's disease. J Cereb Blood Flow Metab (2004). , 24, 7-16.

[23] Huang, C, Eidelberg, D, Habeck, C, Moeller, J, Svensson, L, Tarabula, T, et al. Imaging markers of mild cognitive impairment: Multivariate analysis of CBF SPECT. Neurobiol Aging (2007a). , 28, 1062-9.

[24] Huang, C, Tang, C, Feigin, A, Lesser, M, Ma, Y, Pourfar, M, et al. Changes in network activity with the progression of parkinson's disease. Brain (2007b). , 130, 1834-46.

[25] Jeong, Y, Cho, S. S, Park, J. M, Kang, S. J, Lee, J. S, Kang, E, et al. F-FDG PET findings in frontotemporal dementia: An SPM analysis of 29 patients. J Nucl Med (2005). , 46, 233-9.

[26] Josephs, K. A, Petersen, R. C, Knopman, D. S, Boeve, B. F, Whitwell, J. L, Duffy, J. R, et al. Clinicopathologic analysis of frontotemporal and corticobasal degenerations and PSP. Neurology (2006). , 66, 41-8.

[27] Juh, R, Kim, J, Moon, D, Choe, B, & Suh, T. Different metabolic patterns analysis of parkinsonism on the 18F-FDG PET. Eur J Radiol (2004). , 51, 223-33.

[28] Kalbe, E, Voges, J, Weber, T, Haarer, M, Baudrexel, S, Klein, J. C, et al. Frontal FDG-PET activity correlates with cognitive outcome after STN-DBS in parkinson disease. Neurology (2009). , 72, 42-9.

[29] Lebowitz, E. R, Motlagh, M. G, Katsovich, L, King, R. A, Lombroso, P. J, Grantz, H, et al. Tourette syndrome in youth with and without obsessive compulsive disorder and attention deficit hyperactivity disorder. (2012).

[30] Ma, Y, Tang, C, Spetsieris, P. G, Dhawan, V, & Eidelberg, D. Abnormal metabolic network activity in parkinson's disease: Test-retest reproducibility. Journal of cerebral blood flow and metabolism : official journal of the International Society of Cerebral Blood Flow and Metabolism (2007). , 27, 597-605.

[31] Mayberg, H. S. Frontal lobe dysfunction in secondary depression. (1994).

[32] Mckeith, I. G. Consensus guidelines for the clinical and pathologic diagnosis of dementia with lewy bodies (DLB): Report of the consortium on DLB international workshop. J Alzheimers Dis (2006). , 9, 417-23.

[33] Mckhann, G, Drachman, D, Folstein, M, Katzman, R, Price, D, & Stadlan, E. M. Clinical diagnosis of alzheimer's disease: Report of the NINCDS-ADRDA work group under the auspices of department of health and human services task force on alzheimer's disease 35. Neurology (1984). , 34, 939-44.

[34] Minoshima, S, Foster, N. L, Sima, A. A, Frey, K. A, Albin, R. L, & Kuhl, D. E. Alzheimer's disease versus dementia with lewy bodies: Cerebral metabolic distinction with autopsy confirmation. Ann Neurol (2001). , 50, 358-65.

[35] Moeller, J. R, Strother, S. C, Sidtis, J. J, & Rottenberg, D. A. Scaled subprofile model: A statistical approach to the analysis of functional patterns in positron emission tomographic data. J Cereb Blood Flow Metab (1987). , 7, 649-58.

[36] Mure, H, Hirano, S, Tang, C. C, Isaias, I. U, Antonini, A, Ma, Y, et al. Parkinson's disease tremor-related metabolic network: Characterization, progression, and treatment effects. Neuroimage (2011). , 54, 1244-53.

[37] Nagano-saito, A, Washimi, Y, Arahata, Y, Iwai, K, Kawatsu, S, Ito, K, et al. Visual hallucination in parkinson's disease with FDG PET. Mov Disord (2004). , 19, 801-6.

[38] Poston, K. L, Tang, C. C, Eckert, T, Dhawan, V, Frucht, S, Vonsattel, J, et al. Network correlates of disease severity in multiple system atrophy. Neurology (2012). , 78, 1237-44.

[39] Pourfar, M, Feigin, A, Tang, C. C, Carbon-correll, M, Bussa, M, Budman, C, et al. Abnormal metabolic brain networks in tourette syndrome. Neurology (2011). , 76, 944-52.

[40] Reivich, M, Kuhl, D, Wolf, A, Greenberg, J, Phelps, M, Ido, T, et al. The [18F]fluorodeoxyglucose method for the measurement of local cerebral glucose utilization in man. Circ Res (1979). , 44, 127-37.

[41] Scarmeas, N, Habeck, C. G, Zarahn, E, Anderson, K. E, Park, A, Hilton, J, et al. Covariance PET patterns in early alzheimer's disease and subjects with cognitive impairment but no dementia: Utility in group discrimination and correlations with functional performance. Neuroimage (2004). , 23, 35-45.

[42] Spetsieris, P. G, & Eidelberg, D. Scaled subprofile modeling of resting state imaging data in parkinson's disease: Methodological issues. Neuroimage (2010).

[43] Steele, J. C, Richardson, J, & Olszewski, J. Progressive supranuclear palsy: A heterogeneous degeneration involving the brain stem, basal ganglia and cerebellum with vertical gaze and pseudobulbar palsy, nuchal dystonia and dementia. Archives of Neurology (1964). , 10, 333-59.

[44] Tang, C. C, Poston, K. L, Dhawan, V, & Eidelberg, D. Abnormalities in metabolic network activity precede the onset of motor symptoms in parkinson's disease. J Neurosci (2010a). , 30, 1049-56.

[45] Tang, C. C, Poston, K. L, Eckert, T, Feigin, A, Frucht, S, Gudesblatt, M, et al. Differential diagnosis of parkinsonism: A metabolic imaging study using pattern analysis. Lancet Neurol (2010b). , 9, 149-58.

[46] Teune, L. K, Bartels, A. L, De Jong, B. M, Willemsen, A. T, Eshuis, S. A, De Vries, J. J, et al. Typical cerebral metabolic patterns in neurodegenerative brain diseases. Mov Disord (2010). , 25, 2395-404.

[47] Trost, M, Carbon, M, Edwards, C, Ma, Y, Raymond, D, Mentis, M. J, et al. Primary dystonia: Is abnormal functional brain architecture linked to genotype? (2002).

[48] Wenning, G. K, & Tison, F. Ben Shlomo Y, Daniel SE, Quinn NP. Multiple system atrophy: A review of 203 pathologically proven cases. Mov Disord (1997). , 12, 133-47.

[49] Yong, S. W, Yoon, J. K, An, Y. S, & Lee, P. H. A comparison of cerebral glucose metabolism in parkinson's disease, parkinson's disease dementia and dementia with lewy bodies. Eur J Neurol (2007). , 14, 1357-62.

Chapter 23

Quantitative Mapping of Angiogenesis by Magnetic Resonance Imaging

Teodora-Adriana Perles-Barbacaru and
Hana Lahrech

Additional information is available at the end of the chapter

http://dx.doi.org/10.5772/56492

1. Introduction

Since tumors are commonly associated with angiogenesis and compromised vascular wall integrity, the ability to focus noninvasive imaging techniques on vascular characteristics provides a physiologically-specific approach to tumor delineation which is of utility in guiding the biopsy and in surgical or radiation treatment planning. Hypervascularisation mapped by magnetic resonance imaging (MRI) correlates with histologically-assessed tumor grade [1]. It is also of value in distinguishing residual or recurrent tumor from treatment effects such as radiation induced necrosis [2]. Furthermore, by quantitatively assessing tumor vascularity and endothelial permeability, these approaches allow the evaluation of novel anti-angiogenic therapies, guiding drug development through preclinical stages, and facilitate the inter- and intra-subject comparisons. They also allow the assessment of the biological efficacy of therapies in the clinical setting, before more traditional criteria, such as tumor size change, become apparent. This is particularly important with novel antiangiogenic agents to distinguish potential responders from nonresponders.

This chapter focuses on MRI techniques for angiogenesis assessment. In particular it describes a newly developed quantitative MRI technique for in vivo blood volume fraction mapping for preclinical and above all for clinical applications in neurooncology. The blood volume fraction is a biomarker for angiogenesis and has proven successful in mapping brain dysfunction and in testing drug efficacy. The described technique is compared with other magnetic resonance imaging techniques currently employed in the preclinical and clinical setting. Therefore, this chapter provides an overview of existing quantitative MRI techniques, briefly explains their basic principle, states their acquisition and postprocessing requirements, and compares their advantages and limits. Quantitative results for blood volume fraction measures in laboratory animals and human subjects are presented and compared. Pitfalls and possibilities in neuro-oncological applications are pointed out and discussed.

2. When and why do we need to image angiogenesis?

The vasculature of brain tissue is a complex entity having multiple functions and regulatory mechanisms. One of its functions is to maintain and adjust the blood supply to meet the energy demands of the brain tissue. Most adjustments occur at the microscopic level. Tissues with a high metabolic turnover are generally equipped with a more extensive network of microvessels. Tumor growth and metastasis depend on tumor-induced angiogenesis, i.e. cancer cells with increased metabolism attract and maintain a blood supply [3, 4].

Brain capillaries are composed of a unique and continuous layer of endothelial cells connected by adhesion proteins. In addition, pericytes and foot like processes of astrocytes surround the basal lamina. This forms a regulatory interface between the blood and the cerebral parenchyma: the blood brain barrier (BBB). It is impermeable to many water soluble macromolecules, including many drugs and magnetic resonance contrast agents (CAs). However, the BBB is disrupted in many pathologic processes that involve inflammation or neovascularisation such as tumor growth.

Angiogenesis in malignant tumor tissue is structurally and functionally different from physiologic angiogenesis occurring during fetal development or tissue repair. The microvascular architecture is characterized by tortuous vessels with varying diameter, abnormal branching pattern and blind ending protrusions. Fast growing tumor vasculature is usually immature and lacks the regulatory mechanisms and competent BBB. This leads to a heterogeneous perfusion with parts of the tumor that are hyperperfused due to high microvascular density, and other parts that are hypoperfused with a low proportion of functional vessels. Blood turbulence and stasis as well as endothelial dysfunction lead to thrombosis. Remaining vessels may enlarge in an effort to compensate for the reduced blood flow. The resulting tissue hypoxia triggers secretion of angiogenic factors which maintain the angiogenic process [5]. Hyperpermeability of the incompetent BBB to macromolecules leads to edema and increased interstitial pressure which in turn may impede delivery of therapeutic agents to the tumor tissue.

Figure 1 shows representative vessel sections from healthy rat brain tissue and an experimental brain tumor.

Along with the mitotic index, presence of necrotic areas, invasive potential and cell differentiation, angiogenesis has been recognized as one of the diagnostic criterions of malignancy in the World Health Organization (WHO) classification. Similar to the presence of mitosis and necrosis, vascular proliferation is significantly correlated to survival [6-10]. Although neuroradiologic features can be highly suggestive, diagnosis is based on histologic examination. Neuroradiologic mapping of angiogenesis is important to guide the biopsy needle to sample appropriate tissue. After grading is established neuroimaging techniques help to delineate the

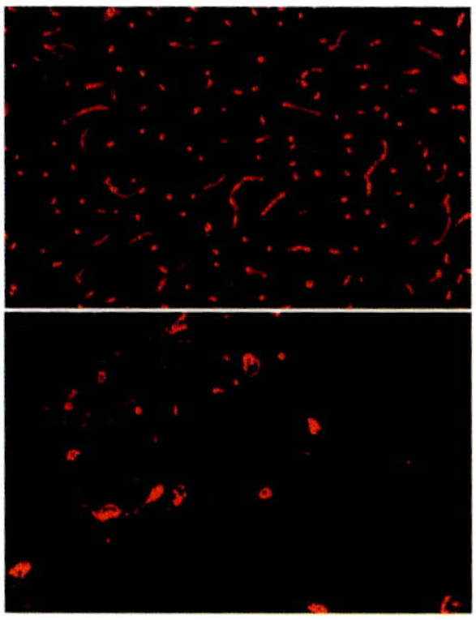

Figure 1. Immunofluorescent staining of collagen IV a component of the basal lamina of the vessel wall. a: Cortical vessels in a healthy rat are delicate, with a narrow distribution of vessel radii around 8 μm and randomly oriented and homogenously distributed. b: Tumor vasculature in a C6 glioma model is composed of sparse irregularly shaped and enlarged vessels. Parts of the tumor are not perfused.

tumor for radiotherapy and/or surgical planning. Magnetic resonance imaging (MRI) capable of multiparametric mapping and yielding high soft tissue contrast is widely used for diagnosis, surgical and radiation treatment planning as well as for treatment follow up. In many imaging facilities, perfusion MRI used to map vascular and hemodynamic parameters is part of the neuroimaging protocol, at least for diagnosis and treatment planning. In the advent of new treatment strategies targeted at the angiogenic process, noninvasive mapping of angiogenesis by MRI will become a requisite to monitor treatment efficacy in follow up studies.

3. What are imaging biomarkers of angiogenesis?

At the microscopic level, several parameters are used to describe and quantify the vascular network. Microvascular density, N_v (cm^{-2}), simply reports the number of vessels per unit area regardless of their shape, orientation or size. Together with the vascular volume density, which is the volume occupied by vascular walls and blood per unit volume of tissue, the microvascular density is the most frequently used parameter for angiogenesis quantification. The microvascular surface S_v is important for exchange processes between blood and interstitium and is approximately 100 cm^2g^{-1} tissue [11]. The length density L_v (cm^{-2}) is the total length of microvessels existing per unit volume of tissue. The vessel radii are important for rheological considerations because they define the cross sectional area that in turn is one of the parameters that determines the blood flow rate. The vascular area density is the ratio between the total area of vessel cross sections and the area of the region of interest (ROI) and correlates with the vascular volume density. The mean intercapillary distance in the human brain is about 40 μm [12] and is an index of the access of an interstitial cell to the exchange processes at the vascular boundary, since in the interstitium transport is mainly governed by diffusion. Other morphological parameters that change under physiologic and pathologic conditions exist, e. g. the tortuosity, interbranching distance, branching angle. Typical microvasculature from mouse cortex and tumor tissue is shown in Figure 12 b.

However MRI and other medical imaging techniques, such as computed tomography (CT) or positron emission tomography (PET) are rather macroscopic techniques. Obviously the above mentioned morphometric parameters of microvessels are not directly measurable. However, some hemodynamic parameters are accessible by these imaging techniques. One of them is the regional cerebral blood volume (CBV), which is the quantity of blood in ml per 100 g tissue that participates in the supply of oxygen and nutrients and in the discharge of toxic metabolites. It is often also expressed as a volume fraction (blood volume fraction, BVf), approximates the vascular volume density reported in microscopy studies and is related to the mean vascular diameter, the microvascular density and length density all of which are altered in the angiogenic process occurring in tumors. The conversion factor between both units is $100\ \lambda/\varrho_{blood} \approx 93.75$ where λ is the brain-blood partition coefficient and ϱ_{blood} is the blood density [13]. CBV mapping has proven successful in assessing angiogenesis to study brain dysfunction and in testing drug efficacy.

Another parameter is the cerebral blood flow (CBF), which is the amount of blood arriving and leaving the tissue of interest in a time interval. The average CBF in humans is approximately 50 ml/min per 100g of brain tissue, while the critical threshold for neuronal function is approximately 20 ml/min per 100g. Another often reported quantity is the mean transit time (MTT), the average time required for blood to pass through the tissue volume of interest. It is related to CBV and CBF by MTT = CBV/CBF. Brain metabolism can be assessed by measuring the cerebral metabolic rate of oxygen ($CMRO_2$) which is about 130 μmol/min per 100g.

The permeability of the microvasculature to a substance is often reported as the product of the diffusional permeability coefficient P (cm min^{-1}) and the surface area S_v. PS_v has the unit of a volume flow per tissue mass (ml min^{-1} g^{-1}). Only values averaged over the volume of the voxel can be obtained without information about the morphology of the vasculature. Clinical studies have demonstrated the utility of this parameter for assessing malignancy and response to therapy in various tumors [14].

However, one MRI technique is sensitive to microvascular architecture, and the parameter obtained is called the vessel size index (VSI). This index is a weighted average of vessel sizes with a strong predominance of larger vessel sizes. It also depends on the vessel orientation which is assumed to be isotropic in healthy gray matter tissue, on the BVf and on the amount of contrast agent used.

Brain pathologies that are accompanied by vascular changes reflected by altered CBV, CBF, BBB permeability or combinations thereof, are brain infarction (ischemia) [15-17], multiple sclerosis [18, 19], infectious and inflammatory diseases [20], some forms of dementia such as Alzheimer's disease [21-23], acquired immune deficiency syndrome associated brain diseases [24, 25], and traumatic brain injury [26]. This chapter focuses on the quantification of tumor angiogenesis, which requires particular methodologic developments, due to the BBB permeability to most CAs.

4. Why are quantitative measures important?

Drugs targeting the angiogenic process such as inhibitors of angiogenic factors bring with them a need for an accurate means of assessing tumor angiogenesis and monitoring response to treatment. In the context of treatment monitoring comparison of values obtained at different time points are necessary. In the context of clinical trials comparisons between patients and centers need to be made.

Unfortunately, the signal intensity from most MR pulse sequences does not relate directly to any physiological parameter. Magnetic field strength, scanner parameters, sequence timing parameters, flip angle as well as image scaling, make the signal scanner dependent and comparisons between serial or multi-center studies difficult.

Procedures for data collection have to be found which are insensitive to scanner, sequence and operator influence, and which are reliable and reproducible over time and between patients. The measured parameters have to be examined for their biological meaning and related to clinically relevant quantities. In this way, changes at the microscopic level such as in cellular or microvascular structures can be detected as changes in MR parameters, such as relaxation times or magnetization transfer ratio, or as changes in diffusion and perfusion parameters at typical MR image resolutions of about 1 mm.

In theory, perfusion MRI techniques can yield quantitative hemodynamic parameters. To do so, they rely on a number of assumptions that are detailed below and require additional measurements that are either time consuming or invasive and therefore difficult in the clinical setting. In routine perfusion imaging, descriptive or semiquantitative parameters are therefore reported, some of which are discussed below. Typically, such values in the tissue of interest are reported relative to the corresponding value in a reference region, or are normalized to an average value taken from the literature. The reference region is chosen in healthy appearing brain tissue, usually in white matter or in the contralateral hemisphere symmetrical to the lesion. This is a pitfall when there is no reference region because the disease affects the whole brain such as a systemic cardiovascular pathology or a generalized infection, or when the "healthy appearing" reference region is affected by the disease, such as might occur with brain tumors that exert a mass effect, or have infiltrated the reference region.

5. What are the available quantitative magnetic resonance imaging techniques?

The perfusion MRI techniques that are presently used in the clinical practice are so called dynamic techniques. Dynamic techniques involve serial acquisition of MR images before, during and after the pass of an intravenously injected exogenous MRI CA through the tissue. As the CA enters into the tissue under investigation, the T_1 and T_2 values of tissue water decrease to an extent that is determined by the concentration of the CA.

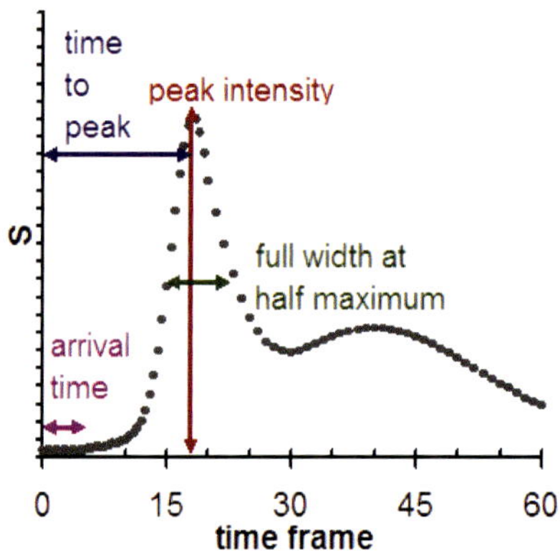

Figure 2. Characteristic signal intensity (S) time course during CA bolus passage. After the first high peak, the second peak corresponds to the second bolus passage after recirculation.

5.1. First pass or bolus tracking techniques

During the first pass of the CA bolus through the brain tissue the signal displays a characteristic intensity time course, which is related to the CA concentration in the tissue. Such a signal intensity time course is illustrated in Fig. 2 as an example of a positive (T_1 weighted) signal change. When changes in transverse relaxivity are exploited this technique is termed dynamic susceptibility contrast (DSC) MRI, which has superior signal to noise ratio (SNR) compared to T_1 weighted techniques. Mixed T_1 and T_2 weighting can complicate the interpretation. Fast imaging techniques with a recommended time resolution below 1.5 s are required, to adequately sample the signal dynamics. Even when using echo planar imaging (EPI) techniques, this requirement imposes limits to the spatial resolution and the number of slices that can be acquired.

Characteristic descriptive parameters measured form the observed signal changes during bolus pass include arrival time of the bolus, peak intensity, time to peak and full width at half maximum (Fig. 2). They generally depend on combinations of physiologic parameters, such as blood flow, fractional blood volume, and CA extravasation. Nevertheless, the peak signal amplitude was shown to correlate with the CBV [27].

For CBV quantification, the signal intensity during bolus pass is converted into a change in R_1 [28], R_2 or R_2^* [29] versus time reflecting the CA concentration. However, the proportionality constant between tissue relaxation rate change and CA concentration not only depends on CA properties and magnetic field strength. In particular the transverse relaxivity also depends on tissue properties such as microvascular architecture, vascular permeability, water exchange rate between intra- and extracellular compartment and blood oxygenation, all of which are spatially variable. The relaxivity is generally assumed to be the same as in plasma or venous blood. Any non-linearity between relaxation rate or signal change and CA concentration in tissue and blood will lead to errors [30].

In clinical routine, the CBV in the tissue of interest is given relative to a reference tissue. Maps of relative CBV are calculated by integrating the area under the CA concentration change during the first pass over time and since the CBV is calculated on the basis of signal recovery to the precontrast baseline, an adequate estimation of the baseline signal by signal averaging is essential. The accuracy of the CBV measure further depends on the ability to separate the first from the second pass of the CA (Fig "2). One approach to correct for CA recirculation is to fit a gamma variate function to the concentration versus time curve [31].

Tracer kinetic analysis [32] of the first bolus passage allows quantification of CBV, CBF and MTT, provided that the arterial CA concentration time course ($C_a(t)$), the so called arterial input function (AIF), is known.

The absolute CBV can be determined from the ratio of the areas under the tissue $C_{tissue}(t)$ and arterial CA concentration $C_a(t)$ versus time curves:

$$CBV = \frac{\int_{-\infty}^{\infty} C_{tissue}(t)dt}{\int_{-\infty}^{\infty} C_a(t)dt}$$

The tissue concentration versus time curve is the convolution of the tissue residue function $\Re(t)$ and the shape of the arterial concentration time curve $C_a(t)$ times the CBF:

$$C_{tissue}(t) = CBF \int_{-\infty}^{t} C_a(\tau)\Re(t-\tau)d\tau$$

$\Re(0)$ is equal to one at $t = 0$ when the CA enters the volume of interest. To calculate the CBF the impulse response CBF × $\Re(t)$has to be determined by deconvolution, and then CBF is obtained as the initial ($t = 0$) height of the impulse response function.

The MTT is obtained by the central volume theorem: MTT = CBV/CBF

The AIF has to be specified from the major feeding artery. The imaging of the time course of the vascular CA concentration requires that the acquisition mode is insensitive to flow, that it has an adequate spatial resolution to identify a vessel and a high temporal resolution to sample the shape of the initial bolus passage. In addition, signal saturation for the very high vascular concentrations during the bolus peak has to be avoided. The AIF is difficult to obtain in a reliable way, and is the major source of error. It can be influenced by variations in injection conditions and by physiologic or morphologic parameters of the vasculature. Delay and dispersion occur from the site of the AIF measurement to the tissue ROI. Dispersion occurring in the larger vessels can be misinterpreted as a low tissue flow, although it is normal [33, 34]. The AIF measure is often affected by partial volume effects or suffers from saturation effects. Deconvolution methods [35, 36] have been proposed to provide more reliable absolute quantifications.

Most clinical studies using bolus tracking techniques report relative/semiquantitative results, because the determination of the AIF is considered too complex or inaccurate. When relative CBV values are reported, in addition to the above mentioned caveats regarding the choice of the reference region, the assumption of identical AIFs and of identical CA relaxivity in the compared tissue ROIs is made.

In the presence of CA leakage, CBV maps computed from T_2* or T_2 weighted dynamic MRI tend to underestimate the CBV values, and may show false negative findings in the event of an active tumor recurrence [1]. Where T_1 weighted sequences are used, the presence of transendothelial CA leakage will act synergistically on signal intensity, causing artefactual CBV increases [37].

5.2. Dynamic contrast enhanced MRI

While with first pass techniques a vascular confinement of the CA is assumed, or models for leakage correction need to be applied, T_1 weighted dynamic contrast enhanced (DCE) MRI is designed to monitor the pharmacokinetics of the CA distribution within different compartments.

A simple qualitative or semiquantitative analysis of the signal enhancement curve with time after CA injection [38] use descriptors such as arrival time of the CA, maximum signal intensity or maximum intensity time ratio [39], initial uptake gradient or washout gradient. These parameters have a link to the underlying tissue physiology and CA pharmacokinetics, but the link is complex and not well defined. Unless the CA concentration versus time curves are used for semiquantitative analysis, they also depend on MR scaling factors.

For quantification, the time-varying signal has to be translated into tissue CA concentration. Pharmacokinetic modeling sets up a simplified description of tissue as a multi-compartment system. Although DCE MRI is used to quantify the microvascular permeability to the CA, appropriate kinetic models also allow quantification of the fractional volumes of the tissue compartments accessible to the CA: the CBV and the extravascular leakage volume assumed to be the extravascular extracellular compartment. CA transport between the compartments may then be modeled in terms of rate constants. Simple approaches model unidirectional CA flux (from intra- to extravascular compartments). More detailed approaches [40] recognize CA reflux in a bidirectional flux model. Kinetic modeling and interpretation is simplified by the assumption of a low extravasation rate compared to vascular flow rate (permeability limited model) preventing a decrease of the intravascular CA concentration [41]. When the CA extravasation rate is in the order of or higher than the blood flow rate in the vessel, the permeability limited model is no longer accurate. Flow limited extravasation is not unlikely in the case of tumor angiogenesis, since blood flow is perturbed and endothelial permeability is high. CAs of greater molecular weight help this limitation to be overcome, because their extravasation rate is lower.

The change in extravascular CA concentration dC_e/dt is proportional to the vascular permeability P (cm/min), the vascular surface area S_v (cm^2/g) and to the difference between the blood plasma concentration $C_p(t)$ (mM) and the extravascular concentration $C_e(t)$ and inversely proportional to the fractional volume of the extravascular compartment:

http://dx.doi.org/10.5772/56492

$$\frac{dC_e}{dt} = \frac{PS_v}{v_e}\left(C_p(t) - C_e(t)\right) \quad (1)$$

where ϱ is the tissue density and approximately 1 g/ml.

The CA concentration in the tissue $C_{tissue}(t)$ is composed of the concentrations in the plasma and in the extravascular compartment:

$$C_{tissue}(t) = v_p C_p(t) + v_e C_e(t) \quad (2)$$

where v_p is the fractional volume of the plasma compartment. The fractional plasma volume is related to the fractional blood volume (BVf) by: v_p = (1-Hct) BVf, where Hct is the capillary hematocrit.

Inserting Eq. 2 into Eq. 1 results in the following differential equation describing the CA flux across the endothelium where equal permeability for the outflux and the backflux is assumed:

$$\frac{dC_{tissue}}{dt} - v_p \frac{dC_p}{dt} = PS_v \varrho\left[C_p(t) - \frac{1}{v_e}\left(C_{tissue}(t) - v_p C_p(t)\right)\right] \quad (3)$$

The tissue concentration is given by the solution to Eq. 3:

$$C_{tissue}(t) = K^{trans}\int_0^t C_p(\tau)\exp\left[-k_{ep}(t-\tau)\right]d\tau + v_p C_p(t).$$

where $K^{trans} = PS_v\varrho$ is the coefficient of endothelial permeability and where the rate constant $k_{ep} = K^{trans}/v_e$ governs the backflux of CA into the vessel. The parameters in this expression can be fitted to the corresponding DCE-MRI data [42].

To derive the physiological parameters K^{trans}, v_e and v_p, the plasma concentration versus time $C_p(t)$ (the AIF) has to be measured or modeled. Tofts and Kermode [41] assumed a typical biexponential decay of C_p, due to rapid leakage into the extravascular extracellular compartment in extracerebral tissues and to the slower filtration by the kidneys. Larsson et al [43] measured it from serial blood samples, while Brix et al [44] included the plasma clearance rate as a free parameter in the fit.

Assumptions common to all models described here are the homogeneity of the compartments with respect to the CA distribution, a CA flux that is proportional to the concentration gradient between compartments, a negligible contribution from diffusion of CA from other voxels and a time invariance of the compartment volumes and permeability coefficients. Further compartmentalization of the CA within the extravascular extracellular space is ignored. Finally the water exchange between compartments is assumed to be fast so that a single relaxation time constant T_1 can be measured for the tissue, although the CA is compartmentalized. The Tofts and Kermode model [41] fails in areas where contrast extraction from the vasculature is extensive (flow limited case) or negligible, such as in normal brain tissue.

5.3. Steady state techniques

The so called steady state approaches for CBV measurement rely on the signal or relaxation rate change induced by a CA after having reached a homogeneous distribution and stable concentration in the intravascular compartment [45, 46]. Since CAs with a long blood half life and high relaxivity or a comparatively high CA dose is needed, they are only used in the research setting.

T_1 [47, 48], T_2 [49] or T_2* weighted acquisitions are performed before and after injection of the CA, to determine the signal difference ΔS or the relaxation rate change ΔR_1, ΔR_2 or ΔR_2^* in the brain tissue before and after injection of a CA. To quantify the CBV with steady state techniques, measurement of the signal change, relaxation rate change or susceptibility difference induced by the CA in the blood compartment is needed. Although limited by the partial volume effect, this information can be obtained from a vascular ROI to avoid blood sampling.

Quantitative CBV is calculated as the ratio of the signal or relaxation rate changes induced by the CA in tissue and blood: $CBV = \Delta S_{tissue} / \Delta S_{blood}$ [47, 48] or $CBV = \Delta R_{i\ tissue} / \Delta R_{i\ blood}$ with i = 1,2 [50].

Other studies [51, 52] have exploited the changes in R_2^* [29]. The CBV quantification by the steady state ΔR_2^* method is based on a simplified geometric model of the brain microvasculature and the approximation of quasi static water protons. The compartmentalization of CAs, such as ultrasmall superparamagnetic nanoparticles of iron oxide (USPIO) characterized by a high magnetic susceptibility, within the randomly oriented capillary network of the brain results in localized microscopic field inhomogeneities in the tissue in which water protons diffuse, inducing a loss of transverse phase coherence with T_2* signal loss in the perivascular space. The component of the magnetic field B(r) which is parallel to B_0 is inversely proportional to the square of the distance r form the vessel $B(r) \propto \Delta M\ (R/r)^2 \sin^2(\Theta)$ and it is a function of the magnetization difference ΔM between the intra- and extravascular compartment induced by the compartmentalized CA, the vessel radius R and the angle Θ between the direction of the main magnetic field B_0 and the axis of the vessel (Fig. 3). A quasi static water proton diffusion regime assumes that the mean diffusion length of the extravascular water proton $d = (D\ TE)^{1/2}$ is short with respect to the vessel radius R. In this case, the water protons situated at different distances r from the vessel experience different magnetic field strengths B(r) and therefore diphase at different rates.

The proportionality factor between the vascular volume fraction and relaxation rate difference ΔR_2^* induced by the presence of the CA depends on the intra-extravascular susceptibility difference $\Delta\chi$. Monte Carlo simulations show good agreement with in vivo results [45, 53]. However $\Delta\chi$ has to be measured from blood samples and is sensitive to differences in hematocrit and oxygenation between the sampled blood and the microvasculature [54, 55].

http://dx.doi.org/10.5772/56492

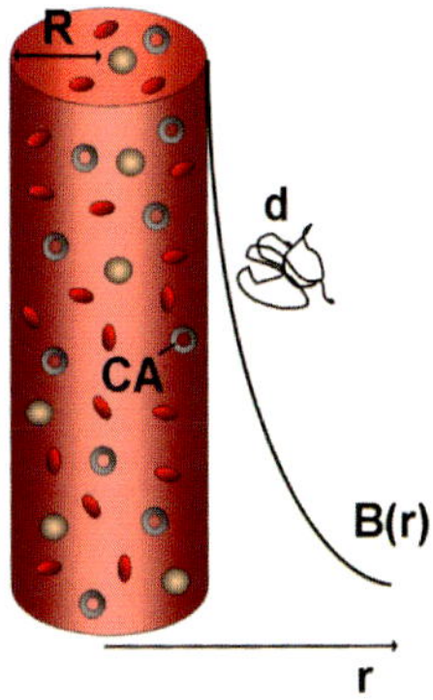

Figure 3. The ΔR_2* method for CBV measurement models the capillary as an infinitely long and homogeneous cylinder containing the CA. The magnetic field gradient around the cylinder is a function of the cylinder radius R, of the magnetization difference between the intra- and extravascular compartment, of the cylinder orientation in the main homogeneous magnetic field B_0 and of the distance from the cylinder r. The diffusion regime is said to be quasi static when the mean water proton diffusion length d is short with respect to R, in such a way that the water protons in the vicinity of the cylinder dephase at a faster rate than those situated further away.

The CBV fraction is obtained in the following way [56]:

$$CBV = \frac{3}{4\pi}\frac{1}{\gamma \Delta X B_0}\Delta R_2^*$$

where γ is the gyromagnetic ratio and B_0 is the static magnetic field strength.

The ratio $\Delta R_2^*/\Delta R_2$ is dependent on the vessel size [45, 57]. ΔR_2 is sensitive primarily to small vessels, while ΔR_2^* is influenced by a broader range of vessel sizes. By measuring $\Delta R_2^*/\Delta R_2$ using gradient echo and spin echo sequences, and the water diffusion coefficient D, it is possible to estimate the VSI: $VSI = 0.424\ (D/\gamma\Delta\chi B_0)^{1/2}(\Delta R_2^*/\Delta R_2)^{3/2}$.

5.4. Vascular space occupancy technique

The vascular space occupancy (VASO) technique [58] is a T_1 weighted technique that uses an inversion recovery sequence with timing parameters optimized to suppress the blood signal, while the extravascular tissue gives rise to a signal, which is not at its equilibrium value. For functional MRI, images are acquired during task performance (regional CBV change) and under rest conditions. It is assumed that the sum of intravascular and extravascular magnetization in a voxel is equal in the rest and in the activated condition and consequently a CBV change would inversely affect the extravascular magnetization. The signal difference between the rest and the activated condition is proportional to the CBV change. A signal decrease of about 0.7% has been detected under task performance consistent with a vasodilation [58]}.

In a quantitative version of this approach [59], the absolute CBV can be determined using the T_1 shortening effect of a CA. The signal before CA injection S_{pre} is only of extravascular origin since the blood signal is suppressed by the inversion recovery sequence using an appropriate inversion time T_{inv}: $S_{pre} = S_{ev}$ where S_{ev} is the extravascular signal. After CA injection, the T_{inv} is sufficiently long to allow full relaxation of the blood water magnetization to thermodynamic equilibrium, and the post-contrast signal S_{post} is given by: $S_{post} = S_{ev} + S_{0\,iv}$ where $S_{0\,iv}$ is the blood signal corresponding to the thermodynamic equilibrium magnetization of the blood compartment. The signals in the difference image are proportional to the blood volume since the extravascular tissue cancels out: $S_{post} - S_{pre} = S_{0\,iv}$.

This method is similar to the steady state T_1 weighted approach except that the equilibrium signal of the blood is acquired directly. For CBV quantification, the resulting blood signal in the difference image is normalized by the signal corresponding to the thermodynamic equilibrium magnetization of the total tissue (intra- + extravascular compartment). The normalization factor is obtained from a ROI containing cerebrospinal fluid on a reference image with sufficiently long acquisition times or from a small ROI containing mainly blood on the postcontrast image.

In humans, mean CBV of 1.4 and 5.5 ml/100 g have been measured with this technique for white matter and cortical gray matter, respectively [59].

The main difficulty encountered with this technique is that the repetition time (TR = 6 s) used is relatively long and therefore the blood T_1 has to be known precisely in order to determine the blood nulling inversion time ($T_{inv} \approx 1$s, depending on the field strength). A slightly inappropriate T_{inv}, reduced inversion efficiency or a change in blood T_1 (e.g. with hematocrit or oxygenation) results in a non negligible negative or positive blood signal before CA injection leading to a misestimation of the CBV in the difference image. Moreover, due to a relatively long T_{inv}, the water exchange between intra- and extravascular compartment will have a large effect. Finally, if the normalization factor is obtained from a vascular ROI affected by a partial volume effect, the CBV might be overestimated.

5.5. The rapid steady state T_1 technique

The Rapid Steady State T_1 ($RSST_1$) technique [60] is a quantitative T_1 weighted MRI technique for cerebral BVf mapping combining features of dynamic and steady state methods. Like the previously described methods it is based on a two-compartment model of the brain (intra- and extravascular) and necessitates the intravenous injection of a CA. It uses an inversion recovery (IR) prepared MRI sequence, but, in contrast to the VASO technique, a short repetition time (TR < 1 s). For such a short TR a dynamic equilibrium of the longitudinal magnetization M_z installs in which slowly relaxing magnetization never reaches its thermodynamic equilibrium value. In addition, for tissues with $T_1 > 1$ s, such as blood without CA and extravascular tissue, M_z crosses the null line at almost the same inversion time T_{inv} (Figure 4 a). The images are acquired using a fast low flip angle gradient echo imaging sequence FLASH [61, 62] and making sure the central k-space line is acquired when the longitudinal magnetization component crosses the null line (Figure 4 b). The signal evolution during this pulse sequence can be modeled [63]. Equation 4 is an approximation for the longitudinal magnetization M_z for low flip angles α, when dynamic equilibrium has installed:

http://dx.doi.org/10.5772/56492

$$\frac{M_z\left(T_{inv},TR,T_1\right)}{M_0}=1-\frac{2\exp\left(-\frac{T_{inv}}{T_1}\right)}{1+\exp\left(-\frac{TR}{T_1}\right)} \tag{4}$$

where M_0 is the longitudinal magnetization at thermodynamic equilibrium and TR the repetition time between two inversion pulses. Suppression of the longitudinal tissue magnetization can be achieved for

$$T_{inv}(TR,T_1)=T_1\ln 2-T_1\ln\left[1+\exp\left(-\frac{TR}{T_1}\right)\right].$$

Figure 4 c shows M_z in function of T_1 for different T_{inv} and TR = 750 ms.

Using a TR/T_{inv} couple such as 750 ms/325 ms or 500 ms/225 ms, the IR-FLASH sequence acts like a T_1 low pass filter suppressing extravascular signals having high T_1 values and selectively acquiring the intravascular signal in the presence of a CA. In particular, a blood signal at thermodynamic equilibrium is acquired when the blood T_1 is below a critical value $T_{1blood} \approx T_{inv}/5$ after CA injection (Figure 4 a), reflecting the quantity of intravascular water protons. To quantify the BVf, the acquired blood signal S is normalized to the thermodynamic equilibrium (proton density weighted) signal of the intra- plus extravascular tissue water S_0 [60] obtained in an acquisition with sufficiently long TR. To eliminate residual signal from extravascular compartments, such as from white matter that has lower T_1, in particular at low magnetic field strength, the average signal acquired before CA injection $\{S_{pre}\}$ is subtracted before normalization. The normalized vascular signal S_{norm} is then given by

$$S_{norm\ i}=\left(S_i-\langle S_{pre}\rangle\right)/S_0$$

where S is the $RSST_1$-signal and i denotes the time frame.

A plot of S_{norm} over time during and after CA injection is shown in Figure 5. For a low CA dose, the signal time course resembles the one in Fig 2 as long as the signal is dependent on the CA concentration in blood. However, when $T_{1blood} \leq T_{inv}/5$ during the first pass the signal is saturated and its amplitude equals the CBV fraction. For a higher CA dose, T_{1blood} can be sufficiently low for the second pass or for a longer time interval. Note that in contrast to steady state techniques, the CA concentration does not need to be in a steady state to result in a steady state signal. The name of the technique "rapid steady state" was chosen to describe the dynamic equilibrium of the signal when it becomes independent of the CA concentration, not the contrast agent concentration in blood itself.

In this way the $RSST_1$ technique bypasses the need for conversion of the signal intensity change into relaxation rate change and the assumption of proportionality between the latter and CA concentration. The concomitant T_2 effect of the CA is minimized by using acquisitions with short TE.

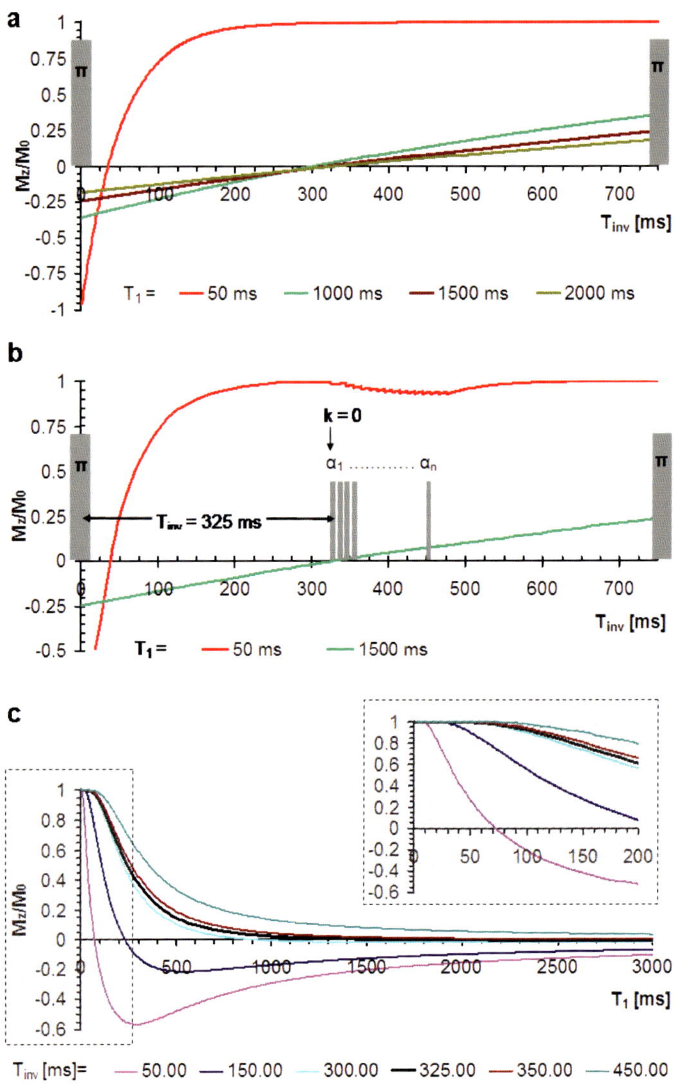

Figure 4. a: The longitudinal magnetization component M_z in an IR sequence with 750 ms repetition time is plotted after dynamic equilibrium has installed. M_z is suppressed and crosses the zero line at almost the same T_{inv} for tissues with long T_1, while for the same T_{inv} M_z is at thermodynamic equilibrium for tissues with short T_1 such as blood in presence of the CA. π = nonselective inversion pulse. b: The FLASH module acquires the image (and in particular the k = 0 line) when M_z of tissues with long T_1 crosses the zero-line and blood magnetization is fully relaxed (due to the T_1 shortening effect of a vascular CA). Here a center-out acquisition scheme is illustrated. α = low flip angle pulse. c: Equation 4 is plotted as a function of T_1 for several T_{inv} and TR = 750 ms. For T_{inv} = 325 ms M_z is suppressed for all $T_1 \geq 1$ s while it relaxes to thermodynamic equilibrium for $T_1 \leq 65$ ms as shown in the zoom.

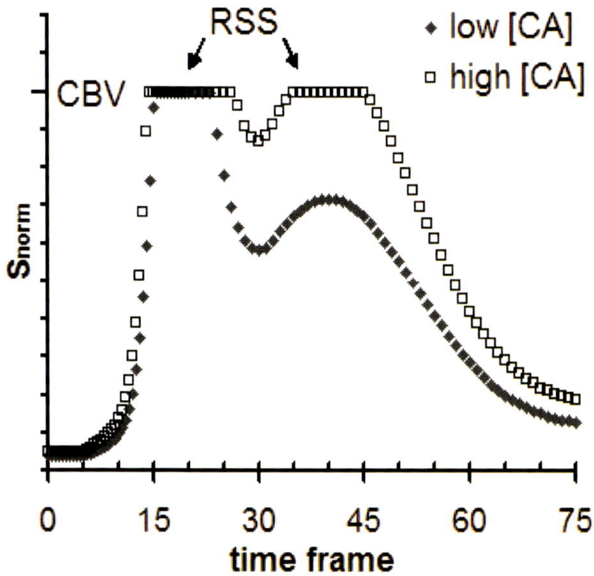

Figure 5. Plot of S_{norm} over time. At a particular CA concentration [CA] during first and sometimes also during the second pass or longer, S_{norm} does not depend on the [CA] any more but reaches a rapid steady state (RSS) value, corresponding to the BVf.

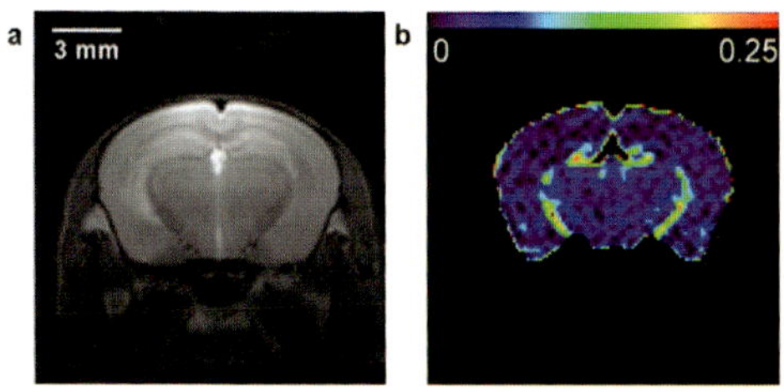

Figure 6. a: Coronal MRI image of a mouse brain showing structural details. b: Corresponding S_{norm} map showing an average cerebral BVf of 0.02 ± 0.004 and demonstrating CA accumulation in the cerebrospinal fluid leading to overestimation of the CBV in periventricular structures.

The $RSST_1$ technique was developed with CAs that remain confined to the vascular space during the measurement such as the clinically approved small molecular size CA Gd-DOTA from Guerbet Laboraories in the presence of an intact blood brain barrier (BBB) [60]. CAs with more convenient properties are available for preclinical applications. The experimental CA P760 from Guerbet Laboratories is an intermediate molecular size CA with higher relaxivities and higher intravascular restriction (molecular weight 5.29 kDa versus 0.55 kDa, mean diameter 2.8 nm versus 0.9 nm, longitudinal relaxivity r_1 = 17.2 $mM^{-1}s^{-1}$ versus 2.9 $mM^{-1}s^{-1}$, transverse relaxivity r_2 = 27.1 $mM^{-1}s^{-1}$ versus 4.8 $mM^{-1}s^{-1}$ at 2.35 T, [64]). A rapid steady state of at least 30 s can be obtained starting at a dose of 0.15 mmol/kg Gd-DOTA and 0.035 mmol/kg P760 at 2.35T. However, quantitative CBV maps were obtained in healthy rats with P760 at a dose of 0.1 mmol/kg and with Gd-DOTA at a dose of 0.2 to 0.3 mmol/kg. These CA doses lead to a RSS interval of up to 5 minutes that can be used for increasing the SNR, the in-plane resolution or the number of slices. Even longer RSS intervals were obtained using a continuous infusion of these CA [60]. Quantitative CBV maps were also obtained in mice at 4.7T [65]. Due to faster hemodynamics in mice and reduced relaxivities of Gd-DOTA at higher magnetic field strength, an intravenous 0.7 mmol/kg dose was used. To lengthen the RSS, the intraperitoneal administration route has been employed in mice using a 6 mmol/kg dose which was well tolerated and lead to a RSS interval of about 30 minutes starting 15 minutes after injection. Quantitatively equivalent CBV measures were obtained using the intravenous and intraperitoneal routes on the same mice. A representative coronal CBV fraction map of a healthy mouse is shown in Figure 6. In studies performed repeatedly (once per month) in the same mice the cerebral BVf was well correlated between time points (Spearman $r = 0.94$, P-value = 0.017), with an intraindividual variability of the BVf measure in the caudate putamen of 0.018 to 0.024 (mean ± standard deviation: 0.022 ± 0.003) demonstrating the reproducibility of the CBV quantification. Intraperitoneal CA administration has the advantage of being less invasive with a lower risk for emboli and hypervolemia than intravenous administration. However, the CBV in cerebral regions close to ventricles might be overestimated due to CA arrival from the cerebrospinal fluid in which the CA accumulates.

The sensitivity of the $RSST_1$ technique to detect CBV changes has been assessed. In rats, the measurement has been repeated under different capnia conditions [60]. Hypercapnia is induced by breathing elevated levels of carbon dioxide and results in vasodilation. In mice the vasodilator acetazolamide has been injected during the long vascular RSS interval obtained after intraperitoneal Gd-DOTA injection [65]. In both experiments, the technique has been found to be sensitive to the BVf change (Figure 7) and the degree of change was comparable with published values using different techniques [66-68].

The quantification of tumor angiogenesis is complicated by the leakiness of the vessels for these CA leading to an overestimation of the CBV in the presence of CA leakage when using

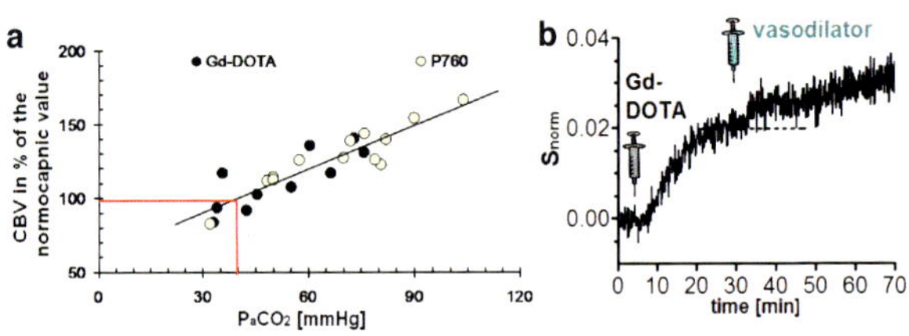

Figure 7. a: A hypercapnia experiment demonstrates CBV increase in healthy rats. b: In healthy mice, the S_{norm} signal during the RSS increases shortly after intraperitoneal injection of the vasodilator acetazolamide.

http://dx.doi.org/10.5772/56492

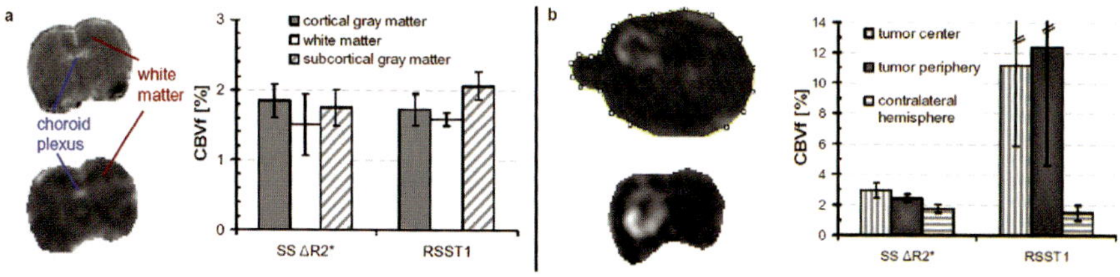

Figure 8.

a T_1 weighted technique. Two strategies are possible: I) Injection of CAs that remain confined to the vasculature despite hyperpermeable endothelium, and II) monitoring the CA accumulation in tumor tissue to be analyzed using an appropriate two compartment model.

USPIO such as AMI 227 (Sinerem, Guerbet Laboratories, Combidex, AMAG Pharmaceuticals) are widely used for their blood pool properties. They have also been used to quantify the blood volume fraction in malignant tumors in preclinical studies [69-72]. AMI 227 has a r^2 relaxivity in the order of 100 $mM^{-1}s^{-1}$ and is mainly used in T^2 or T^{2*} weighted acquisitions. The r1 relaxivity of AMI 227 ($r^1 = 5.4\ mM^{-1}s^{-1}$ at 2.35T) together with its blood pool property, makes it an attractive CA for a T^1 weighted technique. Sequences with ultrashort echo time (TE) need to be used to exploit the T^1 effect. Acquisition schemes starting at the center of k-space such as radial or spiral acquisitions achieve short TE. A 3D projection reconstruction acquisition mode with a TE = 0.7 ms, was used at 2.35T to map the CBV with the $RSST^1$ technique using 0.2 mmol/kg AMI 227 in healthy and tumor bearing rats [73]. The post injection acquisition lasted 24 minutes, for which a steady state CA concentration in blood was assumed. The CBV measurement was compared with a steady state ΔR^{2*} technique in the same animals (Figure 8 a). After correction for transverse relaxation effects, both acquisition techniques yielded comparable results in healthy rat brain and a C6 glioma model. However, in a RG2 glioma model, the RSST1 technique yielded high tumor BVf while in the same ROIs the steady state ΔR^{2*} technique yielded BVfs that were significantly lower than in healthy or contralateral tissue (Figure 8 b). Such a discrepancy can only be explained by loss of CA compartmentalization, which results in underestimation of the BVf with T^{2*} weighted techniques while T1 weighted acquisitions tend to overestimate the BVf. There is also evidence for AMI 227 extravasation in the RG2 tumor model in results published by other authors [69].

In the search for intravascular CA with high r_1 relaxivity for tumor BVf quantification, good results were obtained with a novel preclinical CA based on a modified cyclodextrin [74] in a C6 tumor model [75]. This paramagnetic CA is an inclusion complex of Gd^{3+} with per-(3,6-anhydro)-α-cyclodextrin. It has a molecular weight of 1464 Dalton and the shape of a flat disc. The relaxivities of Gd-ACX decrease with increased concentration, but at a 1.5 mM concentration in normal saline at 2.35T relaxivities are still $r_1 = 8.6\ s^{-1}mM^{-1}$ and $r_2 = 10.4\ s^{-1}mM^{-1}$ about twice as high as for Gd-DOTA [64]. The biodistribution of Gd-ACX (0.05 mmol/kg) and the CBVf were studied using T_1 weighted imaging and the $RSST_1$ technique at 2.35T in healthy and C6 tumor bearing Wistar rats 20 and 21 days after implantation, and compared to

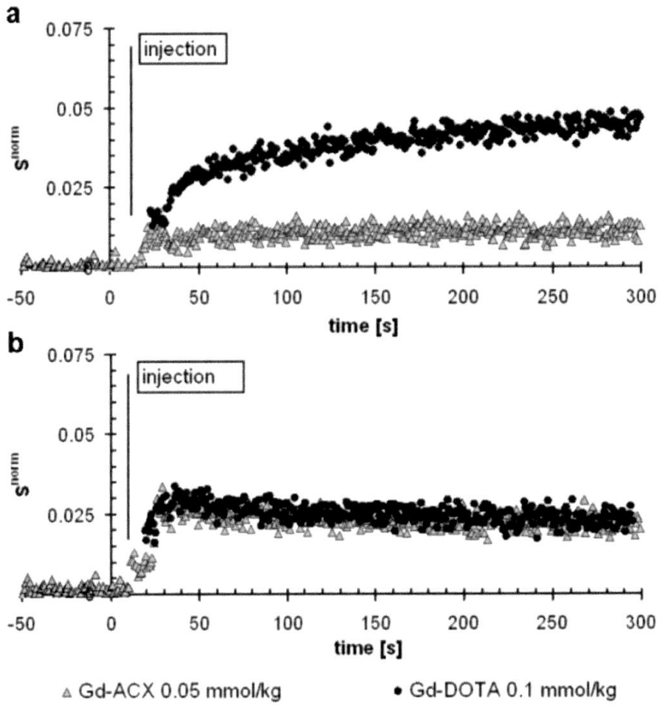

Figure 9. S_{norm} versus time curves after Gd-ACX and Gd-DOTA injection in C6 glioma tissue (a) and contralateral brain tissue (b). There is no evidence of Gd-ACX extravasation during the first 5 minutes after injection enabling BVf quantification in presence of vascular endothelium permeable to Gd-DOTA.

quantitative CBVf maps and the regional signal enhancement obtained after injection of Gd-DOTA. After Gd-ACX injection, the signal enhancement appears immediately in large vessels, but not in the tumor, while injection of Gd-DOTA reveals disruption of the BBB since an extensive signal enhancement is observed inside the tumor area. Representative signal versus time plots from one rat obtained by the $RSST_1$ method in the tumor periphery and in contralateral brain tissue are shown in Fig. 9 a and b respectively. After Gd-ACX injection, S_{norm} remains constant for about 5 min, while after Gd-DOTA injection the signal in tumor tissue increases continuously, reflecting CA accumulation due to a BBB leakage for this CA. Identical signal behavior in cerebral tissue contralateral to the tumor after injection of Gd-ACX and Gd-DOTA is observed (Figure 9 b). The constant signal enhancement obtained with the $RSST_1$ technique during the first five minutes confirms the absence of immediate Gd-ACX Extravasation from tumor vasculature allowing quantification of the tumor BVf using Gd-ACX in presence of vascular permeability to Gd-DOTA. However, the modest thermodynamic stability of Gd-ACX will limit its use to preclinical studies. For clinical applications, tumor angiogenesis needs to be assessed with clinically approved low molecular weight CA such as Gd-DOTA despite CA leakage.

http://dx.doi.org/10.5772/56492

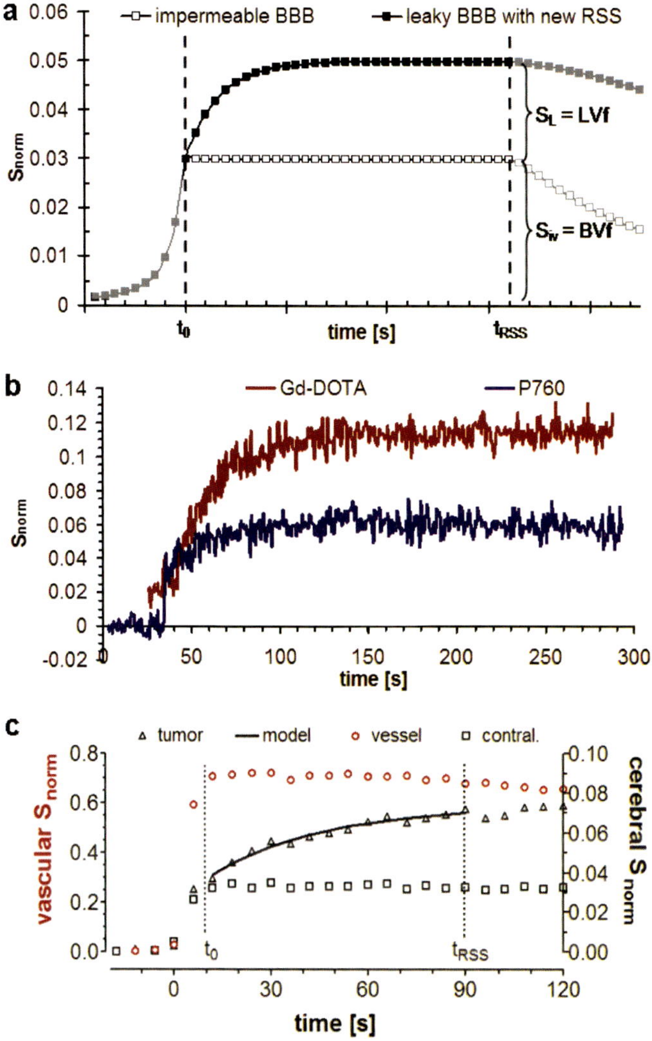

Figure 10. A model of the signal evolution during CA arrival and distribution in the tissue for two ROIs. The lower plot represents the signal in a RSS from a ROI, in which the CA is confined to the blood pool. The upper plot displays the idealized shape of a leakage profile during the vascular RSS time window [t_0, t_{RSS}] attaining a new RSS at a signal amplitude corresponding to the sum of BVf and LVf. CA = contrast agent, RSS = rapid steady state, ROI = region of interest, BVf = blood volume fraction, LVf = leakage volume fraction. b: Typical leakage profiles for a low (Gd-DOTA) and intermediate molecular size (P760) CA in a RG2 tumor model demonstrating that the vascular permeability and the total distribution volume is lower for the larger CA. c: Modeled leakage profile for Gd-DOTA in a C6 tumor model (right axis) along with RSS profiles for signal from a large vessel (left axis) and contralateral brain tissue (right axis) defining the time window [t0, tRSS] for leakage monitoring.

Unlike steady state techniques and similar to DCE-MRI, the high temporal resolution of the $RSST_1$ technique enables monitoring of dynamic signal changes as illustrated in Figure 5.. Due to the use of high relaxivity CA or high doses in preclinical studies, the vascular RSS is maintained over several minutes beyond the first pass. In tissues with permeable vasculature the CA extravasates leading to a continuous signal increase. If the time window for which the vascular signal corresponds to the BVf is known, the CA accumulation in tissue with permeable vasculature can be modeled. The model assumes two compartments accessible to the CA: the blood and the extravascular leakage compartment. The remaining compartments, not attained by the CA, maintain a high T_1 value and do not lead to significant signal. The S_{norm} signal reaches a RSS when the CA reaches a uniform concentration in the distribution compartment leading to a sufficiently low T_1. As illustrated in Figure "10 a, in case of CA leakage the signal time course approaches an asymptote. The maximum signal enhancement is then composed of the BVf and the leakage volume fraction (LVf). The S_{norm} signal is modeled as:

$$S_{model}(t) = S_{iv} + S_L \left\{1 - \exp\left[-\kappa(t - t_0)\right]\right\} \quad (5)$$

where t_0 is the beginning of the RSS time interval which can be obtained from a large vascular structure or brain tissue with intact BBB. The BVf is estimated as S_{iv}, i.e. S_{model} in the beginning of the signal RSS. S_L is the proton density weighted signal of the extravascular leakage compartment approximating the local extravascular distribution volume fraction (i.e. the LVf) of the CA. κ is a parameter related to the leakage rate. The CA leakage is assumed to be permeability limited [41]. Setting BVf = S_{iv} also assumes negligible CA extravasation in the beginning of the first pass of the CA bolus. CA backflow from the extravascular leakage compartment into the blood is not taken into account. A comparison of leakage signal profiles for two CA with different molecular weight in the same tumor tissue are shown in Figure 10 b, showing that the larger CA has a slower leakage rate and a lower distribution volume. Using Gd-DOTA, analysis of the leakage profile can therefore give valuable information about the vascular permeability which is spatially and temporally heterogenous in malignant tumors. Figure 10 c shows how the RSS time window can be determined from tissue containing impermeable vasculature in order to limit the fitting procedure to this time interval. This is not equivalent to the definition of an AIF, since the actual signal intensity is not of importance.

The described methodological development of the $RSST_1$ technique was carried out at magnetic field strengths above 2.35T necessitating injection of high CA doses in order to compensate for the decreasing CA relaxivity with higher field strength and to achieve long vascular RSS intervals for signal averaging to overcome the low SNR in small animal imaging. In the clinical setting, the method is not only limited to Gd-DOTA-like CA, but also to low doses. In routine imaging a dose of 0.1 mmol/kg is administered, but a double or triple dose has been shown to result in higher sensitivity in particular applications. However, gadolinium based CA can result in serious complications such as nephritic systemic fibrosis in susceptible patients, it is therefore cautious to limit the administered dose to a minimum.

A pilot experiment on a 3T Philips Achieva research MRI scanner showed that CBV quantification with the $RSST_1$ technique in the primate (macaque) brain is feasible with a 0.2 mmol/kg

Gd-DOTA dose at this field strength. In order to reduce the Gd-DOTA dose, the RSST$_1$ technique has been implemented on a clinical 1.5T Philips Achieva scanner where it was integrated in the routine imaging protocol for follow up studies of neurooncological patients. The routine imaging protocol necessitated Gd-DOTA administration to look for pathological contrast enhancement on T$_1$ weighted images, but did not include perfusion imaging techniques. A number of 120 RSST$_1$ acquisitions (TR/T$_{inv}$ = 750 ms/315 ms, matrix 64 x 55, flip angle 10º, inter-echo repetition time 4 ms, TE = 1.2 ms) were acquired over 90 s before, during and after CA injection using an automatic injector with an injection rate of 6 ml/s. These acquisitions were normalized to the proton density acquisition acquired before injection using the same sequence without inversion pulse and a TR of 10 s (number of averages = 3). Patients were injected with either 15 ml (= 7.5 mmol) or 30 ml (15 mmol) Gd-DOTA according to their reported or estimated weight as is often done in clinical routine, but weighted after completed examination in order to determine the administered dose precisely. In the feasibility studies, the imaging plane was chosen to include large vessels such as the basilar artery or branches of the circle of Willis and a large dural venous sinus to study the vascular signal with minimal partial volume effect. An example of the S$_{norm}$-signal profile is shown in Figure 11. It can be observed that during the first pass of the CA S$_{norm}$ reaches a value of 1 (one) corresponding to 100% blood when the voxel is placed within the vessel without partial volume effect. Consequently, the S$_{norm}$ amplitude in brain tissue during the first pass reflects the CBV fraction. At 1.5T, a Gd-DOTA dose of 0.13 mmol/kg is necessary for reliable quantitative CBV fraction mapping. Below this dose, a sufficiently high CA concentration in the brain vasculature is only achieved for patients with a relatively low body mass index. The determined optimum dose is 30% higher than the recommended Gd-DOTA dose but still approved and often used in clinical practice. A RSS interval limited to the first pass of the CA has the following advantages: First, extravasation from hyperpermeable vasculature is minimized. When significant CA extravasation occurs, it can be detected as an increasing instead of a constant signal, and algorithms for leakage correction can be applied. Second, hemodynamic information can be derived. Like the mean transit time, the duration of the RSS during the first pass is related to the blood flow, but similar to first pass perfusion techniques it is also determined by the CA injection rate, dispersion and the BVf. As with first pass perfusion techniques the RSS duration relative to a reference region might still have diagnostic value.

6. What are the confounding effects?

To evaluate the accuracy of the RSST$_1$ technique confounding effects need to be taken into consideration. For example, the signal attenuation due to transverse relaxation has been minimized by using short TE. When T$_2$* attenuation was significant as with AMI 227, the blood T$_2$* after injection has been measured to estimate and correct for this effect.

The RSST$_1$ technique is not sensitive to blood flow effects that often affect quantification in dynamic perfusion techniques. First, the inversion pulse is not slice selective, inverting all proton spins whether they are stationary, mobile, in the imaging plane or not. Second, when the blood T$_1$ is sufficiently low after CA injection, the blood flowing into the imaging plane

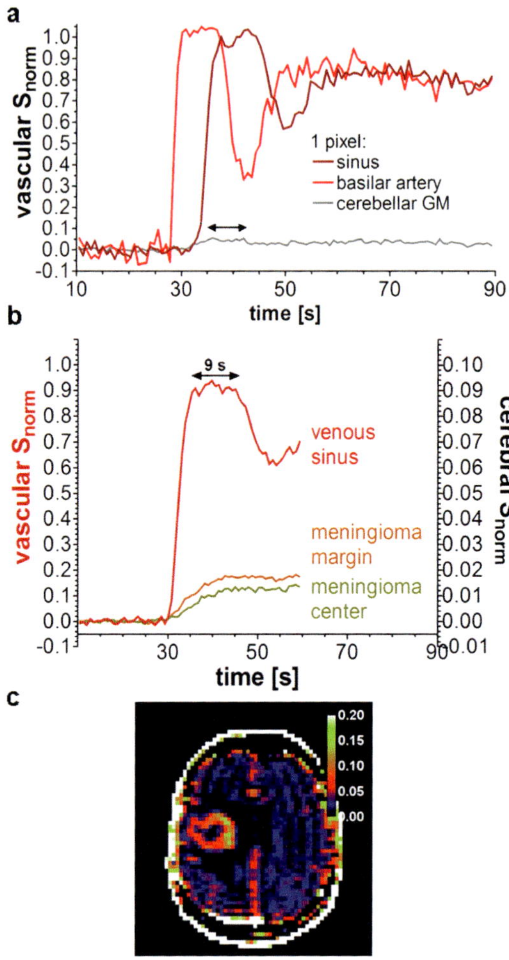

Figure 11. a: After an intravenous Gd-DOTA injection of 0.13 mmol/kg in patients, S_{norm} = 1 is attained during the first pass in large vascular structures without partial volume effect. The S_{norm} amplitude in brain tissue during the first pass (arrow) therefore corresponds to the BVf. S_{norm} = 0.04 in the cerebellar gray matter (GM) voxel. b: While the vascular signal is in a RSS for about 9 s in this patient, a typical CA leakage profile is observed in the meningioma tissue. c: S_{norm} map of a patient with glioblastoma. No leakage correction was applied and the BVf of 8 to 10% in the tumor border might be overestimated if significant CA leakage occurred during the first pass.

between the excitation pulse and the readout arrives with a magnetization at thermal equilibrium such as the blood flowing out of the imaging plane.

However, the $RSST_1$ technique seeks to selectively acquire signal from water molecules that are in contact with the CA. The mobility of water molecules and their exchange across the vessel wall might affect the CBV quantification. For example, water molecules that relax with a short T_1 because they were in contact with the CA in the vascular compartment, but happen to exchange to the extravascular compartment during the inversion time, will reduce the extravascular T_1. This might lead to a signal contribution from the extravascular compartment and therefore to a CBV overestimation. The RSST$_1$ technique is based on a two compartment model and assumes negligible water exchange between these compartments. Whether the exchange regime is fast or slow depends on the water exchange rate and on the difference between the longitudinal relaxation rates of the intravascular and extravascular compartment. An intracapillary residence time of 500 to 650 ms has been reported for healthy brain tissue [76] leading to a transendothelial exchange rate in the order of 2 s^{-1} which is slow compared to the difference of the longitudinal relaxation rates between the two compartments which is in the order of 20 s^{-1} at the peak CA concentration. The exchange effect on the CBV measure was evaluated using the model described in Moran and Prato [77] and showed an overestimation of 10 -12% for a T_{inv} of 325 ms and an assumed vascular T_1 of 50 ms during the RSS. The water exchange effect is more pronounced for higher CA agent doses or relaxivities such as used in preclinical studies. It can be reduced by shortening T_{inv}, allowing the compartments less time to exchange water across the vascular boundary. For example, with the couple of parameters TR = 500 ms and Tinv = 225 ms, the overestimation would be reduced to less than 4% for a vascular T_1 of 45 ms.

Strictly speaking, the blood as well as the extravascular compartment are multi compartment systems. The CA molecules do not enter the cells. However, the blood can be considered as a single compartment because even in the presence of CA molecules in plasma the intra-extracellular difference of the longitudinal relaxation rates is still one order of magnitude lower than the water exchange rate between erythrocytes and plasma ($\tau_{exch}^{-1} \approx 125\ s^{-1}$). In this fast exchange limit, the intracellular water is affected by the presence of the CA, and it is the CBV that is measured and not the plasma volume. It is therefore not necessary to correct for the regional hematocrit.

7. How to validate a quantitative blood volume measure?

When developing new acquisition or analysis techniques the validity of their assumptions and their limits need to be assessed using reference methods ideally on the same brain. This implies either using a MRI technique that does not rely on the same principle or on the same assumptions or a technique that has a different signal origin. Experimental and physiologic conditions need to be kept as similar as possible, which is not straightforward when the subject or animal needs to be moved from one scanner to another or when the measurements are a long time interval apart or relay on CAs with different properties. In particular, comparisons between in vivo and ex vivo techniques have to be interpreted with caution since the "physiologic" conditions are not alike. Nevertheless, histological validation is still the gold standard. When evaluating angiogenesis by histology, surrogate markers such as microvascular density or vascular area density are often used because they can be directly quantified from two-dimensional histological sections. The vascular volume density comes closest to the BVf but necessitates a stereological analysis of vascular morphometric data.

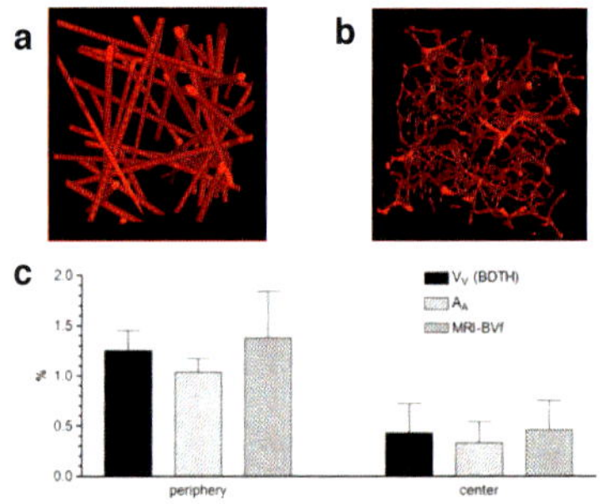

Figure 12. Validation of the C6 tumor BVf measured with Gd-ACX and the $RSST_1$ technique. a and b: Numerical models used to evaluate the stereological approach: cylinder model (a) and cortical mouse vasculature (b). The stereological analysis of vascular morphometry confirms the tumor BVf measured by MRI (c).

To validate the tumor BVf obtained with Gd-ACX by MRI, the vascular volume density was calculated as $V_v = \pi\{d\}^2L_v/4$ where {d} is the mean vessel diameter and L_v is the vascular length density obtained using a stereological analysis technique proposed by Adair [78]. For quantitative analysis of the microvasculature, 20 approximately equally spaced sections of 10 μm thickness were cut from the same location as the MR image (2 mm thickness). The collagen IV component of the vascular endothelium was stained using a fluorescent marker and the intravitally injected Hoechst dye was used to mark vessels which were perfused at the moment of injection. The tissue sections were digitized using a 10× magnification. ImageJ was used for segmentation and vascular morphometry. The stereological technique approximates the vessel sections as elliptical profiles of vessels modeled as randomly oriented straight cylinders. The vessel orientation was determined from the ratio of major and minor ellipse axes in order to derive L_v as described in [78]. However, no gold standard parameter exists that defines the vessels diameter from an irregularly shaped vessel cross section. Therefore, four morphologic parameters were analyzed for their potential utility as descriptors for the vessel diameter: the radius of the inscribed circle, the minor axis of the fitted ellipses, the small side of the bounding box and the breadth. They were evaluated on a simulated idealized cylinder model and on mouse cortical vasculature obtained from two-photon microscopy data (Figure "12). Only the breadth and the minor axis of ellipse yielded reliable and physiologically appropriate diameters. These numeric data was also used to evaluate the minimum number of sections necessary to reliably quantify stereologic parameters such as the L_v. After these optimizations the stereological analysis was applied to healthy rat brain and C6 tumor tissue and yielded vascular volume densities similar to the BVf measured by MRI with Gd-ACX. However, it was shown that only half of the tumor vessels detectable by histology were functional (perfused) vessels that contribute to the BVf measurement by MRI.

In opposite to the RG2 glioma model, the rat C6-glioma model has microvasculature permeable to Gd-DOTA but not to superparamagnetic iron-oxide nanoparticles (USPIO) allowing validation of the BVf derived from the leakage signal time course of Gd-DOTA using a steady state ΔR_2*-MRI method with an USPIO. Figure 13 a shows two BVf maps obtained with the two MRI techniques on the same animal. Despite different spatial resolution both BVf maps reflect almost the same values and heterogeneity in the tumor. The tumor BVf and the contralateral cerebral BVf of 0.034 ± 0.005 and 0.026 ± 0.004, respectively, were confirmed, in the same rats, by ΔR_2*-MRI (0.036 ± 0.003 and 0.027 ± 0.002) and also by immunohistochemical staining (anti-collagen type IV) of perfused vessels (0.036 ± 0.003 and 0.025 ± 0.004) labeled with intravitally injected Hoechst dye. Figure 13 b shows the correlation between the three techniques.

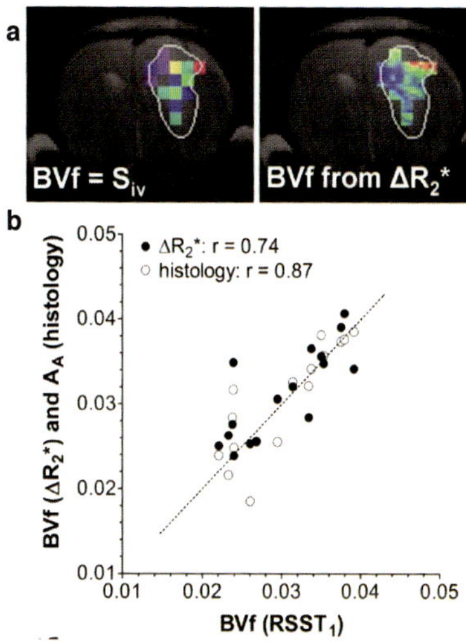

Figure 13. Validation of the BVf obtained in a C6 tumor with the $RSST_1$ technique by modeling the leakage signal profile of Gd-DOTA a: Tumor BVf maps obtained with the $RSST_1$ and a steady state ΔR_2* technique with an USPIO (MoldayION from BioPAL, Worcester, MA)as blood pool agent in the same animal show similar values and heterogeneity. b: Plot demonstrating the good correlation between BVf measured with the $RSST_1$ and the steady state ΔR_2* and with the histological vascular area density.

However, in case of USPIO leakage such as is the case in RG2 tumor tissue, the loss of CA compartmentalization reduces the magnetization difference between intra- and extravascular compartment. The CBV then tends to be underestimated with ΔR_2* methods.

8. What are the quantitative values of the regional blood volume in vivo?

CBV fraction values published for healthy rats are summarized in Table 1. They are in the range of 2 to 4% with regional and technique related differences. Using the $RSST_1$ technique with gadolinium based CA Gd-DOTA, P760 and Gd-ACX, regional CBV from 1.8 to 3.5% were measured in healthy rats (Table 1). When using AMI 227, a lower average CBV was measured (1.6 to 2.1%) and regional differences were less pronounced probably due to the transverse relaxation effect that was insufficiently corrected for and because of a lower spatial resolution. However, steady state ΔR_2^* measures in the same rats confirmed the low CBV (Figure 8). In C6 and RG2 tumor bearing rats, quantitative maps obtained with the $RSST_1$ technique revealed a significantly decreased contralateral CBV compared with healthy rats probably due to compression, edema, or inflammation [75], a finding also observed by other authors [71]. This shows that the vasculature in brain tissue contralateral to the tumor might not be representative of healthy brain vasculature as often assumed when reporting relative values. In a late stage C6 tumor model, a BVf of 0.98 ± 0.34% was measured in non necrotic tumor parts with the RSST1 technique and Gd-ACX, and confirmed by histology when care was taken to account for perfused vessels only.

MRI measurements in mice yield regional CBV fractions in the range of 1.7 to 2.7% including deep brain structures. Using intravital two-photon microscopy with an intravenously injected fluorescent marker, the BVf can be derived from the integrated fluorescence intensity [90]. The results in mouse brain cortex (2 to 2.4%) compare very well with the $RSST_1$ measures, however deeper structures are not measurable in vivo by two-photon microscopy presently limited to a depth of about 600 μm.

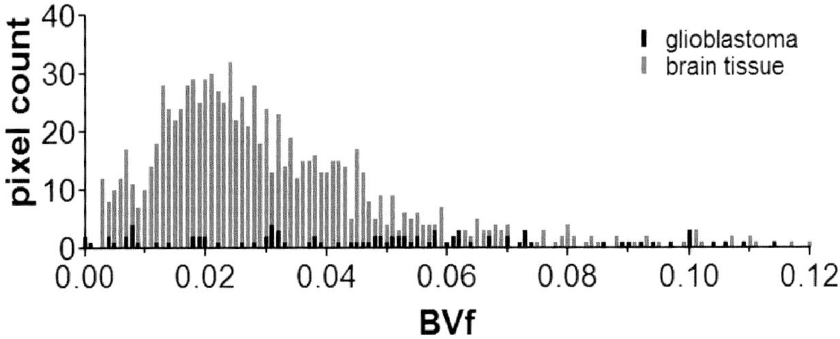

Figure 14.

In humans, BVf of 1.5 to 2.0% were measured in white matter, 3.5 to 4.5% in healthy appearing gray matter and values above 6% in glioblastoma margin. Figure 14 shows the BVf distribution in a healthy brain and in a glioblastoma after correction for CA leakage.

9. Conclusion

Direct quantitative mapping of the cerebral BVf is feasible with clinically approved contrast agents at a well tolerated dose during the first pass. The $RSST_1$ technique is powerful for the

ROI	CBV value	unit	technique	reference
corpus callosum	2.0 ± 0.3%	%	$RSST_1$ [b]	[60]
striatum	2.9 ± 0.6%	%	$RSST_1$ [b]	[60]
cortex	3.1 ± 0.8%	%	$RSST_1$ [b]	[60]
whole brain[a]	2.51	ml/100g	autoradiography[i]	[79]
whole brain[a]	2.96 ± 0.57	ml/100g	autoradiography[i]	[80]
whole brain[b]	2.77 ± 0.24	ml/100g	autoradiography[i]	[81]
whole brain	1.3 ± 0.1	ml/100g	autoradiography[j]	[82]
cortex	3.4	ml/100g	optical bolus tracking	[68]
whole brain[c]	2.40 ± 0.34	%	3D SS T_1 MRI	[48]
whole brain[c]	2.96 ± 0.82	%	3D SS T_1 MRI	[83]
whole brain[b]	3.14 ± 0.32	%	SST_2-MRI	[84]
cortex[b]	1.63 ± 0.18	ml/100g	SST_1-MRI	[85]
corpus callosum[b]	1.22 ± 0.25	ml/100g	SST_1-MRI	[85]
thalamus[b]	3.03 ± 0.36	ml/100g	SST_1-MRI	[85]
whole brain[b]	3.14 ± 0.32	%	$SS\Delta R_2^*$-MRI	[84]
cortex[d]	4.3 ± 0.7	%	$SS\Delta R_2^*$-MRI	[52]
striatum[e]	3.1 ± 0.7	ml/100g	$SS\Delta R_2^*$-MRI	[86]
striatum[f]	2.2 ± 0.6	ml/100g	$SS\Delta R_2^*$-MRI	[71]
cortex[a]	3.01 ± 0.43	%	$SS\Delta R_2^*$-MRI	[51]
striatum[a]	2.94 ± 0.49	%	$SS\Delta R_2^*$-MRI	[51]
cortex[a]	4.07	%	$SS\Delta R_2^*$-MRI	[87]
striatum[a]	2.87	%	$SS\Delta R_2^*$-MRI	[87]
whole brain	1.89 ± 0.39	%	morphometry[k]	[88]
whole brain without MV[g]	1.92 ± 0.32	ml/100g	SRQCT	[89]
whole brain with MV[g]	4.18 ± 1.06	ml/100g	SRQCT	[89]
cortex[g]	2.27	ml/100g	SRQCT	[89]
striatum[g]	2.01	ml/100g	SRQCT	[89]
striatum[h]	5.6	ml/100g	SRQCT	[89]

Reported values for the regional cerebral blood volume obtained with various imaging techniques. Decimal places and standard deviations are given as reported in the original work.

ROI = region of interest, MV = macroscopic vessels, CBV = cerebral blood volume, SST_1-MRI = steady state T_1-weighted magnetic resonance imaging, $SS\Delta R_2^*$-MRI = steady state ΔR_2^* magnetic resonance imaging, SRQCT = synchrotron radiation quantitative computed tomography

[a]rats anesthetized with halothane

[b]rats anesthetized with isoflurane

[c]rats anesthetized with intraperitoneal pentobarbital

[d]contralateral to C6 glioma, under moderate hypoxia, rats anesthetized with halothane

[e]rats anesthetized with intraperitoneal thiopental

[f]contralateral to C6 glioma, rats anesthetized with intraperitoneal thiopental

[g]anesthetized by intraperitoneal infusion of chloral hydrate

[h]contralateral to F98 glioma (n = 1)

[i]^{14}C-dextran labeled plasma and ^{99m}Tc labeled red blood cells

[j]^{125}I- labeled serum albumin and ^{55}Fe labeled red blood cells

[k]with stereo correction for slice thickness, contralateral to 9L tumor

Table 1. Regional cerebral blood volume (healthy regions) in normocapnic, normothermic, anesthetized rats.

clinical practice, because it can quantify the BVf simultaneously for vasculature with or without permeability to the contrast agent, without requiring the AIF and conversion of signal intensity into CA concentration. This technique will play an important role in treatment monitoring and clinical studies in particular for the evaluation of antiangiogenic agents.

Author details

Teodora-Adriana Perles-Barbacaru* and Hana Lahrech

*Address all correspondence to: teodora.perles-barbacaru@univ-amu.fr

Grenoble Institute of Neurosciences (GIN), French National Institute of Health and Medical Research (INSERM U) – University of Joseph Fourier (UJF) – French Atomic Energy Commission (CEA) – University Hospital of Grenoble (CHU), Bâtiment Edmond J. Safra, Chemin Fortuné Ferrini, La Tronche, France

References

[1] Aronen HJ, Gazit IE, Louis DN, Buchbinder BR, Pardo FS, Weisskoff RM, et al. Cerebral blood volume maps of gliomas: comparison with tumor grade and histologic findings. Radiology. 1994 Apr;191(1):41-51.

[2] Sugahara T, Korogi Y, Tomiguchi S, Shigematsu Y, Ikushima I, Kira T, et al. Posttherapeutic intraaxial brain tumor: the value of perfusion-sensitive contrast-enhanced MR imaging for differentiating tumor recurrence from nonneoplastic contrast-enhancing tissue. AJNR Am J Neuroradiol. 2000 May;21(5):901-9.

[3] Folkman J. New perspectives in clinical oncology from angiogenesis research. Eur J Cancer. 1996 Dec;32A(14):2534-9.

[4] Zama A, Tamura M, Inoue HK. Three-dimensional observations on microvascular growth in rat glioma using a vascular casting method. J Cancer Res Clin Oncol. 1991;117(5):396-402.

[5] Folkman J. The role of angiogenesis in tumor growth. Semin Cancer Biol. 1992 Apr; 3(2):65-71.

[6] Abdulrauf SI, Edvardsen K, Ho KL, Yang XY, Rock JP, Rosenblum ML. Vascular endothelial growth factor expression and vascular density as prognostic markers of survival in patients with low-grade astrocytoma. J Neurosurg. 1998 Mar;88(3):513-20.

[7] Assimakopoulou M, Sotiropoulou-Bonikou G, Maraziotis T, Papadakis N, Varakis I. Microvessel density in brain tumors. Anticancer Res. 1997 Nov-Dec;17(6D):4747-53.

[8] Brem S, Cotran R, Folkman J. Tumor angiogenesis: a quantitative method for histologic grading. J Natl Cancer Inst. 1972 Feb;48(2):347-56.

[9] Leon SP, Folkerth RD, Black PM. Microvessel density is a prognostic indicator for patients with astroglial brain tumors. Cancer. 1996 Jan 15;77(2):362-72.

[10] Revesz T, Scaravilli F, Coutinho L, Cockburn H, Sacares P, Thomas DG. Reliability of histological diagnosis including grading in gliomas biopsied by image-guided stereotactic technique. Brain. 1993 Aug;116 (Pt 4):781-93.

[11] Pardridge WM, Triguero D, Yang J, Cancilla PA. Comparison of in vitro and in vivo models of drug transcytosis through the blood-brain barrier. J Pharmacol Exp Ther. 1990 May;253(2):884-91.

[12] Duvernoy H, Delon S, Vannson JL. The vascularization of the human cerebellar cortex. Brain Res Bull. 1983 Oct;11(4):419-80.

[13] Herscovitch P, Raichle ME. What is the correct value for the brain--blood partition coefficient for water? J Cereb Blood Flow Metab. 1985 Mar;5(1):65-9.

[14] Taylor JS, Reddick WE. Evolution from empirical dynamic contrast-enhanced magnetic resonance imaging to pharmacokinetic MRI. Adv Drug Deliv Rev. 2000 Mar 15;41(1):91-110.

[15] Maeda M, Maley JE, Crosby DL, Quets JP, Zhu MW, Lee GJ, et al. Application of contrast agents in the evaluation of stroke: conventional MR and echo-planar MR imaging. J Magn Reson Imaging. 1997 Jan-Feb;7(1):23-8.

[16] Rosen BR. MR studies of perfusion in the brain. Current Practice in Radiology. Thrall, editor. Philadelphia, PA: Mosby Yearbook 1992.

[17] Rother J, Guckel F, Neff W, Schwartz A, Hennerici M. Assessment of regional cerebral blood volume in acute human stroke by use of single-slice dynamic susceptibility contrast-enhanced magnetic resonance imaging. Stroke. 1996 Jun;27(6):1088-93.

[18] Broom KA, Anthony DC, Blamire AM, Waters S, Styles P, Perry VH, et al. MRI reveals that early changes in cerebral blood volume precede blood-brain barrier breakdown and overt pathology in MS-like lesions in rat brain. J Cereb Blood Flow Metab. 2005 Feb;25(2):204-16.

[19] Sibson NR, Blamire AM, Perry VH, Gauldie J, Styles P, Anthony DC. TNF-alpha reduces cerebral blood volume and disrupts tissue homeostasis via an endothelin- and TNFR2-dependent pathway. Brain. 2002 Nov;125(Pt 11):2446-59.

[20] Looareesuwan S, Wilairatana P, Krishna S, Kendall B, Vannaphan S, Viravan C, et al. Magnetic resonance imaging of the brain in patients with cerebral malaria. Clin Infect Dis. 1995 Aug;21(2):300-9.

[21] Harris GJ, Lewis RF, Satlin A, English CD, Scott TM, Yurgelun-Todd DA, et al. Dynamic susceptibility contrast MRI of regional cerebral blood volume in Alzheimer's disease. Am J Psychiatry. 1996 May;153(5):721-4.

[22] Harris GJ, Lewis RF, Satlin A, English CD, Scott TM, Yurgelun-Todd DA, et al. Dynamic susceptibility contrast MR imaging of regional cerebral blood volume in Alzheimer disease: a promising alternative to nuclear medicine. AJNR Am J Neuroradiol. 1998 Oct;19(9):1727-32.

[23] Maas LC, Harris GJ, Satlin A, English CD, Lewis RF, Renshaw PF. Regional cerebral blood volume measured by dynamic susceptibility contrast MR imaging in Alzheimer's disease: a principal components analysis. J Magn Reson Imaging. 1997 Jan-Feb; 7(1):215-9.

[24] Ernst TM, Chang L, Witt MD, Aronow HA, Cornford ME, Walot I, et al. Cerebral toxoplasmosis and lymphoma in AIDS: perfusion MR imaging experience in 13 patients. Radiology. 1998 Sep;208(3):663-9.

[25] Tracey I, Hamberg LM, Guimaraes AR, Hunter G, Chang I, Navia BA, et al. Increased cerebral blood volume in HIV-positive patients detected by functional MRI. Neurology. 1998 Jun;50(6):1821-6.

[26] Garnett MR, Blamire AM, Corkill RG, Rajagopalan B, Young JD, Cadoux-Hudson TA, et al. Abnormal cerebral blood volume in regions of contused and normal appearing brain following traumatic brain injury using perfusion magnetic resonance imaging. J Neurotrauma. 2001 Jun;18(6):585-93.

[27] Cha S, Lu S, Johnson G, Knopp EA. Dynamic susceptibility contrast MR imaging: correlation of signal intensity changes with cerebral blood volume measurements. J Magn Reson Imaging. 2000 Feb;11(2):114-9.

[28] Dean BL, Lee C, Kirsch JE, Runge VM, Dempsey RM, Pettigrew LC. Cerebral hemodynamics and cerebral blood volume: MR assessment using gadolinium contrast agents and T1-weighted Turbo-FLASH imaging. AJNR Am J Neuroradiol. 1992 Jan-Feb;13(1):39-48.

[29] Villringer A, Rosen BR, Belliveau JW, Ackerman JL, Lauffer RB, Buxton RB, et al. Dynamic imaging with lanthanide chelates in normal brain: contrast due to magnetic susceptibility effects. Magn Reson Med. 1988 Feb;6(2):164-74.

[30] Kiselev VG. On the theoretical basis of perfusion measurements by dynamic susceptibility contrast MRI. Magn Reson Med. 2001 Dec;46(6):1113-22.

[31] Thompson HK, Jr., Starmer CF, Whalen RE, McIntosh HD. Indicator Transit Time Considered as a Gamma Variate. Circ Res. 1964 Jun;14:502-15.

[32] Meier P, Zierler KL. On the theory of the indicator-dilution method for measurement of blood flow and volume. J Appl Physiol. 1954 Jun;6(12):731-44.

[33] Calamante F, Gadian DG, Connelly A. Delay and dispersion effects in dynamic susceptibility contrast MRI: simulations using singular value decomposition. Magn Reson Med. 2000 Sep;44(3):466-73.

[34] Ostergaard L, Weisskoff RM, Chesler DA, Gyldensted C, Rosen BR. High resolution measurement of cerebral blood flow using intravascular tracer bolus passages. Part I: Mathematical approach and statistical analysis. Magn Reson Med. 1996 Nov;36(5): 715-25.

[35] Calamante F, Gadian DG, Connelly A. Quantification of perfusion using bolus tracking magnetic resonance imaging in stroke: assumptions, limitations, and potential implications for clinical use. Stroke. 2002 Apr;33(4):1146-51.

[36] Perthen JE, Calamante F, Gadian DG, Connelly A. Is quantification of bolus tracking MRI reliable without deconvolution? Magn Reson Med. 2002 Jan;47(1):61-7.

[37] Hacklander T, Hofer M, Reichenbach JR, Rascher K, Furst G, Modder U. Cerebral blood volume maps with dynamic contrast-enhanced T1-weighted FLASH imaging: normal values and preliminary clinical results. J Comput Assist Tomogr. 1996 Jul-Aug;20(4):532-9.

[38] Parker GJ, Suckling J, Tanner SF, Padhani AR, Revell PB, Husband JE, et al. Probing tumor microvascularity by measurement, analysis and display of contrast agent uptake kinetics. J Magn Reson Imaging. 1997 May-Jun;7(3):564-74.

[39] Flickinger FW, Allison JD, Sherry RM, Wright JC. Differentiation of benign from malignant breast masses by time-intensity evaluation of contrast enhanced MRI. Magn Reson Imaging. 1993;11(5):617-20.

[40] Tofts PS, Brix G, Buckley DL, Evelhoch JL, Henderson E, Knopp MV, et al. Estimating kinetic parameters from dynamic contrast-enhanced T(1)-weighted MRI of a diffusable tracer: standardized quantities and symbols. J Magn Reson Imaging. 1999 Sep;10(3):223-32.

[41] Tofts PS, Kermode AG. Measurement of the blood-brain barrier permeability and leakage space using dynamic MR imaging. 1. Fundamental concepts. Magn Reson Med. 1991 Feb;17(2):357-67.

[42] Daldrup HE, Shames DM, Husseini W, Wendland MF, Okuhata Y, Brasch RC. Quantification of the extraction fraction for gadopentetate across breast cancer capillaries. Magn Reson Med. 1998 Oct;40(4):537-43.

[43] Larsson HB, Stubgaard M, Frederiksen JL, Jensen M, Henriksen O, Paulson OB. Quantitation of blood-brain barrier defect by magnetic resonance imaging and gadolinium-DTPA in patients with multiple sclerosis and brain tumors. Magn Reson Med. 1990 Oct;16(1):117-31.

[44] Brix G, Semmler W, Port R, Schad LR, Layer G, Lorenz WJ. Pharmacokinetic parameters in CNS Gd-DTPA enhanced MR imaging. J Comput Assist Tomogr. 1991 Jul-Aug;15(4):621-8.

[45] Boxerman JL, Hamberg LM, Rosen BR, Weisskoff RM. MR contrast due to intravascular magnetic susceptibility perturbations. Magn Reson Med. 1995 Oct;34(4):555-66.

[46] Rosen BR, Belliveau JW, Vevea JM, Brady TJ. Perfusion imaging with NMR contrast agents. Magn Reson Med. 1990 May;14(2):249-65.

[47] Kuppusamy K, Lin W, Cizek GR, Haacke EM. In vivo regional cerebral blood volume: quantitative assessment with 3D T1-weighted pre- and postcontrast MR imaging. Radiology. 1996 Oct;201(1):106-12.

[48] Lin W, Paczynski RP, Kuppusamy K, Hsu CY, Haacke EM. Quantitative measurements of regional cerebral blood volume using MRI in rats: effects of arterial carbon dioxide tension and mannitol. Magn Reson Med. 1997 Sep;38(3):420-8.

[49] Le Duc G, Peoc'h M, Remy C, Charpy O, Muller RN, Le Bas JF, et al. Use of T(2)-weighted susceptibility contrast MRI for mapping the blood volume in the glioma-bearing rat brain. Magn Reson Med. 1999 Oct;42(4):754-61.

[50] Schwarzbauer C, Syha J, Haase A. Quantification of regional blood volumes by rapid T1 mapping. Magn Reson Med. 1993 May;29(5):709-12.

[51] Payen JF, Briot E, Tropres I, Julien-Dolbec C, Montigon O, Decorps M. Regional cerebral blood volume response to hypocapnia using susceptibility contrast MRI. NMR Biomed. 2000 Nov;13(7):384-91.

[52] Tropres I, Lamalle L, Peoc'h M, Farion R, Usson Y, Decorps M, et al. In vivo assessment of tumoral angiogenesis. Magn Reson Med. 2004 Mar;51(3):533-41.

[53] Turetschek K, Floyd E, Helbich T, Roberts TP, Shames DM, Wendland MF, et al. MRI assessment of microvascular characteristics in experimental breast tumors using a new blood pool contrast agent (MS-325) with correlations to histopathology. J Magn Reson Imaging. 2001 Sep;14(3):237-42.

[54] Bereczki D, Wei L, Otsuka T, Acuff V, Pettigrew K, Patlak C, et al. Hypoxia increases velocity of blood flow through parenchymal microvascular systems in rat brain. J Cereb Blood Flow Metab. 1993 May;13(3):475-86.

[55] Cremer JE, Seville MP. Regional brain blood flow, blood volume, and haematocrit values in the adult rat. J Cereb Blood Flow Metab. 1983 Jun;3(2):254-6.

[56] Yablonskiy DA, Haacke EM. Theory of NMR signal behavior in magnetically inhomogeneous tissues: the static dephasing regime. Magn Reson Med. 1994 Dec;32(6):749-63.

[57] Dennie J, Mandeville JB, Boxerman JL, Packard SD, Rosen BR, Weisskoff RM. NMR imaging of changes in vascular morphology due to tumor angiogenesis. Magn Reson Med. 1998 Dec;40(6):793-9.

[58] Lu H, Golay X, Pekar JJ, Van Zijl PC. Functional magnetic resonance imaging based on changes in vascular space occupancy. Magn Reson Med. 2003 Aug;50(2):263-74.

[59] Lu H, Law M, Johnson G, Ge Y, van Zijl PC, Helpern JA. Novel approach to the measurement of absolute cerebral blood volume using vascular-space-occupancy magnetic resonance imaging. Magn Reson Med. 2005 Dec;54(6):1403-11.

[60] Perles-Barbacaru AT, Lahrech H. A new Magnetic Resonance Imaging method for mapping the cerebral blood volume fraction: the rapid steady-state T1 method. J Cereb Blood Flow Metab. 2007 Mar;27(3):618-31.

[61] Haase A. Snapshot FLASH MRI. Applications to T1, T2, and chemical-shift imaging. Magn Reson Med. 1990 Jan;13(1):77-89.

[62] Larsson HB, Stubgaard M, Sondergaard L, Henriksen O. In vivo quantification of the unidirectional influx constant for Gd-DTPA diffusion across the myocardial capillaries with MR imaging. J Magn Reson Imaging. 1994 May-Jun;4(3):433-40.

[63] Jivan A, Horsfield MA, Moody AR, Cherryman GR. Dynamic T1 measurement using snapshot-FLASH MRI. J Magn Reson. 1997 Jul;127(1):65-72.

[64] Fonchy E, Lahrech H, Francois-Joubert A, Dupeyre R, Benderbous S, Corot C, et al. A new gadolinium-based contrast agent for magnetic resonance imaging of brain tumors: kinetic study on a C6 rat glioma model. J Magn Reson Imaging. 2001 Aug; 14(2):97-105.

[65] Perles-Barbacaru AT, Berger F, Lahrech H. Quantitative rapid steady state T(1) magnetic resonance imaging for cerebral blood volume mapping in mice: Lengthened measurement time window with intraperitoneal Gd-DOTA injection. Magn Reson Med 2013 May;69(5);1451-6

[66] Payen JF, Vath A, Koenigsberg B, Bourlier V, Decorps M. Regional cerebral plasma volume response to carbon dioxide using magnetic resonance imaging. Anesthesiology. 1998 Apr;88(4):984-92.

[67] Perles-Barbacaru TA, Procissi D, Demyanenko AV, Jacobs RE. Quantitative pharmacologic MRI in mice. NMR Biomed. 2012 Apr;25(4):498-505.

[68] Shockley RP, LaManna JC. Determination of rat cerebral cortical blood volume changes by capillary mean transit time analysis during hypoxia, hypercapnia and hyperventilation. Brain Res. 1988 Jun 28;454(1-2):170-8.

[69] Beaumont M, Lemasson B, Farion R, Segebarth C, Remy C, Barbier EL. Characterization of tumor angiogenesis in rat brain using iron-based vessel size index MRI in

combination with gadolinium-based dynamic contrast-enhanced MRI. J Cereb Blood Flow Metab. 2009 Oct;29(10):1714-26.

[70] Bremer C, Mustafa M, Bogdanov A, Jr., Ntziachristos V, Petrovsky A, Weissleder R. Steady-state blood volume measurements in experimental tumors with different angiogenic burdens a study in mice. Radiology. 2003 Jan;226(1):214-20.

[71] Julien C, Payen JF, Tropres I, Farion R, Grillon E, Montigon O, et al. Assessment of vascular reactivity in rat brain glioma by measuring regional blood volume during graded hypoxic hypoxia. Br J Cancer. 2004 Jul 19;91(2):374-80.

[72] Valable S, Eddi D, Constans JM, Guillamo JS, Bernaudin M, Roussel S, et al. MRI assessment of hemodynamic effects of angiopoietin-2 overexpression in a brain tumor model. Neuro Oncol. 2009 Oct;11(5):488-502.

[73] Perles-Barbacaru AT, Lamalle L, Barbier E, Segebarth C, Lahrech H, editors. Rapid Steady State T_1 method for cerebral blood volume fraction mapping using SINEREM as contrast agent and a three dimensional projection reconstruction acquisition mode International Society for Magnetic Resonance in Medicine, 16th Annual Scientific Meeting; 2008; Toronto (Canada).

[74] Gadelle A, Defaye J. Selective halogenation of primary positions of cyclomaltosaccharides and synthesis of per-(3,6-anhydro) cyclomalto-oligosacccharides. Angew Chem Int Ed Engl 1991;30(1):78-80.

[75] Lahrech H, Perles-Barbacaru AT, Aous S, Le Bas JF, Debouzy JC, Gadelle A, et al. Cerebral blood volume quantification in a C6 tumor model using gadolinium per (3,6-anhydro) alpha-cyclodextrin as a new magnetic resonance imaging preclinical contrast agent. J Cereb Blood Flow Metab. 2008 May;28(5):1017-29.

[76] Labadie C, Lee JH, Vetek G, Springer CS, Jr. Relaxographic imaging. J Magn Reson B. 1994 Oct;105(2):99-112.

[77] Moran GR, Prato FS. Modeling (1H) exchange: an estimate of the error introduced in MRI by assuming the fast exchange limit in bolus tracking. Magn Reson Med. 2004 Apr;51(4):816-27.

[78] Adair TH, Wells ML, Hang J, Montani JP. A stereological method for estimating length density of the arterial vascular system. Am J Physiol. 1994 Apr;266(4 Pt 2):H1434-8.

[79] Todd MM, Weeks JB, Warner DS. Cerebral blood flow, blood volume, and brain tissue hematocrit during isovolemic hemodilution with hetastarch in rats. Am J Physiol. 1992 Jul;263(1 Pt 2):H75-82.

[80] Todd MM, Weeks JB, Warner DS. The influence of intravascular volume expansion on cerebral blood flow and blood volume in normal rats. Anesthesiology. 1993 May; 78(5):945-53.

[81] Todd MM, Weeks J. Comparative effects of propofol, pentobarbital, and isoflurane on cerebral blood flow and blood volume. J Neurosurg Anesthesiol. 1996 Oct;8(4): 296-303.

[82] Bereczki D, Wei L, Acuff V, Gruber K, Tajima A, Patlak C, et al. Technique-dependent variations in cerebral microvessel blood volumes and hematocrits in the rat. J Appl Physiol. 1992 Sep;73(3):918-24.

[83] Lin W, Celik A, Paczynski RP, Hsu CY, Powers WJ. Quantitative magnetic resonance imaging in experimental hypercapnia: improvement in the relation between changes in brain R2 and the oxygen saturation of venous blood after correction for changes in cerebral blood volume. J Cereb Blood Flow Metab. 1999 Aug;19(8):853-62.

[84] Dunn JF, Roche MA, Springett R, Abajian M, Merlis J, Daghlian CP, et al. Monitoring angiogenesis in brain using steady-state quantification of DeltaR2 with MION infusion. Magn Reson Med. 2004 Jan;51(1):55-61.

[85] Schwarzbauer C, Morrissey SP, Deichmann R, Hillenbrand C, Syha J, Adolf H, et al. Quantitative magnetic resonance imaging of capillary water permeability and regional blood volume with an intravascular MR contrast agent. Magn Reson Med. 1997 May;37(5):769-77.

[86] Julien-Dolbec C, Tropres I, Montigon O, Reutenauer H, Ziegler A, Decorps M, et al. Regional response of cerebral blood volume to graded hypoxic hypoxia in rat brain. Br J Anaesth. 2002 Aug;89(2):287-93.

[87] Tropres I, Grimault S, Vaeth A, Grillon E, Julien C, Payen JF, et al. Vessel size imaging. Magn Reson Med. 2001 Mar;45(3):397-408.

[88] Pathak AP, Schmainda KM, Ward BD, Linderman JR, Rebro KJ, Greene AS. MR-derived cerebral blood volume maps: issues regarding histological validation and assessment of tumor angiogenesis. Magn Reson Med. 2001 Oct;46(4):735-47.

[89] Adam JF, Elleaume H, Le Duc G, Corde S, Charvet AM, Tropres I, et al. Absolute cerebral blood volume and blood flow measurements based on synchrotron radiation quantitative computed tomography. J Cereb Blood Flow Metab. 2003 Apr;23(4): 499-512.

[90] Verant P, Serduc R, Van Der Sanden B, Remy C, Vial JC. A direct method for measuring mouse capillary cortical blood volume using multiphoton laser scanning microscopy. J Cereb Blood Flow Metab. 2007 May;27(5):1072-81.